S0-ARE-349

Technologies in Vascular Surgery

Technologies
in
Vascular
Surgery

Edited by

JAMES S.T. YAO, M.D., Ph.D.

Magerstadt Professor of Surgery and
Chief, Division of Vascular Surgery
Northwestern University Medical School
Chicago, Illinois

WILLIAM H. PEARCE, M.D.

Associate Professor of Surgery
Northwestern University Medical School
Chicago, Illinois

W.B. SAUNDERS COMPANY

Harcourt Brace Jovanovich, Inc.

Philadelphia / London / Toronto / Montreal / Sydney / Tokyo

W. B. SAUNDERS COMPANY
Harcourt Brace Jovanovich, Inc.

The Curtis Center
Independence Square West
Philadelphia, Pa 19106

Library of Congress Cataloging-in-Publication Data

Technology in vascular surgery / [edited by] James S. T. Yao, William
  H. Pearce.
    p.   cm.
  ISBN 0-7216-4429-5
  1. Blood-vessels–Surgery. I. Yao, James S. T. II. Pearce,
William H.
  [DNLM: 1. Vascular Surgery–methods. WG 170 T257]
RD598.5.T43 1992
617.4'13–dc20
DNLM/DLC   91-33824

Sponsoring Editor: Ray Kersey

TECHNOLOGY IN VASCULAR SURGERY   ISBN   0-7216-4429-5

Copyright © 1992 by W. B. Saunders Company.

All rights reserved. No part of this publication may be reproduced or transmitted in any form or
by any means, electronic or mechanical, including photocopy, recording, or any information
storage and retrieval system without permission in writing from the publisher.

Printed in the United States of America.

Last digit is the print number: 9   8   7   6   5   4   3   2   1

CONTRIBUTORS

R. G. A. ACKERSTAFF, M.D., Ph.D.
Chairman of the Department of Clinical Neurophysiology
University of Utrecht, Utrecht, The Netherlands
The Use of Transcranial Doppler in Carotid Artery Disease

SAMUEL S. AHN, M.D.
Assistant Professor of Surgery, Section of Vascular Surgery, UCLA School of Medicine,
Los Angeles, California
Preliminary Clinical Results of Rotary Atherectomy

CAROL COX ALMGREN, R.N.
Vascular-Thoracic Operating Room Surgical Service Specialist, Northwestern Memorial
Hospital, Chicago Illinois
The Use of Angioscopy in the Saphenous Vein Bypass Graft

GEORGE ANDROS, M.D.
Medical Director, Vascular Laboratory, Saint Joseph Medical Center, Burbank, California
Interventional Technology: Intraoperative Strategies and Techniques

DENNIS F. BANDYK, M.D.
Professor of Surgery, University of South Florida, Tampa, Florida
Real-time Color Doppler in Arterial Imaging

WALTER M. BARKER, Ph.D.
Assistant Director, Clinical Research, Thrombolytics Venture, Abbott Laboratories,
Abbott Park, Illinois
*Advances in Peripheral Vascular Thrombolysis: Recombinant Technology and Methodologies to
Enhance Lysis*

LYNNE D. BARKMEIER, M.D.
Assistant Professor of Surgery, Southern Illinois University School of Medicine, Spring-
field, Illinois
Clinical Application of Color Doppler in Venous Problems

B. TIMOTHY BAXTER, M.D.
Assistant Professor of Surgery, University of Omaha, Omaha, Nebraska
*The Use of Angioscopy in the Saphenous Vein Bypass Graft; A Comparative Study of
Angioscopy and Completion Arteriography after Infrainguinal Bypass*

PHILLIP J. BENDICK, Ph.D.
Director of Surgical Research, William Beaumont Hospital, Royal Oak, Michigan
Noninvasive Follow-up of Endovascular Procedures

JEAN-FRANCOIS BLAIR, M.D., FRCS
Instructor in Surgery, University of Montreal Medical School, Montreal, Quebec, Canada
Real-time Color Doppler in Arterial Imaging

BRUCE J. BRENER, M.D.
Clinical Professor of Surgery, University of Medicine and Dentistry, Newark, New Jersey; Chief of Vascular Surgery, Beth Israel Medical Center, Newark, New Jersey
Peripheral Percutaneous Transluminal Angioplasty with Ultrasound Imaging

SANDRA E. BURKE, PH.D.
Senior Research Pharmacologist, Department of General Pharmacology, Abbott Laboratories, Abbott Park, Illinois
Advances in Peripheral Vascular Thrombolysis: Recombinant Technology and Methodologies to Enhance Lysis

ALLAN D. CALLOW, M.D., PH.D.
Research Professor of Surgery, Washington University School of Medicine, St. Louis, Missouri
Genetic Engineering of an Arterial Bypass Graft

GARY R. CAPUTO, M.D.
Assistant Professor of Radiology, University of California, San Francisco, San Francisco, California
The Evolving Role of Magnetic Resonance in Arterial Disorders

DOUGLAS CAVAYE, FRACS
Clinical Instructor in Surgery, UCLA School of Medicine, Los Angeles, California
Clinical Applications of Intravascular Ultrasound

DOLORES F. CIKRIT, M.D.
Assistant Professor of Surgery, Indiana University Medical Center, Indianapolis, Indiana
Iliac Artery Angioplasty and Stents: A Current Experience

SCOTT R. CLULEY, M.D.
Vascular Fellow, Beth Israel Medical Center, Newark, New Jersey
Peripheral Percutaneous Transluminal Angioplasty with Ultrasound Imaging

MICHAEL D. COLBURN, M.D.
Resident, Department of Surgery, UCLA School of Medicine, Los Angeles, California
Pharmacologic Control of Myointimal Hyperplasia

ANTHONY J. COMEROTA, M.D.
Professor of Surgery, Temple University School of Medicine, Philadelphia, Pennsylvania
Thrombolytic Therapy in Arterial and Graft Occlusion

FRANK J. CRIADO, M.D.
Co-Director, Maryland Vascular Institute, Union Memorial Hospital, Baltimore, Maryland
Long-term Results of Simpson Atherectomy

CHRISTOPHER G. CUNNINGHAM, LCDR, MC, USNR
Bethesda Naval Hospital, Bethesda, Maryland
The Evolving Role of Magnetic Resonance in Arterial Disorders

MICHAEL C. DALSING, M.D.
Associate Professor of Surgery; Chief, Division of Vascular Surgery, Indiana University Medical Center, Indianapolis, Indiana
Iliac Artery Angioplasty and Stents: A Current Experience

ROGER DAMLE, M.D.
Fellow, Cardiology Section/Department of Internal Medicine, Northwestern Memorial Hospital, Chicago, Illinois
Intravascular Ultrasound: Principles and Techniques

RICHARD H. DEAN, M.D.

Professor and Chairman, Department of Surgery, Bowman Gray School of Medicine of Wake Forest University, Winston-Salem, North Carolina
Use of Duplex Scanning in Renovascular Hypertension

SCOTT L. DIAMOND, Ph.D.

Assistant Professor, Department of Chemical Engineering, State University of New York, Buffalo, New York
Regulation of Endothelial Cell Gene Expression by Hemodynamic Forces: Implications for Intimal Hyperplasia and Graft Patency

CARL W. DIEFFENBACH, Ph.D.

Assistant Professor, Department of Pathology, Uniformed Sciences University of the Health Sciences, Bethesda, Maryland
Regulation of Endothelial Cell Gene Expression by Hemodynamic Forces: Implications for Intimal Hyperplasia and Graft Patency

JANETTE DURHAM, M.D.

Assistant Professor, Department of Radiology, University of Colorado Health Sciences Center, Denver, Colorado
Percutaneous Balloon Angioplasty for Arteriosclerosis Obliterans: Long-Term Results

KAREN O. EHRMAN, M.D.

Clinical Assistant Professor of Radiology, Indiana University Medical Center, Indianapolis, Indiana
Iliac Artery Angioplasty and Stents: A Current Experience

BERT C. EIKELBOOM, M.D., Ph.D.

Professor of Vascular Surgery, University of Utrecht, Utrecht, The Netherlands
The Use of Transcranial Doppler in Carotid Artery Disease

BEN EISEMAN, M.D.

Emeritus Professor of Surgery, University of Colorado Health Sciences Center, Denver, Colorado
Technology and Vascular Surgery: A Study in Synergism

SUZANNE G. ESKIN, Ph.D.

Associate Professor of Internal Medicine, University of Texas Medical School at Houston, Houston, Texas
Regulation of Endothelial Cell Gene Expression by Hemodynamic Forces: Implications for Intimal Hyperplasia and Graft Patency

KAREN ETCHBERGER, Ph.D.

JRH Biosciences, Denver, Pennsylvania
Endothelial Cell Seeding: A Technology for Arterial Bypass Grafts

DARWIN ETON, M.D., MSc.

Assistant Professor, University of Illinois, Chicago, Illinois; Visiting Assistant Professor, Section of Vascular Surgery, UCLA School of Medicine, Los Angeles, California
Preliminary Clinical Results of Rotary Atherectomy

STEVEN W. FITZGERALD, M.D.

Assistant Professor of Radiology, Northwestern University Medical School, Chicago, Illinois
Magnetic Resonance Imaging of Venous Disorders

WILLIAM R. FLINN, M.D.
Associate Professor of Surgery, Northwestern University Medical School, Chicago, Illinois
The Use of Angioscopy in the Saphenous Vein Bypass Graft; A Comparative Study of Angioscopy and Completion Arteriography after Infrainguinal Bypass; Excimer Laser Treatment of Femoral Artery Atherosclerosis

THOMAS J. FOGARTY, M.D.
Director of Cardiac Surgery, Sequoia Hospital, Redwood City, California
Angioscopy-assisted Thromboembolectomy

JOHN L. GLOVER, M.D.
Chief of Surgical Services, William Beaumont Hospital, Royal Oak, Michigan
Noninvasive Follow-up of Endovascular Procedures

GREG R. GOODMAN, M.D.
Surgical Resident, University of Utah School of Medicine, Salt Lake City, Utah
Intraoperative Thrombolytic Therapy

ROGER M. GREENHALGH, M.D., MCHIR, FRCS
Professor and Chairman, Department of Surgery, Charing Cross and Westminster Medical School, Charing Cross Hospital, London, England
Genetic Variation on Chromosome 16 and the Growth of Abdominal Aortic Aneuryms

KIMBERLEY J. HANSEN, M.D.
Assistant Professor of Surgery, and Director of Clinical Vascular Laboratory, Bowman Gray School of Medicine of Wake Forest University, Winston-Salem, North Carolina
Use of Duplex Scanning in Renovascular Hypertension

JACK HENKIN, PH.D.
Adjunct Assistant Professor, Department of Biological Chemistry and Structure, The Chicago Medical School, North Chicago, Illinois
Advances in Peripheral Vascular Thrombolysis: Recombinant Technology and Methodologies to Enhance Lysis

GEORGE D. HERMANN, B.S.M.E.
Engineering Manager, Fogarty Research, Portola Valley, California
Angioscopy-assisted Thromboembolectomy

MALCOLM B. HERRING, M.D.
Clinical Associate Professor of Surgery, Indiana University, Indianapolis, Indiana
Endothelial Cell Seeding: A Technology for Arterial Bypass Grafts

CHARLES B. HIGGINS, M.D.
Professor of Radiology, University of California, San Francisco, San Francisco, California
The Evolving Role of Magnetic Resonance in Arterial Disorders

KIM J. HODGSON, M.D.
Assistant Professor of Surgery, Southern Illinois University School of Medicine, Springfield, Illinois
Clinical Application of Color Doppler in Venous Problems

LARRY H. HOLLIER, M.D.
Clinical Professor of Surgery, Louisiana State University Medical Center and Tulane University Medical Center, New Orleans, Louisiana
Peripheral Percutaneous Transluminal Angioplasty with Ultrasound Imaging

JEFFREY M. ISNER, M.D.
Professor of Medicine and Pathology, Tufts University School of Medicine, Boston, Massachusetts
Percutaneous Treatment of Peripheral Vascular Disease: Role of Intravascular Ultrasound

C. JANSEN, M.D.
University of Utrecht, Utrecht, The Netherlands
The Use of Transcranial Doppler in Carotid Artery Disease

GEORGE KOPCHOK, B.S.
Research Associate, Vascular Laser Laboratory, Harbor-UCLA Medical Center, Torrance, California
Clinical Applications of Intravascular Ultrasound

HELENA KUIVANIEMI, M.D., Ph.D.
Research Assistant Professor, Thomas Jefferson University, Department of Biochemistry and Molecular Biology, Jefferson Institute of Molecular Medicine, Philadelphia, Pennsylvania
Identification of Familial Aortic Aneurysms Using DNA Technique

STEPHEN G. LALKA, M.D.
Assistant Professor of Surgery, Indiana University Medical Center, Indianapolis, Indiana
Iliac Artery Angioplasty and Stents: A Current Experience

R. EUGENE LANGEVIN, Jr., M.D.
Tufts University School of Medicine, Boston, Massachusetts
Percutaneous Treatment of Peripheral Vascular Disease: Role of Intravascular Ultrasound

PETER F. LAWRENCE, M.D.
Department of Surgery, University of Utah School of Medicine, Salt Lake City, Utah
Intraoperative Thrombolytic Therapy

JAMES P. LEWKOWSKI, M.D.
Operations Manager, Thrombolytics Venture, Abbott Laboratories, Abbott Park, Illinois
Advances in Peripheral Vascular Thrombolysis: Recombinant Technology and Methodologies to Enhance Lysis

ANDREW W. LITT, M.D.
Assistant Professor of Radiology, New York University School of Medicine, New York, New York
Magnetic Resonance Angiography

GREGG L. LONDREY, M.D.
Virginia Surgical Associates, Richmond, Virginia
Clinical Application of Color Doppler in Venous Problems

DOUGLAS W. LOSORDO, M.D.
Assistant Professor of Medicine, Tufts University School of Medicine, Boston, Massachusetts
Percutaneous Treatment of Peripheral Vascular Disease: Role of Intravascular Ultrasound

JUNJI MACHI, M.D., Ph.D.
Research Assistant Professor, Department of Surgery, Medical College of Pennsylvania Hospital, Philadelphia, Pennsylvania
Intraoperative Use of B-Mode and Color Doppler Imaging

MARK A. MATTOS, M.D.
Vascular Surgery Fellow, Southern Illinois University School of Medicine, Springfield, Illinois
Clinical Application of Color Doppler in Venous Problems

WALTER J. McCARTHY, M.D.
Assistant Professor of Surgery, Northwestern University Medical School, Chicago, Illinois
The Use of Angioscopy in the Saphenous Vein Bypass Graft; Excimer Laser Treatment of Femoral Artery Atherosclerosis

LARRY V. McINTIRE, Ph.D.
E. D. Butcher Professor, Institute of Biosciences and Bioengineering, Rice University, Houston, Texas
Regulation of Endothelial Cell Gene Expression by Hemodynamic Forces: Implications for Intimal Hyperplasia and Graft Patency

DAVID D. McPHERSON, M.D.
Associate Professor of Medicine, Northwestern University, Chicago, Illinois
Intravascular Ultrasound: Principles and Techniques

JOHN T. MEHIGAN, M.D.
Clinical Associate Professor of Surgery, Department of Surgery, Stanford University Medical Center, Stanford, California; Bay Area Cardiovascular Medical Group, Palo Alto, California
Preliminary Clinical Results of Rotary Atherectomy

LOUIS M. MESSINA, M.D.
Assistant Professor of Surgery, University of Michigan Medical Center, Ann Arbor, Michigan
Therapeutic Potential of Genetic Engineering on Vascular Disease

CHERYL D. MEYERS, R.N., R.V.T.
Technical Director, Vascular Studies, Maryland Diagnostic Service, Lutherville, Maryland
Long-term Results of Simpson Atherectomy

WESLEY S. MOORE, M.D.
Professor of Surgery, UCLA School of Medicine; Chief, Section of Vascular Surgery, UCLA Center for Health Sciences, Los Angeles, California
Pharmacologic Control of Myointimal Hyperplasia

JOHN W. NORRIS, M.D.
Professor, University of Toronto, Toronto, Ontario, Canada
Transcranial Doppler: A New Test for Cerebral Embolism?

PEGGY PATTEN, R.N.
Interventional Vascular Specialist, Maryland Vascular Institute, Union Memorial Hospital, Baltimore, Maryland
Long-term Results of Simpson Atherectomy

WILLIAM H. PEARCE, M.D.
Associate Professor of Surgery, Northwestern University Medical School, Chicago, Illinois
The Use of Angioscopy in the Saphenous Vein Bypass Graft; Excimer Laser Treatment of Femoral Artery Atherosclerosis

ANN PIECZEK, R.N., BSN
Cardiovascular Research Coordinator, St. Elizabeth's Hospital, Boston, Massachusetts
Percutaneous Treatment of Peripheral Vascular Disease: Role of Intravascular Ultrasound

RACHEL M. PODRAZIK, M.D.
University of Michigan Medical Center, Ann Arbor, Michigan
Therapeutic Potential of Genetic Engineering on Vascular Disease

JANET T. POWELL, M.D., Ph.D.
Senior Lecturer in Biochemistry and Surgery, Charing Cross and Westminster Medical School, London, England
Genetic Variation on Chromosome 16 and the Growth of Abdominal Aortic Aneurysms

LUIS A. QUERAL, M.D.
Co-Director, Maryland Vascular Institute, Union Memorial Hospital, Baltimore, Maryland
Long-term Results of Simpson Atherectomy

STEPHEN R. RAMEE, M.D., F.A.C.C.
Director, Interventional Cardiology, Cardiac Catherization Laboratory, Ochsner Foundation Hospital, New Orleans, Louisiana
Peripheral Percutaneous Transluminal Angioplasty with Ultrasound Imaging

DON E. RAMSEY, M.D.
Associate Professor of Surgery, Southern Illinois University School of Medicine, Springfield, Illinois
Clinical Application of Color Doppler in Venous Problems

SYED ASIF RAZVI, M.D.
Clinical Professor of Surgery, Tufts University School of Medicine; Chief, Division of Vascular Surgery, St. Elizabeth's Hospital, Boston, Massachusetts
Percutaneous Treatment of Peripheral Vascular Disease: Role of Intravascular Ultrasound

SCOTT W. REAVIS, B.S., R.V.T.
Technical Director, Surgery Vascular Laboratory, Bowman Gray School of Medicine, Winston-Salem, North Carolina
Use of Duplex Scanning in Renovascular Hypertension

THOMAS S. RILES, M.D.
Professor of Surgery, Director, Vascular Training Program, Department of Surgery, New York University Medical Center, New York, New York
Magnetic Resonance Angiography

ROBERT J. RIZZO, M.D.
Assistant Professor of Surgery, Harvard Medical School; Attending Surgeon, Brigham and Women's Hospital, Boston, Massachusetts
A Comparative Study of Angioscopy and Completion Arteriography after Infrainguinal Bypass

ANDREW B. ROBERTS, M.D.
Associate Professor of Surgery, Department of Surgery, Medical College of Pennsylvania Hospital, Philadelphia, Pennsylvania
Intraoperative Use of B-Mode and Color Doppler Imaging

KENNETH ROSENFIELD, M.D.
Assistant Professor of Medicine, Tufts University School of Medicine, and St. Elizabeth's Hospital of Boston, Boston, Massachusetts
Percutaneous Treatment of Peripheral Vascular Disease: Role of Intravascular Ultrasound

DAVID ROSENTHAL, M.D.
Clinical Professor of Surgery, Medical College of Georgia, Atlanta, Georgia
Hot-Tip Laser Angioplasty: A Three-Year Follow-up Study

ROBERT B. RUTHERFORD, M.D.
Professor of Surgery, University of Colorado, Denver, Colorado
Percutaneous Balloon Angioplasty for Arteriosclerosis Obliterans: Long-term Results

CECILIA C. St.MARTIN, M.S.
Clinical Project Manager, Thrombolytics Venture, Abbott Laboratories, Abbott Park, Illinois
Advances in Peripheral Vascular Thrombolysis: Recombinant Technology and Methodologies to Enhance Lysis

ARTHUR A. SASAHARA, M.D.
Professor of Medicine, Harvard Medical School; Senior Physician, Brigham and Women's Hospital, Boston, Massachusetts
Advances in Peripheral Vascular Thrombolysis: Recombinant Technology and Methodologies to Enhance Lysis

ALAN P. SAWCHUK, M.D.
Assistant Professor, Indiana University School of Medicine, Indiana University Medical Center, Indianapolis, Indiana
Iliac Artery Angioplasty and Stents: A Current Experience

GREGORY A. SCHULZ, M.S.
Clinical Project Manager, Pharmaceutical Products Division, Thrombolytics Venture, Abbott Laboratories, Abbott Park, Illinois
Advances in Peripheral Vascular Thrombolysis: Recombinant Technology and Methodologies to Enhance Lysis

JAMES M. SEEGER, M.D.
Associate Professor, Chief, Section of Vascular Surgery, University of Florida, Gainesville, Florida
The Use of Angioscopy in Laser Angioplasty

JOHN B. SHAREFKIN, M.D.
Assistant Professor of Surgery, Tufts University School of Medicine, Boston, Massachusetts
Regulation of Endothelial Cell Gene Expression by Hemodynamic Forces: Implications for Intimal Hyperplasia and Graft Patency

BERNARD SIGEL, M.D.
Professor of Surgery, The Medical College of Pennsylvania, Philadelphia, Pennsylvania
Intraoperative Use of B-Mode and Color Doppler Imaging

MICHAEL B. SILVA, Jr., M.D.
Center for Vascular Disease, Columbus Hospital, Chicago, Illinois
A Comparative Study of Angioscopy and Completion Arteriography after Infrainguinal Bypass

JOHN C. SOBOLSKI, M.D., Ph.D.
Research Assistant Professor of Medicine, University of the Health Sciences/The Chicago Medical School, North Chicago, Illinois; Director, Clinical Research, Thrombolytics Venture, Abbott Laboratories, Abbott Park, Illinois
Advances in Peripheral Vascular Thrombolysis: Recombinant Technology and Methodologies to Enhance Lysis

JAMES C. STANLEY, M.D.
Professor of Surgery, University of Michigan Medical School, Ann Arbor, Michigan
Therapeutic Potential of Genetic Engineering on Vascular Disease

RONALD J. STONEY, M.D.
Professor of Surgery, University of California Medical Center, San Francisco, California
The Evolving Role of Magnetic Resonance in Arterial Disorders

D. EUGENE STRANDNESS, Jr., M.D.
Professor of Surgery and Head, Vascular Surgery Section, University of Washington School of Medicine, Seattle, Washington
New Applications of Ultrasound

DAVID S. SUMNER, M.D.
Distinguished Professor of Surgery; Chief, Section of Peripheral Vascular Surgery, Southern Illinois University School of Medicine, Springfield, Illinois
Clinical Application of Color Doppler in Venous Problems

MARWAN TABBARA, M.D.
Assistant Clinical Professor, UCLA School of Medicine, Los Angeles, California
Clinical Applications of Intravascular Ultrasound

GERARD TROMP, Ph.D.
Research Assistant Professor, Thomas Jefferson University, Department of Biochemistry and Molecular Biology, Jefferson Institute of Molecular Medicine, Philadelphia, Pennsylvania
Identification of Familial Aortic Aneurysms Using DNA Technique

ALEXANDER G. G. TURPIE, M.D., F.R.C.P. (Lond., Glasgow), F.A.C.P.
Professor of Medicine, McMaster University, Hamilton, Ontario, Canada
Thrombolytic Therapy in Acute Venous Thrombosis

FRANK J. VEITH, M.D.
Professor of Surgery, Albert Einstein College of Medicine; Interim Chairman, Department of Surgery, Chief of Vascular Surgical Services, Montefiore Medical Center-Albert Einstein College of Medicine, Bronx, New York
The Impact of Nonoperative Therapy on the Clinical Management of Peripheral Arterial Disease

ROBERT L. VOGELZANG, M.D.
Associate Professor of Clinical Radiology, Northwestern University Medical School, Chicago, Illinois
Magnetic Resonance Imaging of Venous Disorders; Excimer Laser Treatment of Femoral Artery Atherosclerosis

CHRISTOPHER J. WHITE, M.D., F.A.C.C.
Clinical Assistant Professor, Louisiana State University Medical School, New Orleans, Louisiana; Director, Cardiac Catheterization Laboratory, Ochner Foundation Hospital and Clinic, New Orleans, Louisiana
Peripheral Percutaneous Transluminal Angioplasty with Ultrasound Imaging

RODNEY A. WHITE, M.D.
Associate Professor of Surgery, UCLA School of Medicine, Los Angeles, California
Clinical Applications of Intravascular Ultrasound

ANTHONY D. WHITTEMORE, M.D.
Assistant Professor of Surgery, Harvard Medical School; Chief, Division of Vascular Surgery, Brigham and Women's Hospital, Boston, Massachusetts
Urokinase Treatment of Occluded Infrainguinal Grafts

JAMES S. T. YAO, M.D., Ph.D.

Magerstadt Professor of Surgery; Chief, Division of Vascular Surgery, Northwestern University Medical School, Chicago, Illinois

The Use of Angioscopy in the Saphenous Vein Bypass Graft; Excimer Laser Treatment of Femoral Artery Atherosclerosis

C. Z. ZHU, M.D.

Stroke Research Fellow, Stroke Research Unit, University of Toronto, Toronto, Ontario, Canada

Transcranial Doppler: A New Test for Cerebral Embolism?

PREFACE

From the stethoscope and sphygmomanometer to computed tomography scanning and magnetic imaging, technology has played a central role in the diagnosis and treatment of disease. For surgeons, operations on the body presented the earliest opportunities to apply a special instrument in the treatment of a surgical problem. In addition to surgical instruments, various technologies are now available to vascular surgeons for diagnosis and treatment without the need for surgery. The spectacular achievements of high technology in recent years have added a new dimension to the practice of vascular surgery. Dr. Francis D. Moore, in his John B. Rhodes Memorial Lecture, stated that "advances in surgery have resided largely in the growth of effective technology." The purpose of this book is to examine the recent growth of technologies and their effectiveness in the diagnosis and treatment of vascular problems.

Many pioneering surgeons have been involved with the development of technology. Ben Eiseman, a noted innovative surgeon, describes the synergism between vascular surgery and technology. Of all technologies available, nothing is more fundamental and exciting than the application of molecular biology to vascular diseases. Scott Diamond and his group explain the use of molecular technique to extend graft patency. Recently, the identification by Gerard Tromp and Janet Powell of a possible genetic variation in some patients with aneurysms offers new insight into the pathogenesis of the disease. In the future, a simple DNA test may help to identify patients who are at risk to develop an aneurysm. Genetic engineering, a common technique in molecular biology, can now be applied in arterial bypass grafts. The therapeutic potential of such genetic engineering may yet be a breakthrough in the treatment of vascular disease. Allan Callow and James Stanley explain the potential use of these techniques to bypass grafts and arterial occlusive disease. The important functions of the endothelial cell for vascular surgeons are now understood, and Malcolm Herring, a pioneer in endothelial cell research, gives a definitive answer to the role of endothelial cell seeding of bypass grafts as a means to extend graft patency.

For years, physicians and surgeons alike have attempted to improve precision in diagnosis. In an editorial on this subject published in JAMA in 1890, it was stated that "the paramount condition to successful medical practice must ever be that of precision in diagnosis," and precision could only be accomplished by instruments. Fortunately, today, we have many instruments to improve the accuracy of diagnosis. Following the introduction of computed tomography, we now have magnetic resonance imaging to yield diagnostic information unobtainable by arteriography. Better yet, magnetic resonance imaging arteriography may someday replace contrast arteriography. Thomas Riles, Ronald Stoney, and Robert Vogelzang summarize new developments in diagnostic radiology.

In the past decade, refinement of duplex technology has made noninvasive testing a comprehensive examination in patients with a variety of vascular problems. Further developments in this field include color flow mapping and transcranial Doppler, and these new instruments offer more diagnostic information. Chapters on arterial imaging by Dennis Bandyk and the clinical application of color Doppler in venous problems by David Sumner provide an update on the use of color Doppler. Further development of ultrasound is possible, and D. E. Strandness suggests future uses for it. Transcranial ultrasound extends noninvasive examination into the vasculature of the brain. Bert Eikelboom and John Norris explain the role of this modality in patients with cerebrovascular disease. The diagnosis of renal artery stenosis is often difficult, and Richard Dean and his colleagues provide an accurate assessment of duplex scan in the diagnosis of renovascular hypertension. In recent years duplex ultrasound has also found its way into the operating room, and Bernard Sigel and colleagues present their experience in the intraoperative use of duplex ultrasound.

Traditionally, visualization of a vessel is by contrast angiography. With the introduction of fiberoptic technology, surgical practice has changed. For the first time, it is now possible for vascular surgeons to inspect the luminal characteristics of an artery or a bypass graft using angioscopy. Angioscopy not only offers diagnostic information but also can be incorporated with other techniques for therapeutic use. Angioscopy is now an integral part of a variety of diagnostic and therapeutic interventions in patients with arterial problems. William Flinn, William Pearce, James Seeger, and Thomas Fogarty give a summary on the potential clinical application of angioscopy. Another significant development of ultrasound technology is the intravascular ultrasound. This new innovative technique allows examination of a cross-sectional area of an artery. Arterial pathology is easily discernible. Leaders in this field such as David McPherson, Rodney White, and Jeffrey Isner summarize the principle, techniques, and clinical application of these new tools.

Undoubtedly, one significant development in the past decade has been in the area of interventional radiology. Robert Rutherford summarizes the results of balloon angioplasty, and these data offer a standard for the comparison of other new technologies. Interventional endovascular therapy is now available to reopen an occluded artery. Experts in this field such as Walter McCarthy, David Rosenthal, Luis Queral, Michael Dalsing, Samuel Ahn, and Larry Hollier give their experiences in the use of lasers, stents, and atherectomy devices. While these innovations may be useful, pharmacological manipulation of intimal hyperplasia, as described by Wesley Moore, may be necessary to maintain the patency. Surgeons using new technology need to develop strategies for intraoperative use and to understand the impact of this form of nonoperative management. Both George Andros and Frank Veith present an excellent view on this subject.

Finally, renewed interest in thrombolytic therapy with recombinant DNA molecular technology provides surgeons with an alternative or adjunctive treatment of thrombosis of arteries, veins, and bypass grafts. Recombinant urokinase and tissue plasminogen activator (t-PA) as described by Arthur Sasahara offer new alternatives in the management of acute thrombosis. Thrombolytic therapy is an important part of the armamentarium of vascular surgeons, and Peter Lawrence, Anthony Comerota, Alexander Turpie, and Anthony Whittemore summarize their experience in the treatment of thrombotic problems.

Technological innovations are part of the growth of medicine. Any new technology requires analysis, both as a technical development and as an evolution of surgical practice. How these new technologies fare in the future remains to be seen. It is hoped that this book will allow readers to update their knowledge in the rapid growth of high technology with a glimpse into the future of the practice of vascular surgery.

JAMES S. T. YAO, M.D., PH.D.
WILLIAM H. PEARCE, M.D.

CONTENTS

I

BASIC CONSIDERATIONS

1

TECHNOLOGY AND VASCULAR SURGERY: A Study in Synergism

BEN EISEMAN

All clinical specialties are divided into three parts: science, art, and craft. The proportions or mix differ, depending upon the specialty. Craft, which Webster defines as "an occupation, trade, or pursuit requiring manual dexterity or artistic skill, i.e. the carpenter's craft," is more important for some than others. Surgical disciplines inherently emphasize craft, and few would dispute that vascular surgery depends heavily upon manual skills. Unless a vascular surgeon is dexterous, neither his patients nor he will thrive.

Manual dexterity alone has limitations. For example, a door of sorts can be fashioned by moving a rock back and forth at the entrance to a cave using brute force alone. If one wants to substitute a wooden slab for the door, something akin to a saw is required. If a hinge is needed, still more technology is mandatory. Thus, crafts of whatever nature, are technology dependent. This chapter will analyze the relationship between technology and the craft of vascular surgery. I plan not merely to trace the historic synergism between the two disciplines, but to analyze the pattern of their interrelationship to suggest ways that their symbiosis might result in an even more productive future.

VASCULAR SURGERY: THE PAST

History is recorded in two ways. Early historians, such as Herodotus, Thucydides, and Livy, primarily recorded stories of past events such as pestillance, wars, or of the lives of great leaders as had been told to them. They had few means for judging the accuracy of these stories and seldom analyzed the interrelationship between events. These valuable histories provided the data base upon which an understanding of the past depends. Vascular surgery has numerous histories of its colorful past accomplishment, and because of the nature of the craft, technology is prominent in most of these classic stories.[1,2] After many years of dormancy, vascular surgery suddenly underwent an explosive growth, beginning about 50 years ago.

It was the good fortune of those of my generation to have our surgical careers coincide with this exciting "golden era" of vascular surgery. We elders have a tiresome way of overemphasizing the glories of our youth and the past, as though no more heroes of Homeric proportions can possibly match the exploits of ourselves and our colleagues who led the hosts in previous years. Such a solipsistic attitude is nonsense. Those in this audience also live in this golden era. Vascular surgery is, in my opinion, by no means what financial advisors call a "mature industry." It is still in its logarithmic growth phase, with opportunities limited only by the breadth of one's imagination. If you doubt such optimism, merely take a moment to review the list of patients you now have in the hospital, and then critically decide what proportion of them will, in all probability, have to face another operation for a vascular problem before they die.

Because others have adequately documented the mighty deeds of the past 50 years in vascular surgery, I will follow my assigned task by a technique known as historiography.

VASCULAR SURGERY'S HISTORIOGRAPHY

Webster defines historiography as "the synthesis of History into a narrative." This implies identifying themes that run through and connect isolated episodes of the past like the strand that connects the pearls of a necklace. Identifying such themes adds meaning to isolated events and even helps in predicting the future.

Let us use historiographic techniques to explain the remarkable renaissance of vascular surgery that began in the latter half of this century.

Many historians have spent their professional lives identifying the factors that seem to be common to a renaissance, for if we could create such an environment, we might re-create such periods of progress. What was common to Periclean Athens, Elizabethan England, Florence under Medicis, France under Louis the XIV, or England in the 18th and early 19th century? In each, arts and sciences flourished. What caused their rise, and more ominously, what started their decline?[3]

FACTORS THAT CONTRIBUTE TO A RENAISSANCE

Some historians, such as Carlyle, believe that great men shape world events. This seems highly improbable in explaining the sudden emergence of progress in one locality at a single moment in history during which seminal advances in several unrelated disciplines occur. It seems much more likely that times make the man, not the opposite.

A partial list of factors that seem to be common to periods of renaissance might include the following:

Intellectual and personal freedom of thought and expression.

Social and political stability.

The luxury of leisure in which innovative thinkers can contemplate without the need to fight for food or survival during most of their waking hours.

Political power, which characteristically equates with economic power in the country where the renaissance is to occur.

A heritage of individual and social honesty, morality, and discipline.

A critical mass of prior knowledge—which often required many years or even centuries to accumulate, but upon which future discoveries must be based.

The physical means by which new ideas can be modeled, tested, altered, and then applied. This equates with technology.

Each of these prerequisites existed in the United States immediately following World War II, when this country, almost uniquely among industrial powers, was untouched by the ravages of the two World Wars. A strong case can be made that our emerging technology was the spark that ignited the information and craft explosion that constituted the merging of the modern era of vascular surgery—the craft to which you have fallen heir.

It is worth identifying some of the technologies that existed and which were necessary for this vascular surgery renaissance to start in America 50 years ago. It is difficult, in this sophisticated age, to believe they were unavailable when some for the more dramatic events in vascular surgery's history took place.

Anticoagulants. When many of us began our vascular surgical interests, generalized total body anticoagulation was in its infancy. Before use of generalized body anticoagulation we had to hurry through operations in which we had to cross-clamp major vessels, and after reconstituting blood flow, spend much of the rest of the day fishing out clots from the distal vascular bed.

Safe Anesthesia for High-Risk Patients. We now take for granted that there is small risk in performing prolonged operations under general anesthesia on elderly patients with advanced cerebral, cardiac, or renal disease. This was far from the case even 40 years ago, when the significant risk of stroke or a myocardial infarct during operation had to be seriously weighed against the probability of benefiting the patient by operations upon his peripheral arterial tree.

Repair of Block for Atherosclerosis. An important breakthrough was the recognition that atherosclerosis, although a generalized condition, might have as its major limiting manifestations, a localized arterial narrowing or block that was amenable to repair. The breakthrough came with the identification of Leriche's syndrome where great benefit came from opening a localized block in the common iliac artery. This opened the flood gates and surgeons made every localized arterial narrowing fair game for operative repair.

Vascular Surgery Instruments. At the beginning of this renaissance, a short 40 to 50 years ago, we made do with instruments designed for use in gastrointestinal surgery. It soon became evident that special instruments were required. Instruments and sutures had to be miniaturized and changed to keep up with our needs. The ordinary small, curved needle with an eye through which two strands of 4-0 silk had to be pulled through a small-caliber artery caused too much bleeding.

It was at this point that the biomedical engineering industry began its productive relationship with vascular surgeons. Several of the large surgical supply and suture manufacturing houses devoted millions of dollars into development of small-caliber needles with swedged-on fine monofilament sutures which were necessary for precise vascular procedures on small-caliber vessels. Responsible biomedical engineers, salaried by the industry, became our co-workers and allies.

Vascular Prosthetics. A technology essential for development of vascular surgery was the creation of prosthetic tubes capable of transmitting blood without clotting. Fortunately, this need coincided with the emergence of the plastics industry in the United States. The original discovery was made by Voorhees, Jaretzki, and co-workers at Colombia Presbyterian Hospital in New

York, using vinvon.[4] Many of the rest of us tried other materials. I even recall cutting strips of commercially available plastic sponges purchased in the supermarket—welding them together around a mandrill by steam, sterilizing, and then testing the tube as a vascular conduit.

Diagnostic Radiology.   Progress in vascular surgery required precise localization of a vascular block and evaluation of the run-off.

There were a few furious years when x-ray films had to be changed as quickly as possible by hand after the dye injected just proximal to the block flowed past the point of suspected constriction. Outside the radiology suite stood a long, gaunt line of surgical residents and impressed medical students, each clutching a large cassette. At the moment that the last of the radiopaque bolus was pushed in by hand, the injectionist shouted "Fire," and the radiology technician, crouched behind his protective lead shield, pressed the button. A stream of residents then stood to the guns, and each in turn slammed in his cassette beneath the patient, in turn shouted "Fire," withdrew his film, and hastily made way for the next in line who repeated the process for the ensuing 10 seconds. The scene resembled a procedure common on the Western Front of World War I, with Poilu artillerymen serving fast-firing French 75s by ramming home shells into the breach of those venerable field pieces.

Thank God it was not too long before industry came up with automatic film changers and compressors for injecting the dye.

I still recall, when trying to visualize the aortic arch, that we devised a way of sticking a long needle supraclavicularly into the aortic root. One of my residents, Dr. Rainer, who later became a distinguished member of the Thoracic Board and President of the American Association of Thoracic Surgery, by chance injected the dye with such vigor that it streamed under our watchful eyes, which were glued to the fluoroscope, so that it filled the coronary arteries. I was certain it would cause ventricular fibrillation and berated him for his overvigorous injection. Dr. Rainer has subsequently, on several inauspicious occasions, reminded me in public how little foresight I had when he, as far as we knew, for the first time performed a coronary arteriogram, a procedure on which he has subsequently relied heavily in achieving his fame and fortune.

SUBSEQUENT MILESTONES

There have been many subsequent milestones in the development of vascular surgery, almost every one of which was technologically related. It would be highly unwise for me to single-out any one such advance, for fear of hurting the feelings of other colleagues, unmentioned, who each considers his innovation seminal. We were a small band of brothers in those days, and almost every one of us was an innovator by necessity. Walter Lillehei used to say that a surgeon couldn't get on the operating schedule at the University of Minnesota unless he had some new operation to perform.

Let me, however, mention some of the more important ideas that significantly changed the practice of vascular surgery, so as to indicate their dependence on technology and industry.

Vascular Clamps.   In the early days of vascular surgery, the only methods for occluding blood vessels were with encircling tapes or rubber-shod clamps designed for occluding the bowel. I still remember my frustration as I watched a heavy Payr clamp, which I had placed at the base of a large ascending aortic aneurysm, slowly work its way heartbeat-by-heartbeat toward the opened aneurysmal sac. These were, of course, the days before the availability of a pump oxygenator suitable for bypassing the heart.

The Pott's serrated aortic clamp opened the way for many other similar devices of various shapes and sizes. Every surgeon of any vascular pretension designed some variation of a clamp to which he proudly fixed his name. These were weak reeds to lean on, but seemed important at the time.

Flow Meters. Not long after the novelty of opening and closing an artery or vein began to wane, it became clear to thoughtful vascular surgeons of the need to quantitate blood flow through vessels either in evaluating indications for vascular operations or for quantitating results postoperatively. After some highly unsuccessful attempts at using dye and isotope techniques of clearance, we reverted to electromagnetic flowmeters fitted to a C clamp, which partially encircled the vessel. This had the obvious disadvantages of requiring operative isolation of the vessel. Once, in the early 1950s, I gathered a group of petroleum engineers (who were accustomed to measuring fluid flow through pipes) to listen to my story as we sought a noninvasive method of blood-flow measurement. The conversation was most interesting, but we came up with nothing that was applicable for clinical use. This of course had to await advances in ultrasound and Doppler wave-form analysis, plus sensitive pulse recorders—a technology that we all know forms the basis of the vascular laboratories, which is now so important to vascular surgeons. It is such laboratories that still typify the heavy reliance of vascular surgery on technology and the industries that produce these instruments.

Prosthetic Substitutes for Blood Vessels. Devising a nonclotting prosthetic tube that will carry blood was, and still is, a vital part of the interface between vascular surgery and the biomedical engineering industry. The story of how my skiing companion, Bill Gore, demonstrated to me one day after skiing, a tie made of a new material that he (as a chemical engineer) had designed that was both nonwettable and able to transmit gas, is too well documented to recount.[5] The expanded Teflon transmitted gas and yet was impermeable to fluid, so we used it as a membrane in an oxygenator. A few weeks later we asked the Gore company to fashion the material into tubes, which we used experimentally in pigs, and later were the first to use in patients.

To show that Bill Gore and I had our priorities in life straight, we agreed that perhaps the greatest boon of such a unique fabric was the potential for obviating the need for a rain fly on tents. It was Bill who thought of using the material for parkas and gloves. This is what is known in the trade as technology "pull-finding" an unrelated need for an existing technology.

These are but a few examples of the interdependence of progress in vascular surgery with the biomedical engineering industry.

Let us next explore how a surgeon can best prepare himself to contribute to such progress, for every investigator appreciates that good ideas come to the prepared mind.

THE VASCULAR SURGEON'S ROLE IN BIOTECHNOLOGY INNOVATION

Vascular surgery is a full-time job, requiring most of one's waking hours either in operating upon or caring for patients. Much of what time that remains must be devoted to keeping up with progress in this fast-moving field. Those who will aspire to research must steal time from other parts of their lives.

Vascular surgery, and indeed surgery in general, is at best an applied science. It is extremely rare for a surgeon to make significant discovery in pure science. The vascular surgeon can best play his role as an investigator by identifying significant unsolved clinical problems which he brings to the attention of basic scientists and engineers who, working with him, solve the problem. Such a role sounds uninteresting and unimportant, but in fact requires a great deal of imagination and critical training. In the "high-tech" industrial world—this is known as information transfer from a "user" to an industrial producer. This interface is currently, as we shall see, under intense study by industrial managerial analysts.

The compelling force for such innovation can arise either from what is known as "technology push" or "market pull." The vascular surgeon is the origin of the problem that creates the market pull. The engineer seeking a use for a device or material already available in another discipline produces the technology push.

A few examples of the type of problem that a vascular surgeon might currently bring to his industrial scientist coworker for solution might include the following:

A prosthetic lined by living and functioning endothelial cells that could produce cytokines such as prostacyclin.

A noninvasive blood-flow measuring device that could detect occlusion of an aorta coronary bypass in the postoperative recovery room.

Noninvasive methods to destroy atherosclerotic plaques without damaging the surrounding blood vessel.

Substitute venous valves to control postphlebetic syndrome.

Improve noninvasive methods for monitoring blood gases and pH.

The list is endless. In my own experience, the best way for a surgeon to position himself to ask these pertinent questions is by consciously encouraging a critical frame of mind as he reviews the hundreds of daily decisions and actions which are a part of clinical practice. He constantly asks himself if there is not perhaps a better way of doing an operation he has just performed or making a decision that he has made in patient management.

Dr. Carl Walter, the distinguished (and irrascable) Professor Emeritus of Surgery at Harvard and the Brigham Hospital recalls his degrading experience as a young surgical pup when his assignment was to coat the walls of glass containers with paraffin to prevent blood from clotting and then to administer the blood to patients being operated upon by his distinguished chief, Harvey Cushing. Carl Walter's fuse is short and so was that of the professor. In frustration at the clumsiness of then known methods for transfusion, Dr. Walter, in a fury, gave vent to an outburst in the operating room starting with an expletive and ending with the statement, "There just has to be a better way of doing this damn thing." Cushing was outraged, but in dressing down his young colleague following the procedure, started Dr. Walter on a lifetime of invention and innovation to find better and safer ways to store blood and give transfusions. It didn't hurt that Dr. Walter already had a degree in chemical engineering before entering Harvard, but the real key was that he had within him the pent-up rage to demand of himself (and others) that "there has to be a better way."

The would-be surgical innovator keeps an open file in some obscure recess of his mind where he stores all such unsolved problems. There it sits like a part of his guilty conscience, dimly perceived but not recalled on a daily basis.

On occasion, and often at a most unlikely moment, the innovator sees an unrelated fact, or learns of a new technology that suddenly recalls the problem from his subconscious, makes a synapse, and suddenly the idea reaches a conscious level and he says to himself, "Might this be a way of solving this worrisome problem?" This is a moment of pure ecstasy. Never mind that the probability of even one of ten such ideas turns out, on more mature reflection, to be valid. This is what makes surgery (and particularly academic surgery) a profession of lifelong excitement.

One of the primary objectives of a teacher is to create such a self-critical state of mind among his surgical pupils that constantly goads the student to look for better ways of patient management. It is a characteristic that improves patient care, encourages professional humility, and provides for progress. Such an objective has been formalized into the mortality and morbidity conference where every less-than-perfect outcome is brought up for review by one's colleagues.

It is residual from mortality and morbidity conferences that forms the worry list. It is a pity that such a conference has, like so many valuable and fragile ideas, been bastardized by being codified as a prerequisite for approval.

THE ROLE OF INDUSTRY

An industrial manager would classify vascular surgery as just another high-technology industry. Its customers are surgeons whose requirements frequently depend upon research scientists and engineers to produce devices in a highly competitive field where inventions have a discouraging habit of maintaining relatively short periods of applicability. Start-up research and development costs are high and therefore, profit margins must be high when a device is first marketed. As in other high-technology industries, progress depends primarily on successfully bridging the communications gap between the user (who may also be the innovator) and those who will help him bring a new idea to reality.

There is intense current interest in how high-technology industries can most efficiently create productive communication and teamwork involving the wide spectrum of specialists who are required to produce complex, successful technology. Such emphasis obviously stems from the superiority of the Japanese in producing such high-technology products as automobiles and electronics. Indeed, the rush to switch to the Japanese style of management during the past 5 to 10 years has reached almost revolutionary proportions in many large high-technology corporations. It is ironic that these managerial techniques were first developed by three Americans, Deming, Juran, and Cosby, but were largely ignored in this country. It was not until the Japanese adopted them and used these techniques to outproduce the Americans, that we recognized their value.[6]

This is not the place to detail the intricacies of these managerial techniques, but we should appreciate that these radical organizational changes were made precisely to meet the technology demands made by people such as vascular surgeons in developing new products.

Let us cite a few examples of these managerial techniques as they apply to vascular surgery.

Angioscopy is an example of technology push, for it combines two technologies developed for other purposes—fiberoptics and miniaturization of television—to serve a new need in vascular surgery. Another example might be the use of an extremely durable material—pyrollytic carbon, which was developed for the space program—for use in heart valves which must open and close 35 million times a year.[7]

A vascular or cardiac surgeon approaching a biomedical engineering corporation with a potentially new idea for a device may find himself, from the earliest stages of discussions, working with a committee representing many types of business and engineering specialists. There may be various types of basic scientists and engineers, accountants, and financial experts who will have to determine how the project will be funded and financially supervised; developers and managers who will determine how the project will articulate with other ongoing projects; and finally, those who will market the product when it becomes available. Each member of this team will make the project very much a part of his own future and will feel free to enter discussions of the meetings at any time. This is the participatory element in the managerial style.

The surgeon accustomed to the discipline and style of a residency program or the military will find that high-technology industry has altered this classic managerial style. There will be no single authoritarian project manager who is obviously responsible for minor decisions. The classic managerial style is called a functional system. The Japanese system is called a matrix system. In preliminary discussions, the innovator and scientists may provide most of the discussion and, with the engineers, make most of the key decisions. As the project develops, decision-making shifts to the developers and marketing specialists.[8]

The point of this discussion is that industry has found it sufficiently important to reorganize its managerial style and structure to work with users such as vascular and cardiac surgeons in developing new technology. No serious analysis of the relation between vascular surgery and technology should ignore the importance of this managerial revolution which industry has made to meet the challenge of being a partner with us in progress.

PITFALLS IN SYNERGISM

It would be naive to think that a liaison between partners, one of whom is very rich and powerful, and the other, poor, naive, but allegedly virtuous, would be completely trouble free. The unique relationship between the biomedical engineering industry and vascular and cardiac surgeons offers both unique opportunities and some obvious temptations.

The temptations are predictable. By the time industry is ready to market a new device or product, it has made significant investments in the new project which must be made up by a high profit margin. Early obsolescence further drives up costs in a highly competitive industry. Those in charge of marketing must make every possible effort to convince those who make the decision for purchase to buy their product. Such decision makers in cardiovascular surgery are usually surgeons, and they are understandably the focus of intense marketing pressure. The ethical dilemma is well known to every surgeon, to industry, and to ethicists.[9] Where is the line to be drawn? Is a cup of coffee and a donut while discussing the new device with the sales representative acceptable? At the other extreme, it is obviously not appropriate for the clinician to accept a round-trip first-class air ticket to some exotic resort and a weekend for himself and his wife to attend some spurious semiprofessional symposium devoted, presumably, to the discussion of new surgical progress. There is no easy answer to such ethical problems. There seldom is when the line between sin and virtue is involved.

Although these are temptations, there are many totally appropriate advantages for vascular surgeons as they work in partnership with corporations producing the technology on which their craft depends. Both the vascular surgeon and the biomedical industry have in common the objective of producing products that will improve the management of patients with vascular disease. It is of mutual advantage for industry to provide research grants to those who can, with discipline, proper training, and laboratory support, devise and test new devices. In an era when federal funding for clinical research has all but disappeared, such sources of grant money are obviously important.

CONCLUSIONS

The easy way to respond to the challenge of discussing vascular surgery and technology in this opening address would have been simply to recount that some of the dramatic events which have occurred are technology-dependent. From this, neither you nor I would have learned anything. I have instead explored the historiography of progress in a technology-dependent field; in this case, vascular surgery. Because of the recent renaissance in vascular surgery, I have tried to analyze how technology might have played a significant role in such progress.

Because all of us are interested in how we can continue this renaissance in vascular surgery, I have suggested how surgical innovators can best participate in future discoveries. Further, because this is a joint venture between surgeons and industry, I have briefly described how our industrial partners have performed almost revolutionary changes in managerial style to meet the very needs that we know to be important in vascular surgery, but which in fact are common to many other high-technology industries. Finally, both the temptations and the unique opportunities of this liaison between ourselves and industry have been discussed.

REFERENCES

1. Barker WF: A history of Vascular Surgery. *In* Moore W, ed. Vascular Surgery: A Comprehensive Review, 3rd ed. WB Saunders Co, 1991.
2. Kempczinski RF: The Development of Vascular Surgery, vol 1. *In* Kempczinski RF, ed. The Ischemic Leg. Chicago, Year Book Medical Publishers, 1985.
3. Kennedy P: Rise, Fall of the Great Powers. New York, Random House, 1987.
4. Voorhees AB, Jaretski A, and Blakemore WH: The use of tubes constructed from vinyon N cloth bridging arterial defects. Ann Surg 1952; *135*:332.
5. Kelly G, Eiseman B: Development of a new vascular prosthetic Arch Surg 1982; *117*:1367–70.
6. Gabor A: Total Quality Management. New York, Random House, 1990.
7. Collins J: The evolution of the artificial heart valves. N Engl J Med 1991; *324*:624.
8. Morone J, Alben R: Matching R&D business needs. Research Management 1984; *27*:33–59.
9. Doolittle RF: Biotechnology, the enormous cost of success. N Engl Med 1991; *324*:1360.

2

REGULATION OF ENDOTHELIAL CELL GENE EXPRESSION BY HEMODYNAMIC FORCES: Implications for Intimal Hyperplasia and Graft Patency

SCOTT L. DIAMOND, JOHN B. SHAREFKIN, CARL W. DIEFFENBACH, SUZANNE G. ESKIN, and LARRY V. McINTIRE

Maintenance of proper cellular phenotype (or "genetic state") of the endothelial cell and the smooth muscle cell is critical in preventing loss of vessel patency. Intimal hyperplasia is a common cause of obstructive stenosis following many kinds of vascular reconstruction.[1-5] Both intimal hyperplasia and early atherosclerotic lesions occur most often in areas of flow disturbances such as anastomotic sites[1-3] and in areas with low- or oscillatory-fluid shear stress.[6-11] We have carried out experiments to recreate blood flow forces in vitro and to measure the effects of these forces on endothelial cell gene expression.

In the vessel wall, blood factors, cytokines delivered by macrophages or T cells, and platelet-derived products can all cause excessive proliferation of smooth muscle cells. The endothelium may also regulate the phenotype of the smooth muscle cell by releasing mitogens. Molecular biology techniques are particularly powerful in deciphering the many complex events which occur at the cellular level. Studies of cellular phenotype are often used in tandem with cell culture approaches. In vitro techniques allow the study of cell–cell interactions while largely isolating or decoupling hemodynamic, hematologic, and immunologic contributions to the vascular pathology. However, when cells are taken from the body, whether they are derived from normal or diseased tissue, changes can occur in the cultured cell lines. The three-dimensional structure and confinements of the tissue are lost when cells are grown in plastic dishes. The complex nature of the in vivo environment is only approximated by a growth medium. The delicate balance of growth regulatory factors is only partially recreated by addition of growth factors to the cell culture medium.

An additional complication is that the phenotype of the cell in culture is highly dependent on the mode of isolation, the time in culture, the medium and substrate used to culture the cells, and the initial seeding density of the culture. The challenge of studying cells in vitro is to maintain the basic functions of the cell which are important in understanding the disease process.

To understand the process of intimal hyperplasia, it is important to evaluate how strongly particular genes are being transcribed into messenger RNA (mRNA) by cells in the vessel wall. Measurement of mRNA levels in human cells is complicated by the small numbers of cells available (on the order of 10^6 or fewer cells) from early passage cultures. Northern blotting techniques typically require much greater quantities of total cellular RNA isolated from 10^7 to 10^8 cells grown in culture. The detection limit of autoradiography is about 1 pg of nucleic acid. This limit in detection is especially troublesome for investigations of messages which have only a few copies per cell. To obtain large numbers of cultured human endothelial cells requires the use of endothelial cell growth factor, often in combination with heparin, to grow the cells for several passages. It is more desirable to study endothelial cell production of fibrinolytic mediators and smooth muscle cell mitogens without long-term, large-scale cultivation, since phenotypic drift in culture has been documented in human umbilical vein endothelial cells (HUVEC). For example, the urokinase gene, not normally expressed in primary HUVEC or adult vena cava cultures, becomes quite active[12,13] at higher passage numbers. Also, tissue plasminogen activator (tPA) secretion and tPA mRNA is upregulated many-fold with serial passage in culture,[12–14] while plasminogen activator inhibitor 1 (PAI-1) secretion has been shown to decrease 3 to 10-fold with the use of heparin in combination with endothelial cell growth factor.[15] At higher cell passage number, the quantity of the smaller, polyadenylate-free form of the PAI-1 mRNA increases.[13] Additionally, prostacyclin (PGI_2) production is quickly lost and von Willebrand factor production decreases at high passage number.

With the use of the polymerase chain reaction amplification (PCR) technique utilizing recombinant, heat stable *Thermus aquaticus (Taq)* DNA polymerase, mRNA measurements are possible with small numbers (on the order of 10^6 cells) of cells from primary cultures of HUVEC that have not been passaged in culture or exposed to stimulation by growth factors. The PCR-based mRNA assay utilizes the following approach: total cellular RNA is isolated from cells and target mRNA species are reversed transcribed. The complementary DNA (cDNA) synthesized using the reverse transcriptase enzyme is then prepared for PCR amplification. Primers which are specific for the cDNA are added and the PCR amplification is carried out to produce thousands of copies of the original cDNA. The amplified cDNA is then measured using specific radiolabeled oligonucleotide probes (Fig. 2–1) as an indicator of the quantity of input mRNA species into the assay.

This method of analysis of mRNA levels in cells is more sensitive than standard Northern blotting techniques. Northern blotting requires the use of long cDNA probes which are sometimes difficult to obtain and require a plasmid preparation and nick translation of each probe. With the PCR approach, the target signal is much greater than background and small end-labeled oligo probes allow detection of the product. Measurement of up to six genes is feasible with our approach, since it lends itself to automation. To study the many relationships between growth factors, it is desirable to measure the mRNA levels of several genes simultaneously. Our use of an internal amplification standard, glyceraldehyde 3-phosphate dehydrogenase (GAPDH), enhances the

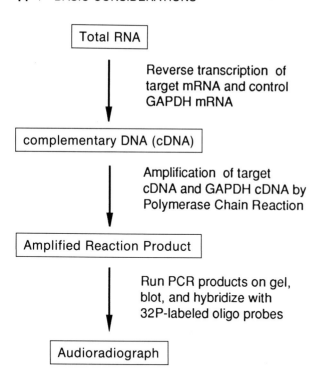

Figure 2–1. Measurements of endothelial mRNA levels in small numbers of human cells is accomplished using a coupled reverse transcription/polymerase chain reaction method. Total cellular RNA is isolated from the cells. The mRNA target and internal control mRNA are then reverse transcribed. The resulting cDNAs are coamplified using PCR and then visualized by standard Southern blotting with radiolabeled DNA probes. The quantity of amplification product serves as an indicator of the amount of the particular mRNA level in the cells.

utility of the technique since the PCR amplification does have some variability from reaction to reaction. As techniques evolve, cRNA constructs added to unknowns[16] may be useful for calibrating our measurements to actual intracellular mRNA copy number. With the internal control gene to normalize for variations in reverse transcription yield and efficiency of amplification, an estimate of the initial mRNA concentration per cell can be made relative to the initial copy number of the GAPDH message.

METHODS

The exposure of monolayers of endothelial cells to defined levels of laminar shear stress used parallel-plate flow channels of known geometry. Replicate primary, confluent monolayers (72 to 86 hours post seeding) of HUVEC were exposed to steady laminar shear stress in individual parallel-plate flow chamber systems with recirculating media driven by a constant hydrostatic pressure head as previously described.[17–19] The cell cultures were mounted on separate parallel-plate flow chambers. The monolayer surface area exposed to shear stress in each chamber was 15 cm^2 with a channel thickness of 200 μm. Flow chambers were connected under sterile conditions to individual flow systems, each filled with 15 ml of medium. The wall shear stress imposed upon the monolayer was evaluated by solution of the Navier-Stokes equation for laminar flow of a Newtonian liquid. The wall shear stress (τ_w = dynes/cm^2) was calculated as follows: $\tau_w = 6\,Q\,\mu/(B^2 W)$ where: flowrate, Q = cm^3/sec; viscosity, μ = 0.01 poise; total gap thickness, B = 0.02 cm; and width, W = 2.49 cm. The entrance length needed for steady parabolic flow to be established was less than 1 mm.[20] The Reynolds number for the flow condition was less than 50, ensuring that the flow was truly laminar with no possibility of turbulence.

For each experiment, control cultures were incubated under stationary conditions. Media samples (1 ml) were taken from each system every 4 to 6 hours and stored at $-80°C$. For PCR analysis of mRNA levels, the flow was stopped and total cellular RNA extracted from the shear stressed monolayers (15 cm^2 of monolayer per slide) within 1 minute after termination of flow. Similarly, RNA was extracted from stationary cultures (15 cm^2 of monolayer per slide). To calculate mean cell density on the slides before RNA extraction, cells were counted in three light micrographs of each monolayer.

Studies of mRNA levels using small numbers of primary human cells were carried out with a reverse transcription/polymerase chain reaction technique (PCR). Isolation of total cellular RNA from small cellular samples was accomplished with a scaled-down adaptation of the guanidine thiocyanate (GTC)/ cesium chloride (CsCl) gradient method[21,22] as previously described.[19] Briefly, monolayers were lysed in 5 M guanidine thiocyanate solution with 25 mM sodium citrate and 0.5 per cent (w/v) sodium N-lauroyl sarcosinate and centrifuged at $20,000g$ for 3 hours over a 5.7 M CsCl cushion. The pellet was dissolved in diethyl pyrocarbonate-treated (DEPC) water (0.2 v/v per cent) and extracted twice with phenol/chloroform/isoamyl alcohol (25:24:1) and once with cholorform/isoamyl alcohol (24:1). Total RNA was precipitated with 3 M sodium acetate (pH 5.4) and 100 per cent ethanol, vacuum dried, and resuspended in 30 μl of DEPC-H_2O. A 2.5 M LiCl precipitation and resuspension was performed prior to the reverse transcription.

To provide an internal standard against experimental variations in the reverse transcription reaction or PCR amplification efficiency, simultaneous reverse transcription and coamplification of the constitutively-expressed mRNA for GAPDH were carried out as previously described.[19] Simultaneous reverse transcription and coamplification of human endothelial cell RNA with primer sets[19,23] for tPA or basic fibroblast growth factor (bFGF) or endothelin-1 (ET-1) and GAPDH produced amplification products of the predicted sizes of 368 bp for tPA, 177 bp for bFGF, 441 bp for ET-1, and 195 bp for GAPDH. Synthesis of tPA (or bFGF or ET-1) cDNA and GAPDH cDNA was carried out simultaneously in 25 μl reactions with 500 U MMLV reverse transcriptase (RT), 0.5 μg of each antisense primer, and 0.5 mM each of all four dNTPs. Each reverse transcription reaction mixture was carried out at 37°C for 20 minutes. The cDNA products were coamplified using the polymerase chain reaction in a total volume of 100 μl. Prior to amplification, a 75 μl volume was added containing 0.5 μg of each sense primer, 0.25 μg of each antisense primer, and 10 mM of each dNTP. Two units of recombinant *Taq* DNA polymerase (AmpliTaq, Beckman) were added to initiate the PCR. Each temperature cycle consisted of 90°C for 1.5 minutes, 50°C for 1 minute, and 72°C for 2 minutes. Amplified products were visualized by Southern hybridization as previously described[19] using T4 kinase ^{32}P end-labeled probes for tPA (or bFGF or ET-1) and for GAPDH.

Immunoreactive endothelin was measured using a radioimmunoassay (Amersham Corporation) employing an ^{125}I-endothelin tracer and antiserum made against synthetic endothelin-1. A calibration curve yielding a LOGIT plot with $r^2 > 0.99$ was generated using synthetic ET-1 added to complete medium (M199 + bovine serum) to control for nonspecific background.

A double antibody enzyme-linked immunosorbent assay (ELISA) technique (American Diagnostica Inc.) using goat antihuman tPA immunoglobin allowed measurement of HUVEC-secreted tPA (free and inhibitor-bound) as previously described.[18] Normal goat IgG was used as a nonspecific blocking agent. Soluble goat antihuman tPA IgG quenched the tPA-specific signal in the blanking well. HUVEC-conditioned media (undiluted) or antigenic standards (Bowes melanoma single-chain tPA) were added to sample wells in triplicate and to blanking wells. The ELISA was calibrated to the limit of its sensitivity (0 to 1500 pg/ml), yielding a linear calibration curve ($r^2 > 0.99$) with a detection limit of 50 pg/ml.

In HUVEC-conditioned media, PAI-1 exists in latent and active forms with only a very small fraction bound to tPA. An ELISA was used to measure uncomplexed (latent and active) PAI-1 antigen (American Diagnostic Inc.). Briefly, mouse antihuman PAI-1 immunoglobin was bound to a 96-well plate. The plate was washed and loaded with samples of conditioned media (diluted 1:10 and 1:25) or standards. The colorimetric reaction (measured at 490 nm) was performed using biotinylated monoclonal mouse antihuman PAI-1 immunoglobin and horseradish peroxidase conjugated streptavidin with a reaction buffer containing orthophenylenediamine and 0.04 per cent (v/v) 30 per cent-H_2O_2.

RESULTS

Our studies of protein production by endothelial cells exposed to shear stress were carried out in experiments lasting over 24 hours. During the first several hours after the onset of fluid flow, the levels of tPA in the circulating medium at all shear stress levels were the same as those of stationary control cultures (Fig. 2–2). Low shear stress (4 dynes/cm²) had no effect on tPA secretion over the entire time course of the experiments. After longer exposure to shear stress of 15 or 25 dynes/cm², however, the level of tPA produced by shear-exposed cells exceeded that of controls (Fig. 2–2). The increase of tPA in the circulating medium was linear with time for over 20 hours, allowing a least-squares fit to determine the steady-state secretion rate. Steady-state tPA secretion rates of cells exposed to 15 and 25 dynes/cm², normalized to matched controls, increased 2.06 ± 0.39 ($n=3$; $p<0.015$)- and 3.01 ± 0.53 ($n=3$; $p<0.015$)-fold over stationary cultures, respectively. The average steady-state secretion rate of tPA by HUVEC in control cultures was 0.168 ± 0.053 ng/10⁶ cells-hr ($n=3$).[18]

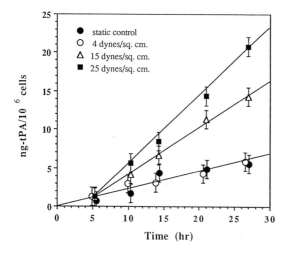

FIGURE 2–2. Cumulative production of tissue plasminogen activator (tPA) by replicate, primary confluent HUVEC monolayers maintained in stationary incubations (●) or exposed to steady laminar shear stress of 4 (o), 15 (△), or 25 dynes/cm² (■) using three independent flow systems. Each point is the average of triplicate ELISA determinations. Steady state production rates were calculated for each monolayer by a least-squares fit of cumulative production between 4 and 24 hours.

The secretion of tPA by control cultures was completely inhibited by cycloheximide (5 μg/ml), suggesting that new protein synthesis was continually required in order to maintain constitutive tPA release. This would indicate that the increase of tPA in the circulating medium was not due to release of intracellular stores of tPA. The greatly enhanced convective mass transport at low stresses of 4 dynes/cm² (compared the natural convection of stationary cultures) had no effect on the production of tPA. Also, the cyclooxygenase inhibitor indomethacin (50 μM) had no effect on shear-stress–stimulated tPA production indicating that the shear-enhanced tPA secretion was not mediated by a cyclooxygenase product.

Shear stress levels ranging from 4 to 40 dynes/cm² caused no significant changes in the PAI-1 secretion rate relative to controls. The average steady-state PAI-1 secretion rate of HUVEC in control cultures was 53 ± 37 ng of PAI-1 per 10⁶ cells per hour ($n = 7$).[18] Measurements of PAI-1 production over the first 200 minutes after the onset of flow demonstrated that the PAI-1 secretion was not affected by shear stress transiently at early exposure times.

Primary HUVEC secreted about 15,000 pg of ET-1 per 10⁶ cells in 24 hours while in stationary culture. Secretion of endothelin was suppressed by laminar shear stress of 25 dynes/cm² within 4 hours after the onset of flow (Fig. 2–3). The suppression of endothelin secretion by high shear stress (25 dynes/cm²) continued for over 20 hours during exposure to flow. In three separate experiments, endothelin production was suppressed only slightly (<15 per cent) by low shear stress of 4 dynes/cm² compared to endothelin production of stationary controls.

To investigate the effect of laminar shear stress on mRNA levels in endothelial cells, replicate HUVEC monolayers were either maintained in stationary culture or exposed to shear stress at 25 dynes/cm² in individual flow systems. In each experiment, secretion of tPA, PAI-1, and ET-1 (per 10⁶ cells) was evaluated for the three individual flow systems and the three matched, stationary cultures. Enhancement of tPA production and suppression of ET-1 secretion were observed after a lag time of several hours of exposure to shear stress (Table 2–1) as was previously observed. In each experiment, the quantity of total cellular RNA isolated from stationary and shear-stressed HUVEC cultures was not significantly different (average variation less than 10 per cent).

FIGURE 2–3. Cumulative production of endothelin by replicate, primary confluent HUVEC monolayers maintained in three separate stationary incubations (□) or exposed to steady laminar shear stress of 25 dynes/cm² (■) using three independent flow systems. Each point is the average of duplicate RIA determinations. Steady state production rates were calculated for each monolayer by a least-squares fit of cumulative production between 4 and 24 hours.

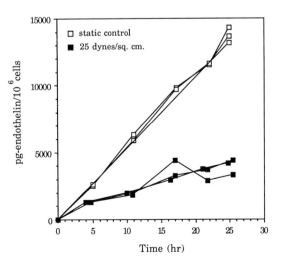

TABLE 2–1. SECRETION RATE OF TISSUE-TYPE PLASMINOGEN ACTIVATOR (tPA), PLASMINOGEN ACTIVATOR INHIBITOR-TYPE 1 (PAI-1), AND ENDOTHELIN-1 (ET) BY HUMAN ENDOTHELIAL CELLS EXPOSED TO LAMINAR SHEAR STRESS OF 25 dynes/cm^2 [a]

Experiment[b]	Cell Density (10^4 cells/cm^2)	tPA Secretion Rate (ng-tPA/10^6 cells/hr)	PAI-1 Secretion Rate (ng-PAI-1/10^6 cells/hr)	ET Secretion Rate (ng-ET/10^6 cells/hr)
1. Control	7.7 ± 0.8	0.170 ± 0.049 ($n = 3$)	70.2 ± 4.97 ($n = 3$)	0.545 ± 0.017 ($n = 3$)
25 dynes/cm^2	7.1 ± 0.9	0.399 ± 0.087 ($n = 3$)	47.8 ± 13.6 ($n = 3$)	0.132 ± 0.026 ($n = 3$)
2. Control	6.7 ± 0.8	0.160 ± 0.039 ($n = 3$)	49.3 ± 3.25 ($n = 3$)	0.485 ± 0.025 ($n = 3$)
25 dynes/cm^2	7.3 ± 0.8	0.527 ± 0.123 ($n = 3$)	26.5 ± 3.04 ($n = 3$)	0.279 ± 0.055 ($n = 3$)
3. Control	5.9 ± 1.0	0.122 ± 0.013 ($n = 3$)	53.0 ± 8.71 ($n = 3$)	0.587 ± 0.057 ($n = 3$)
25 dynes/cm^2	6.2 ± 0.9	0.387 ± 0.073 ($n = 2$)	58.1 ± 7.60 ($n = 2$)	0.335 ± 0.061 ($n = 2$)
Mean rates ± SD				
Control		0.157 ± 0.036 ($n = 9$)	57.2 ± 10.6 ($n = 9$)	0.549 ± 0.046 ($n = 9$)
25 dynes/cm^2		0.453 ± 0.108 ($n = 8$)[c]	42.6 ± 15.5 ($n = 8$)[d]	0.239 ± 0.099 ($n = 8$)[c]

[a] The large induction of tPA secretion is in contrast to the suppression of endothelin secretion. Protein secretion rates were determined by a least-squares fit of antigen production data between 4 and 24 hours. Enzyme-linked immunosorbent assays were used to quantify tPA and PAI-1 production, while endothelin production was evaluated using a radioimmunoassay. Analysis of mRNA levels for experiment 1 is shown in Figure 2–4.
[b] Each experiment was conducted with an independent pool of primary HUVEC.
[c] $p < 0.001$.
[d] Not significant.

Using the RT/PCR method, we found that the tPA mRNA level was elevated in endothelial cells exposed to shear stress (Fig. 2–4, upper left). In contrast, when the same Southern blots were stripped and reprobed for the GAPDH amplification product, the transcript level of GAPDH was constant and independent of shear stress (Fig. 2–4, lower left). When this RNA from

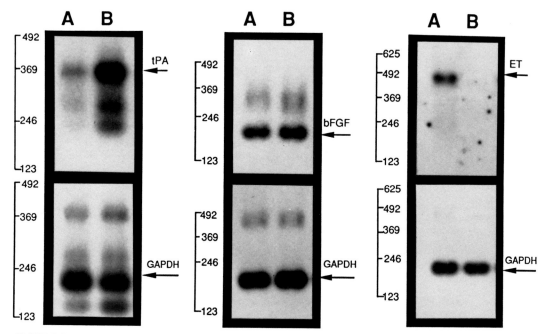

FIGURE 2–4. Analysis of mRNA levels for tissue plasminogen activator (tPA), basic fibroblast growth factor (bFGF), endothelin (ET), and glyceraldehyde 3-phosphate dehydrogenase (GAPDH) in human endothelial cells maintained in control culture (*lane A*) or exposed to 25 dynes/cm^2 (*lane B*). The large induction by shear stress of tPA mRNA is in contrast to the suppression of ET-1 mRNA levels by shear stress exposure. This mRNA phenotyping is in agreement with the protein production data (See experiment 1 in Table 2–1).

control and stressed monolayers was used in a similar coamplification experiment with GAPDH to study the effect of shear stress on levels for bFGF mRNA, no large increase in transcript levels such as that seen for tPA was noted for bFGF (Fig. 2–4, middle). Endothelin-1 mRNA levels were sharply reduced in the endothelial cells exposed to 25 dynes/cm^2 for 24 hours (Fig. 2–4, right). Again, no correspondingly sharp decrease was observed in signal strength for GAPDH product, indicating the uniformity of the coamplification reactions for bFGF and endothelin.

These findings were reproduced in an independent experiment and are unlikely to represent variation in PCR amplification efficiency because of (1) the similar cell numbers in, and RNA amounts extracted from, static and flow-subjected cultures, (2) the comparative constancy of coamplified GAPDH transcript levels observed under different flow conditions, and (3) the observation of increased tPA mRNA levels and increased tPA protein secretion rates detected by the reverse transcriptase/PCR technique in the same RNA and medium samples which showed decreased endothelin secretion and decreased endothelin mRNA levels, indicating opposite flow responses by HUVEC for endothelin and tPA. Our use of the polymerase chain reaction assay technique for quantitative estimates of transcript levels agreed quite well with the results of standard Northern blotting techniques used by Kooistra et al.[24] Those investigators showed that butyrate (1 to 10 mM) can increase HUVEC tPA secretion by a factor of 6- to 25-fold after a lag time of several hours, with slight attenuation of PAI-1 secretion observed at the higher butyrate concentrations. Using Northern blotting techniques, Kooistra et al. found that tPA mRNA levels increase roughly 30-fold during butyrate stimulation of HUVEC, while PAI-1 mRNA levels remain unchanged. Using a butyrate stimulation of HUVEC, we have shown that changes in tPA antigen production correlated with changes in tPA polymerase chain reaction product.[19] Thus, the amount of tPA amplification product can serve as a reliable indication of the tPA mRNA level when compared to the results of more standard methods such as Northern blotting.

DISCUSSION

Several lines of evidence indicate that low shear stress zones in arteries (with reversing flows) are more prone to develop atherosclerotic lesions, intimal hyperplasia, and enhanced thrombogenicity when compared to vascular regions with unidirectional, high shear flow.[6–11] Caro et al.[25] showed that low shear stress zones are prone to develop lesions and implicated poor mass transfer properties of low-flow zones in reducing efflux of lipids out of the vessel wall. In addition to lipid efflux, enhanced concentration of platelet-release products in regions of poor mass transport may play as important a role as reduced lipid efflux.[26]

Examining human carotid bifurcations at autopsy, Zarins et al.[10] found that early atherosclerotic lesions were located in regions of flow separations, low shear stress, and nonuniform directional flow. The outer wall of the carotid sinus (with separating flow and low shear stress) had the most plaques. Few lesions were found near the flow divider where shear stress was high and the flow was primarily axially oriented. Ku et al.[11] have correlated intimal thickening (in 12 autopsy specimens) of the outer wall of the proximal internal carotid with low shear stress (mean shear stress = -0.5 dynes/cm^2) and a high degree of flow reversal (instantaneous shear stress = -7 to 4 dynes/cm^2). The inner walls of the internal carotid (mean shear stress = 17 to 26 dynes/cm^2; no flow reversal) had little intimal thickening. Regions of the vessels downstream of the bifurcation had unidirectional flow, high mean shear stress (14 to 45 dynes/cm^2) and no intimal thickening. Similar work by Friedman et al.[27] with pulsatile flow in human aortic bifurcations demonstrated that intimal thickening was inversely related to the magnitude of the shear stress. Sakata and Takebayashi[28] also found that lesions were localized to the outer wall of the carotid artery. In a similar study, Grottum found lesions in the human left coronary artery bifurcation preferentially on the outer wall where shear stress levels were lowest.[29] In human cerebral arteries, the incidence of lesions was also higher on the outer walls of the daughter vessels.[30]

Loss of vessel patency after vascular graft placement or balloon angioplasty involves excessive smooth muscle cell proliferation and often occurs at vessel injury sites where platelets adhere in the early postinjury period. During these early times, Platelet-derived growth factor (PDGF) released by platelets might act as a potent smooth muscle cell mitogen at the site of injury.[31] However, late postoperative intimal hyperplasia involving vascular prostheses occurs most often at the perianastomotic areas, which are most rapidly resurfaced with endothelium from pannus ingrowth and which obtain the earliest protection against platelet deposition.[1-3,32-35] In addition, late postoperative subendothelial vascular smooth muscle cell proliferation occurs in both 60 μm internodal polytetrafluoroethylene (PTFE) arterial grafts in baboons and in Dacron grafts seeded with autologous endothelial cells in dogs despite confluent endothelial linings free of adherent platelets.[36-40] Both endothelial cells and smooth muscle cells express and release PDGF in vitro,[41-43] and increased PDGF mRNA levels are found in carotid plaques and atherosclerotic lesions[44-46] and in the neointima of healing PTFE prostheses in baboons at sites of abnormal smooth muscle cell proliferation.[38,39]

These data suggest that PDGF from endothelial cells or smooth muscle cells or both might cause intimal hyperplasia. However, PDGF is unlikely to be the only mitogen released by EC. Anti-PDGF antibody can neutralize only 30 to 50 per cent of the mitogenic activity of medium conditioned by cultured endothelial cells or by confluent endothelial cells lining PTFE grafts in baboons.[39,43] In pilot studies employing PCR primers and probes specific for PDGF A-chain, we have found no significant change in PDGF A-chain mRNA level in endothelial cells exposed to high shear stress for 24 hours compared to stationary controls (data not shown). This observation is not inconsistent with recent reports[47] of transient induction of PDGF mRNA at short exposure times (under 6 hours) to laminar shear stress which then return to basal levels. The transient nature of flow disturbances found in vivo, which lead to continually disordered flow at anastomotic sites, however, may continually stimulate endothelial cells to release PDGF.

Although HUVEC express mRNA for PDGF A-chain and PDGF B-chain and synthesize a PDGF-like protein, PDGF produced by endothelial cells is unlikely to have autocrine activity, since normal endothelial cells lack the PDGF receptor.[48] Endothelial cells synthesize bFGF which, when added exogenously to endothelial cells, can stimulate tPA and PAI-1 production[49] and cell migration.[50] However, we found the bFGF mRNA levels in shear-stressed cells were not elevated, which makes this an unlikely mechanism for tPA induction. This is consistent with the lack of any observed increase in PAI-1 secretion which can be induced by bFGF. However, our findings do not exclude the possibility of transient changes of bFGF mRNA at short exposure times.

Non-PDGF factors are likely to account for a significant fraction of EC-secreted mitogenic activity. Endothelin may be an important candidate for the role of a non-PDGF mitogen produced by the endothelium, since the decrease of endothelin gene expression by high shear stress is consistent with the known inverse relationship between fluid shear and intimal hyperplasia. Our results suggest that designing anastomoses to minimize areas of low shear stress or disturbed flow might reduce the severity of intimal hyperplasia.

In the past, observations concerning the geometric localization of hyperplasia at sites of low shear stress have been ascribed to the prolongation of the "residence time" of platelets near the blood/vessel wall interface and possible release of PDGF. In regions of high flow, the concentrations of platelet-released products are reduced by convective mass transport. Since endothelial cells actively participate in thrombotic and fibrinolytic processes and localize these events on or near the cell surface, longer-term alterations of endothelial function by mechanical forces may also play a role in physiological and pathological processes. Blood vessel walls exposed to high flow may have enhanced PGI_2 production[17,51] and enhanced fibrinolytic capacity,[18,19] thus increasing the resistance of high shear zones to fibrin deposition on the vessel wall and platelet-dependent and platelet-independent smooth muscle cell proliferation. Our finding that arterial levels of shear stress suppress endothelin production suggests an additional mechanism whereby reductions in intimal thickening might arise from direct local suppression of endothelial cell expression of the smooth muscle cell mitogen, endothelin. That endothelial cells produce less fibronectin under high flow[52] is also consistent with the in vivo finding of reduced vessel wall thickening in high-flow regions of vessels.

Recently, a molecular mechanism for the suspected link between impaired fibrinolysis and atherosclerosis has been proposed. Lipoprotein(a), which was shown to compete with plasminogen in binding to the endothelial cell surface receptor, may reduce endothelial cell surface-mediated plasminogen activation.[53,51] High serum levels of lipoprotein(a) are correlated with atherosclerosis[55] thus suggesting the link between impaired fibrinolysis at the cell surface and atherosclerosis possibly initiated by enhanced fibrin deposition on the vessel wall. It may follow that attenuated tPA production in low shear stress regions and subsequently reduced fibrinolysis at the endothelial surface may contribute to atherosclerotic plaque development.[56] Fibrin causes disorganization of endothelial monolayers.[57] Fibrin fragment D increases endothelial permeability to albumin, and fibrinopeptide B has been shown to be chemotactic for macrophages in early lesions.[58] In zones of high shear stress, enhanced expression of tPA may protect the vessel wall from shear-induced platelet aggregation[59] with thrombin generation and subsequent fibrin deposition.

SUMMARY

The endothelial cell has been proposed as an ideal vector for human gene therapy, since recombinant proteins can be secreted directly into the blood stream.[60] The seeding of vascular stents and grafts with endothelial cells is currently under study. Several workers using animal models have successfully engineered endothelial cells to express foreign proteins (β-galactosidase, tPA) in vivo.[61–63] The efficacy of gene-therapy approaches using engineered endo-thelial cells may be affected by the intrinsic response of endothelial cells to fluid mechanical forces. The analysis of cellular function and metabolism is particularly important when the hydrodynamics of blood flow may play a critical role in the success of the genetically-modified tissue.

REFERENCES

1. Imparato AM, Bracco A, Kim GFE, Zeff R: Intimal and neointimal fibrous proliferation causing failure of arterial reconstruction. Surgery 1972; 72:1007–1017.
2. LoGerfo FW, et al: Downstream anastomotic hyperplasia. A mechanism of failure in Dacron arterial grafts. Ann Surg 1983; 197:479–483.
3. Echave V, Voornick AR, Haimov M, Jacobson JH: Intimal hyperplasia as a complication of the use of polytetrafluoroethylene grafts for femoropopliteal bypass. Surgery 1979; 86:791–798.
4. Clagett GP, et al: Morphogenesis and pathologic characteristics of recurrent carotid disease. J Vasc Surg 1986; 3:10–23.
5. Liu MW, Roubin GS King SB: Restenosis after coronary angioplasty. Circulation 1989; 79:1374–1387.
6. Morinaga K, et al: Development and regression of intimal thickening of arterially transplanted autologous vein grafts in dogs. J Vasc Surg 1987; 5:719–730.
7. Dobrin PA, Littooy FN, Endean ED: Mechanical factors predisposing to intimal hyperplasia and medical thickening in autogenous vein grafts. Surgery 1989; 105:393–400.
8. Glagov S, Zarins C, Giddens DP, Ku DN: Hemodynamics and atherosclerosis. Arch Path Lab Med 1988; 112:1018–1031.
9. Karino T: Rheologic and geometric factors in vascular homeostasis. In Norman J, ed. Cardiovascular Science and Technology I: Precised Proceedings, Louisville, Oxymoron Press, 1989; 18–20.
10. Zarins CK, Giddens DP, Bharavaj BK, Sottiurai VS, Mabon RF, Glagov S: Carotid bifurcation with flow velocity profiles and wall shear stress. Circ Res 1983; 53:502–512.
11. Ku DN, Giddens DP, Zarins CK, Glagov S: Pulsatile flow and atherosclerosis in the human carotid bifurcation: Positive correlation between plaque location and low and oscillating shear stress. Arteriosclerosis 1985; 5:293–302.
12. van Hinsbergh VWM, et al: Production of plasminogen activators and inhibitor by serially propagated endothelial cells from adult human blood vessels. Arteriosclerosis 1987; 7:389–400.
13. Dichek DA, Quertermous T: Variability in messenger RNA levels in human umbilical vein endothelial cells of different lineage and time in culture. In Vitro Cell Dev Biol 1989; 25:289–292.
14. McArthur MM, et al: The use of human endothelial cells cultured in flat wells and on microcarrier beads to assess tissue plasminogen activator and factor VIII related antigen release. Thromb Res 1986; 41:581–587.
15. Konkle BA, Ginsburg D: The addition of endothelial cell growth factor and heparin to human umbilical vein endothelial cell cultures decreases plasminogen activator inhibitor-1 expression. J Clin Invest 1988; 82:579–585.
16. Wang AM, Doyle MV, Mark DF: Quantitation of mRNA by the Polymerase Chain Reaction. Proc Natl Acad Sci USA 1989; 86:9717–9722.
17. Frangos JA, Eskin SG, McIntire LV, Ives CL: Flow effects on prostacyclin production by culture human endothelial cells. Science 1985; 227:1477–1479.
18. Diamond SL, Eskin SG, McIntire LV: Fluid flow stimulates tissue plasminogen activator secretion by cultured human endothelial cells. Science 1989; 243:1483–1485.
19. Diamond SL, Sharefkin JB, Dieffenbach CW, Frasier-Scott KF, McIntire LV, Eskin SG: Tissue plasminogen activator messenger RNA levels increase in cultured human endothelial cells exposed to laminar shear stress. J Cell Physiol 1990; 143:364–371.
20. Frangos JA, McIntire, LV, Eskin SG: Shear stress induced stimulation of mammalian cell metabolism. Biotechnol Bioeng 1988; 32:1053–1060.
21. Chirgwin JM, Przbyla AE, MacDonald RJ, Rutter WJ: Isolation of biologically active ribonucleic acid from sources enriched in ribonuclease. Biochemistry 1979; 18:5294–5299.
22. Rappolee DA, Wang A, Mark D, Werb Z: Novel method for studying mRNA phenotypes in single or small numbers of cells. J Cell Biochem 1989; 39:1–11.
23. Sharefkin JB, Diamond SL, Eskin SG, Dieffenbach CW, McIntire LV: Fluid flow decreases preproendothelin mRNA levels and suppresses endothelin-1 peptide release in cultured human endothelium cells. J Vasc Surg 1991; 14:1–9.
24. Kooistra T, et al: Butyrate stimulates tissue-type plasminogen activator synthesis in cultured human endothelial cells. Biochem J 1987; 247:605–612.

25. Caro CG, Fitz-Gerald JM, Schroter RC: Atheroma and arterial wall shear: observation, correlation and proposal of a shear dependent mass transfer mechanism for atherogenesis. Proc R Soc Lond [Biol] 1971; *177*:109–159.
26. Folie BJ, McIntire LV: Mathematical analysis of mural thrombogenesis: concentration profiles of platelet-activating agents and effects of viscous shear flow. Biophys J 1989; *56*:1121–1137.
27. Friedman MH, et al: Correlation between intimal thickness and fluid shear in human arteries. Atherosclerosis 1981; *39*:425–436.
28. Sakata N, Takebayashi S: Localization of atherosclerotic lesions in the curving sites of human internal carotid arteries. Biorheology 1988; *25*:567–578.
29. Grottum P, Svindland A, Walloe L: Localization of atherosclerotic lesions in the bifurcation of the main left coronary artery. Atherosclerosis 1983; *47*:55–62.
30. Sakata N, Joshita T, Ooneda G: Topographical study on arteriosclerotic lesions at the bifurcations of human cerebral arteries. Heart Vessels 1985; *1*:70–73.
31. Duel TF: Polypeptide growth factors: Roles in normal and abnormal growth. Ann Rev Cell Biol 1987; *3*:443–492.
32. Chici CC, Klein L, DePalma RG: Effect of regenerated endothelium on collagen content in the injured artery. Surg Gynecol Obstet 1979; *148*:839–843.
33. Edwards WS: Arterial grafts: Past, present, and future. Arch Surg 1978; *113*:1225–1231.
34. Sauvage LR, et al: Interspecies healing of porous arterial prostheses. Arch Surg 1974; *109*:698–705.
35. Hanel KC, et al: Current PTFE grafts: A biomechanical, scanning electron, and light microscopic evaluation. Ann Surg 1982; *195*:456–462.
36. Clowes AW, Kirkman TR, Clowes MM: Mechanisms of arterial graft failure II: Chronic endothelial and smooth muscle cell proliferation in healing polytetrafluoroethylene prostheses. J Vasc Surg 1986; *3*:877–884.
37. Burkel WE, Graham LM, Stanley JC: Endothelial linings in prosthetic vascular grafts. Ann NY Acad Sci 1987; *516*:131–143.
38. Golden MA, Au YP, Kenagy RD, Clowes AW: Growth factor expression by intimal cells in healing polytetrafluoroethylene grafts. J Vasc Surg 1990; *11*:580–585.
39. Golden MA, et al: Platelet derived growth factor activity and mRNA expression in healing vascular grafts in baboons. J Clin Invest 1990; *87*:406–414.
40. Clowes AW, Kirkman TR, Reidy MA: Mechanisms of arterial graft healing. Rapid transmural capillary ingrowth provides a source of intimal endothelium and smooth muscle in porous PTFE prostheses. Am J Pathol 1986; *123*:220–230.
41. Sjolund M, et al: Arterial smooth muscle cells express platelet derived growth factor (PDGF) A chain, secrete a PDGF-like mitogen, and bind exogenous PDGF in a phenotype- and growth state-dependent manner. J Cell Biol 1988; *106*:403–413.
42. Collins T, et al: Cultured human endothelial cells express platelet derived growth factor A Chain. Am J Pathol 1987; *127*:7–12.
43. Limanni A, et al: Expression of genes for platelet derived growth factor in adult human venous endothelium: A possible non-platelet dependent cause of intimal hyperplasia in vein grafts and perianastomotic areas of vascular prostheses. J Vasc Surg 1988; *7*:10–20.
44. Wilcox JN, et al: Platelet derived growth factor mRNA detection in human atherosclerotic plaques by in situ hybridization. J Clin Invest 1988; *82*:1134–1143.
45. Barrett TB, Benditt EP: Platelet derived growth factor gene expression in human atherosclerotic plaques and normal artery wall. Proc Natl Acad Sci USA 1988; *85*:2810–2814.
46. Barrett TB, Benditt EP: (Platelet derived growth factor B Chain) gene transcript levels are elevated in human atherosclerotic lesions compared to normal artery wall. Proc Natl Acad Sci USA 1987; *84*:1099–1103.
47. Frangos JA: Elevation of platelet-derived growth factor in RNA in human endothelial cells by shear stress. Am J Physiol 1991; *260*:H642–646.
48. Kazlauskas A, DiCorleto PE: Cultured endothelial cells do not respond to a platelet-derived growth factor-like protein in an autocrine manner. Biochim Biophys Acta 1985; *846*:405–412.
49. Saksela O, Moscatelli D, Rifkin DB: The opposing effect of basic fibroblast growth factor and transforming growth factor beta on the regulation of plasminogen activator activity in capillary endothelial cells. J Cell Biol 1987; *105*:957–963.
50. Sato Y, Rifkin DB: Autocrinic activities of basic fibroblast growth factor: Regulation of endothelial cell movement, plasminogen activator synthesis, and DNA synthesis. J Cell Biol 1988; *107*:1199–1205.
51. Grabowski EF, Jaffe EA, Weksler BB: Prostacyclin production by cultured endothelial cell monolayers exposed to step increases in shear stress. J Lab Clin Med 1985; *105*:36–43.
52. Gupte A, Frangos JA: Effects of flow on the synthesis and release of fibronectin by endothelial cells. In Vitro Cell Dev Biol 1990; *26*:57–60.
53. Miles LA, et al: A potential basis for the thrombotic risks associated with lipoprotein(a). Nature 1989; *339*:301–303.
54. Hajjar KA, Gavish D, Breslow JL, Nachman RL: Lipoprotein(a) modulation of endothelial cell surface fibrinolysis and its potential role in atherosclerosis. Nature 1989; *339*:303–305.

55. Dahlen GH, et al: Association of levels of liproprotein Lp(a), plasma lipids, and other lipoproteins with coronary artery disease documented by angiography. Circulation 1986; *74*:758–765.
56. Collen D, Juhan-Vague I: Fibrinolysis and atherosclerosis, Semin Thromb Hemost 1988; *14*:180–184.
57. Schleef RR, Birdwell CR: Biochemical changes in endothelial cell monolayers induced by fibrin deposition in vitro. Arteriosclerosis 1984; *3*:14–20.
58. Singh TM, Kadowaki MH, Glagov S, Zarins CK: Role of fibrinopeptide B in early atherosclerotic lesion formation. Am J Surg 1990; *160*:156–163.
59. Moake JL, et al: Shear-induced platelet aggregation can be mediated by vWF released from platelets, as well as by exogenous large or unusually large vWF multimers, requires adenosine diphosphate, and is resistant to aspirin. Blood 1988; *71*:1366–1372.
60. Zwiebel JA, et al: High-level recombinant gene expression in rabbit endothelial cells transduced by retroviral vectors. Science 1989; *243*:220–222.
61. Nabel EG, et al: Recombinant gene expression in vivo within endothelial cells of the arterial wall. Science 1989; *244*:1342–1346.
62. Nabel EG, Plautz G, Nabel GJ: Site-specific gene expression in vivo by direct gene transfer into the arterial wall. Science 1990; *249*:1285–1288.
63. Dichek DA, et al: Seeding of intravascular stents with genetically engineered endothelial cells. Circulation 1989; *80*:1347–1353.

3

IDENTIFICATION OF FAMILIAL AORTIC ANEURYSMS USING DNA TECHNIQUE

GERARD TROMP and HELENA KUIVANIEMI

IDENTIFICATION OF FAMILIAL AORTIC ANEURYSMS USING DNA TECHNIQUE

Aortic aneurysms frequently go undetected until rupture, and therefore are a significant cause of morbidity.[1,2] In the United States, aortic aneurysms are the 13th leading cause of death.[3] The mortality from aneurysms that are repaired electively is low (1 to 7 per cent depending on study cited),[4] whereas the mortality from ruptured aneurysms is as high as 90 per cent[5,6] and depends to a large extent on the time it takes for the patient to reach a medical center and for the condition to be diagnosed correctly. The cost to the health care system per survivor of a ruptured aneurysm is approximately tenfold that of elective repair of an aneurysm. The difference in mortality as well as cost indicates that efficient diagnosis of who is at risk, and who is not at risk, will both save lives and reduce cost to the health care system. If aortic aneurysms were genetic and if the gene or genes that harbor the mutations were identified, the powerful techniques of molecular biology could be used to determine who is, and who is not, at risk for developing aneurysms long before the aneurysm or aneurysms make themselves manifest. Early diagnosis of those at risk could also identify a sufficiently large group of patients to evaluate potential drug therapies, such as those that lower blood pressure.

The premise underlying the use of the DNA techniques of molecular biology is that aortic aneurysms are heritable. It was relatively recently that a familial clustering of aortic aneurysms was recognized. The first report of abdominal aortic aneurysms occurring in several members of the same family was by Clifton in 1977.[7] Since the initial report, a number of studies have been published that expanded on the observation and have estimated that from 6 to 36 per cent of aortic aneurysms are clustered in families.[4,8–15] The incidence of aortic aneurysms that are clustered in families, and specifically the incidence of aortic aneurysms in first-degree relatives within the families, strongly suggests a heritable or genetic cause for many, if not most, aneurysms. There are two general approaches using DNA techniques that can be used to identify the gene or genes harboring the defects (mutations) causing aortic aneurysms. The first approach is linkage studies using markers that have been mapped to a particular locus on the genome and to test whether or not the marker is co-inherited with aortic aneurysms within families. The gene(s) in or near which the markers exist need not be known to determine linkage. Once significant linkage is established, the region of the genome can be mapped, cloned, and sequenced. The information generated can be used to identify the gene(s) in the region. The second approach is analysis of candidate genes for mutations. Both are valid approaches to address the question; however, certain aspects of familial aneurysms present problems for the linkage analysis approach. Here we describe the candidate gene approach to identifying the genetic cause of familial aortic aneurysms.

EVIDENCE FOR THE CLUSTERING OF AORTIC ANEURYSMS IN FAMILIES

A family in which three brothers had abdominal aortic aneurysms that were diagnosed between the ages of 60 and 70 years led to the suggestion that there may be a heritable trait that caused aortic aneurysms.[7] Tilson and Seashore reported on 16 families with abdominal aortic aneurysms in first-degree relatives.[8] From the pedigree data, the authors concluded that the mode of inheritance was either X-linked or autosomal dominant, with the X-linked mode being more common. Subsequently, Tilson and Seashore reported on a collection of 50 families and favored an autosomal dominant mode of inheritance.[9] These reports established that abdominal aortic aneurysms, at least in some cases, did occur in family clusters.

To establish what fraction of abdominal aortic aneurysms were familial, Norrgård et al. surveyed 200 consecutive patients who underwent surgery for repair of abdominal aortic aneurysms over a period of 16 years in Umeå, Sweden.[10] Of the 200 patients, 89 were alive and 87 responded to the questionnaire. Abdominal aortic aneurysms occurred in the families of 16. The familial incidence was therefore 18.4 per cent. Johansen and Koepsell interviewed 250 patients with abdominal aortic aneurysms as well as 250 control subjects and found that 48 (19.2 per cent) of the patients, as compared to 6 (2.4 per cent) of the controls, had a first-degree relative with an abdominal aortic aneurysm.[11] The highest familial incidence of abdominal aortic aneurysms was reported by Powell and Greenhalgh, who interviewed 60 patients and were able to collect family data on 56.[12] They reported a positive family history in 20 patients (35.7 per cent). The lowest familial incidence was reported by Johnston and Scobie in a Canadian study based on the histories of 666 patients that were collected by 72 surgeons.[4] A positive family history was recorded in only 6.1 per cent of the cases. In a second Canadian study, based on telephone interviews of 305 patients who underwent surgery for repair of abdominal aortic aneurysms, Cole et al. reported that 34 patients had positive family history (11.1 per cent).[13] Darling et al. reported that 82 of 542 patients (15.1 per cent) had a positive history for abdominal aortic aneurysms in their families.[14] Most recently, Majumder et al. reported that 13 of 91 patients (14.3 per cent) had a positive history.[15] Summing the number of patients in each of the studies and the number of patients with a positive history in their family, the cumulative value for the familial incidence of abdominal aortic aneurysms is 12.7 per cent (see Table 3–1).

TABLE 3–1. FAMILIAL INCIDENCE OF ABDOMINAL AORTIC ANEURYSMS

Authors	Number of Patients Surveyed	Number of Patients with Positive History	Familial Incidence (%)
Norrgård et al.[10]	87	16	18.4
Johansen and Koepsell[11]	250	48	19.2
Powell and Greenhalgh[12]	56	20	35.7
Johnston and Scobie[4]	666	41	6.1
Cole et al.[13]	305	34	11.1
Darling et al.[14]	542	82	15.1
Majumder et al.[15]	91	13	14.3
Total	1997	254	
Cumulative incidence (%)			12.7

In addition to the above studies, all of which relied on questionnaires and interviews to determine the familial incidence of abdominal aortic aneurysms, there are two studies that used ultrasonography to determine the incidence of undiagnosed aneurysms. Bengtsson et al. found that 13 of 87 siblings (14.9 per cent) in 32 families had dilatation of the abdominal aorta.[16] Not all siblings were screened and no data (with respect to diagnosed aneurysms) was collected on deceased siblings. The incidence of abdominal aortic dilatation according to gender was remarkably skewed to the brothers—10 of 35 brothers (28.6 per cent) as compared to 3 of 52 sisters (5.8 per cent) had dilatations. In the second study, Webster et al. screened first-degree relatives, that were over 40 years old, of 43 patients who underwent surgery for abdominal aortic aneurysms.[17] A total of 103 out of 202 eligible relatives were screened. Seven previously undiagnosed aneurysms (dilatations) were detected. All seven were in the 54 siblings over 50 years old. Five or twenty-four brothers (20.8 per cent) and 2 of 30 sisters (6.7 per cent) had previously undiagnosed aneurysms.

Together, the above two series of studies make an eloquent case for a heritable component in the etiology of abdominal aortic aneurysms; however, until recently, no genetic analysis of familial aortic aneurysms using classical genetic parameters was done. In the first such study, Majumder et al. concluded that abdominal aortic aneurysms are heritable, and that the genetic model that best fits the data is a model with a recessive mode of inheritance and with one major diallelic locus (single locus with a normal allele and a disease-causing allele).[15] The study rejected sporadic incidence in the families and did not support a multifactorial mode of inheritance. Although it did not support a dominant or an additive model for the mode of inheritance, it could not rule these models out.

DIFFICULTIES FACING LINKAGE STUDIES

Linkage is a term in genetics that indicates that a particular marker is co-inherited with a phenotype.[18] The marker may be a biochemical marker such as blood type or histocompatibility antigens, a polymorphic DNA marker, or a phenotypic marker not associated with the disease provided the phenotype is coded for by a single locus. It is important to note that linkage is determined with respect to loci. A locus is a concept in genetics used to represent a region of DNA in the genome. The specific region may, but need not, be physically identifiable (e.g., a locus may be mapped to a band on a chromosome). Also, the locus concept imparts no information about the DNA at the locus, nor does it specify that there is only one gene at the locus. Even if a particular gene that harbors mutations at a locus is identified by cloning and sequencing, there are likely to be many mutations that cause the disease, as has been the case in a large number of diseases.

Linkage of a disease phenotype and a marker means that the two are located closely on the same physical piece of DNA. The closer that two loci occur on a piece of DNA, the less frequent crossovers are, and the more tightly the two are linked. The linkage between the disease phenotype and the marker can be expressed as a distance in genetic map units. Linkage distance (and map units) are measured as a function of the number of meioses (opportunities for crossover). If two loci are tightly linked, they are so close that the frequency of crossover during meiosis is low or undetectable. Therefore, establishing linkage requires families with a large enough number of meioses. The most useful families for linkage studies have at least three generations, with affected individuals in all three generations. The larger the number of offspring in each generation, the more meioses and, therefore, the more reliable the information. In addition to large families, it is necessary to obtain accurate diagnoses of affected individuals, because an undiagnosed individual will result, at best, in data that suggest a larger distance between the marker and the disease locus, and at worst, in data that suggest nonlinkage or exclusion of the gene in that family. A classical genetic analysis to determine the model of inheritance or noninheritance of a disease can make use of information concerning deceased relatives, provided an accurate history is available. In contrast, when using biochemical or DNA markers for linkage studies, it is desirable to obtain samples from as many as possible affected and unaffected individuals being studied, since the status of the two loci (marker locus and disease locus) has to be determined for each individual. Only if samples from affected and unaffected descendants in different branches of the family of a deceased, affected founder are available is the diagnosis of such a deceased family member useful.

The above constraints pose a particular problem for linkage studies of late-onset diseases such as aortic aneurysms. It is rare to find large index families that have more than two generations of living, affected members so that pertinent samples can be obtained. Diagnosis is a problem, since the data on the incidence of aneurysms in the population indicates that few individuals develop aneurysms before the age of 50 and that the incidence increases with age.[17] An individual who is currently between the ages of 50 and 55 may develop an aneurysm by the age of 65. Linkage data obtained from such an individual's family would therefore be skewed toward nonlinkage.

POSSIBILITIES ARISING FROM NEW TECHNOLOGIES

The candidate gene approach involves the characterization of mutations in the candidate gene. As recently as 5 years ago, characterization of mutations in genes was a painstakingly slow process. It took several years to define the mutation in a proband with a heritable disorder even when some protein data clearly indicated that a particular gene harbored the mutation. Several important breakthroughs over the past several years have reduced the time required to characterize a mutation in a gene of known structure and sequence. The first of these was the concept of generating large amounts of a desired region of DNA by replicating the DNA in vitro using the components of the cellular DNA replication machinery.[19] In principle the concept is simple; that is, to cyclically denature DNA into template strands, to hybridize (anneal) short oligonucleotides of defined sequence to the template strands, and to synthesize new strands of DNA using a DNA polymerase (Fig. 3–1). The new-strand synthesis starts at two short pieces of synthetic DNA, called primers. The primers are on complementary strands so that the synthesized DNA is of the same length as the distance between the outer ends of where the primers hybridize to their complementary strands. The sequences of the primers make the reaction specific to those regions between the two primers. In theory, every

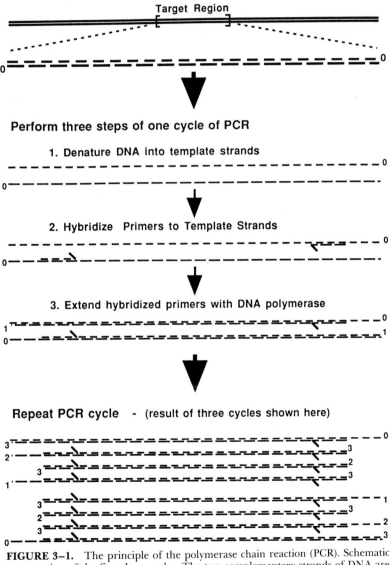

FIGURE 3–1. The principle of the polymerase chain reaction (PCR). Schematic presentation of the first three cycles. The two complementary strands of DNA are shown with different lengths of dashes. Dashed arrows indicate oligonucleotide primers; numbers indicate cycle during which the strand of DNA was synthesized; 0, original template; 1, 2, and 3, strand of DNA synthesized during the first, second, and third cycles, respectively.

cycle doubles the number of copies of DNA. The reaction was therefore named the polymerase chain reaction (PCR). Initially, however, there was one problem: all the available DNA polymerases were denatured by the heat required to denature the DNA into two template strands. Thus, the second technological breakthrough was one related to the PCR—namely, the use of DNA polymerases that were heat stable.[20] Other important breakthroughs were the commercial availability of new enzymes as well as enzymes of greater purity for manipulation and sequencing of DNA, improved chemistry and technology for DNA synthesis, and reduced cost for many of the reagents.

Whereas as recently as 5 years ago it took several years to characterize a mutation in a gene from a proband, the breakthroughs in technology now make it possible to do the same work in as little as a few weeks. Automation of the procedures using robotics is likely to reduce the time even further. If the structure and sequence of a candidate gene is known, it is possible within a short time to sequence the genes from a number of affected individuals to determine if there are any mutations present.

AN EXAMPLE CASE USING THE CANDIDATE GENE APPROACH

In a number of biochemical studies on tissue from abdominal aortic aneurysms, the following changes were found: suggestions of a copper metabolism defect, a decreased content of elastin and collagen, an increased proteolysis by elastase and collagenase, and a decreased level of tissue inhibitor of metalloproteases (TIMP).[21] These studies suggest several candidate genes that may harbor the mutations causing aortic aneurysms. In addition, because aneurysms with medial necrosis have been reported to be associated with heritable disorders of connective tissue such as the Marfan's syndrome[22] and some subtypes of the Ehlers-Danlos syndrome,[22] the genes for types I and III collagen have been considered to be highly likely those that harbor the mutations causing familial aortic aneurysms.

We have been characterizing mutations in the collagen genes of patients with rare, heritable disorders such as osteogenesis imperfecta and the Ehlers-Danlos syndrome.[25] About 3 years ago, a proband came to our attention because she had a remarkable family history of aneurysms.[24] The proband was a 37-year-old female captain in the United States Air Force. Her mother, maternal aunt, maternal grandfather, and a maternal cousin had died of aneurysms at ages 34, 55, 55, and 15 years old, respectively. The proband sought discharge from the Air Force and was required to undergo a physical examination as a standard part of the discharge proceedings. During the physical examination, the proband's remarkable family history of aneurysms came to light, especially as the incidence was underscored by the death of the maternal aunt only shortly before the physical examination. Aside from the history of aneurysms in the proband's family, the proband's physical examination did not reveal anything remarkable. She reported bruising easily, but did not display the stigmata of the type IV or ecchymotic variant of the Ehlers-Danlos syndrome.[25,26] She did not have: (1) characteristic atrophic "cigarette-paper" scars (scars from operation and injury were well-healed); (2) darkly pigmented scars over bony protuberances; (3) an easily visible venous network on the upper torso or on the forehead; or (4) thin skin with a velvety texture. She had some loose-jointedness, but had been a gymnast. The proband also did not display any stigmata of the Marfan's syndrome.

Because of the remarkable history of aneurysms in the proband's family, a skin biopsy was obtained to attempt to find a heritable cause for the aneurysms. Skin fibroblasts were cultured from the biopsy, and RNA and DNA were isolated from the fibroblasts and used to determine the sequence of the type III procollagen triple-helical domain. Initially, cDNA was synthesized and amplified by the PCR in four overlapping fragments. Each fragment was cloned into the bacteriophage vector M13mp18 or mp19 for DNA sequencing by the dideoxynucleotide method.[27,28] Several clones of each fragment were sequenced, and a single base change was found that changed the codon for amino acid 619 of the triple helix from GGA, a codon for glycine, to AGA, a codon for arginine.[24]

During cloning, a single molecule is ligated into a single vector molecule and then transferred into a bacterium by a process called transformation.[18,27] Because a clone is derived from a single molecule, the process of cloning can accentuate isolated artifacts that may have occurred during the PCR or the ligation and transformation steps. Consequently, it was essential to verify that the change that was found was indeed a mutation and not an artifact of the PCR and cloning. To confirm that the change was present in one of the proband's two alleles, the PCR was performed using genomic (nuclear) DNA as the template.[24] The region of the gene that contained the exon with the change was amplified and the PCR products were cloned into M13mp18 or mp19. Several clones were sequenced and the substitution of A for G was present (Fig. 3–2) in 3 of 13 clones.[24] Therefore, the change probably was present in one of the proband's alleles.

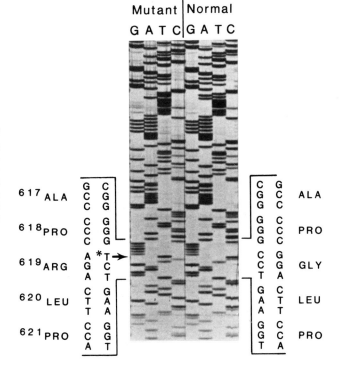

FIGURE 3–2. A DNA sequencing gel of the region with the glycine-619 to arginine mutation in the gene for type III procollagen from a proband with familial aneurysms. The sequences of clones from the mutated and normal alleles from the patient are shown. The arrow and asterisk indicate the site of the mutation. The sequence is in the antisense orientation.

Although it is unlikely that the PCR would generate the same artifact with two different kinds of template, the possibility that the change was an artifact, was not yet ruled out definitively, because both experiments relied on cloning. To definitively rule out that the change was an artifact, we therefore used three independent techniques that give signals proportional to the number of molecules, with or without the change, that are present in the DNA sample. The three techniques are: allele-specific oligonucleotide hybridization,[29] allele-

1. Polymerase Chain Reaction

Amplify DNA - Controls are cloned DNAs: a) Homozygous for normal sequence
b) Homozygous for mutated sequence
      - Samples may be: a) Homozygous for normal sequence
b) Heterozygous for normal and mutated sequence
[for recessive disease c) Homozygous for mutated sequence]

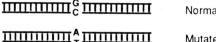 Normal sequence

Mutated sequence

2. Denature DNA and Bind to Solid Matrix
Prepare duplicate blots

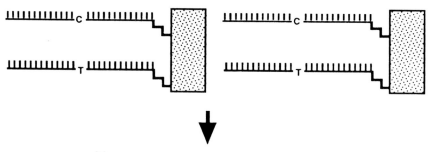

3. Hybridize ^{32}P-labeled Oligonucleotide Probes to Blots

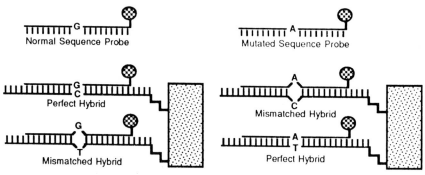

Normal Sequence Probe   Mutated Sequence Probe

Perfect Hybrid   Mismatched Hybrid

Mismatched Hybrid   Perfect Hybrid

FIGURE 3–3. The principle of allele-specific oligonucleotide (ASO) hybridization. The DNA that was amplified by the PCR is attached to a solid matrix (membrane) in duplicate. Labeled oligonucleotide probes are hybridized to the bound DNA. The normal sequence probe is hybridized to one of the duplicate blots and the mutated sequence probe is hybridized to the other blot. Blots are washed at temperatures that remove the mismatched (or imperfect) hybrids. Stippled rectangle indicates solid matrix; checkered circle indicates ^{32}P label on probes; hatched elliptical rectangle indicates surface of membrane that has probe hybridized to bound DNA; open elliptical rectangle indicates surface of the membrane where DNA was bound, but the probe was washed off. (*Figure continues.*)

4. Remove Mismatched Probes by Stringent Washing

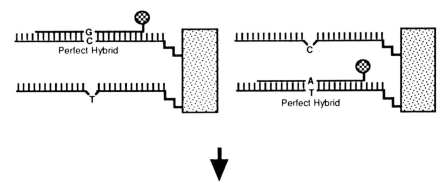

5. Expose Film to Blots and Develop

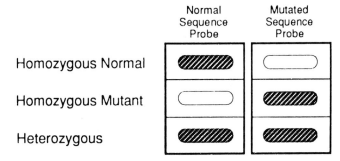

FIGURE 3–3. (*Continued.*)

specific restriction enzyme analysis,[30] and allele-specific primer extension.[31] The principle of allele-specific oligonucleotide (ASO) hybridization is presented schematically in Figure 3–3. Amplified DNA from the proband, an unaffected control subject, as well as from clones with normal and mutated sequences, are denatured and irreversibly bound to a membrane (solid matrix). Membranes with bound DNA are usually referred to as blots. Two oligonucleotides are synthesized that have the same length and the same sequence except for the single-base change that is being assayed for. Some type of marker or label, usually ^{32}P, is attached to the oligonucleotides. The technique relies on the difference between the melting temperature of the perfect hybrids formed by one of the oligonucleotides and the melting temperature of the imperfect hybrids formed by the other oligonucleotide. Perfect hybrids are those in which all the bases are correctly paired, whereas imperfect hybrids have unpaired bases or mismatches in the hybrids. The mismatches destabilize the hybrids and, therefore, cause them to dissociate at lower temperatures than perfect hybrids. At an empirically determined temperature, the mismatched hybrids are therefore washed off, while the perfect hybrids are stable. When an oligonucleotide with a normal sequence (nASO) is hybridized to control DNA with normal sequence (all the molecules have the normal sequence), the hybrids will be perfect and therefore stable at the empirically determined temperature. In contrast, when the same nASO is hybridized to control DNA with mutated sequence (all the molecules have mutated sequence), the hybrids will contain a mismatch and therefore be less stable at the same temperature. The converse is true for the mutated sequence oligonucleotide. By hybridizing the ASOs separately to duplicate blots and washing the imperfect hybrids off at the appropriate temperatures, it is possible to detect the presence of a sequence change in a sample of DNA. Because the resultant signal is dependent on the number of molecules with (and the number of molecules without) the sequence change, it is possible to estimate what fraction of the molecules in the sample have the change by determining the ratio of the two signals.

Allele-specific restriction endonuclease digestion relies on the amazing specificity of restriction endonucleases.[28,30] A particular restriction endonuclease will cleave DNA only if the DNA contains its recognition sequence and, with but a few constraints, most restriction endonuclease will cleave DNA at every occurrence of their recognition sequences. The principle of allele-specific restriction endonuclease digestion is shown in Figure 3–4 for a sequence variant in the gene for type III procollagen. The variant is cleaved by the restriction endonuclease *Hae*III. The recognition sequence of *Hae*III is GG/CC (the / denotes the position where the DNA is cleaved). If as little as a single base in the recognition sequence is altered, the restriction endonuclease will not cleave the DNA. It is therefore possible to assay a sample of DNA for the presence or absence of an allele that has, and an allele that does not have, a restriction endonuclease restriction site. Additional restriction sites within the same piece of DNA that are not variable (i.e., the site is present in almost all individuals), increase the reliability of the assay because they act as internal controls. The additional sites should always be cleaved to completion for the assay to be reliable. If an individual has a sequence variant in one allele (i.e., the individual is heterozygous for the sequence variant), that sequence variant should be present in about one-half of the DNA molecules. Therefore, half the DNA should be cleaved and half should be resistant. The restriction endonuclease that was used to detect the presence or absence of the mutation that converted glycine-619 to arginine was *Nci*I. It has the recognition sequence CC/(CG)GG (the bases in parentheses indicate alternatives, that is, the recognition sequence is CC/CGG or CC/GGG). The glycine-619 to arginine mutation changed the sequence from CCCGG to CCCAG and thereby destroyed the restriction site.

The third technique used to verify that the mutation was not an artifact of the PCR and cloning, was allele-specific primer extension. Figure 3–5 shows the principle of the technique. It relies on the inability of DNA polymerases to extend primers that are mismatched at their 3' ends. DNA polymerases require a template, a primer, deoxynucleotide triphosphates, and the appropriate buffers and ions. The primer has to have a free 3'-hydroxyl group; since it is the group onto which the new deoxynucleotide triphosphate is polymerized. The critical 3'-hydroxyl has to be fully hybridized for the polymerase to catalyze the polymerization (the polymerization process is also called extension of the primer). Therefore, if the primer contains a base at or near its 3' end that will be mismatched when the primer is hybridized to DNA from the mutated allele, the primer will not be extended. The same primer will be extended if it is hybridized to DNA from the normal allele. The converse is true for the primer that contains a mismatch if it is hybridized to the normal allele. Since extension products are separated on a DNA sequencing gel and are detected because of radiolabel that is incorporated during the extension, the intensity of the resulting signal will depend on the number of molecules in the DNA sample that have the normal and mutated sequences.

1. Polymerase Chain Reaction

Amplify DNA - Samples may be:

a) Homozygous for sequence variant C
b) Heterozygous for sequence variants C and T
c) Homozygous for sequence variant T

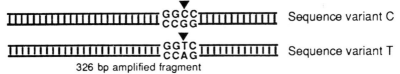

GGCC
CCGG   Sequence variant C

GGTC
CCAG   Sequence variant T

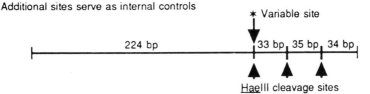

326 bp amplified fragment

2. Cleave DNA with Restriction Endonuclease

Restriction endonuclease does not recognize one of the sequence variants

HaeIII recognition site   GG/CC

C variant cleaved, T variant resistant

Additional sites serve as internal controls

* Variable site

224 bp | 33 bp | 35 bp | 34 bp

HaeIII cleavage sites

Sequence variant C

224 | 33 | 35 | 34

Sequence variant T

257 | 35 | 34

3. Separate Fragments According to Size by Agarose Gel Electrophoresis

M C/C C/C T/T T/T C/T C/T

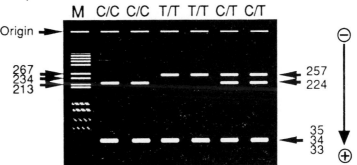

Origin →

267
234
213

257
224

35
34
33

⊖

⊕

FIGURE 3–4.   The principle of allele-specific restriction endonuclease digestion. The DNA from a region of the gene for type III procollagen that contains a C to T variant in exon 33 is amplified by the PCR. The amplified DNA is digested by the restriction endonuclease *Hae*III and the products separated by agarose gel electrophoresis. Asterisk, variable *Hae*III site; origin, wells in the agarose gel; arrows with numbers, sizes of DNA fragments in base pairs (bp); M, DNA size marker lane; C/C, lane of DNA from individual homozygous for the C variant; C/T, lane of DNA from a heterozygous individual; T/T, lane of DNA from an individual homozygous for the T variant; arrow with encircled plus and minus signs, direction of electrophoresis of DNA fragments from cathode to anode.

After determining that the change that converted glycine-619 to arginine was indeed a mutation, the consequence of the mutation on the functional properties of the type III collagen protein was determined. One useful assay determines the consequence of the mutation of the thermal unfolding of the type III collagen triple helix. Type III collagen from the fibroblasts of the proband was subjected to brief protease digestion at different temperatures in the presence of high concentrations of proteases. A fragment containing the first 781 amino acids of the type III collagen triple helix isolated from control fibroblasts was digested above 36°C. A similar fragment of type III collagen

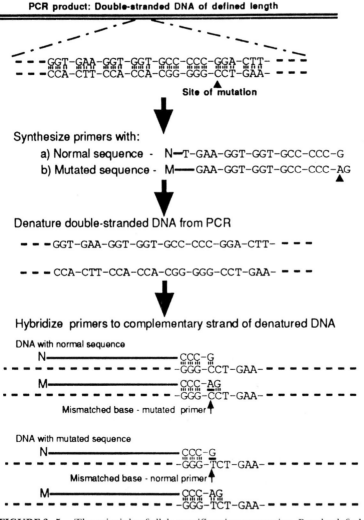

FIGURE 3–5. The principle of allele-specific primer extension. Panel at left shows the hybridization of two oligonucleotide primers, one with the normal sequence and one with the mutated sequence, to DNA with the normal and the mutated sequence. Note that the mismatch need not be at the very 3'-terminal base of the primer. The panel at right shows schematically the extension of fully hybridized primers, and that mismatched primers are not extended. The products of the extension reactions are separated on a sequencing gel (polyacrylamide gel) and the gel exposed to film. Simulated results are shown for individuals that are: homozygous normal, heterozygous, and homozygous mutant. N, normal sequence primer; M, mutated sequence primer; filled elliptical rectangle, presence of label at the position to which the labeled extension product migrated on sequencing gel; open elliptical rectangle, absence of label since the mismatched primer was not extended. (*Figure continues.*)

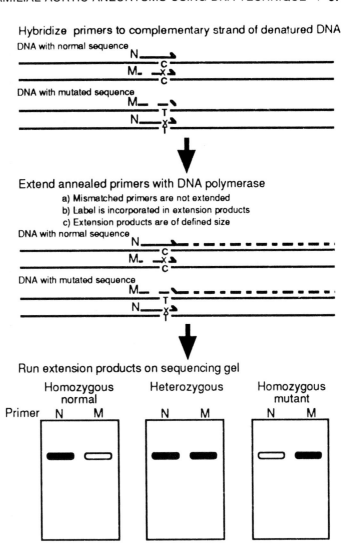

FIGURE 3–5. (*Continued.*)

isolated from the proband's fibroblasts was already partially digested at 20°C. The presence of the mutation destabilized the triple helix.

To determine which relatives of the proband were carriers of the mutation, allele-specific oligonucleotide hybridizations and allele-specific restriction endonuclease digestions were performed on samples from those relatives who wished to participate in the study.[24] Because the relatives were dispersed throughout the United States, and because of the inconvenience to the individuals of obtaining blood samples, we attempted to isolate DNA from other, more conveniently obtainable sample sources. DNA from hair roots had previously been used as template for the PCR,[32] and the PCR products then used for allele-specific assays. We, on the other hand, found that saliva yielded far more DNA and the samples were less likely to be mixed up than were hair roots. Ten of the proband's relatives provided samples and the mutation was found in four.[24] The carriers of the mutation were screened for the presence of an aneurysm. However, since the family members that carried the mutation were relatively young (< 50 years old[17]), none had an aneurysm. All the relatives with aneurysms were deceased. To link the mutation to the disease it was necessary to demonstrate that some of the deceased, affected relatives carried

Biopsy from the proband

⇩

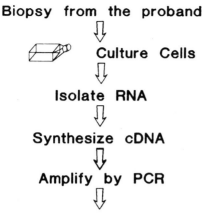 **Culture Cells**

⇩

Isolate RNA

⇩

Synthesize cDNA

⇩

Amplify by PCR

⇩

Sequence PCR products directly

FIGURE 3–6. The strategy of the candidate gene approach to study genetic defects in patients with familial aortic aneurysms. Skin biopsies are collected from patients with aortic aneurysms and a history of aneurysms in their family. Fibroblasts are grown and RNA isolated. The RNA is used to synthesize cDNA that is in turn used as template for the PCR. The coding sequences of candidate genes such as the gene for type III procollagen are amplified and sequenced directly. Direct sequencing not only avoids the problem of accentuating artifacts of the PCR and cloning, but is also much more rapid.

the mutation. Pathological specimens from the proband's mother and maternal aunt were available.[24] The DNA was isolated from the formalin-fixed and stained tissue on a 30-year-old microscope slide (proband's mother) and from 2-year-old tissue that was formalin-fixed and embedded in a block (proband's aunt).[24] The DNA was amplified by the PCR and it was shown that the mutation was present in both the mother and the aunt by allele-specific oligonucleotide hybridization. The mutation could therefore be linked to the disease. In addition, one of the four living relatives that were shown to be carriers of the mutation has, subsequently to the initial screening, developed dilatation of the aorta.

CONCLUSION

We characterized a mutation in the gene for type III procollagen that causes aortic aneurysms in one large family.[24] Subsequently we collected skin biopsies from about 50 patients who had been diagnosed with an aortic aneurysm and who have a family history of aneurysms. Sequencing of the entire triple-helical domain of the type III procollagen genes from six additional patients has not revealed another mutation. We intend to determine what fraction of patients with familial aortic aneurysms have a mutation in the gene for type III procollagen. To this end we have modified and refined some of the DNA techniques of molecular biology to rapidly sequence the regions that code for the type III procollagen gene (Fig. 3–6). We also intend to set up similar strategies for the genes of other extracellular matrix proteins.

Some 15 years after the first report suggesting that aneurysms may be caused by a heritable trait,[7] it is apparent that familial aortic aneurysm is a distant entity and that it is caused by one or more heritable defects. The task at hand is to identify the gene or genes that harbor the mutations causing familial aortic aneurysms.

REFERENCES

1. Collin J: Screening of abdominal aortic aneurysms. Br J Surg 1985; 72:851–852.
2. Bergqvist, D, Bengtsson H: Okat antal patienter dör av bukaorta-aneurysm. Okad diagnostisk skärpa krävs. Lakartidningen 1986; 83:3010–3012.

3. Silverberg E, Lubera JA: Cancer statistics, 1983. New York, American Cancer Society.
4. Johnston KW, Scobie TK: Multicenter prospective study of nonruptured abdominal aortic aneurysms. I. Population and operative management. J Vasc Surg 1988; 7:69–81.
5. Thomas PRS, Stewart RD: Mortality of abdominal aortic aneurysm. Br J Surg 1988; 75:733–736.
6. Johansen K, Kohler TR, Nicholls SC, Zierler RE, Clowes AW, Kazmers A: Ruptured abdominal aortic aneurysm: The Harborview experience. J Vasc Surg 1991; 13:240–247.
7. Clifton MA: Familial abdominal aortic aneurysms. Br J Surg 1977; 64:765–766.
8. Tilson MD, Seashore MR: Human genetics of the abdominal aortic aneurysm. Surg Gynecol Obstet 1984; 158:129–132.
9. Tilson MD, Seashore MR: Fifty families with abdominal aortic aneurysms in two or more first-order relatives. Am J Surg 1984; 147:551–553.
10. Norrgård Ö, Rais O, Ångquist KA: Familial occurrence of abdominal aortic aneurysms. Surgery 1984; 95:650–656.
11. Johansen K, Koepsell T: Familial tendency for abdominal aortic aneurysms. JAMA 1986; 256:1934–1936.
12. Powell JT, Greenhalgh RM: Multifactorial inheritance of abdominal aortic aneurysm. Eur J Vasc Surg 1987; 1:29–31.
13. Cole CW, Barber GG, Bouchard AG, et al: Abdominal aortic aneurysm: Consequences of a positive family history. Can J Surg 1989; 32:117–120.
14. Darling RC III, Brewster DC, Darling RC, et al: Are familial abdominal aortic aneurysms different? J Vasc Surg 1989; 10:39–43.
15. Majumder PP, St Jean PL, Ferrell RE, Webster MW, Steed DL: On the inheritance of abdominal aortic aneurysm. Am J Hum Genet 1991; 48:164–170.
16. Bengtsson H, Norrgård Ö, Ångquist KA, Ekberg O, Öberg L, Bergqvist D: Ultrasonographic screening of the abdominal aorta among siblings of patients with abdominal aortic aneurysms. Br J Surg 1989; 76:589–591.
17. Webster MW, Ferrell RE, St Jean PL, Majumder PP, Fogel SR, Steed DL: Ultrasound screening of first-degree relatives of patients with an abdominal aortic aneurysm. J Vasc Surg 1991; 13:9–14.
18. Davies KE, Read AP: Molecular basis of inherited disease. In Rickwood D, ed: Oxford, IRL Press, 1988.
19. Saiki RK, Scharf S, Faloona F, et al: Enzymatic amplification of β-globin genomic sequences and restriction site analysis for diagnosis of sickle cell anemia. Science 1985; 230:1350–1354.
20. Saiki RK, Gelfand DH, Stoffel S, et al: Primer-directed enzymatic amplification of DNA with a thermostable DNA polymerase. Science 1988; 239:487–491.
21. Reilly JM, Tilson MD: Incidence and etiology of abdominal aortic aneurysms. Surg Clin N Am 1989; 69:705–711.
22. Byers PH: Inherited disorders of collagen biosynthesis: Ehlers-Danlos syndrome, the Marfan syndrome, and osteogenesis imperfecta. In Spittel JA Jr, ed: Clinical Medicine. Philadelphia Harper & Row, 1983; 1–41.
23. Kuivaniemi H, Tromp G, Prockop DJ: Mutations in collagen genes: Causes of rare and some common diseases in humans. FASEB J 1991; 5:2052–2060.
24. Kontusaari S, Tromp G, Kuivaniemi H, Romanic A, Prockop DJ: A mutation in the gene for type III procollagen (COL3A1) in a family with aortic aneurysms. J Clin Invest 1990; 86:1465–1473.
25. Beighton P: The Ehlers-Danlos Syndrome. London, William Heinemann, 1970.
26. McKusick VA: The Ehlers-Danlos syndrome. In Heritable Disorders of Connective Tissue. 4th ed. St. Louis, CV Mosby Company, 1972; 292–371.
27. Sanger F, Nicklen S, Coulson AR: DNA sequencing with chain-terminating inhibitors. Proc Natl Acad Sci USA 1977; 74:5463–5467.
28. Maniatis T, Fritsch EF, Sambrook J: Molecular Cloning, A Laboratory Manual. Cold Spring Harbor, NY, Cold Spring Harbor Laboratory, 1982; 545.
29. Studencki AB, Wallace RB: Allele-specific hybridization using oligonucleotide probes of very high specific activity. Discrimination of the human β^A- and β^S-globin genes. DNA 1984; 3:7–15.
30. Kan YW, Dozy AM: Polymorphism of DNA sequence adjacent to human beta-globin structural gene: Relationship to sickle mutation. Proc Natl Acad Sci USA 1978; 75:5631–5635.
31. Gibbs RA, Nguyen PN, Caskey CT: Detection of single DNA base differences by competitive oligonucleotide priming. Nucleic Acids Res 1989; 17:2437–2448.
32. von Beroldingen CH, Blake ET, Higuchi R, Sensabaugh GF, Erlich H: Applications of the PCR to biological evidence. In Erlich HA, ed. PCR Technology, principles and applications for DNA amplification. New York, Stockton Press, 1989; 209–223.

4

GENETIC VARIATION ON CHROMOSOME 16 AND THE GROWTH OF ABDOMINAL AORTIC ANEURYSMS

JANET T. POWELL and ROGER M. GREENHALGH

"Why did I get an aneurysm?" the patient asks. Should our reply be that it was booked from birth or that environmental factors caused it, or a mixture of the two. Of course we are lucky if there is but a single explanation to offer. The explanation that "it is in your genes" can make the patient relax and feel that the aneurysm is not the result of his wayward lifestyle. But is this explanation true, and what is the evidence for it?

FAMILIAL AORTIC ANEURYSMS

There is an ever-increasing volume of evidence to support the claim that abdominal aortic aneurysms run in families. First, the evidence came from unusual family clustering in some patients.[1] Second, the evidence came from surveys of patients, asking their family histories (their family members had a much higher incidence of aneurysms than the general population).[2-4] Third, screening siblings of patients with aneurysms has indicated that one quarter of the patient's brothers may also harbor an aneurysm.[5,6] Such evidence does not indicate whether genetic or environmental causes contribute to the familial clustering. Further, it may be necessary to separate factors associated with the cause of aneurysms and those associated with the growth of aneurysms.

If your patient is one of the very rare cases with Ehlers-Danlos syndrome type IV, or with the even rarer syndrome recently described by Kontasuuri et al., you can tell them "it is in your genes" and is probably the gene for type III collagen.[7,8] The mutation in type III collagen associated with this second syndrome is not found in the older patient with an "atherosclerotic aortic aneurysm."[9] These are the common aortic aneurysms.

ATHEROSCLEROTIC AORTIC ANEURYSMS

These common aortic aneurysms appear to be getting even commoner.[10] Their repair is one of the most successful vascular reconstructions. The surgeon handles the dilated, thinned, and sometimes friable aorta, the laminated thrombus filling the lumen is shelled out, and atheroma is often conspicuous on the underlying surface. Epidemiological data indicates that we are dealing with a disease caused by cigarette smoking.[11] This association of aortic aneurysm with smoking might depend on the atherosclerotic component. Autopsy evidence indicates that in all age groups, heavy smokers (more than 25 cigarettes per day) have more than twice as much area of the intimal surface of their abdominal aorta covered by raised atherosclerotic lesions as nonsmokers.[12] Aortic aneurysm used to be a nearly all-male disease, but in the 1990s women may constitute 20 per cent of the patients presenting for elective aortic aneurysm repair. This change in sex ratio could be a reflection of the long smoking history necessary for the association with aortic aneurysm. Smoking was not widespread amongst women until after the Second World War, when smoking had already been common amongst men for 30 years. Since smoking may now be more common amongst women than men, the ratio of women to men presenting with aortic aneurysms may increase rapidly.

COLLAGEN AND ELASTIN IN THE ATHEROSCLEROTIC AORTIC ANEURYSM

The histopathologist might often be unable to recognize normal aortic structures in the aneurysm wall. The intima often is replaced by atherosclerotic lesions without trace of the internal elastic lamina. The concentric lamellae of smooth muscle cells and elastic aortic connective tissue of normal aorta have vanished. Few recognizable smooth muscle cells remain, the elastic fibers are disrupted and scant, and there is fibrous replacement of the media with bundles of disorganized collagen. The adventitia is often infiltrated with inflammatory cells.[13] This disruption of the medial architecture with marked loss of elastin appears to be a result of proteolytic degradation.[14]

All enzymes that degrade connective tissue are regulated by inhibitors; elastases are a pertinent example. Genetic variation in α_1-antitrypsin, the inhibitor of leukocyte elastase, has been discussed as a mechanism for susceptibility to aortic aneurysm.[15] In a study of 47 patients, 5 had the unusual MZ phenotype of α_1-antitrypsin, associated with impaired antielastase function.[15] In collaboration with Robert Ferrell (University of Pittsburgh) we have phenotyped 149 consecutive patients with abdominal aortic aneurysm. The distribution of α_1-antitrypsin phenotypes reflected that in a normal population, the frequency of the M, S, and Z alleles being 0.94, 0.04, and 0.02, respectively. There is scant evidence that the disorganization and destruction of connective tissue in the media of aortic aneurysms is under strong genetic control.

Although in a thin patient the pulsatile swelling of the aorta can readily be palpated, the thinned disrupted wall is very inelastic. Not surprisingly, this inelasticity is correlated with loss of elastin from the aneurysmal wall. We have used M-mode ultrasonography to determine the pressure-strain elastic modulus of the aneurysmal wall prior to aortic reconstruction.[9] At resection, a biopsy of the aortic wall was obtained. The relationship between the elastin content of

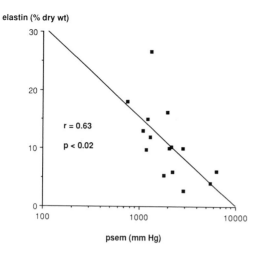

elastin (% dry wt)

r = 0.63

p < 0.02

psem (mm Hg)

FIGURE 4–1. Relationship between pressure-strain elastic modulus of the abdominal aorta and elastin content. The data comes from study of 15 patients, 3 undergoing aortic reconstruction for occlusive disease causing claudication, and 12 patients with aortic aneurysm. The elastin was determined at the same level as pressure-strain elastic modulus.

this biopsy and the pressure-strain elastic modulus is shown in Figure 4–1. There are preliminary indications that the stiffness or inelasticity of the aneurysmal wall may be associated with variation in the type III procollagen gene.[9] This inelasticity of aneurysmal walls is the result, not the cause of dilatation. Currently, there is no evidence to associate aortic dilatation or the destruction of medial architecture with the gene for any connective tissue protein, proteinases, or their inhibitors.

HAPTOGLOBIN AND CLOSELY LINKED GENES ON CHROMOSOME 16

In these atherosclerotic aortic aneurysms, opinion is divided as to whether the atherosclerosis is the primary lesion or a secondary lesion in a damaged aorta. On balance, the evidence (not reviewed here) favors the viewpoint that atherosclerosis is a secondary process in an aorta damaged by dilatation. The pace of atherosclerotic change could hasten aneurysm growth and weakening of the vessel wall. Genetic variation on the long arm of chromosome 16 could influence both aortic aneurysm expansion and atherosclerosis, for here are clustered the genes of haptoglobin, lecithin cholesterol acyltransferase, cholesterol ester transfer protein, and gelatinase. The products of all these genes could influence the growth of abdominal aortic aneurysm in a dilated, damaged aorta.[16–18]

The three common polymorphic variants of the serum protein haptoglobin (Hp^{1-1}, Hp^{2-1}, Hp^{2-2}) have been widely used in genetic linkage and association studies in populations. The terminology of these variants arises from the different alpha-subunits of the $\alpha_2\beta_2$ protein structure, $\alpha_1\alpha_1$ 1-1, $\alpha_1\alpha_2$ 2-1, $\alpha_2\alpha_2$ 2-2. Norrgärd et al.[19] reported an excess of the Hp^{2-1} phenotype amongst patients with abdominal aortic aneurysm. The polymorphic variants of haptoglobin are also readily detected at the gene level.[20] We used this approach to investigate the gene frequencies in two populations of patients, those with abdominal aortic aneurysm ($n = 42$) and those undergoing grafting for aortic stenosis ($n = 32$) and in a control group of healthy subjects ($n = 83$). The results of this genotyping (Table 4–1) indicated that the smaller haptoglobin gene, coding for the Hp^1 protein type, was found significantly more frequently

TABLE 4–1. HAPTOGLOBIN AND CETP GENOTYPES IN PATIENTS AND CONTROLS

| | Haptoglobin Genotypes | | | | CETP Taq I RFLP | |
	$\alpha^1_2\beta_2$	$\alpha^1\alpha^2\beta_2$	$\alpha^2_2\beta_2$	Frequency of α^1 Allele	No.	Frequency of 9.0 Kb Allele
Controls	6	36	24	0.35	83	0.05
Stenosing aortic disease	5	14	13	0.38	32	0.08
Abdominal aortic aneurysm	12	19	11	0.51[a]	44	0.15[b]
Age at aneurysm resection	67.4 ± 4.4	66.2 ± 4.4	72.0 ± 2.6[c]			

[a] Significant difference from controls $p < 0.05$.
[b] $p < 0.01$.
[c] Difference between $Hp^{2\text{-}1}$ and $Hp^{2\text{-}2}$; $p < 0.01$. In some samples insufficient DNA was available to obtain information at both loci.

amongst the patients with aneurysm than in the other two groups ($p<0.05$). The distribution of genotypes between controls and patients with aortic stenosis was very similar.

Such polymorphic variants of haptoglobin may influence directly the pathological processes in aortic aneurysm, or this polymorphism may be a marker for variation in a neighboring gene. Haptoglobin has been in this marker capacity to trace the genetic linkage of "fish-eye disease" or lecithin cholesterol acyltransferase deficiency, associated with premature atherosclerosis.[18] Cholesterol ester transfer protein (CETP) functions in plasma lipid exchange by transferring cholesterol ester from high-density lipoprotein (HDL) to triglyceride-rich lipoproteins. Polymorphisms in the CETP gene modulate plasma HDL levels and also could modulate lipid accumulation in the arterial wall.[21] Several genetic variants of CETP have been described.[21] The frequency of one of these genetic variants, described with the restriction enzyme *Taq*I, was also studied in the two patient groups (aortic aneurysm and aortic stenosis) and in controls. The rare variant of the CETP gene described in this manner generates a DNA fragment of 9.0 Kb after digestion with the enzyme *Taq*I. This rare allele was twice as frequent in patients with aortic aneurysm compared with controls or patients with aortic stenosis (Table 4–1).

This association of specific genes variants (haptoglobin and CETP) with abdominal aortic aneurysm might support a genetic, rather than an environmental, basis for the familial clustering of aneurysms. However, since all the aneurysm patients studied had abdominal aortic aneurysms larger than 6 cm, we could be observing only a genetic influence on aneurysm growth.

Other studies concerning the effect of haptoglobin on degradative enzymes in the aneurysmal wall would argue that the genetic associations observed influence aneurysm growth. Haptoglobins containing the smaller α_1-haptoglobin subunit (both $Hp^{1\text{-}1}$ and $Hp^{2\text{-}1}$) stimulate two- to four-fold the activity of two enzymes which destroy the aortic connective tissue: leucocyte elastase and stromelysin. In contrast, a common form of haptoglobin in the general population, $Hp^{2\text{-}2}$, had no effect.[16] Haptoglobin is not found in the normal aorta but serum proteins leak into the aneurysmal and diseased aorta. The particular variant of haptoglobin which leaks into the aorta could influence how fast the elastic tissue is destroyed and how fast the aneurysm dilates (Fig. 4–2).

The gene for another human enzyme capable of degrading elastin is also found close to haptoglobin and CETP on the long arm of chromosome 16:

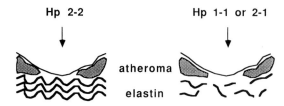

Hp 2-2   Hp 1-1 or 2-1

atheroma

elastin

FIGURE 4–2. The influence of haptoglobin on elastin degradation in diseased aorta. After invasion of the internal elastic lamina by an atherosclerotic lesion, serum proteins leak into the damaged aortic media. The binding of haptoglobin phenotypes Hp[1-1] and Hp[2-1] to the elastic fibrils is proposed to accelerate elastin degradation by rendering it a more suitable substrate for elastases.[16]

gelatinase. This enzyme is abundant in both atherosclerotic and aneurysmal aorta, where it can degrade gelatin, elastin, and collagens type IV and V.[17] In particular, the activities of this enzyme, secreted by inflammatory cells, would allow the establishment of the atherosclerotic plaque or the invasion of the subintima by an encroaching atherosclerotic lesion. In aneurysms, gelatinase is active also in the inflamed adventitia.[17] Polymorphic variants of this enzyme could be associated with modulation of gelatinase activity, thereby influencing the pace of atherosclerotic damage and medial thinning in an aneurysmal aorta. We are now investigating whether polymorphic variation in the gelatinase gene is also associated with aortic aneurysm.

GENES FOR AORTIC ANEURYSMS AND FACTORS INFLUENCING THEIR GROWTH

Most inherited disorders are manifest early in life, but diabetes mellitus type II (adult onset) is another strongly genetically linked disorder that does not become evident until later in life. In this type of diabetes, studies of monozygotic twins have provided some of the strongest evidence for the inherited nature of this disorder. Abdominal aortic aneurysms have been reported in identical twins.[22] This is an important area where vascular surgeons can collaborate to provide a registry of "aneurysm twins" and screen the second twin: ultrasound is quick, painless, cheap, and highly specific and sensitive. Proof that abdominal aortic aneurysms were a genetic disorder would come fast from the study of such twins.

We have used an alternative approach to investigate the frequency of polymorphic gene variants in large groups of unrelated patients. This approach suggests that variations on the long arm of chromosome 16, around the haptoglobin and CETP gene loci, influence the growth of abdominal aortic aneurysms. If atherosclerosis is a secondary pathology to the aneurysmal dilatation, the variations on chromosome 16 discussed here likely are associated with rates of aneurysmal growth. These same variations probably are distinct from those initiating aneurysmal dilatation.

Clinical studies have given information about other factors associated with aneurysm growth, including hypertension, chronic obstructive lung disease, and a small suprarenal/infrarenal aortic diameter. Even so, the growth rate of aneurysms varies widely, from 2 to 8 mm/year.[23–25] A genetic influence on aneurysm growth rates has not been considered previously. The observation that patients with haptoglobin Hp[2-2] presented for aneurysm resection at an older age (Table 4–1) suggests that a genetic influence on aneurysm growth merits further consideration.

CONCLUSION

Current studies give optimism that soon we shall discover the cause, apart from aging, of abdominal aortic aneurysms. This cause is not a unique mutation in the collagen type III gene nor specific mutations on chromosome 16. Discovering the cause of abdominal aortic aneurysms may provide new therapeutic modalities. A very recent publication argues that abdominal aortic aneurysm is a single-gene disorder.[26] The evidence is scanty, since the study used only selected patients and permitted an aortic diameter of more than 2 cm to be considered aneurysmal.[26] Aneurysms do cluster in families, and variations on chromosome 16 probably are associated with the growth rate of aortic aneurysms. Understanding this association could permit the development of strategies to limit aneurysmal dilatation, especially in those unfit for elective aneurysm repair.

So when the patient asks why he has an aortic aneurysm, we have only the epidemiological and autopsy evidence to fall back on. We must tell the patient that smoking probably played a part. We can also tell the patient that with the accelerating pace of research in this area, we soon expect to have more news about the genetic component and how this interacts with environmental factors.

ACKNOWLEDGMENTS: We thank the British Heart Foundation for research support and Drs. S.E. Humphries and A. Henney for fruitful collaboration.

REFERENCES

1. Tilson MD, Seashore MR: Human genetics of abdominal aortic aneurysm. Surg Gynecol Obstet 1984; *158*:129–132.
2. Norrgard O, Rais O, Angqvist K-A: Familial occurrence of abdominal aortic aneurysms. Surgery 1984; *95*:650–656.
3. Johansen K, Koepsell T: Familial tendency for abdominal aortic aneurysms. JAMA 1986; *256*:1934–1936.
4. Powell JT, Greenhalgh RM: Multifactorial inheritance of abdominal aortic aneurysms. Eur J Vasc Surg 1987; *1*:29–31.
5. Bengtsson H, Norrgard O, Angqvist K-A, et al: Ultrasonographic screening of the abdominal aorta among siblings of patients with abdominal aortic aneurysms Br J Surg 1989; 76:589–591.
6. Collin J, Walton J: Is abdominal aortic aneurysm familial? Br Med J 1989; *299*:493.
7. Superti-Fuerga A, Steinmann B, Ramirez F, Byers PH: Molecular defects of type III procollagen in Ehlers Danlos syndrome type IV. Hum Genet 1989; *82*:104–108.
8. Kontusaari K, Tromp G, Kuivanieme H, Romanic AM, Prockop DJ: A mutation in the gene for type III procollagen (COL3A1) in a family with aortic aneurysms. J Clin Invest 1990; *86*:1465–1473.
9. Powell JT, Adamson J, MacSweeney STR, et al: Collagen type III and abdominal aortic aneurysms. Eur J Vasc Surg 1991; *5*:145–148.
10. Fowkes FGR, MacIntyre GAA, Ruckley CV: Increasing incidence of aortic aneurysm in England and Wales. Br Med J 1989; *298*:33–35.
11. Hammond EC, Garfinkel L: Coronary heart disease, stroke and aortic aneurysm: Factors in etiology. Arch Environ Health 1969; *19*:167–182.
12. Strong JP, Richards ML: Cigarette smoking and atherosclerosis in autopsied men. Atherosclerosis 1976; *23*:451–476.
13. Koch AE, Hainier GK, Rizzo JR, et al: Human abdominal aortic aneurysms: Immunophenotypic analysis suggesting an immune-mediated response. Am J Pathol 1990; *137*:1199–1213.
14. Campa JS, Greenhalgh RM, Powell JT: Elastic degradation in abdominal aortic aneurysms. Atherosclerosis 1987; *65*:13–21.
15. Cohen JR, Sarfatti I, Ratner L, Tilson D: Alpha-1-antitrypsin phenotypes in patients with abdominal aortic aneurysms. J Surg Res 1990; *49*:319–321.
16. Powell JT, Bashir A, Dawson SE, et al: Variations on chromosome 16 are associated with abdominal aortic aneurysm. Clin Sci 1990; *78*:13–16.

17. Vine N, Powell JT: Metalloproteinases in degenerative aortic disease. Clin Sci 1991; *81*:233–239.
18. Norum KR, Gjone E: Familial lecithin cholesterol acyltransferase deficiency Scand J Clin Lab Med Invest 1967; *20*:231–235.
19. Norrgard O, Frohlander N, Beckman G, Angqvist K-A: Association between haptoglobin groups and abdominal aortic aneurysm. Hum Hered 1984; *34*:166–169.
20. Bensi G, Raugei G, Klefenz H, Cortese R: Structure and expression of the human haptoglobin locus. EMBO J 1985; *4*:119–126.
21. Kondo I, Berg K, Drayna D, Lawn R: DNA polymorphism at the locus for human cholesterol ester transfer protein (CETP) is associated with high HDL-cholesterol and apolipoprotein levels. Clin Genet 1989; *35*:49–56.
22. Borkett-Jones HJ, Stewart G, Chilvers ASS: Abdominal aortic aneurysms in identical twins. J Soc Med 1988; *81*:471–472.
23. Sterpetti AV, Schultz RD, Feldhaus RJ, Cheng SE, Peetz DJ: Factors influencing enlargement rate of small abdominal aortic aneurysms. J Surg Res 1987; *43*:211–219.
24. Collin J, Araujo L, Walton J: How fast do small abdominal aortic aneurysms grow? Eur J Vasc Surgery 1989; *3*:15–17.
25. Littooy FN, Steffan G, Greisler HP, White TL, Baker WH: Use of sequential B-mode ultrasonography to manage abdominal aortic aneurysms. Arch Surg 1989; *124*:419–421.
26. Majumder PP, St Jean PL, Ferrell RE, Webster MW, Steed DL: On the inheritance of abdominal aortic aneurysms. Am J Hum Genet 1991; *48*:164–170.

5

GENETIC ENGINEERING OF AN ARTERIAL BYPASS GRAFT

ALLAN D. CALLOW

Vascular surgery is the product of the felicitous convergence of seemingly isolated and unrelated events: the discovery and application of the anticoagulant, heparin; the development of arteriography; and the fabrication of biologically nonreactive synthetic fibers into tubular configurations. Of equal importance was the growing recognition that atherosclerotic occlusive disease, heretofore considered untreatable, was most severe at important bifurcations and localized linear segments of long vessels. The predominantly segmental nature of symptomatic lesions made surgical intervention feasible. A similar quantum leap in therapeutics may be attainable by the convergence of vascular surgery with recent enormous advances in cellular and molecular biology. Knowledge of the biology of the vascular wall (specifically, the endothelial cell, the smooth muscle cell, and the extracellular matrix) plus techniques by which the phenotype of these cells can be modulated to express a desired function may result in the development of an entirely new system for disease control, acquired as well as inherited.

By virtue of its location, the vascular endothelial cell may serve as an effective vehicle to deliver peptides and proteins of its own production directly into the bloodstream. By virtue of genetic manipulation, the endothelial cell may be induced to express the needed protein. Manipulation of isolated deoxyribonucleic acid (DNA) in vitro may modify the genome of the endothelial cell.[1] The endothelial cell is also able to modify blood-borne biologically active materials at its surface. Cell types available for genetic manipulation include the fibroblast, the endothelial cell, the lymphocyte, the keratinocyte, glial cells, and mammary cells, the last being of particular interest because of the prodigious amounts of fat and protein it can produce. Any cell capable of division is a candidate. The sole exception appears to be the neurone.

NEEDS

The need for gene therapy and a gene therapy delivery system is illustrated by numerous examples: insulin-dependent diabetes mellitus, cystic fibrosis, Lesch-Nyhan syndrome, antitrypsin deaminase deficiency, several hematologic disorders such as beta-globulin deficiency, responsible for thalassemia, and glucocerebrosidase deficiency, responsible for Gaucher's disease. These last two disorders involve bone marrow progenitor cell types as (in all probability) do severe combined immune deficiency (SCID) and Lesch-Nyhan syndrome. Another candidate is hypercholesterolemia due to insufficient numbers of or ineffective low-density lipoprotein (LDL) receptors on the hepatocyte.[2]

Conventional thinking identifies two approaches to gene therapy: utilization of (1) somatic cells, and (2) the gene cell. For a number of reasons, not the least of which are the ethical and moral issues involved, genetic engineering efforts have been limited to the somatic cell. The germ cell is not presently a candidate. Modification of the somatic cell, sometimes called living-cell therapy, consists of introduction of functional genes into the genetically disabled cell. The disability may be the consequence of heredity, aging, or disease, or may be by intentional disruption of the genome of a normal cell.

Somatic cell utilization has several similarities to organ transplantation. Some of these serve to remove the ethical objections associated with germ cell-line proposals. A change in the phenotype of the somatic cell is confined to that cell population residing in the recipient. By contrast, in germ-line therapy, new or altered genes are distributed in germ cells as well as in somatic cells and therefore may be passed to offspring.

Despite substantial progress in the development of feasible somatic-cell–based gene-therapy technology, more complex problems remain than have been solved. Is it possible to correct a simple single-gene disease with such technology, a task not yet accomplished in an experimental model? Can a suitable experimental animal model be developed? Will the product of the transfected gene lead to an immune response in the recipient? Will a long-term course of immune suppression, now required in organ transplantation, also be required for somatic cell gene-therapy protocols? Are other treatment modalities available or attainable for the relief, if not the cure, of genetic deficiency disorders—modalities which are less expensive, less technology heavy, and less encumbered with theoretical and actual unknowns?

One of the most pressing needs in vascular surgery is prevention of complications which severely and inexorably limit the effectiveness of current surgical and other interventional treatment efforts. The common denominator, the final common pathway leading to failure of all interventional efforts to overcome occlusive arterial disease are the proliferative cellular response and the accumulation of extracellular matrix. This two-component hyperplastic response is largely responsible for bypass graft failure, balloon angioplasty, and indeed, all instrumentation techniques which remove, compress, or ablate the occluding lesion. The after-treatment arterial surface should be nonthrombotic and nonproliferative, two essential characteristics of the normal endothelium. This is not the case in the small-diameter artery or graft where stenosis, early or late, is an all-too-frequent and unpredictable threat.

REQUIREMENTS

For every enzyme, perhaps for every protein a cell produces, there exists a corresponding gene. It is the gene that determines the structure of the protein, and with appropriate gene selection and manipulation, a desirable protein may be created. Necessities of gene therapy implantation are:

1. An appropriate gene must be identified, isolated, and the corresponding regulatory regions described.

2. An appropriate target cell line must be developed.

3. A safe and efficient vector must be provided.

4. The transfected cell must produce a physiologically effective amount of the desired protein.

5. The gene expression of the protein must continue for an appropriate period of time.

6. Neither the foreign gene nor the process by which it is inserted may place the recipient cell or the recipient host in harm's way.[3]

Our interest in genetic engineering emerged from several years of efforts to improve the performance of small-diameter synthetic vascular grafts, in particular, by endothelial cell seeding. Vascular endothelial cells were harvested from a noncritical vein, cultivated in culture medium free of fibroblast and smooth muscle cell contamination, and seeded on a prosthetic graft. We determined the degree of cell retention on the graft in a pulsatile flow circuit

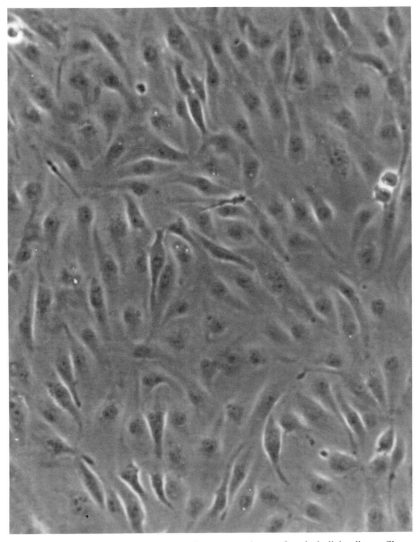

FIGURE 5–1. Appearance of a confluent monolayer of endothelial cells on fibronectin-coated cultureware. The morphology is typical of cultured vascular endothelial cells (100 ×, phase contrast).

as opposed to the static environment of cell-culture flasks. The seeded autologous cell was labeled with a genetic marker, allowed to multiply in culture medium, and then the seeded graft was inserted into the canine carotid artery. This genetic marker, β-galactosidase, was inserted to determine the source and the identity of the cells lining the graft when it was recovered from the dog five weeks later. If the graft was found to be lined with endothelial cells, possible origins included not only those cells that were seeded prior to implantation, but also ingrowth from the host artery endothelial cells, capillaries growing in through the interstices of the graft, and least likely, wandering cells in the bloodstream taking up residence on the graft. Were these recovered grafts lined with the labeled cells that had been implanted? Were they the progeny of those cells? Were they from some other source? The early problems of cell adhesion and retention on a synthetic surface in both a static and a pulsatile flow environment succumbed to the simple measures of providing a fibronectin coat as a graft substrate for the inoculated cells, and growing them on the graft in a tissue culture environment for 72 hours prior to implantation (Figs. 5–1 and 5–2).[4,5]

The desired genetic material can be introduced into somatic cells by a variety of methods. The generic term is transfection, more recently known as transduction. The foreign DNA must cross the cell membrane. This can be accomplished by: (1) precipitation using diethylaminoethyl dextran or calcium phosphate[6]; (2) disruption of the membrane by an electric current, electroporation, referred to by some as "electrocution"[7]; (3) direct injection with a micropipette[8]; and (4) bombardment of the cell with tungsten microparticles coated with bits of genetic material.[9] A fifth method is the use of retroviruses as penetration vehicles.

Prokaryotes (e.g., bacteria) are phylogenetically ancient forms of life. They are distinguished from eukaryotes by, among other things, lack of a genuine nuclear membrane. The hereditary substance of the prokaryote exists as a

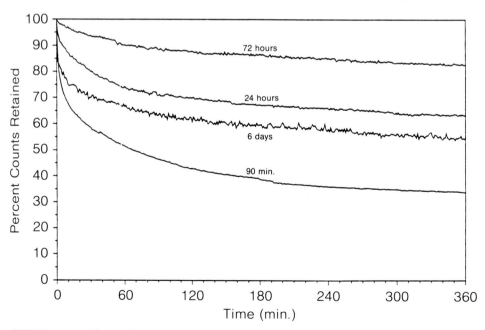

FIGURE 5–2. Effect of flow on cell retention in the canine ex-vivo shunt circuit. 72 hour incubation period is associated with best retention. (Copyright permission pending, Eur J Vasc Surg, 5:311–320, 1991.)

simple tangled coil in the cytoplasm. Circulating freely in the cytoplasm of the prokaryote cell are bits of the genetic material named plasmids. The plasmid may be encapsidated into a recipient cell after cutting of the chromosome of the intended recipient.[10,11] All current methods of gene transfection/transduction have a very low efficiency ratio of transducted-to-nontransducted cells. Baltimore et al.[12] demonstrated that a retrovirus can be used as a packaging vehicle and can be made replication-defective. This made the technique of retroviral transduction safe. In addition, the retroviral transfection or transduction method has a higher efficiency rate than those methods noted above. This technique was selected for our introduction of the marker gene.

A basic requirement of a gene recipient cell is the ability to withstand the process of harvesting, either enzymatically or mechanically, from its normal environment, the traumatic manipulation of transduction, relocation on a synthetic surface, and to pass its newly acquired genetic material to its descendants. Several investigators have confirmed the vascular endothelial cells' ability to survive this biological ordeal.[13,14] We utilized plasmids derived from the prokaryote *Escherichia coli* and the retroviral vectors BAG and BAL. BAG is cell biology jargon for *E. coli*-derived β-galactosidase at the *gag* location of the chromosome. Maloney Mouse Leukemia retrovirus was our selection. The specific steps utilized are to:

1. Convert the natural or wild-type retroviral provirus into a recombinant DNA molecule-defective DNA containing the relevant foreign gene or genes.
2. Make a helper cell to provide functions missing from the transfected DNA, because the cell is unable to make enzymes and other viral proteins necessary to form a complete viral particle.
3. Infect the target cells from the host with a viral vector to enable the cell to produce the protein product of the foreign gene.
4. Return the cell to the host.

The replacement of structural genes, and the transfection of *LacZ* gene are illustrated in Figures 5–3 and 5–4, respectively.

Our studies, using canine endothelial cells transfected with BGAL and the Maloney murine leukemia retrovirus, revealed that:

1. More than 95 per cent of the cells in culture were endothelial cells (based on the expression of an endothelial-cell–specific gene—the acetylated LDL receptor);

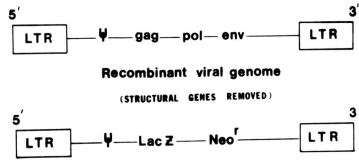

FIGURE 5–3. Replacement of structural genes *gag*, *pol*, and *env* with *LacZ* and *Neo*[r] genes. The packaging complex ψ is retained.

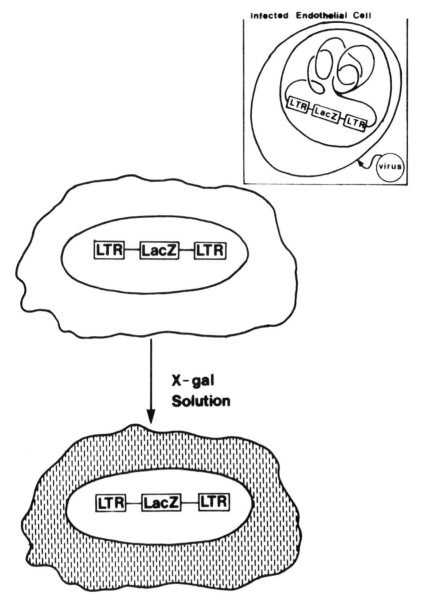

FIGURE 5–4. Transfection of *LacZ* gene into chromosome of the recipient cell and (blue) staining of the recipient cell's cytoplasm and exposure to Y-gal.

2. The efficiency of the retroviral infection based on in situ expression of *LacZ* was approximately 30 per cent (both findings confirmed by 20 independent isolates of canine endothelial cells).

3. Equally effective gene transfer was obtained with primary cultures of remnant saphenous-vein–derived human endothelial cells.[14]

We could not increase the infection rate beyond 5 per cent with the BAG vector and 40 per cent with the BAL. However, the number of genetically modified cells was increased by a three-stage process[15]:

1. The *neo*[r] gene, which confers resistance against the cytotoxic antibiotic G418, was transfected together with BGAL into the endothelial cells.

2. These protected cells were then exposed to various concentrations of G418; the unprotected cells, not successfully transfected, succumbed.

3. The survivors were multiplied in culture to abundance and often confluence (Fig. 5–5).

The final portion of this series of studies was to determine if retrovirally transfected canine endothelial cells, whose structural genomes *gag*, *pol*, and *env*, had been replaced with the *LacZ* and *neo*[r] genes and would survive pulsatile flow in an in vivo model.

The experimental protocol consisted of the following multiple steps:

1. Enzymatic harvest of endothelial cells from the canine external jugular vein;

2. Infecting the endothelial cells with BAG and BAL vectors, and expansion of cell number in culture;

3. Testing the endothelial cells for cell specific functions (e.g., AC-LDL uptake, vWF expression, and prostacyclin production).

4. Seeding 6 cm × 4 mm Dacron grafts with 1.5 million autologous cells per graft and implanting the graft into the left carotid artery.

5. Harvesting the grafts at 5 weeks (to permit sufficient time for cell replication and yet not enough time for the cells to be overgrown by host cells).

6. Aspirin preoperatively and daily for 5 weeks.

7. Explanting and examining the grafts.

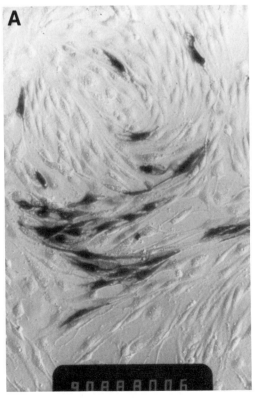 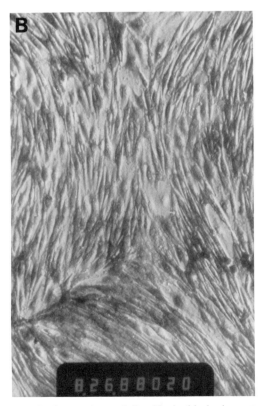

FIGURE 5–5. Endothelial cells, stained and unstained, grown in tissue culture. Cells with the black pigment are actually stained blue from exposure of β-galactosidase to the substrate X-gal. Less that 50 per cent of the cells have been successfully transduced. *A*, without G418 selection. *B*, with G418 selection.

Grafts were divided into three segments: one section was stained for BGAL, the second for scanning electron microscopy to identify cell surface morphology, and the third section for cell harvesting by collagenase of the cells lining its surface. The harvested cells were amplified in culture and tested for β-galactosidase expression, for acetylated LDL uptake, and for vWF response. The recovered cells displayed all functions, stained positively for BGAL, and, on scanning electron microscopy, presented the smooth cobblestone surface typical of confluent endothelial cell monolayer.

SUMMARY

1. The recombinant Maloney murine leukemia retrovirus can be used for efficient transfer of genetic material into cultured canine and human vascular endothelial cells.
2. Genetically modified endothelial cells (GMEC) can repopulate synthetic vascular grafts in vivo.
3. The GMEC persist in vivo for at least 5 weeks and demonstrate stable expression of the transgene.
4. No deleterious effect on the survival and the expression of constitutive functions of the endothelial cell was detected.[14]

To detect the therapeutic feasibility of genetic engineering, an animal model with an easily detectable and correctable single-gene deficiency is needed. Our present goal is to develop such a model. Specifically, we wish to demonstrate that autologous canine external jugular vein endothelial cells can be:

1. Transduced with a retroviral vector containing the gene sequence for human preproparathyroid hormone.
2. That the cells will synthesize and secrete human parathyroid hormone in cell culture.
3. That such cells will continue to do so after seeding on vascular grafts and subsequent implantation into the canine carotid artery.
4. That the hPTH exhibits biological activity in vitro and in vivo.
5. That the secreted hormone will relieve the parathyroid deficiency state in the dog.
6. That the amount of gene product produced in vivo can be amplified as necessary by upscaling the carrier system.
7. That immune system suppression will be unnecessary.

Preliminary observations include:

1. Successful transfection of the PA 317 retroviral packaging cell[a] with the human preproparathyroid gene.
2. Ample production of the hormone by PA 317 retroviral cells as determined by immunoradiometric assay (IRMA), and immunoblot assay of culture supernatant and cell lysate.

---

[a] In collaboration with J. Zweibel, Lombardi Cancer Center, Georgetown University.

3. Successful transfer of the technology to bovine aortic and canine external jugular vein endothelial cells.[16]

The mysteries of the normal anatomy of the human genome and, as a derivative, the morbid anatomy as well, are yielding to gene mapping. Using an alphabet of only four letters, A, C, G, and T[b], the Human Genome Project will write a 3-billion-character message. The potential applications for genetic engineering based on knowledge that will emerge from the genome project are simply staggering. The end product should produce a reference map and sequence, a source book for human biology and medicine for *centuries* to come. Identification of the gene for cystic fibrosis would undoubtedly have been much less expensive if the complete sequence had been available.

"With the full map and sequence, graduate students will be spared the drudgery of cloning and sequencing particular genes before they can get down to the much more interesting and intellectually demanding work of studying variation, function, regulation, and so on."[17]

The laboratory development and clinical application of this new convergence surely require the unique experience and special skills of the vascular surgeon.

ACKNOWLEDGMENT: This work was supported in part by NIH grant number RO1 HL46514-01.

REFERENCES

1. Hood L: Biotechnology and medicine of the future. JAMA 1988; *259*:1837–1844.
2. Nichols EK: Human Gene Therapy. Harvard University Press, Cambridge, MA, 1988.
3. Weatherall DJ: Gene therapy in perspective. Nature 1991; *349*:275–276.
4. Foxall TL, Auger KR, Callow AD, Libby P: Adult human endothelial cell coverage of small caliber Dacron and PTFE vascular prostheses in vitro. J Surg Res 1986; *41*:158–172.
5. Prendiville EJ, Gould KE, Baur W, et al: The effect of anticoagulation and antiplatelet therapy on retention of endothelial cells cultured on fibronectin-coated expanded polytetrafluoroethylene vascular grafts. Eur J Vasc Surg 1991; *5*:311–320.
6. Lopata MA, Cleveland DW, Sollner-Webb B: High level transient expression of a chloramphenicol acetyl transferase gene by DEAE-dextran mediated DNA transfection coupled with a dimethyl sulfoxide or glycerol shock treatment. Nucleic Acids Res 1984; *12*:5707–5717.
7. Potter H, Weir L, Leder P: Enhancer-dependent expression of a human k immunoglobulin genes introduced into mouse pre-B lymphocytes by electroporation. Proc Natl Acad Sci USA 1984; *81*:7161–7165.
8. Capecchi MR: High efficiency transformation by direct microinjection of DNA into cultured mammalian cells. Cell 1980; *22*:479–488.
9. Klein TM, Wolf ED, Wu R, Sanford JC: High-velocity microprojectiles for delivering nucleic acids into living cells. Nature 1987; *327*:70.
10. Fraley R, Straubinger RM, Rule G, Springer EL, Paphadjopoulos D: Liposome-mediated delivery of deoxyribonucleic acid to cells: Enhanced efficiency of delivery related to lipid composition and incubation conditions. Biochemistry 1981; *20*:6978–6987.
11. Kaneda Y, Iwai K, Uchida T: Increased expression of DNA cointroduced with nuclear protein in adult rat liver. Science 1989; *243*:375–378.
12. Mann R, Mulligan RC, Baltimore D: Construction of a retrovirus packaging mutant and its use to produce helper-free defective retrovirus. Cell 1983; *33*:153–159.

---

[b] Adenine, Cytosine, Guanine, and Thymine.

13. Zwiebel JA, Freeman SM, Kantoff PW, Cornetta K, Ryan US, Anderson WF: High level recombinant gene expression in rabbit endothelial cells transduced by retroviral vectors. Science 1989; *243*:220–222.

14. Wilson JM, Birinyi LK, Salomon RN, Libby P, Callow AD, Mulligan RC: Implantation of vascular grafts lined with genetically modified endothelial cells. Science 1989; *244*:1344–1346.

15. Nitzberg R, Gould K, Prendiville E, Allen M, Connolly R, Callow A: The use of gene transfer technology to determine the origin of cells lining a seeded vascular prosthesis. Presented at the 38th Scientific Meeting of the International Society for Cardiovascular Surgery, Los Angeles, CA, June, 1990.

16. Hellerman JG, Cone RC, Potts JT Jr, Rich A, Mulligan RC, Kronenberg HM: Secretion of human parathyroid hormone from rat pituitary cells infected with a recombinant retrovirus encoding preproparathyroid hormone. Proc Natl Acad Sci USA 1984; *81*:5340–5344.

17. McKusick VA: Current trends in mapping human genes. FASEB J 1991; *5*:12–20.

6

THERAPEUTIC POTENTIAL OF GENETIC ENGINEERING ON VASCULAR DISEASE

JAMES C. STANLEY, RACHEL M. PODRAZIK, and LOUIS M. MESSINA

Few areas of research have generated as much interest among the scientific medical community as has recombinant DNA technology. The ability to define molecular mechanisms that control normal physiologic events or cause pathologic states, as well as the ability to manipulate the genetic control of these phenomena, represent the basis of a broad, new form of medicine.[1,2] This general subject only recently has been introduced to the surgical community.[3-5] The role of molecular genetics in treating arterial and venous disease, by eliminating or modifying risk factors such as hypercholesterolemia and diabetes mellitus, as well as altering specific disease states within the vessel wall, such as arteriosclerosis and neointimal hyperplasia, is likely to become of practical importance to the vascular surgeon during the next decade.

MOLECULAR GENETICS AND GENE TRANSFER

Double-stranded deoxyribonucleic acid (DNA) constitutes the substance of the 23 chromosomes located in the nucleus of all somatic cells. Directly and indirectly, DNA regulates cell function by controlling protein synthesis. In fact, all heritable information defining cellular activity is defined by the specific molecular content of DNA in the genes residing within the chromosomes.

Four different nucleotide molecules provide the structure of DNA: two purines, adenine and guanine; and two pyrimidines, thymine and cytosine. These nucleotides are paired on the two strands of DNA such that an adenine and thymine and a guanine and cytosine are always opposite each other. The couplings of these two nucleotides are known as base pairs (bp). The sequence of the bp defines all encoded genetic information. The usual gene is 2000 to 3000 bp in length. Although this may appear to be a rather large structure, it is not when contrasted to the total number of bp within all chromosomes. In fact, there are more than 3 billion bp, or 6 billion of the four individual nucleotide molecules, in the nucleus of each human cell. It is estimated that only 15 per cent of these nucleotides have a direct role in the control of cellular activity, the remaining nucleotides representing genetic material acquired through evolution, but which have no known function in contemporary life.

Transcription is the initial process by which genetic information in DNA is expressed in the cell. DNA, under the influence of the enzyme ribonucleic acid (RNA) polymerase, unwinds preparatory to formation of complementary intermediate messenger RNA (mRNA). This unwinding allows complementary molecules, in a paired fashion, to line up alongside the single strand of DNA. Each nucleotide within the DNA has a pairing with a matching base molecule on the strand of mRNA, except that uracil is substituted for thymine in the mRNA. Further processing of mRNA causes deletion of certain nucleotide segments, introns, that are believed unimportant. This leaves mRNA segments, exons, that contain the essential genetic information for protein formation.

Translation is the process by which mRNA initiates protein synthesis. Translation occurs in the cytoplasm on the ribosomes where mRNA serves as a template upon which specific amino acids become aligned. These amino acids are part of a three-dimensional structure known as transfer RNA (tRNA) which has external exposure of three nucleotides that are complementary to the mRNA nucleotides. A genetic code exists such that a given three-segment nucleotide sequence on tRNA, called a codon, causes alignment on mRNA of one of the 20 amino acid protein building blocks. A total of 64 different arrangements of three-segment nucleotide sequences, (4^3), exist for the 20 amino acids. Thus, some amino acids have more than one codon. The relationship between the codons and amino acids defines the genetic code (Fig. 6–1). These amino acids, two at a time, are subsequently merged to form a polypeptide chain (Fig. 6–2). As this process continues, complex proteins are formed within the cell. Knowledge of a protein's amino acids sequence allows one, with some ambiguities, to work backwards through tRNA, to mRNA, and eventually to identify DNA nucleotide sequences that represent the gene construct responsible for a given protein's production. Because certain amino

1st Nucleotide (5' end)	2nd Nucleotide				3rd Nucleotide (3' end)
	U	C	A	G	
U	Phe	Ser	Tyr	Cys	U
	Phe	Ser	Tyr	Cys	C
	Leu	Ser	-	-	A
	Leu	Ser	-	Trp	G
C	Leu	Pro	His	Arg	U
	Leu	Pro	His	Arg	C
	Leu	Pro	Gln	Arg	A
	Leu	Pro	Gln	Arg	G
A	Ile	Thr	Asn	Ser	U
	Ile	Thr	Asn	Ser	C
	Ile	Thr	Lys	Arg	A
	Met	Thr	Lys	Arg	G
G	Val	Ala	Asp	Gly	U
	Val	Ala	Asp	Gly	C
	Val	Ala	Glu	Gly	A
	Val	Ala	Glu	Gly	G

FIGURE 6–1. The genetic code. Bases are presented as ribonucleotides (U, uracil; C, cytosine; A, adenine; G, guanine). The 64 possible sequences of the three nucleotide molecules (first, second, third) encode for the 20 amino acids (abbreviated in the central portion of the figure) in a specific manner.

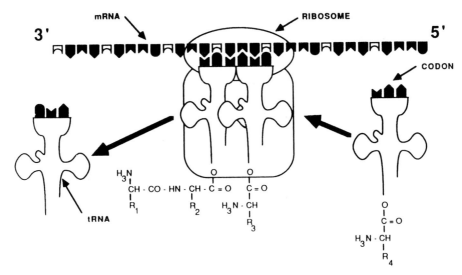

FIGURE 6–2. Translation. The three-dimensional conformation of the midportion of transfer RNA (tRNA) specifically provides external exposure of three nucleotides, known collectively as a codon, that associate with messenger RNA (mRNA) in a complementary fashion. This mRNA-tRNA association occurs on the ribosomes and is restricted to two codons at any one time. This provides approximation of two individual amino acids, and facilitates polymerization and peptide formation. (Modified and reproduced with permission from Brothers TE, Stanley JC: Impact of genetic engineering on vascular disease and biology. *In* Veith FJ, ed: Current Critical Problems in Vascular Surgery, vol 2. St. Louis, MO, Quality Medical Publishers, 1990; 42–50.)

acids have multiple codons, it should be apparent that the exact gene nucleotide sequence may be difficult to predict for proteins containing hundreds of amino acids. Many recent advances in this field have been the result of new micro-chemical technologies, especially protein sequentors and DNA synthesizers.[6]

This simplified description of cellular protein production, in reality, belies a much more complex process. Regulation of gene expression is under the influence of other nucleotide sequences of the chromosome called promoters, located proximal to the gene on the DNA; and enhancer regions, located at more remote distances from the gene, both of which bind proteins that facilitate transcription. Formation of a transcription complex that positions RNA poly-merase at the initiation site of the gene is the result of multiple DNA-protein and protein-protein interactions.[7]

Recombinant DNA technology involves transfer of foreign DNA into a host cell's genomic DNA. This allows very small amounts of a specific gene to be removed and inserted into another cell where the cloned gene may be markedly amplified for study, or used to produce a protein.[8] Essential to this technology has been the discovery of two important enzymes, restriction endonucleases and ligases, which allow cutting and splicing of nucleotides in a predictable manner. Various substances commonly used in clinical practice, such as insulin, growth hormone, erythropoietin, and tissue-type plasminogen activator (tPA), are produced by recombinant means with gene transfer into prokaryotic cells such as *Escherichia coli* bacteria.

Gene transfer may be undertaken in eukaryotic cells and provides the basis for human gene therapy. Gene therapy uses a variety of approaches, with most directed toward gene augmentation. This technology has particular application to a subgroup of the nearly 3500 known genetic diseases associated with deficiencies in specific protein production. Gene augmentation may be achieved by placement of genetic material into the cytoplasmic episomes, a process known as gene introduction. It should be noted that the effectiveness of this type of gene transfer is limited by the cell's longevity, with cell death terminating any effect of such therapy. A second method of gene augmentation is by placement of foreign genetic material directly into the host chromosome through a process known as gene insertion. This approach allows the therapeutic effect to be passed on to the progeny of this cell and holds a distinct advantage if stem cells are the recipients of the new genetic material. The current status of gene insertion does not involve specific site-directed insertion, although specific placement of a foreign gene within the host genome is possible and likely to occur as the science of this technology progresses.[9]

Genetic material may be introduced into eukaryotic cells by techniques using physical or chemical means, fusion carriers, and viral transport. Electroporation, for example, uses electrical currents to facilitate transfer across cellular membranes.[10] Various agents such as calcium phosphate or diethylaminoethyl dextran achieve a similar transfer of genetic material into cells.[11,12] Direct microinjection of DNA, with or without its attachment to microprojectiles,[13–15] and liposomes carrying encapsidated DNA, that subsequently fuse with cell membranes[16–17] also permit introduction of DNA.

Genetic material may also be inserted into eukaryotic cells by the process of transfection, using a number of viral vectors.[18] Included are the transforming DNA viruses, papovavirus and SV-40, as well as certain adenoviruses.[19] Other viruses, including vaccinia,[20] bovine papilloma virus,[21] herpes saimiri virus,[22] herpes simplex 1 virus,[23] cytomegalovirus,[24] and Epstein-Barr virus[25] may also be used for gene transfer. The most important development in viral vectors was the identification and use of appropriate murine and avian retroviruses for the transfer of genetic material.[26–28] These RNA viruses enter the cells, where they reside within the cytoplasm and act as a template for reverse transcription of the genetic information within the virus to form complementary viral DNA. This process is initiated by reverse transcriptase that is incorporated within the viral particle. The newly formed viral DNA then is integrated into the host genome as a provirus, where it may be expressed in protein production. Insertion of a gene of interest into a retroviral carrier provides the basis for gene transfer in many contemporary experiments.

The nucleotides within the normal wild retrovirus contain sequences essential for the production of core proteins (the *gag* region), reverse transcriptase and ligase (the *pol* region), and outer capsule glycoproteins (the *env* region). A ψ segment facilitates later encapsidation of viral RNA into an infective particle.[29] Long terminal repeat (LTR) segments at either end of the central genes within the provirus are necessary for the integration and expression of proviral DNA within the host cell (Fig. 6–3).

A virus must not be able to replicate itself when used for gene therapy. Thus recombinant retroviral particles containing genes of interest are con-

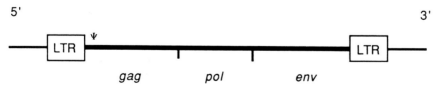

FIGURE 6–3. Wild retroviral provirus genome. Genes for core proteins (*gag*), reverse transcriptase and ligase (*pol*), and outer capsule glycopoteins (*env*) are preceded by the encapsidation signal ψ and flanked by long terminal repeat (LTR) segments.

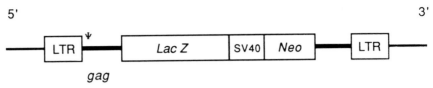

FIGURE 6–4. Retroviral vector. Replacement of the majority of *gag*, *pol*, and *env* regions by genes for β-galactosidase (*Lac*Z), neomycin resistance (*Neor*), and the simian virus (SV-40) early promoter. This represents the BAG (β-galactosidase at *gag*) vector.

structed with only enough native sequences to allow encapsidation and later integration. The removal and insertion of this genetic material is undertaken by conventional DNA cutting and splicing techniques. Under most circumstances, there is a deletion of a considerable portion of native viral genome encoding for the proteins necessary for duplication of the virus. This renders the recombinant viral particles replication incompetent (Fig. 6–4).

Most techniques of inserting foreign DNA into host DNA are very inefficient. Insertion of the neomycin resistance gene, a phosphotransferase gene, transmits cellular protection to the cytocidal antimicrobial agent G418. When this gene is inserted individually or in a cassette fashion with other genes, and the cells are exposed to G418, in vitro, only those that were successfully transduced survive. This provides a means of selecting only those cells carrying the new genetic material.

Integration of the complementary viral DNA strand as a provirus occurs at random sites within the host genomes. Existing technology using viral vectors usually leads to insertion of multiple gene copies into the host genome, with their subsequent expression being unregulated. Such unregulated protein production is called constitutive expression. Single copy integration is more likely to occur with use of retroviral carriers. Although random integration and constitutive expression of genetic material represents the current state of recombinant DNA technology involving gene transfer, site-specific insertion and regulated expression are feasible. The conceptual simplicity of molecular genetics, using recombinant DNA technology as a means of altering a cell's function, makes this form of intervention attractive for application in numerous clinical settings.

APPLICATIONS OF GENETIC ENGINEERING TO THE VESSEL WALL

Genetic modification of the endothelium and smooth muscle of arteries and veins has been successfully accomplished by a number of investigators. Certain unique characteristics of endothelium make it an attractive target organ for expression of foreign genes in vivo. Endothelium's immediate interface with the bloodstream allows luminal release of various proteins having a paracrine effect on local surface thrombotic events, or endocrine effects, such as clot lysis and inhibition of platelet aggregation, along the downstream blood-surface interface. Similarly, because of its close apposition to medical smooth muscle cells, endothelium may influence a number of significant interactions between these two contiguous layers of the vessel wall, especially those involving vasomotion and cellular proliferation. A number of studies have been directed at gene transfer into endothelial cells, both in vitro and in vivo, and the results of these experiments are relevant to applications of genetic engineering as a means of altering vessel wall function. Six recent reports relevant to this topic deserve note, including three in vitro studies and three in vivo studies.

Zwiebel and colleagues at the National Institutes of Health (NIH) were among the earliest to document that endothelial cells in vitro could serve as recipients of functioning recombinant genes.[30] In their experiments, expression of genes encoding for neomycin resistance, human adenosine deaminase, and rat growth hormone occurred in rabbit aortic endothelial cells, using retroviral vectors for gene transfer. In certain of their experiments the transduced endothelial cells were grown in culture on silicone-coated polyurethane vascular prostheses, a study with obvious relevance to vascular surgery.

Dichek and his colleagues, in a second in vitro study at NIH, transferred genes encoding for the production of β-galactosidase and human tPA into cultured sheep endothelial cells.[31] These transduced cells were subsequently seeded onto stainless steel stents of the type applicable for intra-arterial use during angioplasty. In these studies, β-galactosidase was evident in cells that covered the stents. Similarly, measurements of tPA in the culture media used to incubate the stents confirmed that the transduced cells were producing the protein at very high levels (up to 400 times normal) in a constitutive way without conferring any disadvantages to other common functions or the growth of the transduced cells.

In a third in vitro study, Brothers and his colleagues at the University of Michigan assessed the effect of genetic transduction on canine endothelial cell prostacyclin production and cell growth.[3] In these studies, canine venous endothelium was transfected with a retrovirus containing the *LacZ* gene responsible for β-galactosidase production, in combination with the neomycin resistance gene. Transduced cells consistently revealed a slower proliferation rate than normal nontransfected cells in the culture environment. Similarly, basal production of prostacyclin during log-phase growth was less in transduced cells than in nontransfected cells. Once these two cell lines had grown to confluence, the differences in prostacyclin production were absent. Such alterations may become important during the application of clinical gene therapy, and are likely to be different for each transduction event in relation to the particular gene and vector used for transfer.

Nabel and her colleagues at the University of Michigan undertook a series of in vivo studies that documented recombinant gene expression among endothelial cells placed within iliofemoral arteries of Yucatan minipigs after they had been transduced with the *LacZ* and neomycin resistance genes using a retroviral vector.[32] These cells were selected in vitro, and a nearly pure population of genetically modified cells were then transplanted into denuded segments of the pigs' iliofemoral arteries, facilitated by a double balloon catheter specifically designed for the isolation of this vascular segment during the seeding procedure. Arterial tissues examined 2 to 4 weeks following the transplantation of these transduced endothelial cells documented the presence of β-galactosidase production, particularly along luminal surface cells where the transplanted endothelium had proliferated to form a luminal lining. No β-galactosidase activity was observed in iliac artery segments that had been seeded with nontransduced cells.

In a second series of in vivo experiments Nabel and her colleagues documented the presence of site-specific gene expression following a direct gene transfer without a vector. *LacZ* gene expression was documented in excised iliac arteries for as long as 5 months after direct intraluminal exposure to this genetic material.[33] This activity was observed in all three layers of the vessel wall. In the same report, Nabel also documented that DNA transfection was possible using liposomes as vectors, with similar site-specific gene expression noted for up to 6 weeks.

In a third in vivo study, Wilson and his colleagues, at the Whitehead Institute and Tufts University, implanted porous Dacron carotid artery interposition grafts in a canine model that had been seeded with genetically modified endothelial cells.[34] The latter were transduced with the *LacZ* gene alone. Grafts examined up to 5 weeks postimplantation revealed expression of β-galactosidase activity among the seeded cells and their progeny on the surface of the grafts.

Expression of β-galactosidase in transduced cells has been used to document the geographic fate of seeded endothelium in lineage studies in our laboratory. Transduced cells, expressing the *LacZ* gene, exhibit a characteristic blue appearance of the enzyme β-galactosidase when stained with X-gal (Fig. 6–5). Such transfected cells have been seeded on a number of graft substrates, including expanded polytetrafluoroethylene (ePTFE) prostheses placed as thoracoabdominal grafts in dogs. Successful genetic transfer was documented by expression of β-galactosidase in cells harvested from explanted grafts, as

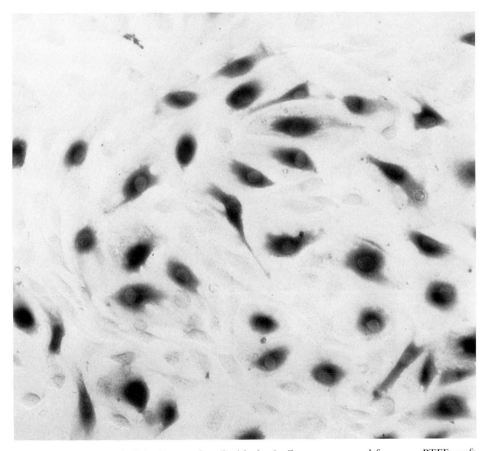

FIGURE 6–5. Endothelial cells transfected with the *LacZ* gene, recovered from an ePTFE graft 6 weeks after implantation in the dog, expressing production of β-galactosidase (dark cytoplastic material). (X-gal stain × 300.)

well as their progeny that spread over graft surfaces over a 6-week period of time (Fig. 6–6 and 6–7).

The potential value of genetic engineering to modify vessel wall and graft tissue will depend on a number of future advances. Currently, the use of retroviral vectors limits the size of the gene that may be inserted to approximately 8000 bp. Similarly, the transfection rate using most retroviral vectors is relatively low and better methods are needed to increase the efficiency of transfection. Unfortunately, certain in vitro methods of increasing the proportion of transfected cells, such as with the use of the neomycin resistance gene with subsequent exposure to G418 to destroy nontransduced cells, may alter other functions of surviving cells. In this regard, the constitutive, unregulated expression of protein production by cells that have had random, rather than site-specific, insertion of genetic material into their genome may alter important cell functions.

Finally, for this technology to be useful in modifying endothelial cell or smooth muscle cell function within the vessel wall, one must clearly understand the molecular basis for many complex phenomena, such as those involving luminal thrombosis and proliferation of abluminal tissues. A major advance will occur when these events are defined and regulatory substances for them

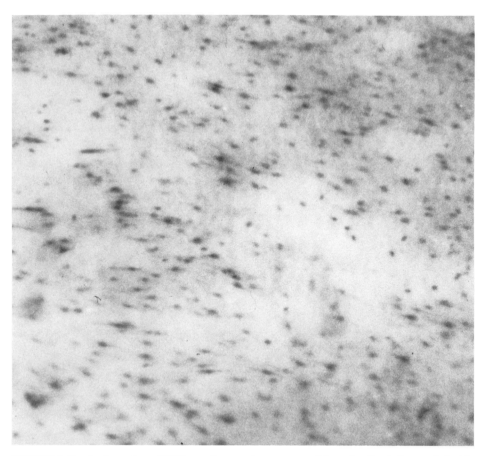

FIGURE 6–6. Surface of an ePTFE vascular prostheses removed 6 weeks after being seeded with selected endothelial cells transfected with the *LacZ* and neomycin resistance genes. The dark areas represent cells containing β-galactosidase as a consequence of successful gene transfer. (X-gal stain × 30.)

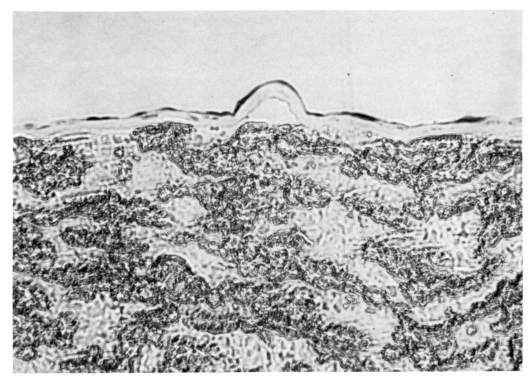

FIGURE 6–7. Cross-section of ePTFE vascular prostheses (same as Fig. 6–6) with evidence of a luminal monolayer of transduced endothelial cells exhibiting production of β-galactosidase. (X-gal stain × 200.)

are determined. If such factors can be related to simple protein production, the nucleotide sequence of the responsible gene may be derived, and by recombinant means, the effect of such gene constructions on cell function may be tested. Clearly, genetic modification of the vascular wall offers considerable potential to our understanding of vessel biology and the treatment of vascular pathology.

APPLICATIONS OF GENETIC ENGINEERING TO VASCULAR DISEASE RISK FACTORS

A lessening of risk factors associated with cardiovascular disease is an important goal of molecular genetic research and gene therapy. Among the major areas of intensive investigative effort are those associated with hyperlipidemic disorders, diabetes mellitus, and hypertension. The vascular surgery community should be aware of this work, not because of its immediate applicability to clinical medicine, but because of the profound effect it will have in the future management of patients with arteriosclerosis.

Markedly elevated serum cholesterol levels are associated with an accelerated arteriosclerotic process. Clearly, in homozygotes with familial hypercholesterolemia, in whom structural and functional defects in hepatocyte low-density lipoprotein (LDL) receptors exist, premature death from cardiovascular events is common. A considerable portion of patients experiencing myocardial infarctions prior to the age of 55 have less-severe genetic defects affecting the expression or function of their LDL receptors. The possibility of gene therapy in these cases exists, in part, because the molecular structure and gene for the LDL receptor have been well characterized. At present, liver transplantation, with an organ that possesses normal LDL receptors, is a relatively radical approach to the management of homozygote disease states associated with severe familial hypercholesterolemia.[35] Genetic engineering, by restoring normal LDL receptor activity, may offer a more reasonable alternative therapy.[36]

Wilson recently has undertaken a series of experiments involving the insertion of the LDL gene into a retroviral vector used for gene transfer.[37–39] Primary cultures of hepatocytes, isolated from Watanabe heritable hyperlipidemic rabbits, have been used in certain of his studies. These rabbits' hepatocytes do not have functional LDL receptor activity because of a specific structural gene deletion. In both in vitro and in vivo studies, functional LDL receptor activity has been observed. In fact, the receptor activity in in vitro studies exceeded normal by four- or fivefold, such that cholesterol metabolism returned toward normal.[39] This therapy will be most useful with the advent of site-directed gene transfer to hepatocytes and extrahepatic tissue, where LDL receptors are responsible for the conversion of this type of cholesterol to HDL.

Diabetes mellitus constitutes another clearly defined risk factor for progression and acceleration of arteriosclerotic cardiovascular disease. The insulin gene was one of the first human genes to be sequenced and cloned,[40] and its recent production by recombinant means in bacteria has been a significant advance in the care of diabetic patients. Recent experiments have been performed using human insulin-synthesizing mouse cell lines that have been constructed using transgeneic methods, employing microinjection of single-cell embryo.[41–42] These mice develop tumors that synthesize insulin and small amounts of glucagon, with clear evidence that the regulatory elements for gene expression are intact. A specific mouse insulin-producing cell line with these elements, beta-TC 1, has been developed by Efrat and his colleagues in transgeneic mice.[43] These cells were implanted intraperitoneally into streptozotocin-induced diabetic athymic nude mice, resulting in the regulated production of insulin and normalization of glucose metabolism.[44] Although this particular line of investigation involved nonautologous transgeneic cells, the possibility of introduction of genetic material responsible for controlled release of insulin in those forms of insulin-deficient diabetes offers significant potential to patients with arteriosclerotic vascular disease. The recognition of genes responsible for increased vasomotor tone and electrolyte disturbances associated with various forms of hypertension awaits further investigation, but is another example of molecular genetic research that clearly will be of major significance to patients with vascular disease.

The Human Genome Project, whose objective of mapping and sequencing the entire human genome will define many heretofore unrecognizable messages encoded in the molecules constituting DNA.[45] Knowledge that is derived from the Human Genome Project will provide the vehicle for gene therapy and an entirely new understanding of the human condition in health and disease.

REFERENCES

1. Friedmann T: Progress toward human gene therapy. Science 1989; *244*:1275–1281.
2. Hood L: Biotechnology and medicine of the future. JAMA 1988; *259*:1837–1844.
3. Brothers TE, Stanley JC: Impact of genetic engineering on vascular disease and biology. *In* Veith FJ, ed: *Current Critical Problems in Vascular Surgery*, vol 2. St. Louis, MO, Quality Medical Publishers, 1990; 42–50.

4. Brown JM, Harken AH, Sharefkin JB: Recombination DNA and surgery. Ann Surg 1990; *212*:178–186.

5. Wong TS, Passaro E Jr: DNA technology. Am J Surg 1990; *159*:610–614.

6. Hunkapiller M, Kent S, Caruthers M, et al: A microchemical facility for the analysis and synthesis of genes and proteins. Nature 1984; *310*:105–111.

7. Echols H: Multiple DNA-Protein interactions governing high-precision DNA transactions. Science 1986; *233*:1050–1056.

8. Sambrook J, Fritsch EF, Maniatis T: *Molecular Cloning: A Laboratory Manual*, 2nd ed. Cold Spring Harbor, NY Cold Spring Harbor Laboratory, 1989.

9. Doetschman T, Gregg RG, Maeda N, et al: Targeted correction of a mutant HPRT gene in mouse embryonic stem cells. Nature 1987; *330*:576–578.

10. Potter H, Weir L, Leder P: Enhancer-dependent expression of human k immunoglobulin genes introduced into mouse pre-B lymphocytes by electroporation. Proc Natl Acad Sci USA 1984; *81*:7161–7165.

11. Graham FL, van der Eb AJ: A new technique for the assay of infectivity of human adenovirus 5 DNA. Virology 1973; *52*:456–467.

12. Lopata MA, Cleveland DW, Sollner-Webb B: High level transient expression of a chloramphenicol acetyl transferase gene by DEAE-dextran mediated DNA transfection coupled with a dimethyl sulfoxide or glycerol shock treatment. Nucleic Acids Res 1984; *12*: 5707–5717.

13. Capecchi MR: High efficiency transformation by direct microinjection of DNA into cultured mammalian cells. Cell 1980; *22*:479–488.

14. Klein TM, Wolf ED, Wu R, Sanford JC: High-velocity microprojectiles for delivering nucleic acids into living cells. Nature 1987; *327*:70–93.

15. Wolff JA, Malone RW, Williams P, et al. Direct gene transfer into mouse muscle in vivo. Science 1990; *247*:1465–1468.

16. Felger PL, Gadek TR, Holm M, et al: Lipofection: A highly efficient, lipid-mediated DNA-transfection procedure. Proc Natl Acad Sci USA 1987; *84*:7423.

17. Fraley R, Straubinger RM, Rule G, Springer EL, Papahadjopoulos D: Liposome-mediated delivery of deoxyribonucleic acid to cells: Enhanced efficiency of delivery related to lipid composition and incubation conditions. Biochemistry 1981; *20*:6978–6987.

18. Gluzman Y, Hughes SH, eds: Viral Vectors. Cold Spring Harbor, NY, Cold Spring Harbor Laboratory, 1988.

19. Morin JE, Lubeck MD, Barton JE, Conley AJ, Davis AR, Hung PP: Recombinant adenovirus induces antibody response to hepatitis B virus surface antigen in hamsters. Proc Natl Acad Sci USA 1987; *84*:4626–4630.

20. Coupar BEH, Andrew ME, Boyle DB: A general method for the construction of recombinant vaccinia viruses expressing multiple foreign genes. Gene 1988; *68*:1–10.

21. Rasmussen CD, Simmen RC, MacDougall EA, Means AR: Methods for analyzing bovine papilloma virus-based calmodulin expression vectors. Methods Enzymol 1987; *139*: 642–654.

22. Desrosiers RC, Kamine J, Bakker A, et al: Synthesis of bovine growth hormone in primates by using a herpesvirus vector. Mol Cell Biol 1985; *5*:2796–2803.

23. Shih M-F, Arsenakis M, Tiollais P, Roizman B: Expression of hepatitis B virus S gene by herpes simplex virus type 1 vectors carrying alpha- and beta-regulated gene chimeras. Proc Natl Acad Sci USA 1984; *81*:5867–5870.

24. Mocarski ES, Manning WC, Cherrington JM: Recombinant cytomegalovirus-based expression vectors. *In* Gluzman Y, Hughes SH, eds: *Viral Vectors.* Cold Spring Harbor, NY Cold Spring Harbor Laboratory, 1988; 78–84.

25. Margolskee RF, Kavathas P, Berg P: Epstein-Barr virus shuttle vector for stable episomal replication of cDNA expression libraries in human cells. Mol Cell Biol 1988; *8*:2837–2847.

26. Cepko CL, Roberts BE, Mulligan RC: Construction and applications of a highly transmissible murine retrovirus shuttle vector. Cell 1984; *37*:1053–1062.

27. Danos O, Mulligan RC: Safe and efficient generation of recombinant retroviruses with amphotropic and ecotropic host ranges. Proc Natl Acad Sci USA 1988; *85*:6460–6464.

28. Tabin CJ, Hoffmann JW, Goff SP, Weinberg RA: Adaptation of a retrovirus as a eucaryotic vector transmitting the herpes simplex virus thymidine kinase gene. Mol Cell Biol 1982; *2*:426–436.

29. Bender MA, Palmer TD, Belinas RE, Miller AD: Evidence that the packaging signal of Moloney murine leukemia virus extends into the gag region. J Virol 1987; *61*:1639–1646.

30. Zwiebel JA, Freeman SM, Kantoff PW, Cornetta K, Ryan US, Anderson WF: High-level recombinant gene expression in rabbit endothelial cells transduced by retroviral vectors. Science 1989; *243*:220–222.

31. Dichek DA, Neville RF, Zwiebel JA, Freeman SM, Leon MB, Anderson WF: Seeding of intravascular stents with genetically engineered endothelial cells. Circulation 1989; *80*: 1347–1353.

32. Nabel EG, Plautz G, Boyce FM, Stanley JC, Nabel GJ: Recombinant gene expression in vivo within endothelial cells of the arterial wall. Science 1989; *244*:1342–1344.

33. Nabel EG, Plautz G, Nabel GJ: Site-specific gene expression in vivo by direct gene transfer into the arterial wall. Science 1990; *249*:1285–1288.

34. Wilson JM, Birinyi LK, Salomon RN, Libby P, Callow AD, Mulligan RC: Implantation of vascular grafts lined with genetically modified endothelial cells. Science 1989; *244*: 1344–1346.

35. Bilheimer DW, Goldstein JL, Grundy SM, Starzl TE, Brown MS: Liver transplantation to provide low-density-lipoprotein receptors and lower plasma cholesterol in a child with homozygous familial hypercholesterolemia. N Engl J Med 1984; *311*:1658–1664.

36. Wilson JM, Chowdhury JR: Prospects for gene therapy of familial hypercholesterolemia. Mol Biol Med 1990; *6*:223–232.

37. Wilson JM, Chowdhury NR, Grossman M, et al: Temporary amelioration of hyperlipidemia in LDL receptor-deficient rabbits transplanted with genetically modified hepatocytes. Proc Natl Acad Sci USA 1990; *87*:8437–8441.

38. Wilson JM, Jefferson DM, Chowdhury JR, Novikoff P, Johnston DE, Mulligan RC: Retrovirus-mediated transduction of adult hepatocytes. Proc Natl Acad Sci USA 1988; *85*:3014–3018.

39. Wilson JM, Johnston DE, Jefferson DM, Mulligan RC: Correction of the genetic defect in hepatocytes from the Watanabe heritable hyperlipidemic rabbit. Proc Natl Acad Sci USA 1988; *85*:4421–4425.

40. Bell GI, Pictet RL, Rutter WJ, Cordell B, Tischer E, Goodman HM: Sequence of the human insulin gene. Nature 1980; *284*:26–32.

41. Hanahan D: Heritable formation of pancreatic β-cell tumours in transgenic mice expressing recombinant insulin-simian virus 40 oncogenes. Nature 1985; *315*:115–122.

42. Selden RF, Skoskiewicz MJ, Russell PS, Goodman HM: Regulation if insulin-gene expression: Implications for gene therapy. N Engl J Med 1987; *317*:1067–1076.

43. Efrat S, Linde S, Kofod H, et al: Beta-cell lines derived from transgenic mice expressing a hybrid insulin geneoncogene. Proc Natl Acad Sci USA 1988; *85*:9037–9041.

44. Stein R, Hicks BA, Demetriou AA: Use of genetically engineered pancreatic β cells in the treatment of experimentally induced diabetes. *In* Hardy MA, ed: Xenograft 25. Amsterdam, Elsevier, 1989, 129–137.

45. Watson JD: The Human Genome Project: Past, present, and future. Science 1990; *248*: 44–51.

7

ENDOTHELIAL CELL SEEDING: A Technology for Arterial Bypass Grafts

MALCOLM B. HERRING and KAREN ETCHBERGER

Endothelial seeding can be defined as a method of transplanting vascular lining cells. Because it is a young technology, endothelial seeding is changing rapidly. Since 1976, experiments with endothelial seeding in the laboratory and in pilot clinical studies have established the basis for formal clinical trials that are now underway. These studies established that endothelial seeding resulted in a cellular lined arterial prosthesis,[1] that the cell linings were made up of endothelium,[2–4] that much of the endothelium came from the transplanted cells,[5,6] that the process may promote resurfacing with other endothelium,[5,6] that the linings were thromboresistant and relatively thin,[1] that platelet consumption on the graft surface was reduced,[7] and that the grafts were less prone to thrombosis under conditions of low flow.[8] If smooth muscle cells were co-inoculated, atherosclerotic changes were seen in the grafts.[9] Sufficiently pure and dense endothelial seeding resulted in endothelialization in patients,[10] and the patency of polytetrafluoroethylene (PTFE) femoral-popliteal bypass grafts was improved by seeding.[11] There was significant improvement in the patency of seeded grafts in patients with cigarette smoking as a risk factor, and patients in one series who did not smoke have thus far had *no* seeded graft occlusions.[11]

The pioneers of this technology have developed several promising methods of endothelial seeding.[1,12,13] Some involve the harvesting of endothelial cells from omental and liposuction fat. Others harvest cells from veins. The derivation of endothelial cells from fat yields many more endothelial cells, but at the cost of contamination with nonendothelial cells. The derivation from veins results in fewer endothelial cells, but reduces the contamination with fibroblasts and smooth muscle cells to an exceptional occurrence. The remainder of this chapter will focus on our preferred method of seeding PTFE arterial prostheses.

OVERVIEW

Endothelial seeding can be performed in the following seven steps:

1. Preclot a PTFE graft.
2. Harvest the donor vein and tie it onto the harvesting catheter.
3. Loosen the endothelial attachments with collagenase enzyme.

4. Remove the excess blood from the PTFE graft.
5. Collect the harvested cells.
6. Apply the cells to the graft.
7. Install the graft.

PRECLOTTING THE GRAFT

Ordinarily, PTFE grafts do not require a "preclotting" step to make them impervious to blood, but preclotting is important to endothelial seeding. Endothelial cells attach to surfaces quite readily. Some investigators estimate that 15 per cent of the endothelial metabolism is devoted to attachment.[14] Polytetrafluoroethylene is electronegative and does not wet very well. These qualities are useful in limiting the attachment of platelets to bare PTFE, but it also limits the attachment of endothelial cells.[15–17]

Even plastics that are well suited to attachment of other kinds of cells do not prove receptive to endothelial cells without the presence of a biologic attachment protein. We tested cell attachment under physiologic shear stress using PTFE and other, more wettable substrates.[18–20] We tested such biologic attachment materials as collagen, laminin, fibronectin, cryoprecipitated plasma-derived fibrin, and whole-blood clot. Fibronectin and whole-blood clot proved the best attachment proteins for immediate endothelial attachment. Not surprisingly, whole-blood clot proved to be a rich source of autologous fibronectin.

Whole-blood clot supports the fibronectin on fibrin strands. During the early minutes after the application of the whole blood, these strands are weakly linked to each other and to the underlying prosthesis. It is important to allow the fibrin formation to mature for at least 20 minutes after it is applied lest the fibronectin and the fibrin be washed out during the inoculation of cells. To accelerate the maturation of the fibrin strands, the graft is filled with the blood, pressurized, clamped, and incubated at 37°C. Furthermore, to anchor

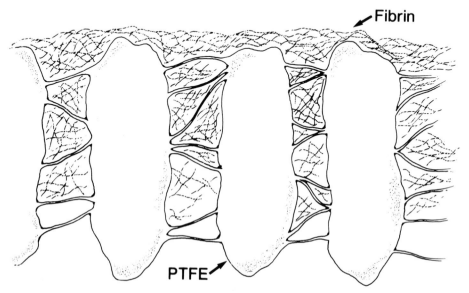

FIGURE 7–1. Preclotting creates a thin network of fibronectin-rich fibrin on the surface of the PTFE. Interlocking fibrin strands also penetrate the air spaces and provide anchorage for the surface network.

the fibrin network onto the surface of the chemically nonadherent PTFE graft, advantage can be taken of the microscopic, interstitial air spaces in the material. Whole blood is introduced under a pressure just sufficient to force small amounts of blood into the interstices of the graft. As the fibrinogen polymerizes to fibrin strands, the strands penetrate the interstices, therapy anchoring the luminal fibrin to the graft (Fig. 7–1).

Occasionally, the blood will fail to clot. A number of clinical situations can be at the root of this problem, such as the premature administration of heparin, the presence of another circulating anticoagulant, or the presence of a coagulation disorder. Except for cases of hypofibrinogenemia, the addition of 30 units of thrombin to the preclot blood (about 1 U/ml) will cause fibrin to form. Thrombin acts quickly; therefore, it is best to add the thrombin *after* the blood is introduced into the graft. If the patient has hypofibrinogenemia, plasma from the blood bank may be introduced into the graft and 30 units of thrombin can be added. The presence of a fibrin surface is critical to seeding on PTFE.

CLEANING EXCESS BLOOD FROM THE GRAFT

While the cells are harvested and the operative sites are exposed, the blood-filled PTFE graft can be kept warm to enhance the polymerization of fibrinogen to fibrin. At the end of this incubation, the blood clot that should have formed inside the graft occupies much of the graft lumen. This excess clot must be removed before the cells are inoculated, and this can be done using a thrombectomy catheter with a Silicone balloon (recall that latex may be toxic to the endothelium).

The purpose of removing the excess clot is not simply to have a wide-open lumen, but to make the fibrin layer on the luminal PTFE surface as thin as possible. Therefore, three passes with the thrombectomy catheter are made. The thin fibrin layer will permit the endothelial cells to develop a closer approximation to the PTFE as the fibrin dissolves in the days after grafting. Thick layers of fibrin may be dislodged along with the attached endothelial cells as a result of shear forces and fibrinolytic activity. Near the anastomoses, smooth muscle cells and fibroblasts from the native artery migrate along the fibrin strands, potentially inviting a neointimal fibrous hyperplastic or atherosclerotic lesion within the graft itself.

HARVESTING CELLS FROM THE VEIN

Autologous vein is the source of the endothelial cells for seeding by this method. A vein should be chosen in which the endothelium is expected to be in good condition. Veins that have been ravaged by phlebitis would be unsuitable, for example. Veins that are too small should also be rejected. However, veins can be used that lack the wall strength for use as a whole-vein graft, since only an intact endothelium is required for a good endothelial cell donor vein. The external jugular vein was used in our clinical trials for most of the procedures, but larger branches of the saphenous vein can often be identified, and theoretically *any* vein will do.

Practically speaking, the vein should be at least 3 mm in diameter, or large enough to accommodate the harvesting catheter (Endotech Corporation, Indianapolis, IN). The surface area of the vein lumen determines the number of endothelial cells that can be derived. The concept of the "minimum inoculum" came from canine studies.[21] Endothelialization of a prosthesis in vivo occurred only if the number of inoculated cells exceeded a threshold which was called the "minimum inoculum." The most convenient way for surgeons to characterize the minimum inoculum is by using a ratio of the surface area of the donor vein to the surface area of the graft to be inoculated.

Based on the clinical histology of grafts seeded by this method, a ratio exceeding 1:20 is needed to achieve endothelialization.[22] Consequently, we recommend a ratio exceeding 1:13, or a donor area equal to 7.5 per cent of the graft surface area. The standard minimum inoculum was established by measuring the length of the veins with a simple vinyl ruler. The diameters were measured before the veins were manipulated because dissection commonly induces spasm, which results in an erroneous measurement. Once the dimensions are determined, the minimum vein length can be determined using a nomogram (Fig. 7–2). However, the longer the donor vein, and the greater its diameter, the better.

As the vein is removed, the branches are secured as though the vein were to be used for a graft, because during the subsequent steps the vein should be water-tight. Glove starch should be cleansed before starting the procedure. Starch proved toxic to suspended endothelial cells in the laboratory, presumably because some unidentified product of latex rubber vulcanization is taken up by starch particles.[23]

A final technical note on the removal of the donor vein is that grasping or clamping the vein damages the endothelium on the inside. Any break in the endothelium allows the digesting enzymes to act on the subendothelial fibroblasts

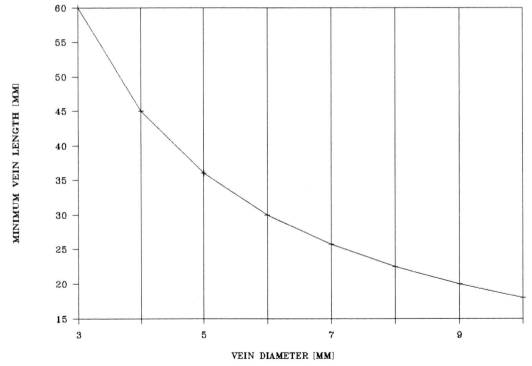

FIGURE 7–2. To determine the minimum length of donor vein to remove for harvesting, measure the diameter. Find the diameter on the X-axis and determine the length on the Y-axis. Use a vein as long as practicable, but at least as long as the minimum length.

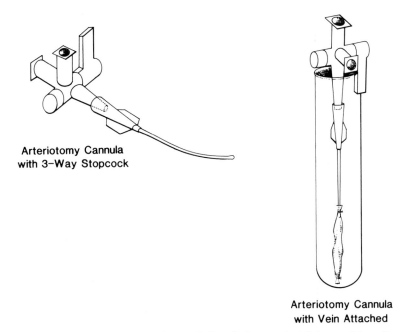

Arteriotomy Cannula
with 3-Way Stopcock

Arteriotomy Cannula
with Vein Attached

FIGURE 7–3. The harvesting catheter (Endotech Corporation) is inserted into the donor vein and secured with a ligature. The flush solutions and the collagenase enzyme solution can be delivered through it.

and smooth muscle cells. These subendothelial cells will then contaminate the cells that are transplanted onto the graft. These cells will respond to atherogenic stimuli once the graft is implanted.[9] The vein can be manipulated by grasping the loose adventitial material or by using a Silastic rubber loop to retract gently. Next, the vein is cannulated with a harvesting catheter (Fig. 7–3), which has a bulb tip. The vein is tied onto the tip of the harvesting catheter.

LOOSENING THE CELLS WITH COLLAGENASE

Endothelium is removed from the vein lining by exposing it to a series of three solutions. The vein is flushed with tissue culture medium 199 (M199) to wash out blood products. To prepare the endothelium for the harvesting enzyme, the vein is flushed again with calcium-free saline solution. A small volume of collagenase solution is used to flush out the saline solution. The distal end of the vein is occluded with a tie or clip to create a water-tight enclosure within the vein, and the vein is filled with 0.1 per cent collagenase (Endotech Corporation, Indianapolis, IN).

The enzyme exposure is critical. The collagenase that we use is a mixture of enzymes, and its capacity to harvest viable endothelium is certified by the manufacturer. Purified collagenases will *not* remove the endothelium. The concentration of collagenase, the 15-minute exposure time, and the incubation temperature of 37°C have been adjusted to optimize the yield of endothelial cells and minimize contamination by nonendothelial cells. Generally, the use of higher concentrations of collagenase, longer exposure times, and higher incubation temperatures than the standard increase the contamination by nonendothelial cells and reduce the viable endothelial yield. Reducing these parameters will reduce the number of harvested endothelial cells. A very small reduction in the exposure time may result in no yield at all.

COLLECTING THE CELLS

With the fibrin-coated PTFE surface prepared, the cell suspension is made by severing the vein near the distal tie and allowing the excess collagenase to drain out. A collection tube is placed under the vein and harvesting catheter assembly. The M199 is flushed through the vein and collected. The mechanical effect of this flush is to dislodge the cells that were loosened by the action of the collagenase enzyme treatment.

The cells are collected in a test tube, often in large sheets containing hundreds of cells. To achieve a good distribution of endothelium on the graft, the cell clusters ideally should have three to five cells each. The large sheets of endothelium are broken up easily by aspirating the suspension three times through a 4-inch pipetting needle (Endotech Corporation, Indianapolis, IN).

APPLYING THE CELLS TO THE GRAFT

The density of endothelial seeding refers to the number of cells that are seeded per unit area of graft surface. The necessary cell density is achieved by inoculating only the length of graft to be used for the bypass operation. The suspension is introduced into the graft lumen with a syringe, and two atraumatic vascular clamps are used to isolate the inoculated segment of graft, thereby containing the cell suspension in the graft (Fig. 7–4).

The graft must rest on its side undisturbed for optimum sedimentation of the endothelial cells from the suspension and attachment to the fibronectin-rich, fibrin-coated PTFE graft. Motion in the graft agitates the cells and tends to resuspend them. At least 10 minutes are required for the cells to sediment and attach.[24] The initial attachment is strengthened in the ensuing hours as

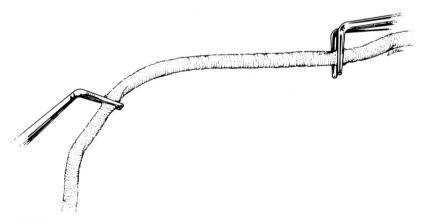

FIGURE 7–4. The endothelial cell suspension is inoculated into the preclotted PTFE graft. To maintain a high inoculation density, vascular clamps are used to sequester the inoculum only within the portion of the graft to be installed.

the cells change from a rounded configuration to a flattened shape that brings more of the cell surface into apposition with the graft.[25] The attachment is further strengthened in the ensuing days as basement membrane substances, such as collagen and laminin, are added to the fibronectin attachment sites by the endothelium.[26,27]

In round-tube grafts, a single inoculation results in initial cell attachment to 25 to 35 per cent of the circumference of the graft.[24] Unsupported PTFE can be flattened somewhat during inoculation, thereby increasing the covered circumference to nearly 50 per cent. To achieve circumferential endothelial healing, two sequential inoculations are used, rotating the graft 180 degrees between inoculations.[24] Ten minutes after the second inoculation, the graft is ready for installation.

INSTALLING THE GRAFT

The installation of the graft differs in only a few ways from the installation of an ordinary PTFE graft. Unless the patient has heparin-associated antibodies, the patient is systemically heparinized. In femoral-popliteal bypass grafting, it is helpful to perform the femoral anastomosis first simply to help retain the M199 in the lumen of the graft. Air exposure can desiccate the endothelial cells, and the assistant should moisten the lumen every 30 to 60 seconds with M199 during the construction of the anastomoses.

Like the endothelium of the donor vein, the newly seeded endothelial cells can be removed with minor mechanical trauma, such as grasping with forceps or the simple passage of a catheter along the wall. The passage of inflated balloon catheters effectively removes all of the endothelial cells from newly seeded surfaces and removes *most* of the endothelium from more mature seeded surfaces.[10] Synthetic grafts differ from the vein grafts in that there are neither vasa vasorum nor branches in the synthetic from which an endothelial outgrowth onto the flow surface can develop.

Endothelial attachment to fibronectin may be modulated in part through heparan sulfate, an endothelial glycosaminoglycan.[28] The reversal of systemic heparinization with protamine during the first hour after inoculation may interfere with endothelial attachment as has been demonstrated in tissue culture experiments. A second effect of heparin reversal is unopposed thrombin activity on the graft surface. Thrombin digests part of the fibronectin molecule which binds the endothelium to the PTFE,[29] stimulates platelet activating factor (PAF)-release by endothelium,[30] and increases the neutrophil-specific adhesiveness of the endothelium.[31] In turn, PAF stimulates neutrophil attack on the endothelium,[30,32] resulting in detachment of the seeded cells.

We therefore recommend that protamine reversal of heparin be deferred until at least 1 hour after graft inoculation. If bleeding is a problem from needle holes, anastomoses, or the wound, topical thrombin can be used with good results. Needle-hole bleeding seems to be minimized by using a suture diameter that is large compared to the needle.

Postoperative anticoagulation was practiced in our studies using low molecular weight dextran followed by a course of aspirin 80 mg and dipyridamole 50 mg twice daily for 3 months; however, a brief course of aspirin is probably sufficient.

SUMMARY

Endothelial seeding is the transplantation of vascular lining cells to another site in the body. The technique of endothelial seeding involves seven steps: 1. Preclot a PTFE graft. 2. Harvest the donor vein and tie it onto the harvesting catheter. 3. Loosen the endothelial attachments with collagenase enzyme. 4. Remove the excess blood from the PTFE graft. 5. Collect the harvested cells. 6. Apply the cells to the graft. 7. Install the graft. Seeding should prove easy to accomplish and should reduce the occlusion rates in synthetic grafts.

ACKNOWLEDGMENTS: The authors thank Rebecca Comptom, C.S.T., C.S.A., for her help in the preparation of this chapter.

REFERENCES

1. Herring MB, Gardner AL, Glover J: A single-staged technique for seeding vascular grafts with autogenous endothelium. Surgery 1978; 84(4):498–504.
2. Dilley R, Herring M, Boxer L, et al: Immunofluorescent staining for Factor VIII related antigen. J Surg Res 1979; 27(3):149–155.
3. Herring MB, Dilley R, Jersild RA Jr, et al: Seeding arterial prostheses with vascular endothelium; the nature of the lining. Ann Surg 1979; 190:84–90.
4. Baughman S, Herring M, Glover J: The peroxidase antiperoxidase staining of factor VIII related antigen on cultured endothelial cells. J Biomed Mat Res 1984; 18:561–566.
5. Nabel EG, Plautz G, Boyce FM, et al: Recombinant gene expression in vivo within endothelial cells of the arterial wall. Science 1989; 244:1342–1344.
6. Wilson JM, Birinyi LK, Salomon RN, et al: Implantation of vascular grafts lined with genetically modified endothelial cells. Science 1989; 244:1344–1346.
7. Sharefkin J, Latker C, Smith M, et al: Early normalization of platelet survival by endothelial seeding of Dacron arterial prostheses in dogs. Surgery 1982; 92(2):385–393.
8. Hunter T, Schmidt S, Sharp W, Malindzak G: Controlled flow studies in 4 mm endothelialized Dacron grafts. Trans Am Soc Artif Intern Organs 1983; 29:177–182.
9. Herring MB, Gardner AL, Glover JL: Seeding of human arterial prostheses with mechanically derived endothelium: The detrimental effect of smoking. J Vasc Surg 1984; 1:279–289.
10. Herring MB, LeGrand DR: The histology of seeded PTFE grafts in humans. Ann Vasc Surg 1989; 3(2):96–103.
11. Herring MB, Compton RS, LeGrand DR, et al: Endothelial seeding of polytetrafluoroethylene popliteal bypasses. J Vasc Surg 1987; 6:114–118.
12. Graham LM, Burkel WE, Ford JW, et al: Immediate seeding of enzymatically derived endothelium on Dacron vascular grafts: Early experimental studies with autogenous canine cells. Arch Surg 1980; 115:1289–1294.
13. Jarrell BE, Williams SK, Carabasi RA, Hubbard FA: Immediate vascular graft monolayers using microvessel endothelial cells. In Herring MB, Glover JL, eds: Endothelial Seeding in Vascular Surgery. New York, Grune & Stratton, Inc., 1987; 37–55.
14. Jaffe EA, Minnick CR, Adellman B, et al: Synthesis of basement membrane collagen by cultured human endothelial cells. J Exp Med 1976; 144:209–225.
15. Lucas JH, Czisny LE, Gross GW: Adhesion of cultured mammalian central nervous system neurons to flame-modified hydrophobic surfaces. In Vitro Cell Dev Biol 1986; 22:37–43.
16. van Wachem P: Interactions of cultured human endothelial cells with polymeric surfaces. Doctoral Thesis, 1987.
17. Hasson JE, Wiebe DH, Abbott WM: Adult human vascular endothelial cell attachment and migration on novel bioabsorbable polymers. Arch Surg 1987; 122:428–430.
18. Herring MB, Gardner A, Glover J. Seeding endothelium onto canine arterial prostheses: The effects of graft design. Arch Surg 1979; 14:679–682.
19. Campbell JB, Lundgren C, Herring M, et al: Attachment and retention of indium 111 labeled endothelial cells onto polyester elastomer. JASAIO 1985; 8:113–117.
20. Kesler KA, Herring MB, Arnold MP, et al: Enhanced strength of endothelial attachment on polyester elastomer and polytetrafluoroethylene graft surfaces with fibronectin substrate. J Vasc Surg 1986; 3(1):58–64.
21. Herring M, Dilley R, Cullison T, et al: Seeding endothelium on canine arterial prostheses: The size of the inoculum. J Surg Res 1980; 28:35–38.
22. Herring M, Baughman S, Glover J: Endothelium develops on seeded human arterial prostheses: A brief clinical note. J Vasc Surg 1985; 2(5):727–730.

23. Sharefkin JB, Fairchild KD, Albus RA, et al: The cytotoxic effect of surgical glove powder particles on adult human vascular endothelial cell cultures: Implications for clinical uses of tissue culture techniques. J Surg Res 1986; *41*:463–472.
24. Kesler KA, Herring MB, Arnold MP, et al: Sequential inoculation for optimal cell distribution on tubular grafts. *In* Herring MB, Glover JL, eds: Endothelial Seeding in Vascular Surgery. New York, Grune & Stratton, Inc., 1987; 103–118.
25. Young WC, Herman IM: Extracellular matrix modulation of endothelial cell shape and motility following injury in vitro. J Cell Sci 1985; *73*:19–32.
26. Madri JA, Williams SK: Capillary endothelial cell cultures: Phenotypic modulation by matrix components. J Cell Biol 1983; *97*:153–165.
27. Martin GR, Timpl R: Laminin and other basement membrane components. Am Rev Cell Biol 1987; *3*:57–85.
28. Ruoslahti E, Engvall E: Immunochemical and collagen-binding properties of fibronectin. Ann NY Acad Sci 1978; *312*:178–191.
29. Galdal KS, Evensen SA, Nilsen E: The effect of thrombin on fibronectin in cultured human endothelial cells. Thromb Res 1985; *37*:583–593.
30. Zimmerman GA, McIntyre TM, Prescott SM: Thrombin stimulates neutrophil adherence by an endothelial cell-dependent mechanism: Characterization of the response and relationship to platelet-activating factor synthesis. Ann NY Acad Sci 1986; *485*:349–368.
31. Cavender E, Saegusa Y, Ziff M: Stimulation of mononuclear cell binding to human endothelial cell monolayers by thrombin. Fifth International Symposium on the Biology of the Vascular Endothelial Cell, July 26–30. Toronto, Ontario, Canada, 1988; 4.
32. Zimmerman GA, McIntyre TM, Prescott SM: Thrombin stimulates the adherence of neutrophils to human endothelial cells in vitro. J Clin Invest 1985; *76*:2235–2246.

II

NEW RADIOLOGIC DIAGNOSTIC TECHNOLOGY

8

MAGNETIC RESONANCE ANGIOGRAPHY

THOMAS S. RILES and ANDREW W. LITT

Since the introduction of human magnetic resonance imaging (MRI) a decade ago, the application of this technology to the diagnosis of vascular disease has progressed at a phenomenal rate. The first use of MRI for vascular surgeons was for the assessment of the size of abdominal and thoracic aneurysms.[1-4] In addition to the transverse images of the vessels which are of similar quality to computed tomographic (CT) scans, MRI also provided coronal and sagittal images of the large vessels without the necessity of contrast media.

As experience increased, it became apparent that MRI could be used to image blood vessels and measure the velocity of blood flow.[5,6] The observation that blood moving from an area unaffected by the magnet and radiofrequency waves could be easily distinguished as it passed into an area already activated made it possible to calculate the transit time of the blood. Development of this concept led to the imaging of flowing blood without visualization of any of the tissues that were stationary within the "slab" that was presaturated with pulsed radiofrequency waves. Since these images of the flowing blood are similar to those obtained by the injection of intravenous contrast, the technique is termed "magnetic resonance angiography" (MRA).

Over the past few years, reports have appeared demonstrating the ability of MRA to image blood vessels in all parts of the body, including the aorta, vena cava, major branch vessels of the aorta, the femoral arteries, the carotid and vertebral arteries, and the circle of Willis.[7-13] The potential advantages of MRA over conventional contrast angiography are clear. If the quality of the studies is sufficient to accurately assess the normal as well as diseased vessels, it may soon be possible to obtain the necessary diagnostic information without the risks of catheterization, contrast injection, and radiation. To date, clinical correlations using MRA are few and involve small numbers of patients. It is clear from the early data, however, that MRA will soon play a significant role in the diagnosis of vascular disease.

Along with the rapid emergence of MR technology, an MR vocabulary has evolved which is unfamiliar to most surgeons. Anticipating that this chapter may serve as a starting point for the clinician interested in understanding the basic concepts of MRA and following the future literature, we have included a brief overview of the relevant aspects of MRI and MRA with an explanation of the technical jargon commonly used. A complete review of the basic physics of MRI is clearly beyond the scope of this chapter. For those who wish to pursue that topic further, we recommend several excellent references.[14-17]

PRINCIPLES OF MAGNETIC RESONANCE IMAGING

Magnetic resonance imaging is a method of imaging the soft tissues of the body by taking advantage of inherent differences among tissues in how they respond to the presence of a magnetic field and to the introduction of energy in the form of radiofrequency (RF) waves. Although all atoms, such as carbon, sodium, phosphorus, etc., are affected by MRI, clinical MRI examines only the hydrogen atoms (protons) within the tissue of interest.

When tissue is placed in a strong magnetic field and exposed to an appropriate RF pulse, a signal is reflected from the tissue and detected by an array of sensors around the tissue. The "signal intensity" is the amplitude or strength of the signal emitted from the tissue. With the help of computer manipulation, the signal intensity of the various points within the tissue can be mapped on a point-by-point basis to create an image of the structure within a given space.

With CT, the whiteness or blackness of a structure only depends on its x-ray attenuation coefficient. With MR, the relative difference in signal intensity (i.e., the whiteness or blackness of a point on the image) depends on the inherent tissue properties, as well as on the chosen imaging parameters such as frequency, duration, and interval between RF pulses. It is important to note that while the true inherent properties of the tissue cannot be changed, the appearance of that tissue in the image can be greatly modified by the operator of the MRI device through the choice of imaging parameters.

TISSUE PROPERTIES AFFECTING SIGNAL INTENSITY

The proton density is the number of mobile "resonating" protons in hydrogen nuclei per unit volume in the sample examined. In biological tissues, the proton density depends strongly on the water content, and secondarily on the lipid content; hence, MR images are essentially images of body water and fat. Imaging parameters can be chosen to produce an image in which the signal intensity is primarily, but not totally, proportional to proton density. These are called "proton density weighted," "spin density weighted," or "balanced" images. Because the number of protons in air and cortical bone is extremely small,

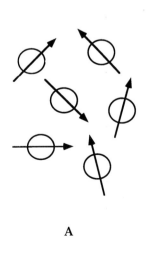
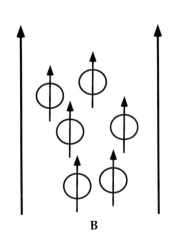

A   B

FIGURE 8–1. Outside the magnet *(A)* the protons are randomly positioned, while inside the magnet *(B)* the protons align with the magnet field lines (large arrows).

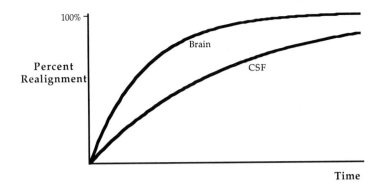

FIGURE 8-2. Proton realignment versus time for tissues with 2 different T1s. Note how the magnetization regrows exponentially.

these tissues appear black on MR images. Proton-dense tissues appear white on these images.

All protons have a magnetic moment which can be considered to have a direction of positioning. In the normal state, the vectors of the magnetic moments of protons are randomly arrayed. When a patient is lying within the MRI device, the protons of the hydrogen atoms are all aligned, and are all at the same energy state (Fig. 8-1). When an RF pulse is produced, energy is imparted from the radiofrequency wave to the hydrogen atoms, causing them to be "tipped" so that they are no longer aligned with the main magnetic field. The tipped hydrogen atoms are said to be in an "excited" energy state. These nuclei lose energy over time as they realign with the magnetic field and return to the original energy state. "T1 relaxation" is the time constant which is used to mathematically describe this realignment and loss of energy. T1 relaxation is an exponential growth process (Fig. 8-2).

The energy is actually lost to the surrounding molecules or "lattice." Small molecules such as water tend to release their energy more slowly, resulting in longer T1 relaxation. Medium- to large-size molecules have tumbling rates that result in a more rapid release of energy to the lattice and, therefore, have shorter T1 times.

The hydrogen molecules interact not only with the lattice as a whole, but with one another. Because there are differences in the chemical environment within tissues, the magnetic field throughout the patient being imaged is not uniform. This nonuniformity leads to a rapid transfer of energy from one molecule to another. The time constant that describes this energy loss is T2 relaxation. Whereas T1 relaxation describes an exponential growth process, T2 relaxation describes a process of exponential decay (Fig. 8-3). Pure water has a long T2 time, whereas complex fluids and tissue solids have shorter T2 times.

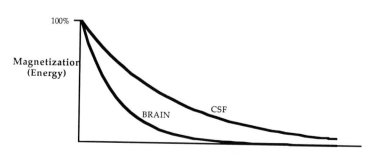

FIGURE 8-3. Loss of magnetization (energy) over time secondary to T2 decay. Note the exponential loss.

T1 and T2 relaxations are occurring both simultaneously and independently. T2 relaxation occurs at a much faster rate than T1 relaxation. Different tissues have characteristic and different T1 and T2 relaxation times.

Moving protons can dramatically alter the signal intensity of structures within the body, such as blood vessels. Parameters that affect the appearance of these structures are extremely complex and are related not only to the intrinsic characteristics of proton density, T1 and T2, as discussed above, but also to the imaging parameters employed, and, most importantly, to the properties of flow itself. While much of the flow within the blood vessels of the body is laminar, the many areas of turbulent flow at normal structures such as bifurcations, as well as at areas of pathology such as aneurysms and stenosis, result in a wide range of signal intensities for flowing blood. While rapid blood flow in arteries is often black (signal void) on routine MR images, blood flow can be everything from bright white to black, or any shade in between.

IMAGING PARAMETERS AFFECTING SIGNAL INTENSITY

As previously noted, the signal intensity within MR images is dependent on both the inherent characteristics of the tissue being imaged and the technical parameters chosen by the operator. The most important operator-chosen parameters are repetition time (TR) and echo time (TE) of the radiofrequency pulse. These parameters, along with other factors such as the application of special magnetization gradients, constitute the pulse sequence.

Repetition Time

The TR is the time between the onset of two successive RF pulses. For the most common clinically used pulse sequence, the spin-echo sequence, the TR ranges from 300 to 3000 msec. If a short TR is employed, tissues with a short T1 will be bright on the image, because only those tissues will have realigned with the main magnetic field in the time between pulses. This constitutes a T1-weighted image. In this form of weighting, fat with its very short T1 is bright, water with its long T1 is black, and muscle is gray. With a long TR, the image will be less sensitive to T1 weighting because all the protons will have a chance to realign. Depending on the echo time chosen, these images will either be proton-density or T2-weighted.

Echo Time

The echo time (TE) is the time after the RF pulse that the signal is received by the radio antenna. In spin-echo sequences, this time depends on the generation of a special 180-degree RF pulse to generate an "echo" of the signal. The duration of TE times generally vary between 15 and 150 msec. If the chosen TE is long, then tissues with a short T2, such as muscle, will have lost their energy by the time the signal is received and will appear dark, whereas water, with its long T2, will appear bright. Thus images obtained with a long TR and a long TE are T2-weighted. If the TR chosen is long but the TE chosen is short, then the image will be largely proportional to the proton density of the tissue. It cannot be overstated that in all imaging sequences, the signal intensity depends on all four factors: T1, T2, proton density, and flow. There are no pure T1 or T2 images; hence the terminology, "T1- or T2-weighted."

PRINCIPLES OF MAGNETIC RESONANCE ANGIOGRAPHY

Magnetic Resonance Angiography results from the application of the principles discussed above to the study of vasculature in the body.[7,10,11,18,19] In general, MRA techniques do not study the vessel or its wall; rather, MRA forms an image of the vessel based on the flow of blood within the vessel lumen. In this way it is similar to conventional contrast angiography. As previously mentioned, the appearance of flowing blood on MRI can be complex and extremely variable. This variability comes from two groups of properties of flowing blood: phase effects and time-of-flight effects.

Phase Effects

Since the hydrogen atoms within the bloodstream are moving with respect to the effects of magnetic gradients and RF pulses, each will respond to these energy forces differently. The variability in response results in a loss of coherence, or "dephasing." The amount of dephasing depends upon the distance and direction moved. Since stationary tissue maintains coherence, one can take advantage of the difference in coherence (i.e., phase) between the moving and stationary tissues to create subtraction images of flowing blood. This technique is finding some limited applications in the study of intracranial vessels, but is not widely used and will not be further discussed here.

Time-of-Flight Effects

Time-of-flight (TOF) effects come from the flow of blood into and out of the volume of tissue being imaged. Magnetic resonance angiography based on these effects is most commonly used clinically, and has proven extremely efficacious in the study of the extracranial carotid arteries and bifurcation, as will be described below. For MRA, the important TOF effects are "partial saturation" and "flow-related enhancement."

If the TR is chosen such that it is extremely short (e.g., 40 to 80 msec), much shorter than the T1s of the tissue being imaged, then the tissue will never be allowed to completely or even largely realign with the main magnetic field. Thus the signal intensity of that tissue in the image produced will be very low. This is referred to as "saturation" of the tissue. Because the tissue will always have some signal intensity, it is "partially" saturated (Fig. 8–4).

If blood flows into the slice being imaged such that it is only present there for one or even two TRs, the hydrogen nuclei will never become saturated,

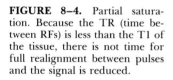

FIGURE 8–4. Partial saturation. Because the TR (time between RFs) is less than the T1 of the tissue, there is not time for full realignment between pulses and the signal is reduced.

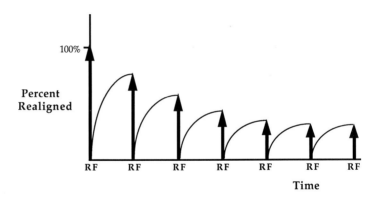

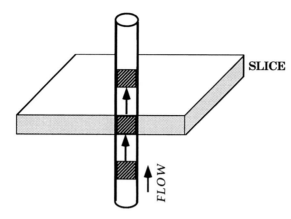

SLICE

FLOW

FIGURE 8–5. Flow-related enhancement. The stationary protons within the slice have been partially saturated (stippling) and give little signal, but the protons flowing into the slice in the vessel (cross-hatched) enter fully magnetized at each TR and produce considerable signal.

☐ Saturated stationary tissue in slice

▨ Flowing blood moving into slice with each TR

even if the TR is short. Therefore, the signal intensity of the blood will be high on the resulting image. This phenomenon of a bright vessel within a uniformly low-signal (dark gray) background is called "flow-related enhancement" (Fig. 8–5).

A limitation of any technique based on flow-related enhancement is the competing effect of spin dephasing. When the flow is extremely fast (e.g., in a stenotic region) and/or turbulent (e.g., poststenosis) there will be loss of phase coherence as discussed above. This will produce signal loss in those areas and may lead to overestimation of the stenosis in a MRA study. It has been found that shorter TEs and thinner slices may help to overcome this dephasing in many, but not all, cases.

MRI Pulse Sequences

In order to obtain the short TRs necessary to produce flow-related enhancement, the classical spin-echo pulse sequence referred to above was replaced by a "gradient-echo" pulse sequence. This uses additional magnetic gradients, instead of the 180-degree RF pulse, to create the echo detected by the radio antenna.

The MRA sequence used will produce a series of tomographic slices oriented in the axial, the sagittal, or the coronal plane, in which the vessels are bright and the surrounding stationary tissues are of low signal. These slices can be obtained in either a two-dimensional (2D) or a three-dimensional (3D) acquisition sequence. In the 2D sequence, the slices are obtained consecutively, with each slice imaged independently. In the 3D sequence, a volume of tissue comprising many slices, (e.g., 64 or 128 slices), is imaged at one time, and later mathematically separated into its individual slices. The former has the advantage of better flow-related enhancement and is generally employed in studies of the extracranial carotid arteries in the neck. The latter allows for thinner slices to be obtained and is often applied to studies of the intracranial vasculature.

In the acquisition of the flow-sensitive slices based on flow-related enhancement, it is often useful to image blood flowing in only one direction. For example, in an examination of the neck, one is primarily interested in the carotid arteries, which are flowing caudal to cranial, rather than in the jugular veins, which are flowing cranial to caudal. It is possible to eliminate visualization

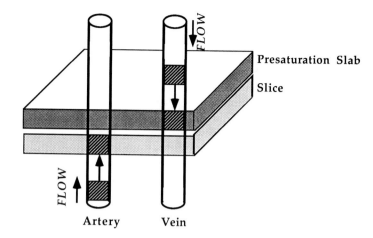

FIGURE 8–6. Presaturation. An RF pulse is given to a slab of tissue above the slice of interest saturating the venous blood flowing into that slice. Only the arterial blood coming from below reaches the slice being fully magnetized and gives any signal.

☐ Saturated stationary tissue in slice

▨ Flowing blood moving into slice with each TR

of flow in the less desired direction by use of a presaturation slab. In the application of this sequence in the neck, the tissue above the slice of interest receives an additional strong RF pulse prior to the routine pulses that affect the slice being imaged. This saturates that tissue, including the blood within it which will soon flow into the imaging slice. Once within that slice, the venous blood remains saturated and gives off no signal, so that it appears gray, similar to the stationary tissue (Fig. 8–6).

Image Processing

Once the tomographic slices are obtained, they are processed by the computer into projections, or views, that are similar to the standard angiographic films. Typically, this is performed by the application of a maximum-intensity

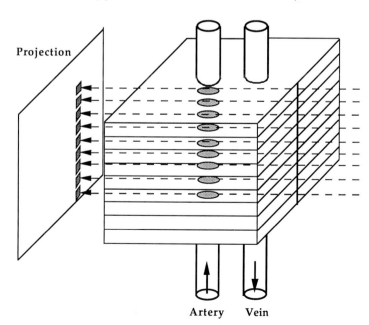

FIGURE 8–7. Maximum intensity projection. The computer draws a ray through the stack of axial slices, finding the brightest point and projecting that onto an image that is perpendicular to the stack.

projection (MIP) algorithm to the slice data. In this method, the slices are stacked to form a volume, and multiple lines (or rays) are drawn through the slice data to the projected image. The brightest signal intercepted by each line becomes the signal intensity of the corresponding pixel in the image (Fig. 8–7). Typical processing times are 10 to 20 seconds per projected image, with projections obtained "around" the patient, beginning at 0 degrees (facing the patient. The data can be segregated so that only one carotid is visualized on each projection. This reduces the overlap of vessels and makes interpretation easier. The set of projections per carotid can be filmed in the usual manner, or can be viewed as a cine movie loop on the computer or on a video recorder.

CLINICAL APPLICATION OF MAGNETIC RESONANCE ANGIOGRAPHY

Experimental studies have demonstrated the potential for MRA to image almost any major blood vessel in the human body. At this time the major interest has been in the imaging of the carotid arteries and the intracranial vessels (Fig. 8–8). There are several reasons for this. First, the carotid vessels are especially suited for evaluation by current MRA technology. The arteries are in straight-line configuration, with flow in a predictable direction. Also, the pathologic process generally involves a short segment at the carotid bifurcation. The length of artery one must image is more limited than in the leg, for example. Most important, however, is the inherent risk of stroke from conventional contrast angiography of the extracranial and intracranial circulation. This factor alone is a compelling reason to develop a reliable noninvasive technique for imaging these vessels.

Although many investigative teams have demonstrated remarkably clear MRA images of the carotid vessels, relatively few have had a sufficiently large experience with comparing MRAs to conventional contrast angiograms to assess the overall accuracy of the technique. Ross et al. reported on their experience using a 3D technique to visualize the carotid bifurcations.[11] Of 27 patients studied, 21 also had intra-arterial digital subtraction angiography (DSA). Of the 42 bifurcations studied by DSA, MRA successfully visualized 39. Compared to the DSA studies, the MRA correctly identified 7 of 7 carotids as being normal, 8 of 8 as having minimal disease, 7 of 7 as having moderate disease, and 2 of 2 as having total occlusion. In the category of severe stenosis, 13 of 15 were correctly identified. The authors point out some of the problems associated with MRA. First, if the patient is not properly positioned or if the carotid bifurcation is unusually low, the area of interest may be outside the area of imaging. Although they did not elaborate, the authors also noted that there was a tendency to overestimate the severity of stenosis.

In a similar study by Peters and associates, 52 patients were prospectively evaluated by MRA and DSA.[20] Of the 38 stenoses of the carotid bifurcation seen on DSA, only 33 were seen on MRA; four were outside the area of imaging. Sixteen of seventeen occlusions were correctly diagnosed by MRA. Of the 33 stenoses, the MRA overestimated the severity in 15, and underestimated it in two.

FIGURE 8–8. Comparison of conventional angiograms of the carotid artery (left) with magnetic resonance angiograms (right) in the same patient.

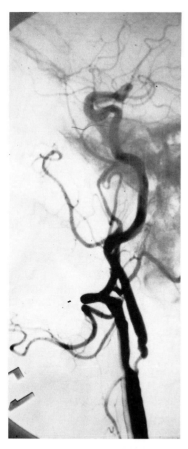

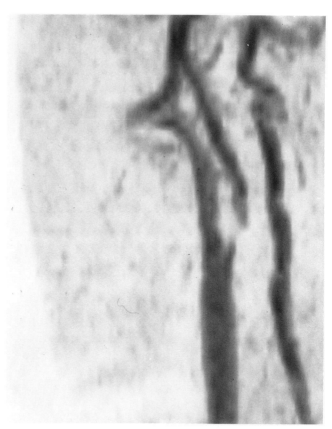

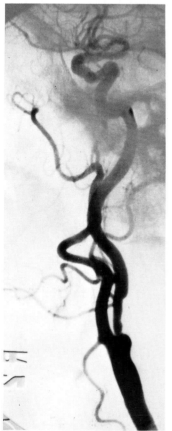

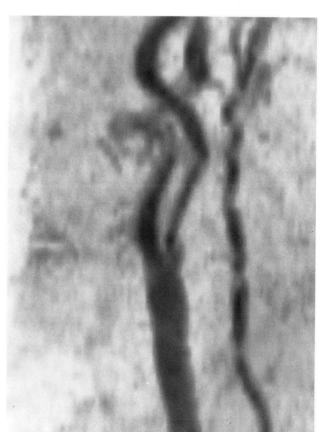

TABLE 8–1. COMPARISON OF READINGS OF THE DEGREE OF STENOSIS AT THE CAROTID BIFURCATION BY CONVENTIONAL CEREBRAL ANGIOGRAPHY (CCA) AND MAGNETIC RESONANCE ANGIOGRAPHY (MRA)

MRA	CCA				
	0–15%	16–49%	50–79%	80–99%	Occluded
Normal 0–15%	1				
Mild 16–49%	5	10			
Moderate 50–79%		6	6		
Severe 80–99%		3	19	20	3
Occluded					2

Our group performed a validation study on MRA in 42 patients.[21] A total of 75 carotid arteries were visualized by MRA, conventional contrast angiography (CCA), and Duplex scanning (DS). The residual lumen at the carotid plaque was measured on the CCAs and used as a basis for evaluating the MRA readings and Duplex interpretations. Our findings were similar to that of other authors. In general, the MRA tended to overread the degree of stenosis (Table 8–1). For the most part, the MRA was off by only one category. Three vessels which had only mild (16 to 49 per cent) stenosis on CCA, however, were interpreted as having severe stenosis on MRI. Another major error involved three patients who were believed to have severe stenosis on the MRAs, but in fact were totally occluded. It was noted that the Duplex scan, which also was not entirely accurate in reading the exact amount of stenosis at the carotid bifurcation, always correctly distinguished between severe stenosis and total occlusion. Another important observation from the paper was that two patients in the study sustained strokes while having their conventional cerebral angiogram.

MISREADINGS WITH MRA AND THEIR SIGNIFICANCE

From these studies, one can reach several conclusions regarding the role of MRA in assessing the carotid bifurcation. First, there is a tendency to overread the severity of the stenosis on the MRA. Unlike a conventional angiogram where the contrast entirely replaces the blood in the vessel lumen to give an accurate outline of the inner vessel wall, with MRA the image is a function of the blood velocity and flow pattern. As long as all the blood is moving at the same velocity, the image intensity of the column of blood is uniform. Slow blood flow and turbulence will result in distortions or loss of the signal. With irregular surface of the lumen there tends to be both slowing and turbulence at the periphery of the column of flowing blood (Figure 8–9). If that blood along the artery wall does not register as contrast, the artery will appear to be more narrow that it actually is.[12]

For related reasons, the MRA may misinterpret a severe stenosis as having complete occlusion of the artery. As blood flow passes through a severe stenosis, there is extreme turbulence which results in the blood moving in many different vectors at once. The appearance on the MRA is a signal void and absent signal at the point of the stenosis and a few millimeters beyond (Fig. 8–10). If one is fortunate enough to image the carotid more distal to the stenosis, there is a reconstitution of the image with reestablishment of laminar flow. In the case

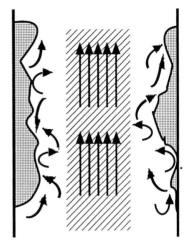

FIGURE 8–9. This diagram indicates the changes in vector and velocity of blood flow as it passes through an area of stenosis within an artery. These changes result in loss of MRA signal. The result is the appearance of more severe stenosis or occlusion than actually exists.

 Atherosclerotic Plaque

 Region of Signal

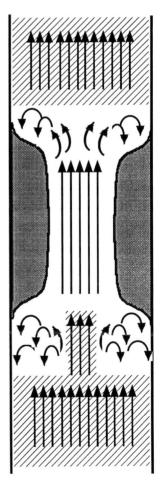

FIGURE 8–10. This diagram indicates the effect of marked irregularity along the surface of the arterial wall. The turbulence caused by the irregularity results in changes in the vector and velocity of the blood flow. As a result, these areas do not emit a signal and, therefore, are not visualized on the MR angiography. The result is the appearance of a more severe stenosis than actually exists.

 Atherosclerotic Placque

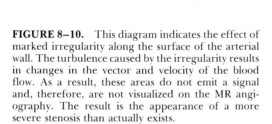 Region of Signal

of total occlusion at the bifurcation, a branch of the external carotid may be misread as a continuation of the occluded internal carotid. If there is a reading of total occlusion of an internal carotid artery with an MRA, one should follow with a Duplex scan or conventional angiogram to be sure that the artery is, in fact, occluded, rather than severely stenosed.

Clinicians that have access to MRA are eager to use this technique to select patients for carotid surgery. Although the clinical correlation studies show MRA to be generally accurate for identifying carotid stenosis, the potential exists for making decision errors in some cases. If, for example, a patient with a symptomatic high-grade stenosis of the internal carotid is misread on the MRA as being totally occluded, surgery may be denied and the patient may remain at risk for a stroke. Conversely, if a total occlusion is believed to be a severe stenosis, an unnecessary exploration of the carotid may result.

For patients with asymptomatic carotid stenosis, there is yet disagreement regarding the indications for carotid endarterectomy. Many surgeons recommend prophylactic surgery for patients with greater than 80 per cent reduction in the transverse diameter of the lumen at the carotid bifurcation. This is based on natural history studies that indicate there is a 5 to 10 per cent annual risk of stroke for patients with asymptomatic high-grade stenosis.[22–24] These studies also show that there is little risk of stroke for asymptomatic lesions with less than 80 per cent stenosis. If one were to rely entirely on MRA for the evaluation of asymptomatic lesions, it is likely that many more patients would be advised to have surgery than if conventional angiography were used for preoperative evaluation, since MRA tends to overread the severity of stenosis. In our study, or the 42 carotid bifurcations judged to have greater than 80 per cent stenosis on MRA, 22 (52 per cent) were found to have less than 80 per cent stenosis on conventional angiography; three of the patients had less than 50 per cent stenosis.[21] It is hopeful for patients, as well as clinicians, that MRA will eventually become accurate in evaluating asymptomatic patients, since it is this group that one is least willing to expose to the risk of conventional angiography.

MRA AND DUPLEX SCANNING

We considered the possibility that the combination of two noninvasive tests, MRA and Duplex, would be more accurate than either test alone. Of the 75 carotid arteries evaluated, the Duplex and MRA agreed in only 49 cases.[21]

TABLE 8–2. AMONG THE CASES WHERE THE DUPLEX SCAN AGREED WITH THE MAGNETIC RESONANCE ANGIOGRAM (MRA), THIS TABLE COMPARES THE READINGS OF THE BIFURCATION STENOSIS BY THE NONINVASIVE TESTS WITH THOSE OF THE CONVENTIONAL CEREBRAL ANGIOGRAM (CCA)

Duplex and MRI Agree	CCA				
	0–15%	16–49%	50–79%	80–99%	Occluded
Normal 0–15%					
Mild 16–49%	3	8			
Moderate 50–79%		2	6		
Severe 80–99%			11	17	
Occluded					2

Assuming that we would be more likely to use the MRA and Duplex information for making clinical decisions if the two tests agreed than if they disagreed, we compared those 49 cases with the conventional angiography readings (Table 8–2). Of the 49, the severity of stenosis was overread in 16 cases by both MRA and Duplex. Eleven overreadings were vessels judged to have 80 to 99 per cent stenosis, but in fact had greater than 80 per cent stenosis on conventional angiography. In review of these 11 studies, all were "borderline" cases, or at the upper end of the 50 to 79 per cent category. There were no instances of misreading severe stenosis for occlusion or vice versa when the Duplex agreed with the MRA.

THE CURRENT ROLE FOR MRA IN EVALUATING PATIENTS WITH CAROTID DISEASE

Over the past 5 years, there has been much debate regarding the operative morbidity and mortality of carotid surgery. The recent North American Symptomatic Carotid Endarterectomy Trial (NASCET) demonstrated that the operative risk was 2.3 per cent, far less than had been predicted by most critics (Barnett HJN, personal communication). Some groups are now reporting large series with even lower risks of stroke and death. As the risks of surgery decrease, the risk of stroke from conventional angiography receives more attention. Depending upon the types of patients being studied, the risks of cerebral angiography vary from 1.4 to 23.2 per cent.[25,26]

Clearly, there is a need to provide a safe, noninvasive outpatient method of assessing arteries and veins throughout the body. Ultrasonography, particularly with the Duplex technology, has proven to be a simple and relatively inexpensive means of screening patients for vascular diseases. Some have felt that Duplex scanning of the carotid arteries is sufficient evaluation before performing carotid endarterectomy.[27-30] There are several factors that have fostered this trend. The disease in the carotid vessels, in contrast to the lower extremities, for example, tends to occur in a predictable location. The Duplex technology is particularly suited to evaluation of the vessels in the neck, and the risk of a cerebral angiogram with contrast is greater than angiograms of the extremities. All who advocate carotid surgery without cerebral angiography are quick to say that the quality of Duplex scans varies considerably from one laboratory to another,[31] and that surgical decisions should not be based upon those tests unless the accuracy of the laboratory has been determined by a proper validation study comparing their readings to those of conventional angiograms.[32,33] Only a handful of the thousands of laboratories throughout North America have actually performed validation studies, and it is doubtful that many laboratories achieve the 90 to 95 per cent accuracy reported by a few centers. For most surgeons, Duplex data alone is insufficient for selecting patients for carotid endarterectomy.

At present, MRA suffers some of the same problems associated with Duplex scanning; that is, inaccuracy in reading the severity of the stenosis at the bifurcation and occasional major errors in distinguishing between severe stenosis and occlusion. On the other hand, unlike the Duplex, MRA does produce a hard-copy image of the carotid bifurcation that can be read by the surgeon. Also, the technique is reproducible and less technician-dependent.

At its present state of development, we feel MRA is reliable for evaluating some of the patients referred for carotid surgery. The patient with multiple hemispheric transient ischemic attacks (TIAs) and a Duplex scan indicating 50 to 95 per cent stenosis of the ipsilateral carotid would be an ideal candidate for MRA. In this situation, the goal is primarily to confirm the Duplex findings before surgery. For the patient with nonfocal neurologic symptoms, or basi-vertebral symptoms with minimal stenosis of the carotids on Duplex scan, the MRA would be of little value. The resolution of the image would be insufficient to survey the arch vessels, vertebrals, and intracranial vessels where atypical lesions could exist that would explain the symptoms. Since the issues regarding asymptomatic stenosis have not yet been resolved, the usefulness of an MRA depends much upon one's philosophy regarding surgery for these patients. If surgery is to be reserved for greater than 80 per cent stenosis, the MRA could be used to confirm the presence of such a plaque suggested on Duplex. One must expect, however, that both Duplex and the MRA will tend to overread the lesion.

Given the rapid development of MRA technology over the past few years, it is certain that we will see many more changes in the next decade. Newer, more powerful MRA machines are now available. Radiologists continue to experiment with the many variables of MR to improve the resolution of the images. Also as experience reading MRA images increases, undoubtedly we will become more confident in the reliability of the interpretations. It is likely that, in the near future, surgeons will depend upon MRA images of the arterial tree for much of their reconstructive surgery.

REFERENCES

1. Dinsmore, RE, Liberthson, RR, Wismer, GL, et al.: Magnetic resonance imaging of thoracic aortic aneurysms: Comparison with other imaging methoids. AJR 1986;146:309.
2. Evancho, AM, Osbakken, M, Weidner, W: Comparison of NMR imaging and aortography for preoperative evaluation of abdominal aortic aneurysms. Magn Reson Med 1986;2:41.
3. Flak, B, Li, DKB, Ho, BYB, et al.: Magnetic resonance imaging of aneurysms of the abdominal aorta. AJR 1986;144:991.
4. Vale, PE, Hale, JD, Kaufman, L, et al.: MR Imaging of the aorta with three-dimensional vessel reconstruction: Validation by angiography. Radiology 1985;157:721.
5. Walker, MF, Souza, SP, Dumoulin, CL: Quantative flow measurement in phase contrast MR angiography. J Comput Assist Tomogr 1988;as(2):304–313.
6. Crooks, LE, Kaufman, L: NMR imaging of blood flow. Br Med Bull 1984;40:167.
7. Duloulin, CL, Souza, SP, Walker, MF, Wagle, W: Three-dimensional phase contrast angiography. Magn Reson Med 1989;9:139–149.
8. Wendt, RE III, Nitz, W, Morrisett, JD, Hedrick, TD: A technique for flow enhanced magnetic resonance angiography of the lower extremities. Magn Reson Imaging 1990;8(6):723–728.
9. Edelman, RR, Mattle, HP, O'Reilly, GV, et al.: Magnetic resonance imaging of flow dynamics in the circle of Willis. Stroke 1990;21:56–65.
10. Eidelman, RR, Mattle, HP, Atkinson, DJ, Hoogewound, HM: MR angiography. AJR 1990;154:938–956.
11. Ross, JS, Masaryk, TJ, Modic, MT, et al.: Magnetic resonance angiography of the extracranial carotid arteries and intracranial vessels: A review. Neurology 1989;39:1369–1376.
12. Masaryk, TJ, Ross, JS, Modic, MT, Lenz, GW, Haache, EM: Carotid bifurcation: MR imaging: Work in progress. Radiology 1988;166:461–466.
13. Rapp, JH, Hahrohk, Z, Hale, J, et al.: Angiography by magnetic resonance imaging: Detailed vascular anatomy without radiation or contrast. Surgery 1989;105(5):662–667.
14. Fullerton, GD: Magentic resonance imaging signal concepts. Radiographics 1987;7:579–597.
15. Stark, DD, Bradley, WG, eds.: Magnetic Resonance Imaging. St. Louis, MO, CF Mosby Company, 1988.
16. Young, SW: Nuclear Magnetic Resonance Imaging: Basic Principles. New York, Raven Press, 1984.
17. Atlas, SW, ed.: Magnetic Resonance Imaging of the Brain and Spine. New York, Raven Press, 1991.
18. Axel, L, Morton, D: MR flow imaging by velocity-compensated/uncompensated difference images. J Comput Asssit Tomogr 1987;11:31–34.

19. Keller, PJ, Drayer, BP, Fram, EK, et al.: MR angiography with two-dimensional acquisition and three-dimensional display. Radiology 1989;*173*:527–532.

20. Peters, PE, Bongartz, G, Drewz, C: Magnetic resonance angiography of the arteries supplying the brain. (German) ROFO 1990;*152(5)*:528–533.

21. Riles, TS, Eidelman, EM, Litt, AW, Pinto, RS, Oldford, F: Comparison of magnetic resonance angiography, conventional cerebral angiography and duplex scanning in the evaluation of patients with carotid bifurcation disease. Presented before the Stroke Council of the American Heart Association, February 1991, San Francisco. (Stroke, accepted for publication.)

22. Roederer, GO, Langlois, YE, Jager, KA, et al.: The natural history of carotid arterial disease in asymptomatic patients with cervical bruits. Stroke 1984;*15*:605–613.

23. Hertzer, NR, Flanigan, RA, O'Hara, PJ, Beven, EG: Surgical vs. nonoperative treatment of asymptomatic carotid stenosis. Ann Surg 1986;*204*:163–171.

24. Chambers, BR, Norris, JW: Outcome in patients with asymptomatic neck bruits. N Engl J Med 1986;*315*:860–865.

25. Hass, WK, Fields, WS, North, RR, Kricheff II, Chase, NE, Bauer, RB: Joint study of extracranial arterial occlusion. II. Arteriography, techniques, sites and complications. JAMA 1968;*203*:961–968.

26. Faught, G, Trader, SD, Hanna, GR: Cerebral complications of angiography for transient ischemia and stroke: Prediction of risk. Neurology 1979;*29*:4–15.

27. Kenagy, JW: Comparison of duplex scanning and contrast arteriography: A community hospital experience. J Vasc Surg 1985;*2*:591–593.

28. Ricotta, JJ, Holen, J, Schenk, E, et al.: Is routine angiography necessary prior to carotid endarterectomy? J Vasc Surg 1984;*1*:96–102.

29. Goodson, SF, Flanigan, P, Bishara, RA, Schuler, JJ, Kikta, MJ, Meyer, JP: Can carotid duplex scanning supplant arteriography in patients with focal carotid territory symptoms? J Vasc Surg 1987;*5*:551–557.

30. Comerata, AJ, Cranley, JJ, Katz, ML, et al.: Real-time B-mode carotid imaging: A three-year multicenter experience. J Vasc Surg 1984;*1*:84–95.

31. Howard, G, Jones, AM, Chambless, L, et al.: A multicenter validation of Doppler ultrasound vs. angiogram: The Asymptomatic Carotid Athersclerosis Study experience. Presented at the 16th International Joint Conference on Stroke and Cerebral Circulation, San Francisco, CA, February 22, 1991.

32. Jacobs, NM, Grant, EG, Schellinger, D, Byrd, MC, Richardson, JD, Cohan, SL: Duplex carotid sonography: Criteria for stenosis, accuracy and pitfalls. Radiology 1985;*154*:385–391.

33. Geuder, JW, Lamparello, PJ, Riles, TS, Giangola, G, Imparato, AM: Is duplex scanning sufficient evaluation before carotid endarterectomy? J Vasc Surg 1989;*9*:193–201.

9

THE EVOLVING ROLE OF MAGNETIC RESONANCE IN ARTERIAL DISORDERS

RONALD J. STONEY, CHRISTOPHER G. CUNNINGHAM, GARY R. CAPUTO, and CHARLES B. HIGGINS

The spectrum of arterial disorders that present to the vascular surgeon for definitive diagnosis may require accurate information about blood flow, the diseased arterial segment itself, the paravascular space, as well as organs supplied by the involved artery. Technological advances in imaging have always been fundamental to the diagnosis of arterial disease, beginning with arteriography. This defined the configuration of the patent but diseased arterial lumen, and the collateral flow patterns beyond an occlusion of the axial vessels. The introduction of the arterial catheterization technique by Seldinger has more recently been expanded for precise catheter placement for introduction of contrast material into the arterial tree and, therapeutic agents which can be administered at desired arterial sites. The dimensions of arterial walls, important mainly in dilating, dissecting, and aneurysmal disease, was initially suspected by plain roentgenographic findings; however, ultrasound and computerized axial tomography with and without contrast have now become important imaging modalities.

To this list of diagnostic technologies, we can now add magnetic resonance imaging (MRI) which offers unique characteristics for imaging the vascular system.[1-4] The arterial circulation provides striking inherent contrast between blood flowing within the arterial lumen and the extraluminal environment (Figs. 9–1 through 9–3). This allows acquisition of images of the arterial and para-arterial region, without exogenous contrast. The only limitation is the unstable patient who requires life support apparatus that is incompatible with the magnetic fields required.

This chapter will describe the technique of MRI, which is a precise imaging modality for the vascular system. It will detail the applications of MRI for lesions of the cerebrovascular system, the thoracic and abdominal aorta, the detection of healing complications of prosthetic arterial repairs, and the definition of arteriovenous malformations. The technique for measuring blood flow, velocity encoded cine (VEC), which is unique to MR, will also be reviewed.

MRI TECHNIQUE

Several MRI techniques are used for imaging the vascular system. Tomographic images of high spatial resolutions are acquired using the spin-echo technique. For imaging the thoracic aorta, the spin-echo images are obtained with electrocardiographic (ECG) grating (Figs. 9–1 through 9–3). The images are obtained in the transaxial plane from above the arch to the diaphragm or lower. Images are also done parallel to the long axis of the aorta; this oblique sagittal plane usually displays the ascending aorta, arch, and proximal descending aorta, along with the origin of the arch vessels on a single or two adjacent planes. For imaging the abdominal vessels, ECG gating of the image acquisition is usually not done. Spin-echo images with a prolonged repetition time (TR) or echo delay time (TE) is used for examining possible graft infection, because fluid surrounding a graft causes high signal on images using these parameters (Fig. 9–4).

Using the spin-echo technique, the intravascular region (blood pool) shows little or no MR signal; however, slow-flow situations can cause intraluminal signal. Another MRI technique is the gradient-echo sequence; in which the flowing blood produces bright signal. On the gradient-echo images, intraluminal pathology appears as a filling defect (thrombus) (Fig. 9–5) or linear lucency (intimal flap) within the bright signal of the blood pool. High-flow velocity or turbulence in disturbed flow situations also cause a signal void; such a signal void is observed at the site of and beyond vascular stenoses.

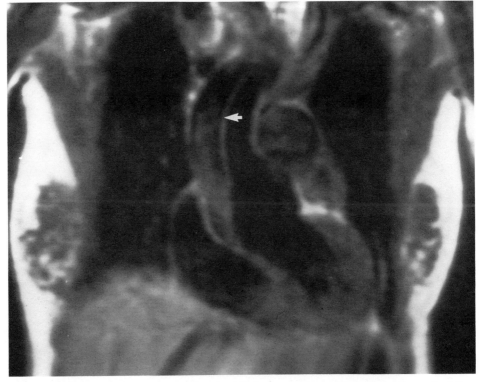

FIGURE 9–1. ECG-gated coronal spin-echo MR image displays an intimal flaw (arrow) of the ascending aorta in a type A aortic dissection. Because of slow flow, there is intraluminal signal in the false channel.

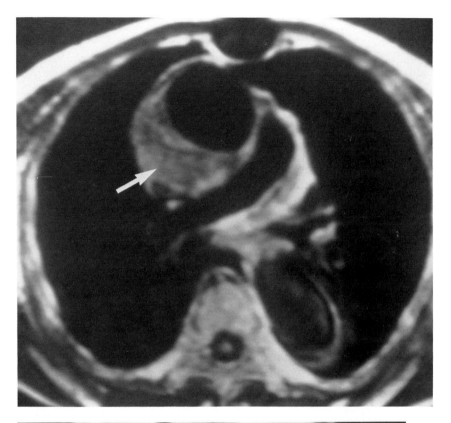

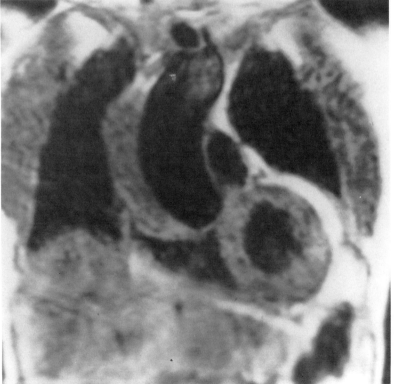

FIGURE 9–2. ECG-gated transaxial (top) and coronal (bottom) MR images demonstrate compression of the aortic true lumen by a thrombosed false channel (arrow).

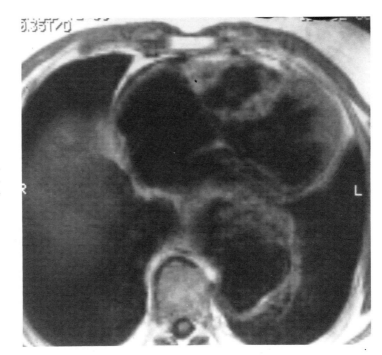

FIGURE 9–3. ECG-gated transaxial MR image of a large thoracic aortic aneurysm which compresses the left atrium.

It is now possible to measure blood-flow velocity and volume flow using a newly introduced technique called velocity-encoded MRI. This technique is based upon the principle that the velocity of blood flow is directly related to the phase shift which MR-sensitive nuclei experience during the imaging sequence when they flow along a magnetic gradient. This technique, termed

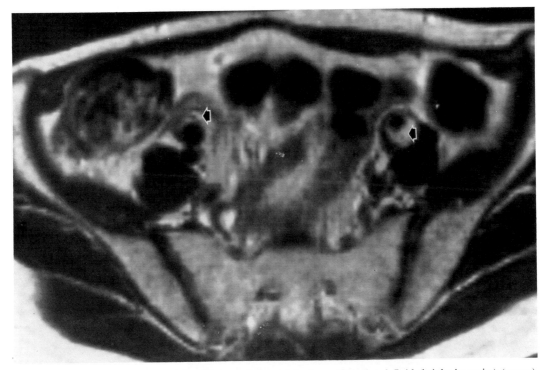

FIGURE 9–4. Transaxial T2-weighted image of the pelvis shows high-signal fluid (bright intensity) (arrow) surrounds the right and left limbs of an aortofemoral graft.

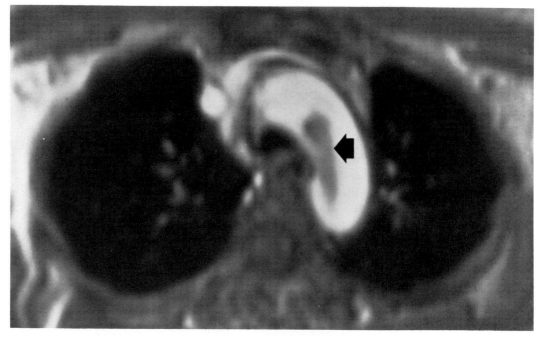

FIGURE 9–5. Gradient-echo MR image at the level of the aortic arch shows a mural thrombus of the arch. The thrombus (arrow) appears as a "filling defect" in the high signal of the blood pool.

velocity encoded cine MR (VEC) has been applied for quantifying blood flow under a variety of pathological conditions including the differential flow velocity in the true and false channels of aorta dissection, and the flow distal to arterial stenosis.[5,6] With this technique, velocity is encoded in the direction of flow (long axis of vessel), and imaging is performed perpendicular to long axis of the vessel.

The most recent MRI technique available for the vascular system is magnetic resonance angiography (MRA) (Fig. 9–6). There are several techniques for

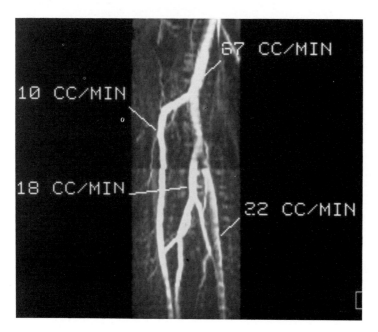

FIGURE 9–6. MR angiogram (two-dimensional time-of-flight technique) of the popliteal artery and trifurcation. Flow measured by velocity encoded cine MR is shown for each artery.

MRI including two- and three-dimensional time-of-flight and phase-contrast sequences.[6,7] Reconstruction of these images produces a projectional image of a vascular bed, and consequently is called a magnetic resonance angiogram.

CEREBROVASCULAR DISEASE

Among the earliest uses of magnetic resonance in carotid disease was its role in identifying and following the natural history of spontaneous and post-traumatic internal carotid dissection. The inherent difference in signals of flowing blood in the narrowed lumen and nonmoving blood (thrombus) within the dissected media provides an intense, bright image of the dissecting hematoma that contrasts with the dark image of the flowing blood in the arterial lumen. The application of MRA for the definition of intracranial and extracranial carotid and vertebral arterial disease has allowed noncontrast angiography to develop rapidly. Modifications of computer software programs are now allowing development of similar applications in other peripheral arteries. Clearly, MR has extraordinary abilities to image the brain and eye, the target organs for extracranial arterial disease. Ischemia and infarction are distinct vascular events that are precisely recognized by MR, and sequential imaging can define resolution of these ischemic events accurately, over time.

Finally, the extravascular environment is important in extracranial lesions. Transaxial MR images define the extent and relationship of paragangliomas to the native arteries as well as adjacent nerve and soft-tissue structures. The features of both carotid and vagal body tumors can now be routinely assessed in this manner.

THORACOABDOMINAL AORTA

Dissection of the thoracic and abdominal aorta, although unusual, is a vascular catastrophe with the gravest consequences. Accurate definition of the proximal extent of a thoracic aortic dissection is crucial to effective management. Ascending aortic intimal tears (type A) are surgically managed using prosthetic conduit replacement to prevent retrograde dissection with aortic valvular incompetence, myocardial ischemia, and pericardial tamponade. Descending thoracic aortic dissections (type B) are usually managed conservatively using the Wheat regimen, unless progressive dissection threatens critical organ function or the patient's life owing to aneurysm enlargement of frank rupture.

The distal extent of the aortic dissection must be known when intervention is planned to restore compromised organ or limb perfusion. Luminal definition by MR can clearly identify the pattern of the dissection (Figs. 9–1 and 9–2), a dilemma that may remain after computed tomography (CT) or aortographic studies.

Primary dissection of a major aortic branch, specifically the visceral and renal arteries, are unusual, but can be accurately defined by MRI. Intestinal and renal ischemia can be recognized by MR, as well as the nature of the aortic branch lesion which causes impaired perfusion to the target organ. Dilation or frank aneurysm formation of the thoracic or thoracoabdominal aorta is demonstrated easily by MR (Figs. 9–3 and 9–7). The size and extent of the aneurysm, the presence of luminal thrombus or atherosclerotic debris, and the relationship of the aneurysm to other structures and neighboring aortic branches

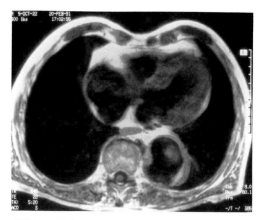 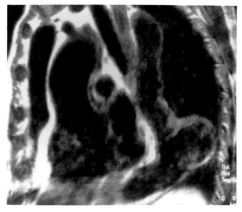

FIGURE 9–7. Transverse (left) and sagittal (right) MR images display a large thoracoabdominal aneurysm. There is mural thrombus in the aneurysm.

are important requirements met by MRI. Although CT is capable of depicting the external zone of the aneurysm, the size of the residual lumen, and the presence of luminal thrombus or intimal disease, it may be less precisely identified unless luminal opacification with intravenous contrast bolus is added.

Takayasu's aortitis can be detected by abnormal concentric thickening of the wall involved segments of the aorta and major branches. These thickened walls are seen as a medium-intensity signal sharply contrasting with surrounding high-intensity fat and low-intensity luminal blood.

ABDOMINAL AORTA

The distribution of arterial lesions thought to affect the lower abdominal aorta is clearly changing as a better definition of the disease is now possible. Computed tomography and now MRI are unmasking disease of the juxta and pararenal aorta, which requires significant modifications in exposure and control of the aorta in order to affect a repair. The left renal vein, which used to be considered a landmark separating the lower and upper abdominal aorta, has become an obstacle to our now expanded understanding of diseases of the abdominal aorta and its branches. The major aortic branches arise from the upper abdominal aorta and provide nearly 40 per cent of the cardiac output to the abdominal viscera and kidneys. Atherosclerosis, although the most common disorder of this region, is only one of a spectrum of arteriopathies that affect this portion of the aorta and its branches. The advent of more complete multiplanar aortography for luminal definition, collateral flow patterns and soft-tissue imaging now include MR, allowing the vascular surgeon to accurately define the extent of abdominal aortic disease precisely, before operation rather than during surgical exploration (Figs. 9–8 and 9–9).

Magnetic resonance can assess the course, configuration, and dimensions of the aorta (Figs. 9–5 and 9–6). The lumen can be defined transaxially; however, spatial relationships between major aortic branches are most clearly shown with biplaner aortography. These combined modalities now provide state-of-the-art imaging to precisely define any suspected aortic disease.

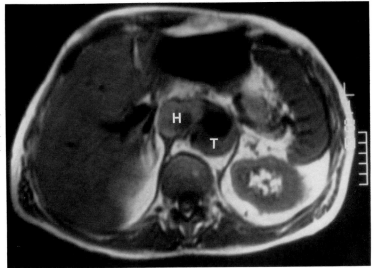

FIGURE 9–8. Transaxial MR image of the upper abdomen demonstrates a suprarenal aneurysm with thrombus (T) and periaortic hematoma (H).

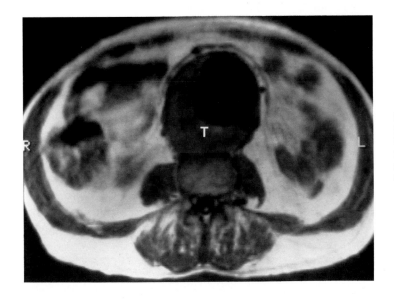

FIGURE 9–9. Transaxial MR image of the abdomen displays a huge aneurysm with mural thrombus (T). The aneurysm has caused severe extrinsic compression of the inferior vena cava.

COMPLICATIONS OF HEALING FOLLOWING PROSTHETIC ARTERIAL REPAIR

The precise method by which humans incorporate (heal) a prosthetic arterial substitute remain a mystery. True rejection of foreign material is not recognized following prosthetic graft implantation, but sterile graft "reactions" with seroma formation are well described. All too commonly, perigraft infection occurs, which represents the gravest complication to the patient and the greatest challenge to the vascular surgeon who undertakes management of the affected patient. Abnormal attempts to regenerate a new intimal flow surface on the graft may lead to myointimal fibrosis, causing narrowing or occlusion at anastomotic sites. Thrombus may adhere to the luminal surface of the graft and accumulated layers may progress to complete thrombosis or distal embolization. Distraction, distention, and dehiscence of the graft artery anastomosis may be the precursors of anastomotic false aneurysm. Any of the above complications threaten the vascular bed supplied by the graft, the continued function of the graft itself, and, in some instances, the life of the patient.

The vascular surgeon requires specific information about each complication in order to accurately define the problem and develop a solution. Magnetic resonance imaging can demonstrate the size of the residual lumen, the dimensions of the prosthetic and arterial segments, and the perigraft environment. The presence of extraluminal abnormalities may be differentiated as blood, purulent material, or fibrotic scar (Fig. 9–7). Luminal thrombus may be detected by an absence of signal void within the graft limb when compared to the presence of a signal void in the patient's contralateral patent graft limb.

Anastomotic false aneurysms are suspected by finding aneurysmal dilation at anastomotic sites. Some changes extend from the area of aneurysmal dilation into surrounding tissues and may suggest an underlying infectious etiology. The changes in the contour of the flow channel in a suspected anastomotic false aneurysm may be the result of layered thrombus, which can be easily detected using MR. Although luminal anatomy and contour may be defined accurately with conventional arteriographic visualization, the abundance of information about the vascular bed where a complication is suspected makes MRI the method of choice to complete the investigation of the vascular complication and the adjacent perivascular environment.

ARTERIOVENOUS MALFORMATIONS

The management of arteriovenous malformations (AVM) is a challenge both to the vascular surgeon and the interventional radiologist. Interruption of flow to the lesion through ligation, or more recently, transarterial embolization, offer palliation of the lesion but not cure. Excision is applicable to those certain lesions that can be accurately defined as localized to resectable structures. Previous techniques of arteriography and soft-tissue imaging using ultrasound and CT have not provided this critical preoperative assessment. Magnetic

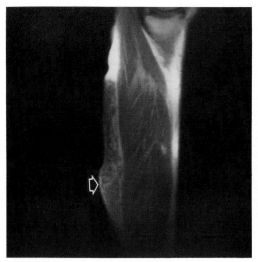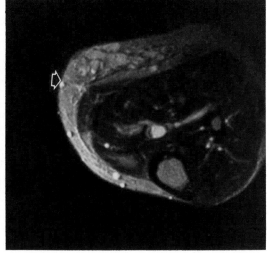

FIGURE 9–10. Coronal MR image of extensive superficial AV malformation (left). Transaxial MR image (right) shows the well-defined margin of this lesion which correctly predicted its safe and complete surgical excision.

resonance imaging provides remarkable contrast between the vascularized lesion and adjacent or involved structures. The resulting image, Figure 9–10, shows the true extent of the lesion, which may allow excision and cure localized malformations. The expanded use of MRI in these vascular lesions will more clearly define the true utility of this technology for imaging AVMs.

SUMMARY

This chapter has reviewed our experiences to date with MR for arterial imaging. We believe the initial results are revolutionary, since they add another dimension to the assessment of vascular disease, with very little downside risk. Newer technology will refine this modality, which is the state of the art in arterial imaging today. When combined with MR angiography, it will likely become the imaging method of choice for all arterial disease.

REFERENCES

1. Kersting-Sommerhoff, BA, Higgins, CB, White, RD, Sommerhoff, CP, Lipton, MJ: Aortic dissection: Sensitivity and specificity of MR imaging. Radiology 1988;*166*:651–655.
2. Amparo, EG, Higgins, CB, Hoddick, W, et al.: Magnetic resonance imaging of aortic disease: Preliminary results. AJR 1984;*143*:1203–1209.
3. Auffermann, W, Olofsson, P, Stoney, R, Higgins, CB: MR imaging of complications of aortic surgery. JCAT 1987;*11(6)*:982–989.
4. Auffermann, W, Olofsson, P, Rabahie, GN, Tavares, NJ, Stoney, R, Higgins, CB: Incorporation versus infection of retroperitoneal aortic grafts: MR imaging features. Radiology 1989;*172*:359–362.
5. Chang, J-M, Friese, K, Caputo, GR, Higgins, CB: MR measurement of blood flow in the true and false channel in chronic aortic dissection. J Comput Assist Tomogr 1991;*15*:418.
6. Caputo, GR, Masui, T, Higgins, CB: Two dimensional time of flight MR angiography and phase velocity mapping of the popliteal and tibioperoneal arteries: Feasibility study. Radiology 1991 (In Press).
7. Edelman, RR, Wentz, KV, Mattle, H, et al.: Projection arteriography and venography: Initial clinical results with MR. Radiology 1989;*1732*:351.

10

MAGNETIC RESONANCE IMAGING OF VENOUS DISORDERS

ROBERT L. VOGELZANG and STEVEN W. FITZGERALD

Magnetic resonance imagine (MRI) has enjoyed a rapid expansion as a primary imaging tool and as a supplementary study in a wide range of disease states. The increasing application of MRI to body and musculoskeletal disease has resulted in an opportunity to evaluate both suspected and unexpected vascular disease. Because MRI can provide both static structural information, as well as dynamic physiologic information, MR is becoming recognized as a valuable noninvasive modality to evaluate blood vessels and flow. In this chapter, we will provide a basic discussion of the appearance of flow and flow-related phenomenon on MR images. We will also discuss common artifacts observed in vascular imaging, MR venography, and the clinical value of MRI in venous disorders.

APPEARANCE OF FLOW

Conventional MR studies are primarily composed of spin-echo pulse sequences. These imaging sequences make use of precise radiofrequency pulses, the so-called 90-degree and 180-degree pulses, to excite hydrogen protons within body tissues. As these nuclei relax to the equilibrium state, a detectable signal is emitted. This signal contains information which can be spatially encoded by frequency, phase, and intensity to produce an image. Flowing blood, depending upon its orientation within the slice and its velocity, may not experience all of the necessary radiofrequency pulses to produce an MR signal, resulting in a demagnetization and washout of signal intensity. This results in the loss of MR signal, or "flow void" typically associated with flowing blood on MR images. Other, more complex mechanisms including phase shifts are also important, but are beyond the scope of this chapter. This flow void is most reliably observed in rapidly flowing vessels and when flow is oriented perpendicular to the imaging plane (i.e., the abdominal aorta on transverse images) (Fig. 10–1). The presence of intravascular signal could, therefore, at least naively be interpreted as evidence of occlusion or thrombus. Unfortunately, in a variety of commonly encountered situations, intravascular signal can be observed on spin-echo sequences.[1]

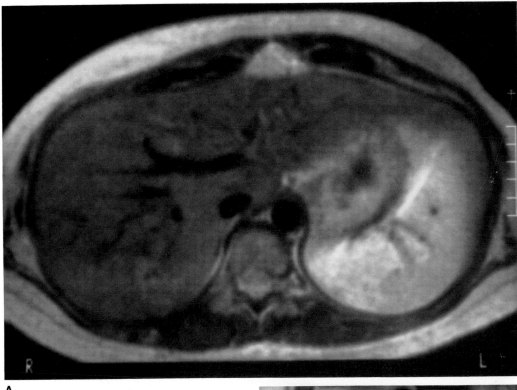

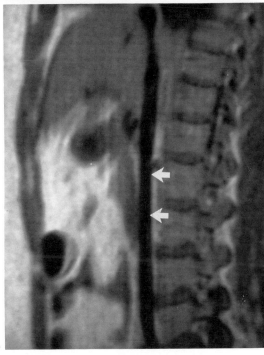

FIGURE 10–1. Flow-void phenomenon. *A*, Transverse spin-echo image (TR = 650/TE = 20) demonstrating complete absence of intravascular signal within the abdominal aorta, inferior vena cava, and intrahepatic veins. *B*, Sagittal image (TR = 650/TE = 20) demonstrating extrahepatic and intrahepatic compartments of the inferior vena cava (arrows).

Although blood flowing out of an imaging slice or volume results in a signal void, fresh blood flowing into a slice is unsaturated and produces signal of greater intensity than adjacent stationary tissue and results in flow-related enhancement. This effect varies with blood velocity, slice thickness, and imaging parameters. It is most commonly observed on slices at the periphery of the imaging volume, where fresh blood can enter. For veins, this entry-slice phenomenon tends to occur over one to three slices (Fig. 10–2). A second situation resulting in intravascular signal occurs under special conditions. Typically, most MR studies are performed without cardiac gating and triggering and data acquisition occurs randomly across the cardiac cycle. If data acquisition happens to coincide with diastole when flow is minimal or absent, high intensity will be observed. This is known as "diastolic pseudogating," and because of its

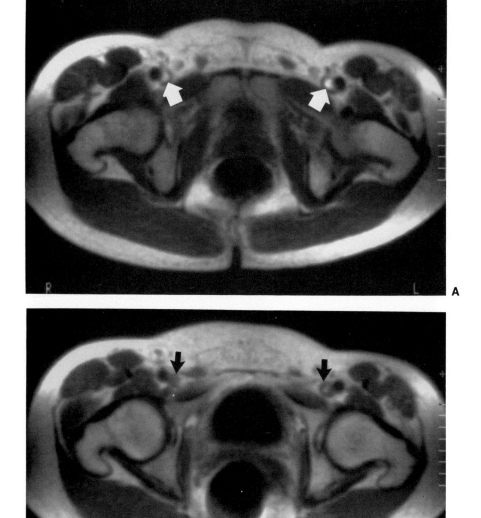

FIGURE 10–2. Entry-slice phenomenon. *A*, Transverse image (TR = 500/TE = 20) demonstrating absence of intravascular signal within the common femoral arteries bilaterally. Hyperintense signal is seen within the common femoral veins (arrows) resulting from inflow of unsaturated blood on this first slice of the imaging volume. *B*, Transverse image obtained more cephalad within the imaging volume demonstrating a decrease in the intensity of the inflow phenomenon (arrows) owing to partial saturation effect. *C*, Transverse image at the top of the imaging volume demonstrating hyperintense intravascular signal within the descending aorta (A) as a result of entry-slice effect. (*Figure continues.*)

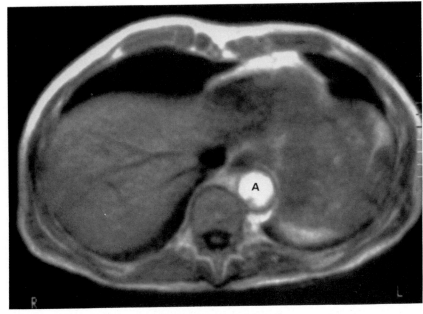

FIGURE 10–2. *(Continued.)*

random occurrence, can result in confusing and potentially misleading images. A third, more commonly encountered mechanism is related to the pattern of flow within vessels. As the flow profile within a vessel creates shearing and boundary layers, the phase of the MR signal is dispersed. This loss of MR signal is maximal at the vessel wall while faster flow centrally produces more intravascular signal (Fig. 10–3). This appearance can be problematic because this

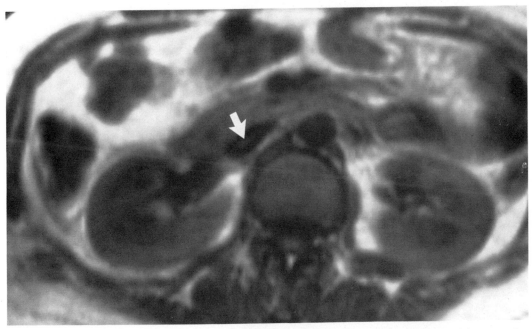

FIGURE 10–3. Doughnut sign. Transverse image (TR = 500/TE = 20) demonstrating central intravascular signal within the inferior vena cava (arrow) as a result of phase shift occurring at the flow boundary layers. This appearance can mimic partially recanalized thrombus. Note the expected signal void within the abdominal aorta and mesenteric vessels.

pattern, the "doughnut" or "target" sign, mimics the appearance of partially recanalized thrombus. All of the above effects can be observed on both T1- or T2-weighted sequences. A fourth mechanism of intravascular signal is unique to T2-weighted sequences. T2-weighted studies are typically composed of multiple echoes. The signal intensity of stationary tissues demonstrates a decrease in intensity on later echoes related to the T2 decay process. However, for the unique cases of flow at a constant velocity (i.e., venous flow), phase dispersion is minimal on the even-numbered echoes and an increase in signal intensity can be observed. This usually does not result in diagnostic confusion and can occasionally be used to confirm the presence of thrombus (Fig. 10–4).[2]

In addition to potentially confusing patterns of intravascular signal, flow within vessels can also produce ghost or pulsation artifacts which may degrade the appearance of adjacent structures.[3] Because these artifacts are proportional to the intensity of intravascular signal, special radiofrequency pulses can be applied to regions of tissue and blood outside the imaging volume.[4] This results in presaturation of these tissues and a loss of magnetization and signal. When presaturated blood flows into the slice, it results in less intravascular signal and, therefore, less ghosting. Ghost artifacts are also the result of pulsation and may require cardiac gating to completely eliminate them. Presaturation techniques

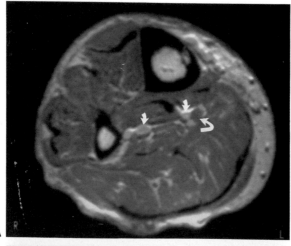

A

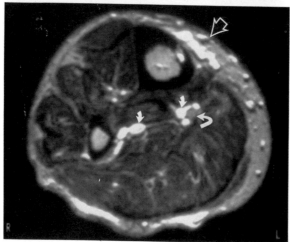

B

FIGURE 10–4. Even-echo rephasing. *A,* Transverse image through the calf (TR = 1800/TE = 40) demonstrating intravascular signal within the posterior tibial and peroneal veins (small arrows). Less intense intravascular signal is also identified within the posterior tibial artery (curved arrow). *B,* Second echo image at the same level (TR 1800/TE 80) demonstrating marked increase in signal intensity within the peroneal and posterior tibial veins (small arrows). There is no equivalent increase of intravascular signal within the posterior tibial artery (curved arrow). Also note the abnormal collection of vessels within the anterior subcutaneous tissues from the patient's venous angioma (open arrow).

will also suppress entry-slice effects and other problems resulting from flow-related enhancement.

The previous discussion has been related to spin-echo pulse sequences. A newer group of imaging sequences has found an increasingly wider application in MR studies. These techniques are referred to as gradient-recalled or gradient-echo imaging and may be termed "bright blood" studies. These studies typically employ a single radiofrequency pulse and an excitation angle of less than 90 degrees. A gradient is than employed to generate the echo. These gradient studies can typically be obtained faster than spin-echo sequences. Also, instead of the signal void observed on spin-echo images from washout effects, flow on gradient images is characterized by bright intensity from "wash-in" and flow-related enhancement. The signal intensity related to flow can vary with the flip angle and other imaging parameters, but will typically always be greater than stationary tissues (Fig. 10–5). While this can be exploited on single slices to document vessel patency, this process can be extended to produce MR angiograms. First, imaging parameters are manipulated to maximize intravascular signal and to minimize signal from stationary tissue. Postprocessing of the acquired data is performed by a maximum-intensity rendering. This profile does not provide much useful information for a single slice, but when applied to a stack of slices or a three-dimensional (3D) imaging volume, a maximum-intensity projection (MIP) can be produced that can demonstrate intravascular flow without the need for intravascular contrast agents (Fig. 10–6). By combining these gradient-echo techniques and presaturation pulses, flow from a certain direction can be eliminated and can produce either MR angiograms or MR venograms.[5]

Magnetic resonance imaging can be useful in a wide variety of venous disorders. By combining anatomic information and patency from conventional and venographic studies, MR can diagnose venous occlusions, thrombus, varices, vascular malformations, and shunt patency. Comparative studies on the relative accuracy of MRI to contrast venography or Doppler studies are beginning to appear, and suggest that MR is competitive and may offer unique information in some settings.

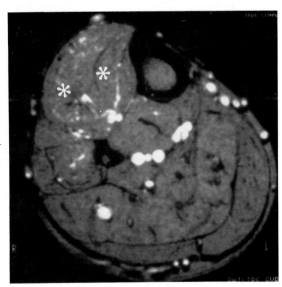

FIGURE 10–5. Gradient-echo image. Transverse image through the calf (TR = 550/TE = 25/flip angle = 25 degrees) demonstrating intense intravascular signal within both small arteries and veins of the calf, as well as subcutaneous veins. Also note the high signal intensity within hemangioma of the anterior compartment (asterisk).

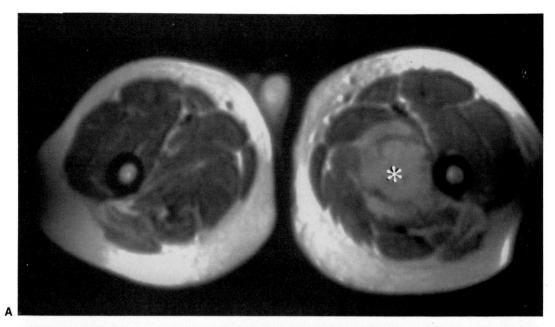

A

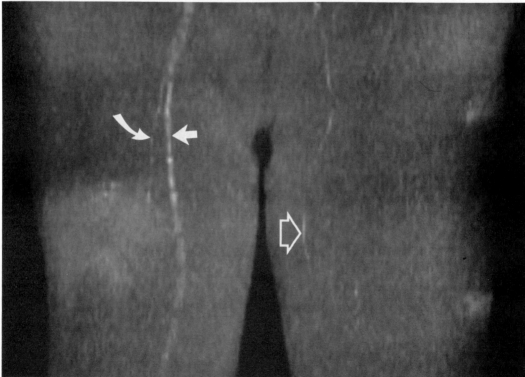

B

FIGURE 10–6. Use of MR venography. *A*, Transverse spin-echo image (TR = 1800/TE = 30) demonstrating soft tissue mass (asterisk) within the adductor compartment of the thigh. The expected profunda femoral vessels are not identified. *B*, Coronal maximum intensity projection from multiple thin-sliced gradient-echo images obtained in the axial plane. This coronal projection demonstrates the normal profunda femoris vein (curved arrow) and superficial femoral vein (short arrow) on the unaffected side. The side of the patient's sarcoma demonstrates complete absence of flow within the profunda femoris vein and superficial femoral vein and a small amount of flow within the medial saphenous vein (open arrow). Color Doppler sonography confirms completed tumor thrombosis involving these vessels.

Probably the most important role of MR in venous disease is to distinguish patent veins from thrombus. As has been indicated, the presence of intravascular signal alone is not sufficient to rule in thrombus, although a pure signal void on spin-echo sequences or the presence of flow-related enhancement on gradient sequences is sufficient to document venous patency. Venous thrombosis can be distinguished from the broad group of physiologic and spurious causes of intravascular signal, in many cases by using a variety of criteria. True thrombosed vessels will not be affected by changes in imaging orientation, while flow can vary from axial to coronal scans.[6] Thrombosed vessels cannot produce pulsation or ghost artifacts and will not be affected by saturation techniques. Even echo rephasing only occurs in flowing vessels and should not be seen with thrombus, although the signal intensity of thrombus can vary. Entry-slice phenomenon are limited to a few slices and can be eliminated by presaturation techniques, while thrombus will usually be more extensive and not be altered by presaturation.

CLINICAL APPLICATIONS

Imaging of the large central veins of the body has, until the recent past, relied upon the performance of venography, usually via catheter techniques. These techniques have a certain degree of risk associated with them (hemorrhage, hematoma, and thrombosis), and may be prone to misinterpretation through the production of flow defects and artifacts as can be seen with inflow of unopacified blood and production of what can appear to be thrombosis. The problem is even more pronounced when the mesenteric venous circulation is investigated, because it must be studied by injection of large doses of contrast into the arteries supplying the venous bed.

Sectional imaging techniques such as Doppler color-flow ultrasound, CT and MRI are currently the imaging procedures of choice for noninvasive visualization of large central veins. Each technique has its unique advantages and disadvantages (e.g., CT requires the intravenous injection of contrast material and Doppler ultrasound is thwarted by the presence of air or gas, thus preventing visualization of a large percentage of the veins of the chest and abdomen). Magnetic resonance imaging should, in theory, be the most optimal imaging technique of the three mentioned. It possesses inherent advantages over CT in terms of absolute contrast resolution and, as we have indicated, is intrinsically flow sensitive and should not generally require the injection of potentially toxic contrast agents. Magnetic resonance imaging has no limitations in terms of scan plane, since the plane of section is not reliant upon mechanical tilting of the scanning apparatus as in CT. Magnetic resonance imaging, however, is also far more complex and more dependent upon appropriately used pulse sequences, many of which are recently developed or in development. The technique is also heavily reliant upon the use of surface coils for examinations of many parts of the body; these coils are currently in an extremely active stage of design, testing, and manufacture. Thus, any comparison between CT, ultrasound, and MRI must take into account the fact that MRI is comparatively less mature than the other modalities. In fact, MRI has made astonishing progress and is used in virtually every area of the body, most notably in neuroimaging, where it has largely supplanted CT as the primary imaging technique for most intracranial and intraspinal disease processes. It has also proven remarkably effective in the field of orthopedic imaging where it is the technique of choice for most bone and joint disorders. In the arena of cardiovascular imaging, MRI has begun to be broadly used in cardiac and aortic imaging, including the identification and follow-up of aortic aneurysms and dissections. In venous imaging, MRI has not yet been as widely applied, but an increasing number of scientific and clinical papers attest to the fact that MRI can and will be an important imaging modality. Exceptional work in the production of magnetic resonance arteriograms using sophisticated new pulse sequences and image reconstruction algorithms promises very exciting developments in the near future, such that most workers in the field anticipate replacement of some routine arteriography by these techniques. In this section, we will review some of the current applications of venous MRI and discuss some areas of future development.

Chest

Magnetic resonance imaging of the chest is frequently used for the identification of cardiac abnormalities, and is an important diagnostic tool in the identification of a variety of congenital and acquired lesions of the heart and great vessels, including the mediastinal veins and conditions such as total anomalous pulmonary venous return with or without atrial septal defects. Theissen and his colleagues were able to detect an atrial septal defect in all 31 patients studied with the technique; gradient-echo scans were the most reliable in this regard.[7] Other congenital abnormalities of pulmonary veins including return to the azygos vein and drainage into the inferior vena cava ("scimitar syndrome") have been imaged with MRI.[8–10] Pulmonary blood flow has also been accurately assessed with the use of a variety of techniques including cine gradient-recalled imaging. Hatabu and his colleagues at the Hospital of the University of Pennsylvania have used high-resolution techniques to accurately depict sixth- and seventh-order pulmonary artery branches.[11] Use of such techniques in pulmonary thromboembolic disease readily comes to mind. Gefter et al. were able to note characteristic disorders of the pulmonary venous signal in patients with mitral valvular disease; other workers have been able to quantitate pulmonary blood flow in patients with mitral valvular stenosis.[12,13] Magnetic resonance imaging has also proven to be of great benefit in presurgical planning for the Fontan procedure; extracardiac veins and the pulmonary circulation were identified correctly with accuracies between 95 and 98 per cent.[14] The possible uses for MRI in and around the heart and pulmonary circulation appear to be virtually limitless as new body coils, pulse sequences, and cardiac gating techniques (including the use of fast scanning) come into clinical practice.

The mediastinal veins, including the great veins and superior vena cava, are, or course, very accurately depicted with MRI. Congenital and acquired abnormalities are generally imaged with excellent clarity. For example, Hansen et al. recently evaluated 31 patients with suspected thoracic venous obstruction secondary to a variety of causes including coagulopathy, tumor, and catheter injury. Magnetic resonance imaging depicted central venous abnormalities very accurately; clot and obstruction or compression of the superior vena cava was seen in all 16 patients with that finding; in the jugular veins, 6 of 6 cases were accurately diagnosed. Evaluation of the veins of the shoulder was slightly less precise; 10 of 12 with subclavian or axillary vein thrombosis had diagnostic MRI studies. Overall, MR correctly identified abnormality in 32 of 34 vessels, and in all cases, a negative MR study was found to be a true-negative (100 per cent specificity).[15] Other authors have noted similar findings in superior vena cava obstruction and mediastinal venous occlusions. Weinreb and colleagues studied both CT and MRI in 14 patients with superior vena caval obstruction and found them comparable in all regards; in 2 patients MR was able to better differentiate residual flow through a narrowed caval lumen.[16] We have had similar clinical experiences (Figs. 10–7 and 10–8). It remains to be seen, however, what the precise role of MRI will be in thoracic venous obstructions. From the above as well as anecdotal experience reported elsewhere, it would seem that MRI is quite accurate. However, recent work from the University of Nebraska indicates that MRI may have limitations in focal lesions of the proximal left subclavian vein and in nonocclusive subclavian venous thrombi. Magnetic resonance imaging was only able to detect 2 of 8 nonocclusive subclavian clots and missed 1 of 5 totally occlusive left subclavian thrombi. The authors conclude that in cases of suspected subclavian vein thrombosis, MRI should not be the sole diagnostic test.[17]

In congenital anomalies of the superior vena cava, MRI has at least anecdotally been reported to be accurate in identifying the nature of the anomaly[18]; this would certainly be anticipated given the relative ease with which MR is able to visualize large vascular structures.

It appears that MRI is as accurate, and probably more accurate, than CT in accurately assessing the mediastinal venous anatomy. Certainly MRI is far more accurate than CT in cardiac and pulmonary vascular problems. Increasing clinical experience should lead to broad acceptance of this modality as the imaging tool of choice in many pathological conditions.

Abdomen

Magnetic resonance imaging has not achieved as much acceptance and utilization in the abdomen as was predicted for it. Undoubtedly this is because respiratory or bowel-motion artifact can obscure visualization of a structure or cause production of an image that is perceived to be less "sharp" or detailed than other modalities. Solving the problem of motion-induced image degradation has not been easy. Unlike cardiac motion, respiratory and bowel movement artifacts cannot be easily eliminated through gating, and the length of time needed to acquire conventional spin-echo images has generally precluded the use of breath holding. There has, however, been significant progress in the development of fast scans, which can be obtained in a few seconds; these would obviously be of great utility in eliminating the problem. Nevertheless, most major intraabdominal venous structures can be imaged with good clarity and resolution. In the following sections we will discuss some of the modern applications of MRI in the large intraabdominal veins.

Mesenteric Veins

Magnetic resonance imaging has been used for the detection of splanchnic vein thrombosis, including that in the portal vein, in which a study by Levy and Newhouse found that portal vein occlusion is seen as well on MRI as on CT or Doppler ultrasound[19] (Fig. 10–9). In general, the portal venous system has been found to be reliably imaged, although artifacts can occasionally be generated owing to such phenomenon as slice-entry and even-echo rephasing.[20]

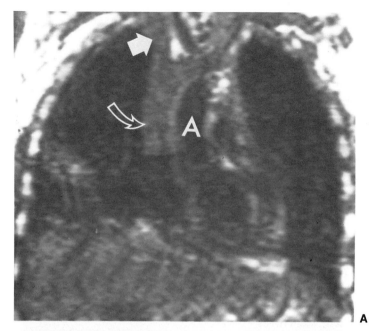

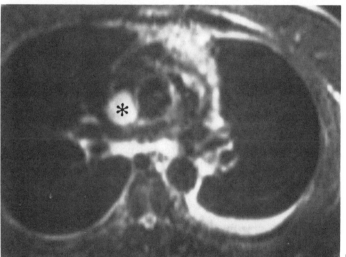

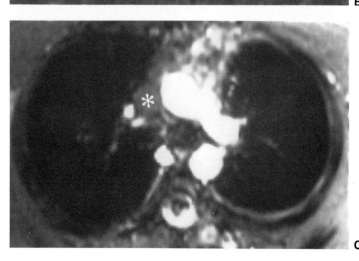

FIGURE 10–7. Superior vena caval occlusion. *A*, Coronal spin-echo image (TR = 550/TE = 20) demonstrates increased intravascular signal within the superior vena cava (curved open arrow) and right innominate vein (short white arrow). Intravascular flow void is seen within the ascending aorta (A). *B*, Transverse spin-echo sequence (TR = 2000/TE = 80). There is intravascular signal void demonstrated within the ascending and descending aorta, right main pulmonary artery, and azygous vein. High signal intensity is identified within the superior vena cava (asterisk). This appearance is consistent with thrombus; however, as previously demonstrated, increased signal intensity can be seen in a variety of normal flow conditions. *C*, Transverse gradient-echo sequence (TR = 60/TE = 13/flip angle = 25 degrees) demonstrating the expected intense intravascular signal from flowing blood within the patent aorta, left main pulmonary artery, and azygous vein. Thrombus within the superior vena cava (asterisk) is confirmed by the lack of hyperintensity on this sequence. (Case courtesy of Scott Erickson, M.D.)

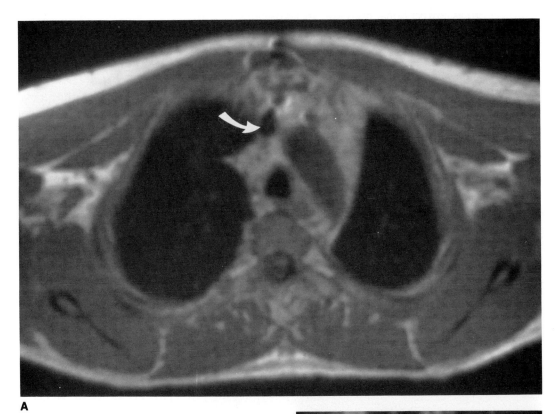

A

FIGURE 10–8. *A,* Thoracic veno-occlusive disease. Transverse spin-echo image (TR = 600/TE = 20) in a patient with previously documented occlusive disease of the upper extremity and thorax. This image demonstrates obliteration of the superior vena cava and flow void within the patient's right sided jugulo-atrial graft (curved arrow) indicating patency. *B,* Coronal, oblique maximum intensity projection MR flow study demonstrating a normal appearance of the aortic arch (Ao) and the great vessels (small arrows). The patient's jugulo-atrial graft is visualized descending along the right side of the mediastinum (large white arrows) to the right atrium. Note the absence of intravascular signal from the expected location of the subclavian, jugular, and innominate vessels in this patient. Upper extremity venography confirmed obliteration of these vessels.

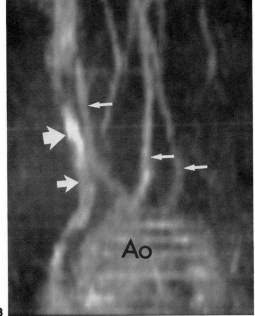

B

Significant progress has also occurred in actual measurement of portal velocities by MRI techniques. Tamada et al. were able to achieve close correlation with Doppler ultrasound measurements (r = 0.968) using a technique they referred to as "direct bolus imaging" in 14 normal individuals. They were also to observe changes in portal velocity in a variety of systemic conditions.[21] Such work holds great promise for future developments in vascular imaging with MRI.

In portal hypertension and cirrhosis, MRI has been found to be of great value in preoperative and postoperative evaluation. Using fast-scan techniques, Finn and his colleagues were able to reliably assess the patency of the portal vein in 26 of 27 patients and depict pathological conditions such as portal vein thrombosis, reversal of portal flow, and assess the extent and location of varices and portosystemic collateral vessels[22] (Fig. 10–10). Postoperatively, the same group found MRI very useful for noninvasively identifying portosystemic shunt patency. This valuable use of MRI has also been confirmed by several other groups[23,24] (Fig. 10–11).

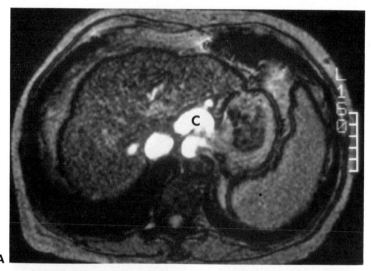

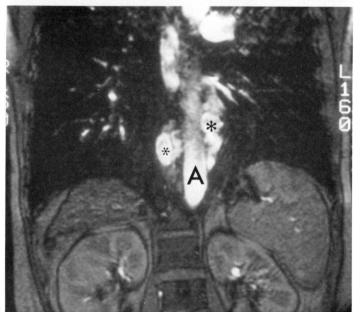

FIGURE 10–9. Portal hypertension and portal vein thrombus. *A*, Transverse gradient-echo image (TR = 60/TE = 13/flip angle = 25 degrees) demonstrating hyperintense intravascular signal within the inferior vena cava, intrahepatic veins, and large periaortic collaterals (C). The expected hyperintensity from the intrahepatic portal vein is not identified. *B*, Coronal gradient-echo image in the same patient demonstrating intravascular signal within the descending aorta and in the large periaortic collateral veins (asterisks). (Case courtesy of Scott Erickson, M.D.)

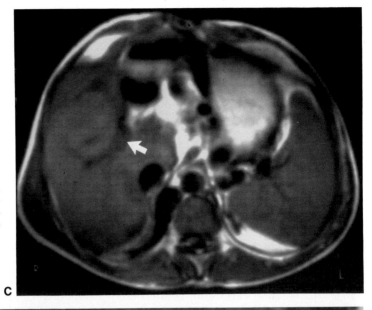

FIGURE 10–10. Portal vein thrombus and collateral vessels. Transverse spin-echo image (TR = 600/TE = 20) demonstrating normal flow void within the inferior vena cava and descending aorta as well as multiple large collateral vessels identified within the gastrohepatic ligament and splenic hilum. Note the intravascular signal intensity within the main portal vein (white arrow) indicating portal venous thrombus. Portal vein thrombus was confirmed by color Doppler sonography.

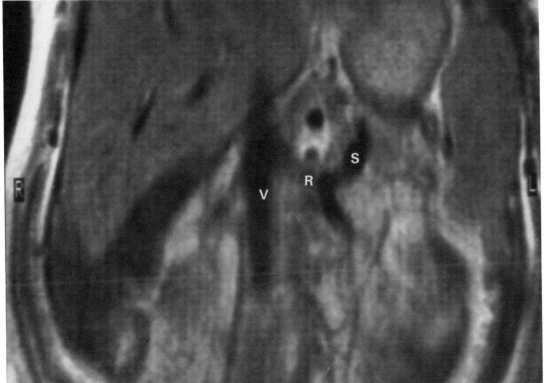

FIGURE 10–11. Evaluation of portosystemic shunt. Coronal spin-echo sequence (TR = 600/TE = 20) demonstrating cirrhotic liver and ascites. Flow void is identified within the splenic vein (S) descending to the anastomosis with the left renal vein (R). Flow void within the abdominal vena cava (V) is also noted.

Hepatic Veins

In hepatic vein occlusion (Budd-Chiari syndrome) MRI provides a characteristic picture with higher signal intensity in the central portion of the liver and lower signal intensity in the periphery as a result of relative congestion and slow blood flow.[25,26] In fact, MRI may be more reliable than CT in this disease, since imaging of the hepatic veins can be more easily done with the multiplanar capabilities of MRI. Stark claims that preoperative planning is aided by the use of MRI, particularly when it is used to evaluate the anatomy of the upper cava and right atrium, when congenital webs or tumors are the cause of obstruction.[27]

Renal Veins

Staging of renal-cell carcinoma always involves assessment of the patency of the renal vein and inferior vena cava. For many years, venography was the preoperative test of choice, but in the past 10 years, CT has been found to reliably image the presence or absence of tumor invasion. Magnetic resonance imaging has also been fairly widely used for this purpose; when compared to CT, MRI is not able to detect the primary neoplasm as well, but according to Hricak and her colleagues, it is more accurate in evaluating the presence of vascular extension. In their study evaluating 104 patients, MRI had 95 per cent sensitivity and 100 per cent specificity in detecting venous tumor extension. This figure compares favorably with reported corresponding figures for CT of 78 and 96 per cent, respectively.[28,29]

Other groups have also attempted to evaluate the role of MRI in renal-cell carcinoma staging. Horan and his co-workers prospectively compared venacavography and MRI in 44 patients with renal-cell carcinoma and found that the two tests were equally accurate in that determination; they observed that the combination of the two resulted in higher diagnostic yield than either test alone and recommended the use of both in difficult cases such as large, bulky lesions with considerable adenopathy.[30]

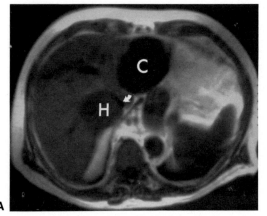 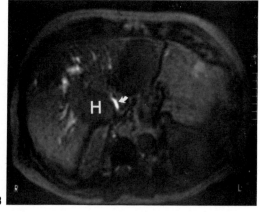

A   B

FIGURE 10–12. Intrahepatic vena caval occlusion. *A,* Transverse spin-echo image (TR = 550/TE = 20) in a patient with color Doppler diagnosis of vena caval occlusion. This image demonstrates a mass (H) compressing the intrahepatic vena cava (curved arrow). A small flow void within the cava is identified. Note is also made of a large hepatic cyst (C). *B,* Transverse gradient-echo image (TR = 60/TE = 20/flip angle = 25 degrees) at the same level demonstrating a normal hyperintense signal within the compressed but not occluded intrahepatic vena cava. Subsequent workup indicated that the intrahepatic mass (H) represented a hepatic hemangioma. Vena caval sarcomas can have a similar appearance.

Magnetic resonance imaging has also been used to identify the presence of benign, bland thrombus within the renal vein and cava in adults and newborns.[22,23]

Inferior Vena Cava

As one would anticipate, the largest vein in the abdomen can be well imaged with MRI. In fact, coronal MR or sagittal plane MR or both are particularly useful in visualizing the superior extent of caval clot. Venous

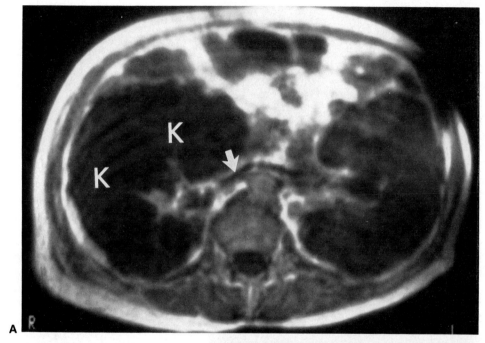

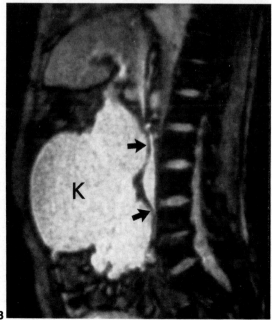

FIGURE 10–13. Abdominal vena caval compression. *A,* Transverse spin-echo image (TR = 600/TE = 20) in a patient with adult polycystic kidney disease and lower extremity swelling. This image demonstrates compression of the abdominal vena cava (white arrow) at the level of the renal vein inflow. This compression appears to result from the patient's enlarged kidney (K). *B,* Sagittal gradient-echo image (TR = 550/TE = 30/flip angle = 25 degrees) demonstrating compression of the abdominal vena cava (arrows) by the patient's enlarged kidney (K).

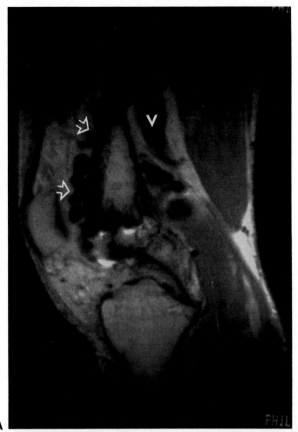

FIGURE 10–14. Lower extremity vascular malformation. *A,* Sagittal spin-echo sequence (TR = 2000/TE = 30) demonstrating multiple abnormal vascular channels (open arrows) surrounding the distal femor. An enlarged popliteal vein (V) is identified. *B,* Multiple axial gradient-echo scan (TR = 50/TE = 13/flip angle = 65 degrees) demonstrating enlarged popliteal artery and vein, as well as abnormal vascular channels in the affected thigh. (*Figure continues.*)

A

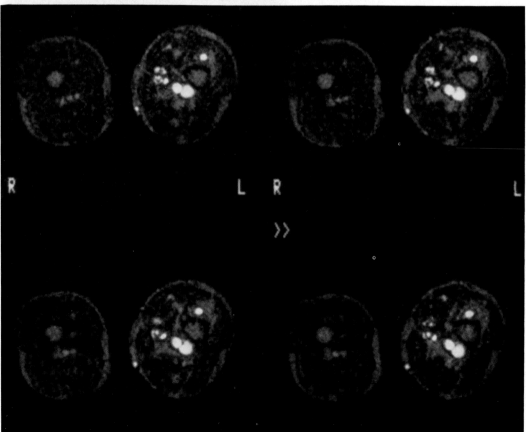

B

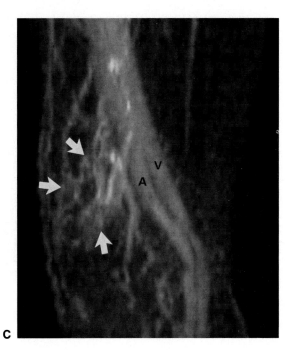

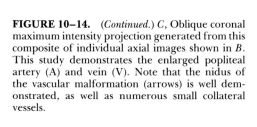

FIGURE 10–14. (*Continued.*) *C*, Oblique coronal maximum intensity projection generated from this composite of individual axial images shown in *B*. This study demonstrates the enlarged popliteal artery (A) and vein (V). Note that the nidus of the vascular malformation (arrows) is well demonstrated, as well as numerous small collateral vessels.

collaterals can also be differentiated from lymphadenopathy with greater ease. As we indicated above, tumors that secondarily involve the cava are well seen with MRI; primary caval neoplasms have also been observed.[32] Vena caval anomalies are generally well seen with MRI; we have been impressed with the usefulness of the technique in obtaining multiplanar views of some of these anatomic variants (Figs. 10–12 and 10–13).

One of the most novel and useful applications of MRI has been in the study of vena caval filters for follow-up of the presence of caval occlusion or propagation (or both) of clot above the filter. Most of the commercially available filters produce some magnetic artifact in the vicinity of the cava; the stainless steel Greenfield filter produces the most and the Simon Nitinol filter produces none at all.[33,34]

Extremities: Iliofemoral and Popliteal Veins

Obviously, MRI is not and will not become the technique of first choice in identifying deep venous thrombosis of the lower extremities, but there is evidence that the technique can be helpful in certain circumstances. Gehl et al. found that MR was very useful in identifying the cephalad extent of lower-extremity thrombosis in 8 or 32 patients.[35] Others have confirmed the utility of MRI in specific situations, predominantly when venography or ultrasound fails to precisely determine the morphology or location of the thrombosis.[36,37] We have used MRI to evaluate the appearance of the iliocaval system in cases of chronic caval occlusion; collateral veins and the presence of unusual anatomy has been well displayed.

We and others have also found MRI to be of great assistance in identifying and localizing arteriovenous malformations (AVM). Magnetic resonance imaging consistently has supplied detailed information about the flow into and location of these lesions (Figs. 10–14 and 10–15).

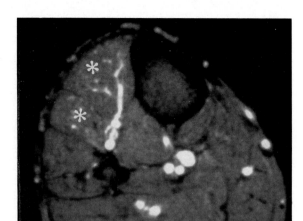

FIGURE 10–15. Intramuscular hemangioma. Transverse gradient-echo image (TR = 550/TE = 30/flip angle = 25 degrees) previously shown in Figure 10–5 demonstrating an enlarged vessel and numerous small vessels in the anterior compartment (asterisk). Arteriography demonstrated an intramuscular hemangioma.

Other pathology which has been seen with MRI includes popliteal-vein entrapment and a variety of vascular malformations.[38,39]

CONCLUSION

Without question, MRI will become the cross-sectional imaging technique of choice for imaging of a large number of vascular abnormalities. It seems clear that the expanding use of new pulse sequences as well as the coming revolutionary use of three-dimensional display of data from entire tissue volumes rather than simple slices will ensure an ever-increasing role for MRI in the investigation of vascular diseases.

REFERENCES

1. Bradley, WG, Waluch, V, Lai, KS, et al.: The appearance of rapidly flowing blood on MR images. Am J Roentgenol 1984;*143*:1167–1174.
2. Axel, L: Blood flow effects in magnetic resonance imaging. Am J Roentgenol 1984;*143*:1157–1166.
3. Perman, WH, Maan, PR, Moran, RA, et al.: Artifacts from pulsatile flow in MRI. J Comput Assist Tomogr 1986;*10*:473–484.
4. Felmlee, JP, Ehman, RL: Spatial presaturation: a method for suppressing flow artifacts and improving depiction of vascular anatomy in MRI. Radiology 1987;*164*:559–564.
5. Edelman, RR, Wentz, KU, Mattle, H, et al.: Projection arteriography and venography: Initial clinical results with MR. Radiology 1989;*172*:351–357.
6. Rapport, S, Softman, HD, Pope, C, et al.: Venous clots: Evaluation with MRI. Radiology 1987;*162*:527–530.
7. Theissen, P, Sechlem, U, Mennicken, U, Hilqer, HH, Schicha, H: Noninvasive diagnosis of atrial septal defects and anomalous pulmonary venous return using magnetic resonance tomography. Nuklearmedizin 1989;*28*:172–180.
8. Hsu, YH, Chien, CT, Hwany, M, Chiu, IS: Magnetic resonance imaging of total anomalous pulmonary venous drainage. Am Heart J 1991;*121*:1560–1565.
9. Thorsen, MK, Erickson, SJ, Mewissen, MW, Youker, JE: CT and MR imaging of partial anomalous pulmonary venous return to the azygos vein. J Comput Assist Tomogr 1990;*14*:1007–1009.
10. Baxter, R, McFadden, PM, Gradman, M, Wright, A: Scimitar syndrome: Cine magnetic resonance imaging demonstration of anomalous pulmonary venous drainage. Ann Thorac Surg 1990;*50*:121–123.

11. Halabu, H, Gefter, WB, Kressek, HY, et al.: Pulmonary vasculature: High-resolution MR imaging. Work in progress. Radiology 1989;*171*:391–395.
12. Gefter, WB, Hatabu, H, Dinsmore, BJ, et al.: Pulmonary vascular cine MR imaging: A noninvasive approach to dynamic imaging of the pulmonary circulation. Radiology 1990;*176*:761–770.
13. Mohiaddin, RH, Amanuma, M, Kilner, PJ, et al.: MR phase-shift velocity mapping of mitral and pulmonary venous flow. J Comput Assist Tomogr 1991;*15*:237–243.
14. Julsrud, PR, Elman, RL, Hagler, DJ, Ilstrup, DM: Extracardiac vasculature in candidates for Fontan surgery: MR imaging. Radiology 1989;*173*:503–506.
15. Hansen, ME, Spritzer, CE, Sostman, HD: Assessing the patency of mediastinal and thoracic inlet veins: Value of MR imaging. Am J Roentgenol 1990;*155*:1177–1182.
16. Weinreb, JC, Mootz, A, Cohen, JM: MRI evaluation of mediastinal thoracic inlet venous obstruction. Am J Roentgenol 1986;*146*:679–684.
17. Haire, WD, Lynch, TG, Lund, GB: Limitations of magnetic resonance imaging and ultrasound-directed (duplex) scanning in the diagnosis of subclavian vein thrombosis. J Vasc Surg 1991;*13*:391–397.
18. Gefter, WB: Chest applications of magnetic resonance imaging: An update. Radiol Clin North Am 1988;*26*:573–588.
19. Levy, HM, Newhouse, JH: MR imaging of portal vein thrombosis. Am J Roentgenol 1988;*151*:283–286.
20. Davy-Miallou, C, Guinet, C, Bellin, MF, et al.: MRI of the normal portal system: The artefacts. J Radiol 1990;*71*:339–343.
21. Tamada, T, Moriyasu, F, Ono, S, et al.: Portal blood flow: Measurement with MR imaging. Radiology 1989;*173*:639–644.
22. Finn, JP, Edelman, RR, Jenkins, RL, et al.: Liver transplantation: MR angiography with surgical validation. Radiology 1991;*179*:265–269.
23. Baunin, C, Quesnel, C, Vaysse, P, et al.: Value of magnetic resonance imaging in the follow-up of children operated for portal hypertension. Chir Pedatr 1988;*29*:161–164.
24. Williams, DM, Eckhauser, FE, Aisen, A, et al.: Assessment of portosystemic shunt patency and function with magnetic resonance imaging. Surgery 1987;*102*:602–607.
25. Stard, DD, Han, PF, Trey, C, et al.: MRI of the Budd-Chiari syndrome. Am J Roentgenol 1986;*146*:1141–1146.
26. Betti, A, Vittori, O, Vezzoli, G: Diagnostic imaging of Budd-Chiari syndrome in adults and children. Radiol Med 1990;*79*:70–76.
27. Stark, DD: Liver. *In* Start, DD, Bradley, WG Jr, eds.: Magnetic Resonance Imaging. St. Louis, MO, CV Mosby Company, 1988;934–1059.
28. Hricak, H, Thoeni, RF, Carroll, PR, et al.: Detection and staging of renal neoplasms: A reassessment of MR imaging. Radiology 1988;*166*:643–649.
29. Johnson, CD, Dunnick, NR, Cohan, RH, Illescas, FF: Renal adenocarcinoma: CT staging of 100 tumors. Am J Roentgenol 1987;*148*:59–63.
30. Horan, JJ, Robertson, CN, Choyke, PL, et al.: The detection of renal carcinoma extension into the renal vein and inferior vena cava: A prospective comparison of venacavography and magnetic resonance imaging. J Urol 1989;*142*:943–947.
31. Honda, H, Yuh, WT, Lu, CC: Magnetic resonance imaging of renal vein and inferior vena cava thrombosis in a patient with glomerulonephritis: A case report. J Comput Tomogr 1988;*12*:147–149.
32. van Rooij, WJJ, Martens, F, Verbeeten, B Jr, et al.: CT and MR imaging of leiomyosarcoma of the inferior vena cava. J Comput Assist Tomogr 1990;*14*:479.
33. Teitelbaum, GP, Bradley, WG Jr, Klein, BD: MR imaging artifacts, ferromagnetism, and magnetic torque of intravascular filters, stents, and coils. Radiology 1988;*166*:657.
34. Vinitski, S, Clark, RA, Watanabe, AT, et al.: Optimization of gradient-echo imaging parameters for intracaval filters and trapped thromboemboli. Radiology 1990;*174*:1013.
35. Gehl, HB, Bolmodorf, K, Gunther, RW: MR-angiography (MRA) in deep leg and pelvic venous thrombosis: A comparison with phlebography. ROFO 1990;*153*:654–657.
36. Totterman, S, Francis, CW, Foster, TH, et al.: Diagnosis of femoropopliteal venous thrombosis with MR imaging: A comparison of our MR pulse sequences. Am J Roentgenol 1990;*154*:175–178.
37. Erdman, WA, Jayson, HT, Redman, HC, et al.: Deep venous thrombosis of extremities: Role of MR imaging in the diagnosis. Radiology 1990;*174*:425.
38. Lemme-Plaghos, L, Kucharczyk, W, Brant-Zawadzki, M, et al.: MRI of angiographically occult vascular malformations. Am J Roentgenol 1986;*146*:1223.
39. Fermand, M, Houlle, D, Cormier, JM, et al.: Popliteal vein entrapment shown by MR imaging (letter). Am J Roentgenol 1990;*155*:424–425.

III

NONINVASIVE DIAGNOSTIC TECHNOLOGY

11

REAL-TIME COLOR DOPPLER IN ARTERIAL IMAGING

JEAN-FRANCOIS BLAIR and DENNIS F. BANDYK

Rational planning for endovascular or direct surgical intervention in patients with peripheral arterial disease requires accurate depiction of anatomic and hemodynamic derangements. While a careful history and physical examination are typically all that are required to establish a diagnosis of arterial occlusive disease, additional testing using noninvasive methods is necessary to accurately screen patients for suspected aneurysms, vascular trauma, or postimplantation lesions which can develop following arterial surgery. Since many of these conditions are asymptomatic, vascular imaging coupled with hemodynamic testing permits detection, grading severity, and timing of intervention. In symptomatic patients, especially those with critical limb ischemia, a comprehensive vascular evaluation is paramount because of the likelihood of multilevel (e.g., aortoiliac, femoropopliteal, infrageniculate, digital) disease. Failure to identify lesions or quantify hemodynamic abnormalities within each arterial segment can result in persistence of limb ischemia following intervention, or jeopordize patency of an arterial repair.

Arteriography has been the standard method of evaluating peripheral arterial disease, and in many surgeons' practices, remains the "gold standard" diagnostic test and a prerequisite prior to intervention. With the development of color flow technology, it is now possible to map the arterial system in a manner analogous to an angiography in nearly all areas assessible to interrogation by ultrasonic energy. Importantly, both vascular anatomy and hemodynamics can be assessed. The drawbacks of arteriography such as patient discomfort, arterial injury, and the potential toxicity of contrast agent administration can be avoided, thus permitting widespread clinical applications such as patient screening and serial examinations. Detailed mapping of the extracranial cerebral, abdominal/visceral, and peripheral arteries is possible with color Doppler imaging.[1,2] Advances in probe technology and software data processing have improved ultrasound image resolution, which have further enhanced the clinical usefulness of this diagnostic method compared to both arteriography and conventional duplex instruments. Duplex ultrasonography has emerged as a valued clinical and research tool, in particular by expanding our understanding of the natural history of vascular lesions. The recent recognition that atherosclerotic disease progression in the internal carotid artery (ICA) to a high-grade stenosis as a risk factor for stroke would not have been possible without duplex scanning.[3,4] Clinicians frequently have to be reminded of the diagnostic limitations of arteriography, particularly when grading the severity of occlusive lesions. Atherosclerotic plaques typically develop in an eccentric fashion, and a single planar image is subject to gross underestimation or overestimation of severity.[5-7] In both experimental and clinical validation studies with arteriography, the capability and accuracy of duplex scanning to grade lesions has been confirmed.[8] Diameter reduction and hemodynamic significance (flow reduction, pressure gradient) can be accurately predicted using diagnostic criteria based on changes in the B-mode images and center-stream velocity spectra. The high diagnostic accuracy of duplex scanning has resulted in it becoming an accepted method for the evaluation of the peripheral and cerebrovascular arterial system. The introduction of color Doppler to duplex instrumentation has added a new dimension to the noninvasive evaluation of arterial disease. This feature permits spatial and temporal information of blood flow patterns to be superimposed on the B-mode grey-scale image. Real-time assessment of vessel anatomy, patency, and flow hemodynamics facilitates the diagnosis of disease, as well as details of lesion morphology, extent, and severity. There are valid concerns regarding the cost of color flow technology, but if applied appropriately and if the information gleaned is used for clinical decision-making, it would prove to be cost-effective compared to arteriography.

It is the intent of this chapter to review the unique diagnostic features and current clinical applications of color Doppler in peripheral arterial imaging. Since its introduction in 1988 at the Medical College of Wisconsin, we have found the detailed anatomic and hemodynamic data provided by color Doppler imaging to greatly facilitate vascular diagnosis, and in selected patients, allowed for medical treatment, endovascular intervention, or direct surgical repair or bypass without a preceding angiographic study.

BASIC PHYSICS OF REAL-TIME COLOR DOPPLER IMAGING

The application of duplex ultrasonography diagnosis has required vascular surgeons, radiologists, and internists to become more sophisticated in their understanding of ultrasound physics and arterial hemodynamics. A solid data base in these disciplines is particularly important when utilizing color Doppler for arterial imaging. Complexities in the instrumentation, video display format, scanning technique, and computed blood flow patterns can easily result in misleading and erroneous conclusions owing to artifacts, aliasing, or improper Doppler beam angle correction.[9-11] Familiarity with the instrumentation reduces the majority of the interpretation errors. Briefly, color duplex instrumentation employs an electronically steered multigated pulsed Doppler transducer coupled to an autocorrelation processor which enables rapid analysis of echoes returning to the transducer along a known Doppler angle line for phase, amplitude, and frequency content. Stationary soft tissue structures, which lack phase- or frequency-shift compared to the previous scanline, are assigned an amplitude value and displayed in a standard grey-scale B-mode image. Areas of tissue motion, such as blood flow, can be detected from the estimation of the mean frequency-shift of moving red blood cells (RBC). The image generated is then superimposed on the B-mode image and updated up to 18 times per second. It is incorrect to conclude that color Doppler generated flow images are equivalent to an arteriogram or that blood flow is displayed in real time.[11] When injected contrast moves along the arterial tree in sequential angiographic images, it is correct to conclude that the blood has moved from the first location to the second. In color Doppler, no such relationship exists because of space and time distortions inherent to the instrumentation.

Color assignment depends on direction of blood flow with respect to the transducer and RBC velocity (Fig. 11–1). Color saturation or hue reflects the magnitude of the mean Doppler frequency-shift for each range cell (pixel) and depends on both RBC velocity and Doppler beam angle. Less saturation of colors (red, blue) indicate regions of higher blood flow velocities, deeper colors indicate slower flow, with the absence of flow coded as black. It should be emphasized that computation of the digital blood flow data to generate color Doppler images varies with manufacturer, and in general, differs from maximum frequency shift obtained by pulsed Doppler spectral analysis. In color Doppler, a single representative number, usually the mean RBC velocity, is assigned to each pixel, while discrete spectral analysis provides for interpretation of the full spectrum of back-scattered frequency shifts recorded from a sample volume. Of note, it is the responsibility of the operator to select color assignment (direction of flow) and the color map (dynamic range). For example, the color red is used to indicate flow toward the transducer or flow in an artery, and the color blue to indicate flow in the opposite direction, away from the transducer, or blood flow in veins. Because of sensitivity and gain limitations of the instruments, color Doppler imaging must be performed using optimal beam angles. Vessels should be insonated at a Doppler beam angle of 60 degrees or less.[12] When the Doppler beam angle approaches 90 degrees to the axis of blood flow, little or no Doppler frequency shift will be detected and the color black will be displayed, erroneously indicating no flow (Fig. 11–2). If the direction of blood flow is parallel to the scanlines (beam angle = 0 degrees), Doppler frequency-shifts are increased and color encoding of flow will dem-

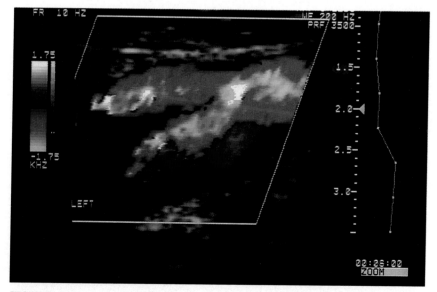

FIGURE 11–1. Color Doppler image of normal carotid bifurcation recorded at peak systole. Red to orange colors indicate flow away from the transducer, while blue to white colors indicate flow toward the transducer. A region of boundary layer separation in the carotid bulb is noted by the blue color, which signifies that reverse flow is present.

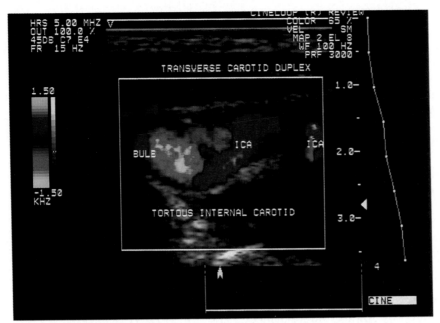

FIGURE 11–2. The color changes seen in a tortuous internal carotid artery represent change in the direction of flow relative to the angle of the incident sound beam. A zone of black in the distal erroneously coded as "no flow" due to beam angle of 90 degrees.

onstrate less color saturation. If the dynamic range of the color map selected is less than the computed mean Doppler frequency shift, aliasing occurs. This artifact of Doppler data processing results in erroneous depiction both of direction and magnitude of blood flow (Fig. 11–3). The aliasing which occurs in color Doppler is identical to that observed with conventional pulsed Doppler spectral analysis when one half of the pulse-repetition frequency (PRF), also referred to as the Nyquist limit, is exceeded. Many of the commercially available color duplex scanners allow the Doppler scanlines to be electronically steered for flow data acquisition. This feature aids in imaging vessel segments at or near 60 degrees, the angle best suited for duplex scanning. Use of a mechanical wedge (angle of 18 to 24 degrees) interposed between the transducer and the skin surface is an alternate method of steering Doppler scanlines to facilitate accurate color-encoding of flow within the B-mode image. An inherent limitation of color Doppler not frequently appreciated is the degradation in the resolution of the B-mode image which occurs when vascular structures are imaged at scanlines other than 90 degrees.

Variations in acoustic impedance of tissues encountered during color Doppler imaging require the operator to constantly adjust the instrumentation so the color-coded flow column fills the vessel lumen but does not "bleed" into the adjacent structures. This calibration can be accomplished by adjustment of the frame rate, color sensitivity, and PRF. Both frame rate and the sensitivity of the color-coding algorithm vary as a function of the width and depth of the region of interest. The larger the size of the color flow image, the longer the data acquisition time is, which results in less frequent image update (e.g., decreased frame rate). The PRF of the instrument must also be varied, unless done automatically by the system, in relation to the depth of the posterior boundary of the color flow image. For example, evaluation of deeply positioned vascular structures (renal arteries, profunda femoris and peroneal arteries,

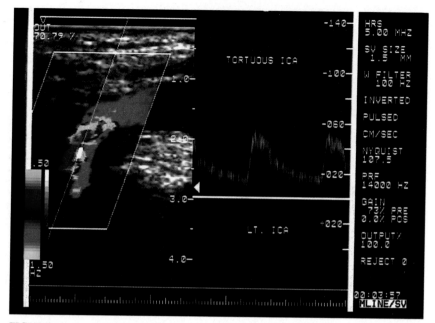

FIGURE 11–3. Angled distal internal carotid artery can be recognized by color Doppler. The changes in color do not signify velocity change or flow abnormality, but reflect changes in beam angle and artifact produced by aliasing. Normal velocity spectra recorded from site of color changes.

distal internal carotid artery, middle cerebral artery) or veins in which low RBC velocities are expected, mandates a scanning strategy that includes a lower transmitting frequency and thus PRF, and slower frame rate to ensure optimum color imaging.[9,11]

NORMAL COLOR DOPPLER ARTERIAL FLOW PATTERNS

The pattern of blood flow in an individual artery segment is influenced by the driving arterial pressure waveform, vessel wall anatomy (diameter, luminal irregularity, elasticity), and the resistance to flow of the distal arterial tree and microcirculation. Even under normal laminar flow conditions, the magnitude and direction of RBC velocity vectors vary greatly across the vessel cross-section (velocity profile) and change constantly during the cardiac cycle. Viscous and inertia forces of blood result in the lowest RBC velocities adjacent to the artery wall and highest in the centerstream of flow, often referred to as "plug flow", and produce a blunted rather than parabolic velocity profile. Anatomic configurations, such as dilatations, bifurcations, and anastomoses dramatically alter laminar flow patterns by producing regions of flow separation, helical flow, and boundary layer formation.[9,13] Blood flow patterns in the carotid bifurcation have been studied in greatest detail because of the importance of this artery segment in the pathogenesis of stroke and its easy access for ultrasound imaging. The low peripheral resistance of the brain results in antegrade flow throughout the cardiac cycle, also referred to as "quasi-steady" flow, in the common (CCA) and internal carotid arteries (ICA) and vertebral arteries. Consequently, the color flow images of these arteries maintain a red hue throughout the pulse cycle, with less saturation (light red to white) of centerstream flow due to higher

RBC velocities. In the region of the bulb, the pattern of blood flow becomes more complicated. Opposite the flow divider, which separates the origins of the internal and external carotid arteries, an area of reversed flow develops in early systole and persists into diastole (Fig. 11–1). This region of boundary layer separation in the "normal" carotid bulb is depicted in the color flow image by a variable layer of blue (reversed flow) or black (no flow) adjacent to the outer wall of the bulb.[2,13]

The pattern of blood flow in the external carotid artery is analogous to that seen in peripheral arteries with a multiphasic pulsatile waveform due to a high basal outflow resistance. During systole, the vessel lumen fills with red-coded pixels of uniform saturation, indicating a narrow range or RBC velocities and laminar undisturbed flow. At peak systole, a region of lighter hue appears in centerstream, which is followed in early diastole by incomplete luminal filling with blue-coded pixels indicating reversal of flow. In late diastole, the vessel lumen may be incompletely filled with color-coded pixels due to low RBC velocities.[2]

COLOR DOPPLER IMAGING OF ARTERIAL LESIONS

Arterial Stenosis

Stenoses produced by trauma, atherosclerosis, myointimal hyperplasia, or vessel entrapment produce characteristic color flow images.[14–17] Regions of increased RBC velocities that persist throughout the cardiac cycle (i.e., "flow jet") develop in the inlet of the stenotic segment and propagate downstream for a varying (one to three vessel diameters) distance depending on the severity and geometry of the lesion. The color image demonstrates a zone of color desaturation (increased whiteness) and typically, aliasing of the color-coded flow due to the high RBC velocities (Fig. 11–4). The persistent increased hue of the blood flow jet throughout the cardiac cycle compared to immediately proximal and distal arterial segments greatly facilitates localization of stenoses with color flow imaging compared to conventional duplex scanning.[14,18] Other color Doppler characteristics of flow through stenotic lesions include: flow reversal along vessel walls downstream from the lesion, and turbulent flow which is depicted in the video display as a mosaic of colors due to random RBC velocity vectors and aliasing. The extent and duration of flow disturbances produced by stenosis increase with severity (diameter reduction). A disturbed flow pattern with high velocity vectors (greater than 125 to 150 cm/sec) and spectral broadening that persists throughout systole and diastole indicates greater than 50 per cent diameter reduction and correlates with a pressure-reducing lesion in the peripheral and cerebrovascular arterial circulation.[2,8,15,18] Several investigators have attempted to quantify the severity of stenotic lesions using the real-time color Doppler image alone.[16,17] Using a green-tag method to estimate the maximum RBC velocities during systole, Landwehr et al.[17] were able to grade stenoses in a pulsatile flow model with an accuracy comparable to pulsed Doppler spectral analysis. In clinical practice, the examination of long, tortuous segments of arteries (e.g., abdominal aorta, iliac and lower limb arteries) is commonplace. Such complicated anatomic configurations limit the use of color Doppler alone to quantify disease. A beam angle of 60 degrees cannot always be obtained, or wall calcification obscures the site of maximal frequency shift; two potential and important sources of error when duplex

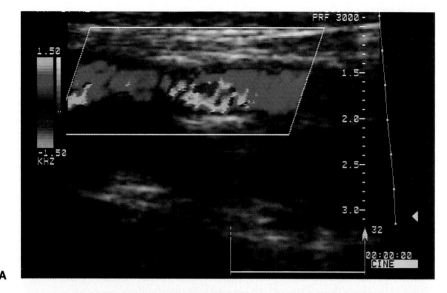

A

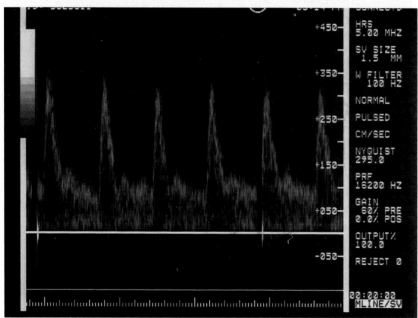

B

FIGURE 11–4. *A,* Color image of arterial stenosis with focal reduction in flow channel and localized color changes indicating increased RBC velocities. Color coding produced by aliasing in the color map. *B,* Velocity spectra recorded from site of maximum "flow jet" confirm systolic velocities to 350 cm/sec and end-diastolic velocities of 100 cm/sec indicative of high-grade (>75%) diameter reduction stenosis.

scanning is used to classify stenosis severity. The examining technologist and interpreting physician must be aware of these pitfalls since they introduce potential sources of variability if the degree of stenosis is based on color changes in the image alone. A more appropriate use of color flow imaging is to use the video display to localize stenotic lesions and guide the placement of a pulsed Doppler sample volume at a Doppler beam angle of 60 degrees or less. Quantification of the stenoses should be based on analysis of recorded velocity spectra identical to the scheme used with conventional duplex scanning.

Arterial Occlusion

Vessel occlusion is readily apparent by color flow imaging by the absence of flow within the lumen of a properly imaged vessel. Caveats which must be heeded to diagnose occlusion with confidence include: (1) use of a slow-flow mode to exclude the possibility of a "string sign" and a patent vessel distal to a high-grade stenosis, (2) scanning the vessel in multiple planes (sagittal, transverse) particularly if wall calcification with acoustic shadowing is identified, and (3) identifying reduced RBC velocities proximal to the occlusion.[18] In peripheral arteries, the configuration of the velocity waveform changes from triphasic to biphasic, with loss of the reversed flow component in diastole.[8,19] If collaterals are not well developed around the occlusion, or none exist, a "staccato" flow pattern immediately proximal to the occlusion can be demonstrated by an abrupt antegrade and retrograde color flow pattern in systole. In patients with chronic occlusions, particularly involving peripheral arteries such as the superficial femoral artery, both exit and reentry collateral vessels can be imaged directly. The flow pattern of collateral vessels is one of low resistance with antegrade flow throughout the pulse cycle. Distal to an obstruction, the magnitude of RBC velocities is reduced compared to the proximal segment or collateral vessels, and flow is antegrade in both systole and diastole. Accurate measurement of the length of an occlusion requires identification of its origin, typically by the presence of exit collaterals, and the site where flow returns to the lumen via a reentry collateral.[18] Color flow imaging using a sensitive slow-flow mode (flow rate of 1 to 5 cm/sec) has been demonstrated to be more accurate than arteriography in predicting the length of superficial femoral artery occlusion and assessing patency of tibial arteries in limbs with critical ischemia. In the carotid system, occlusion of the internal carotid artery can be suspected by the indirect hemodynamic findings such as low flow velocity in the common carotid artery compared to the contralateral side, and the conversion from a low- to high-resistance flow pattern in the ipsilateral common carotid artery with flow to zero or flow reversal during early diastole.[20]

Arterial Aneurysm and Pseudoaneurysm

The use of real-time B-mode ultrasonography to evaluate the abdominal aorta and peripheral arteries for aneurysmal degeneration is well established. The method is rapid, versatile, and accurate with a sensitivity and specificity approaching 100 per cent for the diagnosis of aneurysms involving the infrarenal abdominal aorta or peripheral (brachial, femoral, popliteal) arteries.[21] The precision of ultrasound diameter measurements are within 0.5 cm of the maximal diameter of the operative specimen. Similarly, with interobserver and intraobserver variability in diameter measurement of less 5 mm, ultrasonic imaging is well suited for the detection of aortic aneurysm expansion by serial examinations. B-mode ultrasonic imaging does not provide sufficient anatomic definition of abdominal aneurysms to plan operative repair, such as cephalo-caudad extension, relationship of the visceral arteries to the aneurysmal segment, or identification of concomitant occlusive disease in visceral and iliac arteries. By contrast, real-time color Doppler imaging with its ability to visualize flow can accurately diagnose the presence of intraluminal thrombus, determine the location and patency of visceral arteries, and identify occlusive lesions.[22-24] Accurate abdominal duplex scanning requires skill and careful patient preparation, since examination of visceral (celiac, superior and inferior mesenteric, renal) and iliac arteries can be hampered by a variety of factors including obesity, vessel tortuosity, bowel gas, and peristalis. In patients in whom complete examination is possible, we have found color Doppler can replace arteriography prior to elective abdominal aortic aneurysm repair. Computed tomography of the abdomen is also included in the preoperative evaluation of these patients because of its ability to assess other intraabdominal organs and the suprarenal aorta for abnormalities.

Pseudoaneurysms of the arterial tree can be accurately diagnosed with color Doppler as an extravascular collection of blood with a persistent communication with the arterial system (contained rupture). This lesion most commonly develops following invasive procedures, such as angiography, cardiac catheterization, or percutaneous balloon angioplasty, but can also occur as a healing complication at a graft-artery anastomosis due to aneurysmal degeneration, infection, or suture failure. Color Doppler imaging of pseudoaneurysms demonstrate a "whirlwind" flow pattern within the aneurysm cavity with swirling of red and blue colors throughout the cardiac cycle (Fig. 11–5). During systole, the higher pressure in the artery forces blood into the pseudoaneurysm, while during diastole, pressure in the artery decreases relative to the pseudoaneurysm, permitting blood flow back into the native circulation. This "to-and-fro" flow pattern can also be demonstrated by pulsed Doppler spectral analysis, but recognition of the lesion is facilitated by color Doppler.[25] An important consideration in planning therapy for pseudoaneurysm is the precise localization of the neck or communication between the artery and the cavity. This site can be identified in the majority of patients as a systolic flow jet at the base of the pseudoaneurysm. Recently, color Doppler has been advocated as a continuous monitoring technique for manual obliteration of pseudoaneurysms recognized following percutaneous vascular procedures.[26] Utilizing a linear probe, extrinsic

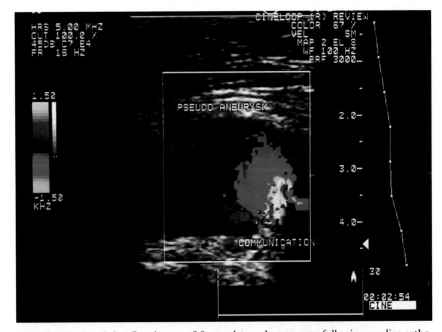

FIGURE 11–5. Color flow image of femoral pseudoaneurysm following cardiac catheterization with swirling flow (red and blue color changes) in the cavity and localization of the communication with the native artery recognized by a "flow jet" and aliasing color changes.

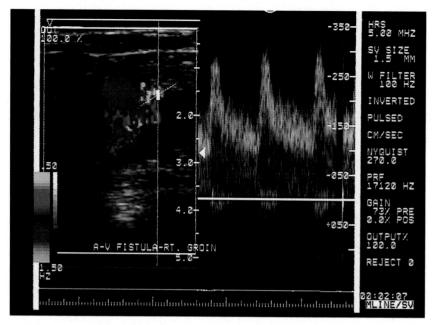

FIGURE 11–6. Color flow image and velocity spectra recorded from a traumatic arteriovenous fistula in the groin. A tissue bruit can be recognized by color pixels seen outside the walls of the vessels.

pressure is applied at the site of the arterial communication until no Doppler shift is demonstrated. The ability to simultaneously monitor anatomic and flow data permits the precise amount of pressure of the pseudoaneurysm cavity to be applied to obliterate flow and facilitate thrombosis.

Uncommon Lesions

Other flow abnormalities which can readily be documented using real-time color flow imaging include arterial dissection and arteriovenous fistula.[27–30] The latter abnormality is characterized by simultaneous visualization of pulsatile flow in the artery and proximal vein. Additionally, a flow jet (high Doppler frequency shifts throughout pulse cycle) from the artery into the venous lumen can be readily identified. A universal color Doppler characteristic of an arteriovenous fistula is demonstration of a "tissue bruit" due to transmitted wall vibration produced by turbulent flow (Fig. 11–6). Tissue motion is erroneously coded flow as transient speckles of color without any specific pattern in tissues adjacent to the vessels. Identification of a "tissue bruit" should alert the diagnostician to the presence of turbulent flow and an area of increased blood-flow velocity. These hemodynamic characteristics can also occur at an arteriovenous fistula or a high-grade (greater than 50 per cent diameter reduction) arterial stenosis. The tissue bruit produced by turbulent flow of a stenosis may be perceptible only during systole. Importantly, this artifact of color flow imaging can obscure ultrasound details of underlying vascular anatomy.

CLINICAL APPLICATIONS IN ARTERIAL IMAGING

Cerebrovascular Disease

The development of duplex ultrasonography has revolutionized the noninvasive diagnosis of extracranial carotid disease. Using established criteria based on pulsed Doppler spectral analysis, duplex scanning has been shown to be both cost-effective and accurate compared with arteriography for the detection of quantification of occlusive lesions. Sensitivities and specificities ranging from 85 to 99 per cent, and overall accuracies of 90 to 95 per cent have been reported for differentiation of stenoses with greater than 50 per cent diameter reduction.[2,20,25,31] The impact of color Doppler imaging on diagnostic accuracy were readily apparent in our laboratory when compared to conventional duplex scanning. Vessel identification was facilitated, especially the vertebral arteries, as well as the carotid bifurcation and its branches, and tortuous distal ICA configurations. The time required for examination decreased owing to rapid vessel identification and localization of sites of disturbed flow. Vessel kinks, coils, and occlusion are easily recognized. Importantly, the complex flow patterns in the normal carotid bulb can now be identified, which has resulted in improved confidence that minor lesions are not being missed or their severity overclassified.[2] With rapid vessel identification, examination time is now used to record spectral waveforms rather than trying to map complicated vessel anatomy, such as tortuous ICAs or carotid endarterectomy sites closed by patch angioplasty. The varied and often acute Doppler beam angles encountered when scanning tortuous segments can produce color flow images which mimmick stenoses, primarily by aliasing of the color map. Discrete spectral analysis and assessment of vessel diameter from the color image are helpful in confirming the absence of an occlusive lesion. Similarly, following carotid endarterectomy, disturbed flow is routinely seen in the vein-patch segment, with a zone of flow separation and increased velocities at the distal endpoint of the angioplasty. Careful attention to the diameter of the vessel lumen, particularly on transverse scanning, is important in avoiding overestimation of stenosis in these situations, or when a contralateral ICA occlusion and compensatory ipsilateral collateral flow is present.

Color Doppler has theoretical advantages compared with conventional duplex in diagnosis of low-grade (less than 50 per cent diameter reduction) stenoses or nonocclusive but ulcerated plaques in the carotid bulb. Real-time analysis of the flow patterns at and downstream of abnormal or irregular luminal surfaces improves specificity of the examination. Although there exists a controversy regarding the ability of any imaging technique to reliably diagnose plaque ulceration, color Doppler imaging is more likely to demonstrate abnormal flow patterns adjacent to plaques before an ulceration becomes apparent on the B-mode image. Paradoxically, the absence of a zone of flow reversal in the carotid bulb may indicate presence of a nonocclusive carotid bulb plaque.[2] At the opposite end of the disease spectrum, ICA occlusion can be recognized with an accuracy approaching 95 per cent as compared to angiography.[31] Key components in this determination were previously discussed. The presence of an ICA stump (as well as its length) can be readily noted by the presence of simultaneous forward and reversed flow immediately proximal to the occluded segment. The finding of a long ICA stump in a patient with ipsilateral symptoms may localize a potential site of embolization via the remaining patent external carotid artery. A persistent ICA cul-de-sac has correlated with an increased incidence of ipsilateral transient ischemic attack or stroke in patients with ICA occlusion. Despite the increased ability to diagnose complete ICA carotid occlusion by color Doppler imaging, we continue to advocate confirmation by angiography in the patient with recent hemispheric symptoms referable to the side of suspected occlusion. In selected patients with proximal common carotid occlusion, color Doppler can document patency of the carotid bifurcation.

Reversed (blue) flow is identified in the external carotid artery with simultaneous antegrade (red) ICA flow.

The extracranial portion of the vertebral arteries can be visualized in greater than 90 per cent of patients. Although the accuracy of color Doppler imaging to define and grade vertebral artery stenoses is not as well defined and reproducible as in the carotid system, its major role is in the detection of flow and direction. In the subclavian steal syndrome, proximal subclavian stenosis or occlusion results in diversion of blood flow by the ischemic arm (especially during exercise) from the posterior circulation via retrograde flow in the ipsilateral vertebral artery. Using color Doppler, this condition is identified by the detection of reversed flow (blue) in the vertebral artery compared to antegrade (red) flow in the ipsilateral CCA. The subclavian steal phenomenon may be incomplete at rest, with retrograde flow in systole but antegrade flow in diastole, or occult with detection of reversed vertebral artery flow only after provocative maneuvers (arm exercise, reactive hyperemia testing).

Although evaluation of the extracranial cerebral circulation for atherosclerotic disease has received the most attention, color Doppler has been of value in the diagnosis of ICA dissection, carotid body tumors, and neoplastic invasion of the carotid bifurcation. Carotid artery dissections can occur spontaneously, can be associated with fibromuscular arterial disease, or can result from blunt cervical trauma. On color-flow imaging, the abberant channel can demonstrate a "to-and-fro" flow phenomenon previously described in pseudoaneurysms.[25] Carotid body tumors are a type of paraganglioma that develop as well-encapsulated lesions at the carotid bifurcation. These tumors often contain arteriovenous communications which are readily recognized by color Doppler imaging. Spaying of the external and internal carotid arteries is readily apparent on imaging, as is the size of the tumor (Fig. 11-7).[29] The extent of tumor

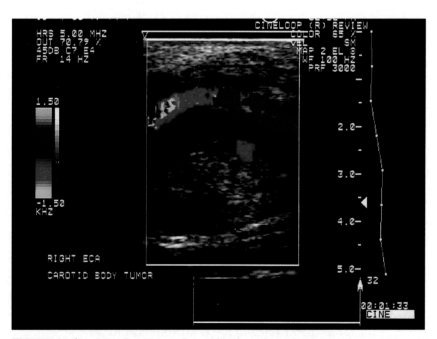

FIGURE 11-7. Color flow image of carotid body tumor with spaying of external carotid artery superiorly and flow visualization in the tumor produced by arteriovenous communications.

invasion into the vessel wall and patency can be assessed, but experience is still limited due to the low prevalence of the tumor.

Lower Limb Occlusive Disease

The extent and sequence of patient evaluation will vary based on the severity of limb ischemia and its etiology. Use of diagnostic testing sufficient to address the problem at hand is the ideal. In patients with multilevel disease, angiography will not identify hemodynamically abnormal segments in up to 30 per cent of patients.[5-7,32,33] The addition of pressure measurements to angiography improves diagnostic accuracy for aortoiliac disease, but add to the complexity and length of the procedure, and importantly, are not applicable for infrainguinal evaluation. Several investigators have confirmed the accuracy of duplex scanning in classifying peripheral arterial disease compared to angiography.[8,18,32-34] A major drawback to its widespread application is the need for an experienced technologist, the length of time necessary to perform a complete evaluation (1 to 2 hours per patient), and reluctance of surgeons to institute treatment based on the findings. Our experience using color Doppler imaging for "mapping" the lower extremity arterial system has demonstrated that examination time is significantly reduced, diagnostic accuracy is high, and confidence is sufficient that, in selected patients, no angiographic procedure is obtained prior to intervention. An agreement of over 90 per cent with angiography in grading lower limb occlusive disease has been reported for color Doppler in recent studies of patients undergoing endovascular or direct surgical repair.[18,32,34] Incomplete examination and misinterpretation of color images occurs in a number of patients, and the reasons are varied, including: (1) nonvisualization of the iliac system secondary to bowel gas, obesity, or the presence of long calcified segments, and below the inguinal ligament; (2) difficulties in imaging the popliteal trifurcation (inadequate studies in over 25 per cent of patients) not visualized; and (3) the presence of a proximal occlusion which alters downstream arterial hemodynamics.

Endovascular techniques have expanded treatment options in patients with disabling claudication objectively documented by pressure measurements and/ or treadmill testing. Most surgeons would agree that transluminal balloon angioplasty (PTA), laser-assisted PTA, or percutaneous atherectomy are suitable approaches for treating focal lesions in peripheral arteries.[34,35] The technical success rate exceeds 90 per cent, and long-term patency is comparable to bypass grafting if residual stenosis at the PTA site is avoided. To determine if a patient is a candidate for an endovascular procedure, the physician must know the location of the offending occlusive lesion, the lesion's morphology (occlusion versus stenosis), lesion length, whether multiple segments are affected, and the status of distal arterial tree. Using color Doppler, the aortoiliac and femoropopliteal arterial segments can be imaged for short (less than 10 cm) stenotic or occluded segments, which may be ideal lesions for endovascular therapy. Such lesions occur more often in claudicators, and correction of single-segment disease in this patient population can return functional status to normal. Use of angiography to screen claudicants for PTA is not appropriate, but rather should be reserved for patients with appropriate lesions as documented by duplex scanning or in whom extensive nature of the disease mandates bypass grafting. In a recent study that evaluated the results of laser-assisted PTA, segmental limb pressure measurements and angiography were used to screen 195 patients with symptomatic lower limb ischemia. Of the 130 patients who underwent angiography, 84 patients were excluded because of inappropriate lesions for the procedure.[36] This observation underscores the need to eliminate unnecessary angiography and its attendant risks in evaluating patients with limb ischemia. Using duplex scanning as a screening method prior to angioplasty, 50 of 122 patients evaluated were considered as suitable candidates for angioplasty based on duplex criteria, and 47 patients underwent a successful procedure.[34] Cossmann et al.[18] also reported excellent correlation with angiography and predictive value of color Doppler imaging in selecting the type of (percutaneous versus surgical bypass) intervention necessary to correct symptomatic limb ischemia.

Our policy is to grade the severity of limb ischemia with resting ankle-brachial systolic pressure measurements, and if indicated, perform treadmill exercise testing to establish the diagnosis of claudication. If the patient is considered to be a candidate for revascularization based on a clinical evaluation and pressure measurements, color duplex imaging from the aorta to tibial arteries is performed on the symptomatic limb(s). The intent of the study is to define the pattern of disease, localize lesions, and decide whether the patient should undergo an angiographic evaluation. If a lesion appropriate for PTA is identified, the risks and benefits of the procedure are discussed with the patient prior to the angiogram, and the interventionalist can select an appropriate angiographic approach. For example, if a focal superficial femoral artery stenosis/occlusion is to be treated, an ipsilateral antegrade puncture may be selected. In patients not deemed candidates for PTA because of long-segment occlusions or multilevel disease, the risks of bypass grafting are explained to the patient prior to angiography and medical treatment elected in those patients judged to be a prohibitive risk for direct surgical intervention. This approach minimizes unnecessary angiography and permits clinical decision-making based on noninvasive testing, the pattern of disease, and physician assessment of risk-versus-benefit variables of each patient.

Color Doppler imaging has a more limited but still useful role in the evaluation of patients with critical limb ischemia manifest by rest pain and/or tissue loss. Patients with this degree of ischemia will have multilevel disease, with the most common pattern being a long segmental occlusion of the superficial femoral artery (SFA) and concomitant aortoiliac or infrapopliteal arterial disease. Uncommonly (less than 20 per cent incidence) will the patient be a candidate for PTA alone. In this patient group, color flow imaging is used primarily to document SFA occlusion at its origin, assess the aortoiliac segment for significant (greater than 50 per cent diameter reduction) stenoses, and assess the popliteal and tibial arteries for continuous patency to the ankle. Patients identified to have focal iliac artery stenosis can undergo PTA prior to infrainguinal bypass.

Based on the excellent graft patency and limb salvage rates following lower extremity bypass procedures for critical ischemia, no patient with an acceptable operative risk profile should be denied a high-quality angiographic evaluation based on the results of color Doppler imaging. Although sensitivity for predicting patency exceeds 90 per cent for the anterior and posterior tibial arteries, the peroneal artery patency is more difficult to assess (sensitivity of 69 per cent), and acceptable runoff arteries at the ankle may not be visualized due to low flow. Problems with popliteal trifurcation imaging, vessel wall calcification, and obesity frequently confound the examiner and make angiographic evaluation prior to femorodistal bypass a prequisite. At the present time, we utilize color Doppler imaging in patients with critical ischemia to exclude occult inflow lesions in the iliac or SFA (if a short distal bypass is contemplated) and to evaluate specific arterial segments whose hemodynamic significance is not clear, even following angiography.

Aneurysmal Disease

The role of color Doppler imaging in aneurysmal disease of the aorta is limited at present to screening high-risk patient populations or confirming abnormalities found on physical examination. Despite the reported efficacy of duplex scanning in the evaluation of visceral artery abnormalities, it remains to be proven that sufficient anatomic information can be obtained in patients with abdominal aortic aneurysm (AAA) using color Doppler imaging so that an additional angiographic examination would be redundant. In approximately 80 per cent of our patients, we have been able to confirm the status of the renal arteries relative to the neck of aneurysm, exclude stenosis of visceral arteries, and identify aneurysmal involvement of the iliac and hypogastric arteries. Examination of obese patients or those with large (greater than 7 cm) aneurysms is difficult. By contrast, diagnosis of peripheral (femoral, popliteal) artery aneurysms is possible in essentially all patients using color flow imaging (Fig. 11–8).[37] Planning operative therapy of popliteal aneurysm is aided by preoperative color Doppler, since SFA dilatation and luminal thrombus formation may not always be appreciated by inspection of the angiogram, and this clinical situation usually requires SFA exclusion and construction of a long bypass graft. An important role of duplex scanning in patients with confirmed aneurysmal disease is screening for concomitant contralateral popliteal artery (greater than 50 per cent incidence) or abdominal aortic (over 30 per cent incidence) aneurysm. Following an exclusion-bypass procedure of an aneurysm, color flow imaging can be used to confirm thrombosis of the aneurysm, and if residual flow is identified, its source can be localized.

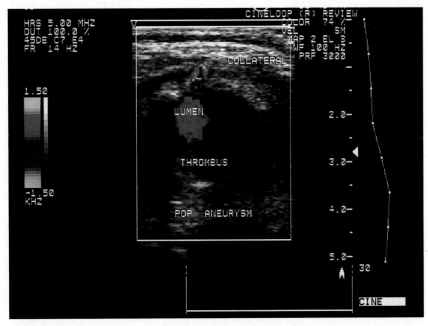

FIGURE 11–8. Transverse color flow image of popliteal aneurysm demonstrating luminal thrombus and an eccentrically positioned flow channel.

Evaluation of Bypass Grafts and PTA Sites

The surveillance of arterial repairs and correction of significant occlusive or aneurysmal lesions following carotid endarterectomy or limb revascularization before occlusion develops in an accepted principle of vascular surgery.[37–41] Particularly following infrainguinal vein bypass, the low sensitivity of ABI measurements in the detection of the hemodynamically failing bypass mandate use of a vascular imaging technique for graft surveillance. Multiple investigators have confirmed the utility of duplex scanning in the postoperative evaluation of bypass graft hemodynamics and identification of graft stenosis.[39–41] As in other clinical applications, a major advantage of color Doppler imaging is the reduction of examination time required to completely map a femorodistal bypass graft. The visual feedback afforded by the color flow imaging enables areas of flow abnormalities to be rapidly identified. Long graft and arterial segments can be assessed in minutes, and color coding of flow facilitates identification of anastomoses and runoff arteries. In a recent experience, color Doppler improved our ability to completely image femorodistal saphenous vein bypass prior to patient discharge from 15 to 69 per cent of grafts studied. Later in the postoperative period, over 90 per cent of the grafts, including anastomotic sites, were successfully imaged and interrogated by spectral analysis (Fig. 11–9). Color imaging of the femoral anastomosis following in situ saphenous bypass grafting typically demonstrated disordered flow patterns with simultaneous forward and reversed flow pixels, consistent with flow-separation phenomena seen at bifurcations and dilated arterial segments. To accurately evaluate the vein conduit for stenosis, RBC flow velocities immediately proximal (inflow artery) to and distal to the zone of disturbed color flow must be compared using pulsed Doppler spectral analysis. A velocity ratio greater than 2.0, or

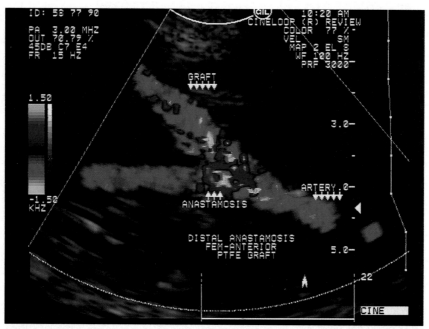

FIGURE 11–9. Color flow image of a normal graft-anterior tibial artery anastomotic site. Color changes do not represent turbulent flow but rather changes in flow direction relative to the angle of the incident sound beam.

peak systolic velocity in excess of 150 cm/sec is evidence that a stenosis is present (Fig. 11–10).

The identification of other postimplantation lesions can also be made with confidence using color Doppler. Arteriovenous communications following in situ bypass grafting are easily noted by demonstrating high-velocity flow in a

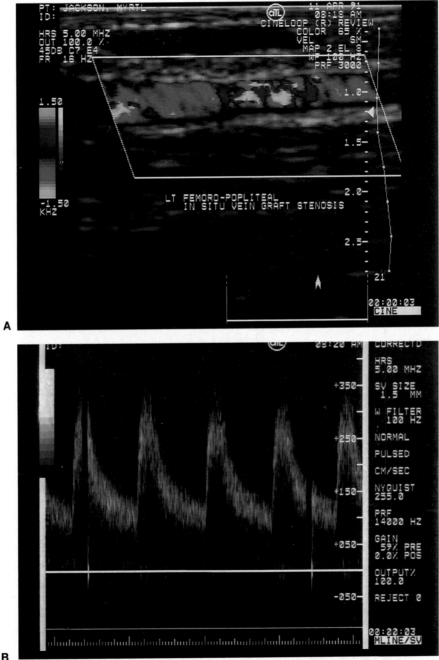

FIGURE 11–10. Abnormal color flow image *A* and velocity spectra *B* recorded from an in situ saphenous vein graft demonstrating a localized region of increased Doppler frequency-shifts due to a retained valve leaflet. Velocity spectral analysis confirm the presence of a high-grade stenosis with end-diastolic velocities greater than 100 cm/sec.

persistent side branch rather than the conduit itself. Groin masses and perigraft fluid collections are easily differentiated from aneurysms by noting the presence of absence of extravascular blood flow. Lastly, myointimal lesions can be differentiated from residual technical errors by serial examinations with the initial color Doppler study occurring in the operating room or prior to discharge from the hospital.

Color Doppler imaging has also demonstrated benefit in assessing the technical adequacy of PTA. To determine the durability of these procedures, a rigorous, objective evaluation identical to direct surgical repairs is required. Not unlike bypass grafts, failure following PTA occurs for multiple reasons including residual stenosis, recurrent disease at the angioplasty site, or disease progression in a remote arterial segment. Duplex ultrasonography is the only noninvasive method capable of evaluating a specific arterial segment for degree of stenosis.[8] We evaluate patients undergoing PTA prior to the procedure and within 1 week of PTA using a combination of ankle pressure measurements and color Doppler imaging. In a prior study, PTA failure and restenosis developed in 89 per cent of limbs if persistent greater than 50 per cent diameter reduction stenosis was identified at the angioplasty site.[42] By contrast, 80 per cent of PTA sites with none or less than 50 per cent diameter reduction stenosis remained patent and did not restenose during a 2-year follow-up period. Color Doppler studies can identify patients with residual stenosis who should be considered for a secondary endovascular procedure. With serial (3 to 6 month intervals) examinations, diagnosis of recurrent PTA stenosis, prior to occlusion, is also possible, and a repeat PTA would be indicated, particularly if the initial procedure demonstrated long-term patency and no disease progression was demonstrated at other locations.

Evaluation of Iatrogenic Vascular Lesions

The femoral artery has become the preferred access route for arteriography and percutaneous endovascular procedures (coronary and peripheral) due to its size and superficial location. The reported incidence of iatrogenic complications following femoral artery puncture has varied between 0.2 to 1 per cent depending on the catheter size, use of anticoagulation or thrombolytic therapy, presence of concomitant occlusive disease, and the expertise of the angiographer.[43-45] Color Doppler imaging has served a valuable function in our institutions in the diagnosis and treatment of vascular complications following these procedures. Lesions which warrant surgical intervention (pseudoaneurysm, vessel thrombosis) are easily distinguished from lesions which may be more appropriately managed by expectant treatment (arteriovenous fistula, hematoma). Operative intervention can be based on the information provided by color flow imaging; for example, size of the pseudoaneurysm, site of communication, patency of distal arterial tree, associated arteriovenous fistula, and presence of luminal thrombus/intimal flap. In a recent study, color flow imaging was used to study the natural history of pseudoaneurysm following cardiac catheterization.[44] All lesions with well-defined borders, smaller than 3.5 cm in diameter, and not associated with an arteriovenous fistula were asymptomatic and thrombosed within 6 weeks of observation. Color Doppler monitoring of pseudoaneurysm thrombosis by probe pressure was successful in 27 of 29 attempts.

Miscellaneous Applications

The full range of clinical applications of color Doppler in arterial imaging is only beginning to be explored. The technology has demonstrated value in the evaluation of abdominal and pelvic organs, tumor vascularity, and intra-operative assessment of vascular reconstructions.[14,45] Diagnosis of hepatic and renal transplant dysfunction based on charges in perfusion patterns has shown promise in differentiating between correctable vascular lesions and parenchymal changes associated with rejection, ischemia, or toxic reaction to drugs.[46,47] Whether clinicians utilize color Doppler in these areas depends on their mastering the complex technology of the instrumentation, and gaining confidence in the diagnostic components of arterial evaluation, such as recognition of normal and diseased characterization of abnormal flow patterns.

SUMMARY

The ability of real-time color Doppler imaging to simultaneously process anatomic and hemodynamic information of the arterial system makes it a powerful noninvasive diagnostic modality. The method has limitations, but these are few in number and most can be overcome with experience and proper patient preparation. An important caveat is that the images generated by color Doppler instruments are not analogous to contrast angiography. The sonographer must be knowledgeable of basic ultrasound physics, arterial anatomy, and hemodynamic changes produced by disease to avoid misinterpretation of the color images, and thus an erroneous diagnosis. For the present time, the best application of color Doppler in arterial imaging is to display the anatomy and assist the user in recognizing sites of flow abnormality, selection of appropriate Doppler angle correction, and precise placement of the pulsed Doppler sample volume to record velocity spectra changes. In selected patients, such as those with focal arterial aneurysms or stenoses, color flow imaging can provide sufficient information that treatment can be instituted without the need for arteriography.

REFERENCES

1. Meritt CR: Doppler color flow imaging. J Clin Ultrasound 1987;*15*:591–597.
2. Zierler RE, Phillips DJ, Beach KW, et al: Noninvasive assessment of normal cartoid bifurcation hemoynamics with color-flow ultrasound imaging. Ultrasound Med Biol 1987;*13*:471–746.
3. Roederer GO, Langlois YE, Jager KA, et al: The natural history of carotid arterial disease in asymptomatic patients with cervical bruits. Stroke 1984;*15*:605–613.
4. Moneta GL, Taylor DC, Nicholls SC, et al: Operative vs nonoperative management of asymptomatic high-grade internal carotid stenosis: Improved results with endarterectomy. Stroke 1987;*18*:1005–1010.
5. Thiele BL, Strandness DE Jr: Accuracy of angiographic quantification of peripheral athero-sclerosis. Prog Cardiovasc Dis 1983;*26*:223.
6. Thiele BL, Bandyk DF, Zierler RE: A systemic approach to the assessment of aortoiliac disease. Arch Surg 1983;*118*:447–450.
7. Flanigan DP, Gray B, Schuler JJ, et al: Utility of wide and narrow blood pressure cuffs in the hemodynamic assessment of aorto-iliac occlusive disease. Surgery 1982;*92*:16–20.
8. Jager KA, Ricketts HJ, Strandness DE Jr: Duplex scanning for the evaluation of lower limb disease. *In* Bernstein EF, ed: Noninvasive Diagnostic Techniques in Vascular Disease. St Louis, MO, CV Mosby Co, 1985;619–631.
9. Taylor KJW, Holland S: Doppler ultrasound, part I. Basic principles, instrumentation, and pitfalls. Radiology 1990;*174*:297–307.

10. Mitchell DG: Color Doppler imaging: Principles, limitations, and artifacts. Radiology 1990; *177*:1–10.
11. Beach KW: Physics and instrumentation of ultrasonic duplex scanning. *In* Strandness DE Jr, ed: Duplex Scanning in Vascular Disorders. New York, NY, Raven Press, 1990;196–227.
12. Phillips DJ, Beach KW, Primozich J, Strandness DE Jr: Should results of ultrasound Doppler studies be reported in units of frequency or velocity. Ultrasound Med Biol 1989;*15*:205–212.
13. Ku DN, et al.: Hemodynamics of the normal human carotid bifurcation: In vitro and in vivo studies. Ultrasound Med Biol 1985;*11*:13–26.
14. Bandyk DF, Govostis D: Intraoperative color flow imaging of "difficult" arterial reconstructions. Video J Color Flow Imaging 1991;*1*:13–20.
15. Erickson SJ, Mewissen MW, Foley DW, et al: Stenosis of the internal carotid artery: Assessment using color Doppler imaging compared with angiography. AJR 1989;*152*:1299–1305.
16. Steinke W, Kloetzch C, Hennerici M: Carotid artery disease assessed by color Doppler flow imaging: Correlation with standard Doppler sonography and angiography. AJR 1990;*154*:0161–1068.
17. Landwehr P, Schindler R, Heinrich U, et al.: Quantification of vascular stenosis with color Doppler flow imaging: In vitro investigations. Radiology 1991;*178*:701–704.
18. Cossman DV, Ellison J, Wagner W, et al: Comparison of contrasst arteriography to arterial mapping with color-flow duplex imaging in the lower extremity. J Vasc Surg 1989;*10*:522–529.
19. Kohler TR, Nance DR, Cramer M, et al: Duplex scanning for diagnosis of aortoiliac and femorpopliteal disease: A prospective study. Circulation 1987;*76*:1074–1080.
20. Middleton WD, Foley WD, Lawson TL: Color flow Doppler imaging of carotid artery abnormalities. AJR 1988;*150*:419–425.
21. Maloney JD, Pairolero PC, Smith BF Jr, et al: Ultrasound evaluation of abdominal aortic aneuryms. Circulation 1977;*56*(suppl 2):11–80.
22. Taylor DC, Moneta GL: Duplex scanning of the renal and mesenteric circulation. *In* Rutherford RB, ed: Seminars in Vascular Surgery. Philadelphia: WB Saunders Co, 1988;*1*:23–31.
23. Hansen KJ, Trible RW, Reavis SW, et al: Renal duplex sonography: Evaluation of clinical utility. J Vasc Surg 1990;*12*;227–236.
24. Villemarette PA, Kornick AL, Rosenberg DML, et al: Color flow Doppler evaluation of the pulsatile mass. J Vasc Tech 1990;*14*:18–24.
25. Abu-Yousef MM, Wiese JA, Shamma AR: The to-and-fro sign: Duplex Doppler evidence of femoral artery pseudoaneurysm. AJR 1988;*150*:632–634.
26. Fellmeth BD, Roberts A, Bookstein JJ, et al: Post angiographic femoral artery injuries: Nonsurgical repair with us-guided compression. Radiology 1991;*178*:671–675.
27. Carroll BA: Carotid sonography. Radiology 1991;*178*;303–313.
28. Bluth EI, Shyn PB, Sullivan MA, Merritt CRB: Doppler color flow imaging of carotid artery dissection. J Ultrasound Med 1989;*8*:149–153.
29. Steinke W, Hennerici M, Anlick A: Doppler color flow imaging of carotid body tumors. Stroke 1989;*20*:1574–1577.
30. Mulligan S, Matsuda T, Lanzer P, et al: Peripheral arterial occlusive disease: Prospective comparison of MR angiography and color duplex ultrasound with conventional angiography. Radiology 1991;*178*:695–700.
31. Londrey GL, Spadone DP, Hodgson KJ, et al: Does color-flow imaging improve the accuracy of duplex carotid evaluation. J Vasc Surg 1991;*13*:659–662.
32. Polak JF, Mitchell KI, Meyerovitz MF: VAlue of color Doppler sonography in predicting the severity of peripheral arterial disease. Radiology 1990;*177*;(supp):124.
33. Foley DW, Erickson JJ, Mewissen M: Color Doppler sonography: Utility in extremity arterial disease. Radiology 1990;*177*;(supp):176.
34. Edwards J, Coldwell D, Goldman M: The role of duplex scanning in the selection for transluminal angioplasty. J Vasc Surg 1991;*13*:69–74.
35. Veith F, Gupta SK, Wengerter KR, et al: Changing arteriosclerotic patterns and management strategies in lower limb-threathening ischemia. Ann Surg 1990;*212*;402–414.
36. Sanborn TA, Cumberland DC, Greenfield AJ, et al: Peripheal laser-assisted balloon angioplasty. Arch Surg 1989;*124*:1099–1103.
37. Dawson I, Hajo van Bockel J, Brand R, et al: Popliteal artery aneurysms: Long-term follow up of aneurysmal disease and the results of surgical treatment. J Vasc Surg 1991;*13*:408–411.
38. Bergamini TM, Towne JB, Bandyk DF, et al: Experience with in situ saphenous vein bypasses during 1981 to 1989: Determinants of long term patency. J Vasc Surg 1991;*13*:137–149.
39. Bandyk DF, Schmitt DD, Seabrook GR, et al: Monitoring functional patency of in situ saphenous vein bypasses: The impact of a surveillance protocol and elective revision. J Vasc Surg 1989;*9*:286–296.
40. Londrey GL, Hodgson KJ, Spadone DP, et al: Initial experience with color-flow duplex scanning of infrainguinal bypass grafts. J Vasc Surg 1990;*12*:284–290.
41. Sladen JG, Reid JDS, Cooperberg PL, et al: Color flow duplex screening of infrainguinal grafts combining low- and high-velocity criteria. Am J Surg 1989;*158*:107–112.

42. Kinney EV, Bandyk DF, Mewissen ME, et al: Monitoring functional patency following percutaneous transluminal angioplasty. Arch Surg 1991;*126*:743–747.
43. Kresowik TF, Khoury MD, Miller BV: A prospective study of the incidence and natural history of femoral vascular complications after percutaneous transluminal coronary angioplasty. J Vasc Surg 1991;*13*:328–336.
44. Oweida SW, Roubin GS, Smith RB, et al: Postcatheterization complications associated with percutaneous transluminal coronary angioplasty. J Vasc Surg 1990;*12*:310–315.
45. Merritt CR: Real-time Doppler color-flow imaging: Other applications. *In* Berstein EF, ed: Recent Advances in Noninvasive Diagnostic Techniques in Vascular Disease. St Louis, MO, CV Mosby Co, 1990;42–56.
46. Rigsby CM, Burns PM, Wetlin GG, et al: Doppler quantification in renal allografts: Comparison in normal and rejecting transplants with pathologic correlation. Radiology 1987;*162*:39–42.
47. McGee GS, Paterson-Kennedy L, Astleford P, Yao JST: Duplex assessment of the renal transplant, Surg Clin N Am 1990;*70*:133–141.

12

NEW APPLICATIONS OF ULTRASOUND

D. EUGENE STRANDNESS, Jr.

Since the introduction of continuous-wave Doppler to clinical practice in the 1960s, dramatic advances have been made both in the development of new technology and its application to clinical practice. The evolution of the technology from the simple hand-held systems to the modern duplex scanning devices has been a remarkable process. For those of us interested in vascular disorders and who saw a pressing need for better noninvasive methods, many of our goals have been met by the new technology and its improvements. It appears that the new duplex scanning systems are now in the phase of improving image quality and Doppler performance. These will not result in major changes in our approach to vascular disease. They will in all likelihood simply make the methods easier to use and perhaps more accurate. Whether these improvements will lead to new applications is a legitimate question, which is difficult to answer.

With regard to vascular disease, the questions that needed an answer (from a diagnostic standpoint) were rather straightforward. In reality, all we need to make a diagnosis and plan therapy is to document the location and extent of the disease (its anatomy) and its effect on function (its physiology). The arteriogram gave us the anatomy of disease, but by itself, did not provide information on its effect on function. The functional effects of the disease were left for the physician to interpret based on patient presentation and performance. While this aspect of patient evaluation is of paramount importance, collecting objective data to confirm the physicians impressions was a goal worthy of pursuit. Many indirect tests were introduced to provide physiologic data that would complement the standard clinical evaluation.

From a practical standpoint, the major bits of information that have been most useful to the surgeon include the precise location of the disease, and its effects on distal pressure and flow. Duplex scanning has provided us information on disease location along with an accurate estimate of the effects of the disease on velocity of flow. Systolic pressure, which is the most reliable index of the functional effects of arterial stenosis and obstruction in the resting state, has been obtained by noninvasive methods such as continuous-wave Doppler. In fact, it is remarkable that it took physicians as long as it did to appreciate the importance of pressure as an index of perfusion and how it was modified by progression of disease, improvements in collateral flow, and direct arterial surgery.

It is always dangerous to predict the future in any field without taking stock of where we are and the changes that will affect our direction. The approach that I will use in this chapter is to examine each area of the circulation that is relevant to the practice of the vascular surgeon and ask the following questions: (1) What is the current status? (2) What information is lacking? And (3) what are the likely directions that new developments will take?

THE CAROTID ARTERY

It is not surprising that duplex scanning was first applied to the carotid artery and that this is where it is most commonly used today. This critical artery was the most accessible to ultrasonic energy, was of immense clinical importance, and was frequently investigated by arteriography. The liberal use of arteriography permitted documentation of the accuracy of duplex scanning. It is also clear that duplex scanning has had a major impact on what we know about the disease and how we handle it.

Current Status

There is little argument that a well-performed duplex scan of the carotid artery can provide accurate data on the degree of narrowing produced by an atherosclerotic plaque. This has been successful because of the documentation of the effects of arterial narrowing on the velocity within the diseased segment of the artery. As the disease progresses and the artery becomes increasingly narrowed, the velocity in the diseased area will increase in a predictable manner. The ability of a well-performed duplex scan to accurately and reproducibly estimate the extent of narrowing has great practical value. For example, now that the North American Symptomatic Carotid Endarterectomy Trial (NASCET) has been in part concluded with the observation that lesions that narrow the carotid bifurcation by 70 per cent or greater are best treated by endarterectomy, the role of duplex scanning becomes even more important.

If a patient presents with transient ischemia attacks (TIA) or a stroke and is found by scanning to have a high-grade stenosis, the plan of action is clear. The patient will have an arteriogram to confirm the degree of narrowing. This will be followed by endarterectomy unless there are other reasons not to do so. For lesser degrees of narrowing, the best therapy remains to be addressed. If during follow-up with duplex scanning the lesion progresses to the 70 per cent stenosis or greater, the patient should by current evidence be offered carotid endarterectomy.

It is also clear that duplex scanning is a satisfactory method of documenting the natural history of the carotid bifurcation atheroma. In fact, it was due to the availability of ultrasound that the relationship between the degree of narrowing, its progression over time, and outcome became better understood.

What Information is Lacking?

A major problem that remains to be evaluated is: Which of the carotid bifurcation plaques pose a real risk to the patient? While there is a definite relationship between the degree of narrowing and clinical events, it is not yet possible to precisely predict which patients are most likely to have a stroke. It is clear that the majority of the "dangerous" carotid artery lesions will never cause a problem. There must be something unusual or unique to the plaque that becomes the cause of a clinical event. There are two changes within the complicated plaque that must be of importance. First, local release of emboli; and second, sudden occlusion due to acute thrombosis. While the processes that lead to both of these problems are similar, this has not yet been proven with any degree of certainty.

This message has not been lost on the surgical community, as evidenced by the attempts to use ultrasound to categorize the changes in the lesions and relate them to clinical events. The factors thought to be important include loss of surface covering (ulceration), intraplaque hemorrhage, necrosis, calcification, and local thrombosis. While these factors singly or in combination are of importance, it has been difficult to relate them in a specific instance to clinical events or projected outcome.

Likely Directions for the Future

Given the advances in computer memory and software, it is now feasible to carry out three-dimensional reconstructions of any object from which accurate data on the X, Y, and Z coordinates can be obtained. This can be obtained with repetitive "slicing" of the carotid artery low in the neck to past the bifurcation. Each of these planar images can then be put together in a three-dimensional format, which in theory should provide information on the nature of the surface, the homogeneity or heterogeneity of the plaque, and a rough estimate of the types of materials within the lesions. This type of data can then be confirmed by performing similar scanning when the plaque is excised and in a more favorable environment (from an ultrasound standpoint).

Once these two procedures have been carried out, it is then possible to carry out similar reconstructions of the gross and microscopic pathology of the lesion as viewed by the pathologist. With this type of data, another three-dimensional reconstruction can be done comparing the results with those obtained with ultrasound. By using this format, it may be possible to not only identify the major constituents of the plaque by their location, but to also assess their volume.

This work is underway and it is much too early to provide any certain results other than to indicate that it is feasible within certain limits that will undoubtedly become apparent but also may change as the research proceeds. It will be necessary to not only verify the accuracy of ultrasound in documenting the pathology of the plaque, but to also relate the pathologic findings to the clinical status of the patient. This will require comparing the findings from subsets of patients who are operated upon for symptoms, versus those who are asymptomatic. It must be admitted that this is a difficult and possibly impossible task, but it appears to be worthy of the effort. The payoff could be important and could add to our ability to predict the clinical course of patients when first encountered with carotid artery disease.

ACUTE DEEP VEIN THROMBOSIS

Next to carotid artery disease, the use of duplex scanning to detect the presence of deep vein thrombi has rapidly become the standard diagnostic method. The method permits both the precise localization of the thrombus and its effects on flow. In addition, it is suitable for follow-up studies to assess the effects of therapy.

Current Status

It now is clear that compared to venography, duplex scanning is accurate in establishing the presence or absence of venous thrombi. While the plethysmographic studies were able to detect thrombi in the proximal deep veins (popliteal to inferior vena cava) precise localization of the thrombi was not feasible. With the advent of duplex scanning, the diagnosis of acute deep vein thrombosis (DVT) depended upon one or more of the following findings: visualization of the thrombus, the lack of compressibility of the imaged vein, and the appearance of abnormal flow of patterns that develop when the venous system is obstructed.

Another desirable feature of the method is that it can be used to document the rate of lysis of the thrombus and its effect on venous valve function. This is very important, since for the first time we are able to document the natural history of the disorder and how this is influenced by therapy.

What Information is Lacking?

While the patient who presents for the first time with an episode of deep vein thrombosis is not a problem in most cases, this is not true with those patients who have had a previous episode and again present with symptoms or signs. In this setting, it may be nearly impossible to determine from an ultrasonic standpoint whether some of the observed changes are new or old. What is urgently needed is firm information on how to predict the age of a thrombus from the changes seen by ultrasound. While it has been my impression that the early thrombi are uniformly echogenic, this has not been widely accepted.

Another problem that urgently needs attention is the relationship between venous thrombi confined to the veins below the knee and their natural history. Are these thrombi confined to the veins below the knee of clinical significance? Are these thrombi indeed benign or do they have the potential to lead to changes in the venous valves that will lead to the development of the post-thrombotic syndrome? This should be possible to determine if this patient population can be identified and followed prospectively.

Likely Directions for the Future

For ultrasound to become the complete method for the evaluation of acute deep vein thrombosis, it will be necessary to develop criteria for thrombus age. While the work that has been done would suggest that the early thrombi are the most echogenic, this will require further confirmation using a model that is both suitable and realistic in terms of what is seen in the human. When this becomes feasible, we will be in a strong position to accurately evaluate all patients with acute, chronic, and acute recurrent symptoms to assess the basis for their presenting complaints.

The one area that has been most difficult to evaluate, with regard to the presence of acute venous thrombi, has been below the knee. This is due to the fact that "black and white" scanning is not always successful in identifying all the major paired veins in this region. It may be that color Doppler may play a very key role in this regard. The ability to immediately visualize the paired veins would be very helpful in the detection of acute thrombi.

PERIPHERAL ARTERIAL DISEASE

The greatest amount of experience has been in the use of continuous-wave (CW) Doppler in the lower limbs. This device has been used as a method for the evaluation of arterial velocity signals at all levels of the upper and lower limbs. In addition, CW Doppler has been very useful for the measurement of limb systolic blood pressures. These measurements can be made to document the effect of arterial disease when the patient is at rest or following a period of exercise or reactive hyperemia. In fact, this simple device has become the standard for the evaluation for nearly all patients with suspected or confirmed peripheral arterial disease. With increasing use of duplex scanning, during the past few years, it has become apparent that this method may also play an important role in the evaluation of peripheral arterial problems. Several applications have emerged that are of demonstrated value, along with some new approaches that will require considerably more time and effort to evaluate.

Current Status

At the present time, one application that appears to have been well accepted is the surveillance of vein grafts to document sites of stenosis that may be responsible for graft failure. It has been established that during the first year, myointimal hyperplasia may develop and can be detected at relatively early stages by duplex scanning.

Since it is possible to scan the entire limb from the level of the abdominal aorta to the pedal arteries, it should be possible to use the method for selection of patients for both angioplasty or direct arterial surgery or both. In the studies done to date, it appears to be feasible as long as the laboratory is experienced in the procedure.

What Information is Lacking?

As with most new applications of technology, a major problem that needs to be solved is the more widespread testing of the procedure for an intended application. This is not a simple matter, since the study technique has to be mastered, and the study criteria developed and carefully controlled to ensure that bias does not play a role in the data analysis. The major step that is most difficult is the implementation of a new approach such as this to daily practice. To perform direct arterial surgery without the preoperative use of arteriography is such a major step and deviation from the standard of care, that it is likely to take many years to implement.

Likely Directions for the Future

It would appear certain that wider use of duplex scanning will continue to occur, and with the passage of time, this will become the standard for the evaluation of patients with peripheral arterial disease.

Since ultrasound has the capability of making measurements of interfaces with differing acoustic impedance, it may be feasible to use the method for the sequential monitoring of atherosclerosis to document progression/regression. While the most attractive use of the method would be to monitor the changes in the fully developed atherosclerotic plaque, this presents several problems, some of which are as follows:

1.   The lesion is three-dimensional, making measurements in a single plane at best suspect as representing changes in the entire lesion.

2.   It is difficult to be certain that the sampling is being done at the same site from time to time.

3.   The degree of stenosis and its change over time is best estimated by the measurement of the velocity changes in the narrowed segment.

4.   Calcification within the lesion by the producing acoustical shadowing may make the estimation of changes within the lesion difficult if not impossible.

One possible way of using ultrasound to monitor the progression/regression of atherosclerosis is to make measurements of arterial wall thickness at sites that do not frequently calcify or progress to the stage of the fully developed complicated plaque. This presumes that the changes in wall thickness at these alternate sites accurately reflect the underlying disease process.

In using ultrasound to interrogate arteries, it is clear that for most locations, it is impossible to make an estimate of wall thickness due to the fact that the adventitial interface with surrounding tissue is not sharp enough to permit any measurements to be made. However, there are sites where the artery can be examined using the vein wall as well. A major assumption that has to be made is that atherosclerosis does not affect the vein, so that any changes in wall thickness that are observed are occurring in the artery alone. This appears to be a reasonable assumption.

Preliminary studies are underway to document the changes in arterial wall thickness at the following sites—common carotid, proximal mid and distal superficial femoral artery, and the brachial artery. These sites were chosen for the following reasons:

1.   The brachial artery, for reasons that are not understood, rarely develops atherosclerosis. It could be a good test site for documenting the effects of aging alone on wall thickness.

2.   The common carotid artery is rarely the site for the development of the complicated plaque, but does develop severe intimal thickening as is well known by surgeons who perform carotid endarterectomy. The transection of the proximal intimal-medial segment often reveals the extent to which this artery has developed the thickening of the arterial wall. What is not known are the factors that lead to this process developing in the first place—hypertension, elevations of lipoproteins, diabetes mellitus, and cigarette smoking; all of which may be present either singly or in combination.

3.   The superficial femoral artery is the most common site in the lower limb for the development of atherosclerosis. It is also known that the adductor canal region is where most of the complicated far-advanced lesions develop. While intimal thickening frequently occurs in the other segments of the superficial femoral artery, it is unusual to see the far-advanced complicated plaques in the proximal superficial femoral artery with the same frequency. This might be an ideal site for study, since atherosclerosis resulting in an increase in wall thickness can be studied over time.

The procedures for making the measurement here are currently being developed, but basically revolve around the detection of the "edge interface" between the artery wall and the flowing blood. The accuracy of the method will depend upon the type of image that can be obtained and the reproducibility of the measurements. It appears that the images obtained from the common carotid artery are good enough to permit accurate measurements to be made.

Image quality for the deeper segments of the superficial femoral artery are not as good, but may be satisfactory for the purposes of this study.

VISCERAL CIRCULATION

Until duplex scanning appeared, it was impossible to study the blood supply to the gut and the kidneys by any noninvasive means. This left only the use of arteriography as a suitable method for documenting the status of the inflow to these important organs. Mesenteric arterial disease can lead to the development of intestinal angina, and in later stages, infarction of the gut. Renal arterial stenosis is a major cause of hypertension and renal failure. Detection of renal artery stenosis is important because it may lead to the use of procedures to correct the stenosis and cure the hypertension. In addition, progressive, bilateral renal artery stenosis can lead to "ischemic renal failure" requiring dialysis.

Current Status

From an ultrasonic standpoint, the study of the mesenteric blood supply is relatively straightforward when the goal is the detection of high-grade (greater than 50 per cent) stenoses which can be the cause of intestinal angina. It is now accepted that in order to have this problem, it is necessary to have involvement of the superior mesenteric, celiac, and inferior mesenteric arteries. If any one of these arteries is not involved, the collateral circulation that develops is sufficient to provide adequate blood flow to the small bowel and prevent the development of chronic mesenteric angina.

For the study of the renal arteries, it is necessary to document not only the presence of arterial narrowing, but to relate this to its role in the activation of the renin-angiotensin system. While this has been successfully done, the examination is difficult to do, requiring an expert and dedicated technologist. Even given the difficulties in the examination, the information obtained is very important, since it either rules in or out disease of the renal arteries as the cause of the problem.

What Information is Lacking?

For the mesenteric circulation, it is yet uncertain at what stage the extent of narrowing will limit the blood-flow response to an ingested meal. While it would appear intuitively obvious that one could use a meal as an intestinal stress test to uncover underlying lesions in the blood supply to the gut, this has not yet proven to be true. If a pattern did appear, it could prove to be very important as a diagnostic test for those patients who have abdominal pain with chronic mesenteric ischemia as one of the potential causes.

In the renal circulation, it is not yet clear what role the intrarenal circulation and changes at this level play in the pathogenesis of hypertension or renal failure or both. For example, while it may be possible to detect a renal artery stenosis, how could one detect a change in the resistance within the kidney as a possible factor contributing to the hypertension. While it is possible to examine the resistance to flow by measurements of ratios that include changes in the end-diastolic velocity, it has not yet been clear how useful these changes will be in quantifying renal parenchymal changes. Another factor that complicates the validation of the noninvasive studies is the lack of tissue that might be helpful in documenting the changes taking place within the kidney itself.

Likely Directions for the Future

For the future, it is clear that continued study and refinement of the methods will take place. The recent improvements in image quality and the availability of color will make the study procedures easier and perhaps more accurate as well. It will also be necessary for more studies to look at the problem of renal artery stenosis over time to define its natural history. This is of critical importance, since without this natural history data it will be difficult to determine the optimum therapy when patients are first seen.

DISCUSSION

It has been remarkable that in the short span of 10 years duplex ultrasound has become such an important diagnostic test for the evaluation of vascular disease wherever it occurs. In its initial testing and application, most efforts were concentrated on the carotid circulation. While this remains the most commonly test done with duplex scanning, the applications have widened considerably.

While it would be nice to predict the future applications of ultrasound, this is very risky because of the appearance of new technology. For example, when duplex scanning was being applied to the carotid artery, it was not possible to obtain useful information from other sites such as the legs or the abdomen because of the limitations in the technology that was available.

There were two developments that were essential for the more widespread application of duplex scanning. The first was the recognition of the clinical need. For example, when the issue of peripheral arterial scanning was first discussed, it was not clear that the method would ever have an application here because of the great length of the arteries that might be involved and the time it might take to scan these arteries. Yet when the technology was sufficiently developed to permit the use of duplex scanning to the arteries from the level of the abdominal aorta to the tibial-peroneal arteries, progress accelerated.

The procedures employed in testing a new diagnostic test are quite simple. It is necessary to first demonstrate how often the normal subject can be successfully studied. If the important information can be regularly obtained, it is then necessary to determine those parameters that might be of diagnostic importance to establish a normal range of values for the test. In doing such studies, it is necessary to work from both ends of the spectrum of involvement— those with clinically evident disease, back to those who are known to be free of disease. However, even when this process is completed, there will always be a "gray zone" where some uncertainty remains.

It is at this stage where refinements in the diagnostic approach may take place. For example, in the evolution of carotid artery testing, it was noted early in our experience that the specificity of the test was poor, being in the range of 37 per cent. This was unsatisfactory, since it meant that 63 per cent of normal patients would be labeled as having carotid artery atherosclerosis. In examining the data, it became clear that the problem was not in classifying normal subjects as having high-grade stenoses, but rather those with minimal degrees of disease. It soon became evident that the reason for the poor specificity was in the interpretation of the flow changes in the bulb of normal subjects that we now know is secondary to boundary layer separation. In the early phases of our studies, we did not recognize this as being a normal finding and thus classified many normals as having minimal disease. Once it was noted that boundary layer separation was a normal finding, the specificity of the procedure rose to over 90 per cent.

Another area where test results confirming the accuracy of the testing has revealed problems that will need to be solved in the future is with deep vein thrombosis. As noted earlier, one of the major problems that will need to be resolved is the patient with a history of previous deep vein thrombosis who appears with recurrent symptoms. At the present time it is difficult to separate the findings associated with acute occlusion from those seen in patients with chronic venous obstruction.

For the forseeable future, most new developments will represent new wrinkles from existing technology. For example, all ultrasound companies are always in the process of improving both their B-mode image and their Doppler component, and more recently, their color presentation. While these improvements, from a commercial standpoint, are designed to increase their companies' share of the market, the impact on the daily or projected use of ultrasound will be of marginal benefit.

The reasons for only marginal benefit from a clinical standpoint are quite simple. For example, will the imaging component become so much better that all the necessary answers that have been asked will be immediately answered? The answer is obviously no. This is due to the fact that the improvements will not be of the scale necessary to be considered such an advance. The same would appear to be true for the Doppler component of the systems. Color will undoubtedly fall into the same category.

In considering the future of the field, it is important to consider alternative forms of diagnosis that could impact on the field of ultrasound. At the moment, the only potential competitor appears to be magnetic resonance imaging (MRI). The imaging component of the system is indeed impressive, providing the kind of detail that has never been seen before. It is also clear that the method can be used for real-time imaging of blood vessels. There is good early evidence that it may be feasible to perform MRI arteriography of the large and medium sized arteries with a resolution at present that is equal to that obtained by intravenous digital subtraction arteriography. While this is unsatisfactory for many applications, it is also clear that this will undoubtedly improve.

If progress with MRI continues, it may well be that this method could become a replacement for standard arteriographic studies. While this might appear to be a worthwhile goal, its realization may be impossible from time and economic standpoints. At present, MRI systems are so fully utilized that they would be virtually impossible to use as a method to handle the arteriography cases that need to be done. It also appears that most institutions would be unable to defray the costs of additional MRI systems to meet this need.

While standard arteriographic procedures do not lend themselves for follow-up studies due to their cost and invasive nature, many of these same problems are presented by MRI. Since unlimited space and funds are not available, it is likely that ultrasound will continue to play an important role in this field.

In conclusion, while new developments will continue to appear, it is not likely that they will be of the revolutionary nature that had its beginning in the 1970s. This will be a time of refinement with extended applications of existing technology.

13

THE USE OF TRANSCRANIAL DOPPLER IN CAROTID ARTERY DISEASE

C. JANSEN, R.G.A. ACKERSTAFF, and BERT C. EIKELBOOM

During the last decades, many invasive and noninvasive diagnostics have been developed to reveal atherosclerosis of the cerebral vasculature and to evaluate the hemodynamic sequelae of stenoses and occlusions. Although arteriography is still preferred by many institutions to demonstrate morphological changes of the cerebral arteries, ultrasonic duplex scanning now is generally accepted as a reliable noninvasive technique to assess extracranial atherosclerosis. Since Aaslid in 1982 described a pulsed Doppler technique with a relatively low emitting frequency of 2-MHz to investigate the cerebral arteries, many studies have reported the usefullness of transcranial Doppler (TCD) sonography in patients with cerebrovascular disorders. With TCD it is possible to directly investigate the intracranial segments of the cerebral vasculature. In combination with carotid artery compression, the collateral pathways and in particular the circle of Willis can also be evaluated.

Moreover, transcranial Doppler has been used in combination with induced hypercapnia to estimate the vasomotor reactivity of the cerebral arterioles in patients with hemodynamically significant lesions. In several studies, an interrelationship between the extent of disease, adequacy of collaterals, vasomotor reactivity, and clinical state of the patient have been demonstrated.

Finally, transcranial Doppler sonography is the only technique to continuously noninvasively register the blood-flow velocities in the middle cerebral artery. It is therefore increasingly used as a monitoring function during surgical procedures, as for example, during carotid endarterectomy.

ASSESSMENT OF INTRACRANIAL STENOSIS

Since the introduction of duplex scanning in our laboratory, the assessment of extracranial atherosclerosis is mainly performed by noninvasive diagnostics. Intra-arterial angiography is only used in a minority of the patients. Although the risk of stroke is high if significant intracranial lesions are present,[2] the incidence of such lesions is relatively low and, therefore, screening arteriograms are frequently negative. This makes clinicians hesitant to apply invasive techniques only for the evaluation of the intracranial arteries. We feel, on the contrary, that this attitude bears the risk of missing the correct vascular diagnosis. Thus, a reliable noninvasive estimation of intracranially located hemodynamically significant stenoses and occlusions has now achieved major importance. Transcranial Doppler has opened perspectives for such detections as of obstructive disease of the carotid syphon and main stem of the middle cerebral artery. For the assessment of stenotic lesions in these segments of the cerebral vasculature, sonographic criteria such as local increase of blood-flow velocities, a spectrum distribution with increased low-frequency components, and the occurrence of "musical murmurs" have been used by several authors. As blood-flow velocities vary with age, sex, carbon dioxide tension, and cerebral vascular resistance,[3-5] it is not prudent to use rigid average velocity values for the diagnosis of vascular obstructive disease. However, validation of the results with angiographical data is described in only a few studies.[6-8] In a group of 133 consecutive patients, Ringelstein et al[9] reported remarkably good agreement between the findings of TCD and selective cerebral arteriography. The accuracy for the detection of stenosing or occluding lesions was presented in terms of sensitivity, specificity, positive and negative predictive values, and a chance-corrected measure of agreement (kappa). For both the carotid syphon and the main stem of the middle cerebral artery, the values of these parameters were mostly higher than 90 per cent and kappa was close to +1. In several studies, however, differentiation from vasospasm or high blood-flow velocities in a collateral pathways such as the anterior or posterior cerebral arteries (by means of TCD only) still remained difficult.[10,11] This is one of the main reasons the sonographer has to be aware of the extent of extracranial disease to correctly understand and identify cross-filling phenomena. In general, for the assessment of significant stenoses in the intracranial segments of the cerebral arteries, transcranial Doppler is a valid method when this technique is used in combination with selective arteriography. The combined use of these two methods may result in the delineation of otherwise unrecognized lesions.

EVALUATION OF COLLATERAL PATHWAYS

Although during the past 20 years surgical treatment for carotid artery disease has been performed on a large scale,[12,13] it is not known exactly which patients really need carotid endarterectomy. Until recently, the decision as to whether carotid surgery should be recommended or not was made according to individual patients. With respect to symptomatic patients, the indications have now been narrowed to cases with documented internal carotid artery stenosis of 70 per cent linear reduction or more.[14,15] This group of patients will benefit from surgery, according to the announcement of the collaborators of the North American Symptomatic Carotid Endarterectomy Trial (NASCET) and the European Carotid Surgery Trial (ECST) in 1991.[16]

Knowledge of the natural history of asymptomatic internal carotid artery stenosis is also increasing. In general, patients with asymptomatic carotid stenosis have a remarkably low overall risk of stroke,[17-19] However, widespread application of noninvasive testing has indicated that a subgroup of patients with hemodynamically significant lesions have an annual stroke risk of 4 to 12 per cent.[20-22] In these studies, many of the neurologic events were unheralded strokes. Nevertheless, it is still not yet known if such a stroke rate is high enough to justify carotid surgery. Our discussion will focus on what may be an important factor of progressive extracranial obstructive disease: namely, the presence or absence of sufficient collateral circulation. In other words, the clinical outcome of significant cerebral atherosclerosis may be partially linked to differences in available collateral circulation and vasomotor reactivity. Simple noninvasive tests such as electroencephalogram (EEG), occuloplethysmography (OPG), and TCD can be used to evaluate a patient's collateral system.[23-25] Evaluation of the periorbital collateral circulation between the external and internal carotid arteries can now be employed with transcranial Doppler as well. Through the transorbital approach, the ophthalmic artery itself is an easily accessible vessel which reflects hemodynamic alterations due to cerebrovascular disease. There is a direct relation between the ophthalmic systolic pressure as measured with OPG and the ophthalmic artery blood flow velocity.[26] Therefore, this technique may enhance our understanding of the role of the ophthalmic artery in cerebrovascular obstructive disease. Furthermore, the TCD technique has also shown promise in the identification of hemodynamically significant intracerebral collaterals.[27,28] Combining transcranial Doppler sonography with carotid compression provides information on the functional status of the circle of Willis or, more specifically, on the anterior and posterior communicating arteries. Finally, TCD in combination with hypercapnia or intravenous acetazolanide (Diamox) tests whether the cerebral precapillary vessels are able to dilate, which is a normal phenomenon of autoregulation.[29-31] However, when vasodilatation is already maximal as in the case of significant cerebrovascular disease with insufficient collateral circulation, increase of the intra-arterial carbon dioxide pressure will not lead to further vasodilatation. The so-called vasomotor reactivity (VMR) is then reduced. Thus, the VMR is a reflection of the reserve capacity of the cerebral vasculature and is usually expressed as the percentage change in blood-flow velocity of the middle artery per absolute change in end-tidal carbon dioxide. In a study of 86 patients with unilateral occlusion of the internal carotid artery, Keunen[32] evaluated the relation between the degree of contralateral disease, the functional state of the circle of Willis, the direction of periorbital blood flow, the vasomotor reactivity, and the clinical outcome of the patient. In this study, four types of Willis circulation were identified: a complete type with functioning anterior and posterior communicating arteries, the anterior and posterior types with only one of the two communicating arteries functioning, and the incomplete type without and functioning communicating artery. Reversal of the periorbital blood-flow direction occurred if the ipsilateral internal carotid artery had a linear stenosis of 65 per cent or more. Compared to patients with a complete circle of Willis, a significant decrease of VMR was noted in patients with a partial or incomplete type of the circle. Ipsilateral to an occluded internal carotid artery, a physiological periorbital blood flow was indicative of a complete circle of Willis and a normal VMR, and vice versa. In patients with an incomplete circle of Willis, occlusion of the internal carotid artery resulted mostly in cerebral deficit, whereas in patients with a complete circle, the occlusion remained asymptomatic. For the maintenance of adequate cerebral circulation, the basilar and posterior communicating arteries were more important than the anterior communicating or ophthalmic arteries.[26,32]

INTRAOPERATIVE MONITORING DURING CAROTID ENDARTERECTOMY

The complication rate of carotid endarterectomy varies greatly between centers[33,34] and should be held to an absolute minimum to ensure that this prophylactic operation is superior to conservative nonsurgical treatment. The most important cause of cerebral damage during carotid surgery is probably thromboembolism.[35] Another risk ensues from carotid artery cross-clamping, which reduces cerebral perfusion and may give rise to ischemia when the collateral cerebral circulation is not sufficient; for example, when there is contralateral carotid artery stenosis and an incomplete circle.[25] In selected cases, the risk of a low-flow state during clamping is reduced by shunting.[36,37] Unselected use of a shunt, however, carries the risk of embolization during shunt insertion.

The phenomenon of hyperperfusion has been discussed recently.[38-40] High cerebral blood-flow velocities occurring immediately after endarterectomy and restoration of physiological vascular resistance in the extracranial vessels potentially endangers the ipsilateral hemisphere. In some patients this hyperperfusion causes intracerebral hematomas.

To control intraoperative cerebral function and manifestations of low flow, thromboembolic events, and hyperperfusion, we use both an EEG monitoring system[41] and a transcranial Doppler monitoring unit. The EEG is recorded from frontoparietal and temporo-occipital lobes on both sides. The EEG monitoring system provides automatic acquisition and recording of the EEG as well as data concerning the blood pressure and anesthetics used. Relevant features are extracted from these data and abnormal activity results in automatic alarm, which is directly transmitted to the surgeon, the anesthesiologist, and the neurophysiologist. Asymmetry between the hemispheres is numerically displayed. The neurophysiologist compares the data (which are graphically displayed) with the on-line EEG, which is important in ruling out EEG artifacts. Asymmetry is calculated by using the formula: (Nleft − Nright / Nleft + Nright) × 100 per cent, in which N is the number of zero crossings of the EEG signal measured during the last 15 seconds. Asymmetry greater than 15 per cent is considered severe, and when it emerges during cross-clamping, is a sign of hemodynamic insufficiency and poor collateral circulation. In such cases the use of a shunt is advocated. In a series of 230 carotid endarterectomies performed with this EEG system before the introduction of TCD monitoring, a shunt was used in 35 (15.2 per cent) cases. Eleven strokes were noticed immediately after surgery (4.8 per cent), five major and six minor strokes. Four of these major strokes were heralded by persistent severe EEG asymmetry. One major and all minor strokes ran their course undetected by the EEG monitoring. With transcranial Doppler the hemodynamic state of the brain and the collateral circulation can be investigated before and during carotid surgery.[42,43] Reduction of blood-flow velocity in the middle cerebral artery on the operated side during cross-clamping depends on the degree of stenosis of the operated vessel and the intracranial collateral circulation. Another important application of TCD is the detection of emboli dislodged in the bloodstream during surgery. Emboli may be detected by Doppler ultrasonography not only in the laboratory,[44,45] but also in clinical practice. Cerebral embolism has been documented in diver's illness and during cardiovascular and carotid surgery.[46-48] In our institution we use a pulsed Doppler transducer gated at a focal depth of 45 to 60 mm which is placed over the temporal bone to insonate the main stem of the middle cerebral artery. Ipsilateral carotid artery compression tests confirm that the middle cerebral artery is being insonated. The transducer is fixed with a head strap, and video recordings of the Doppler spectra and audio signals are registered from the time the patient is intubated until the end of anesthesia. The Doppler audio signal is audible in the operating theater throughout the entire procedure. Signals of embolization, which have a very characteristic crisping, chirping quality[21] exert a direct influence on the surgical team. In the course of carotid endarterectomy, several moments of embolization can be expected. During manipulation of the artery in the first phase of the operation, small emboli can be dislodged from the vessel wall when the vessel is tilted or retracted with a clip, a vessel loop, or a pair of tweezers. These emboli probably consist of small atheromatous particles from the atherosclerotic vessel wall. We frequently observe that detection of emboli in this phase influences the technique of the surgeon. After the endarterectomy and flushing of the vessel, emboli are often detected during release of the internal carotid artery clamp. These signals probably represent small air bubbles, platelet thrombi, or both. In case of an external-internal collateral circulation via the ophthalmic artery, emboli can be detected in the middle cerebral artery even after release of the external carotid artery clamp. Introduction of a needle for measurement of stump pressure is often accompanied by short embolization signals.

A decrease of blood-flow velocities on cross-clamping of more than 75 per cent probably reflects to impending ischemia. Following restoration of flow, a marked increase in blood-flow velocities must alert the physician to take measures in order to prevent hyperperfusion injury.

In our institution, embolization is detected in 39 per cent of all carotid endarterectomies. After surgery in most of these cases, there are no new neurological deficits or brain infarcts on the computed tomographic (CT) scanning. In a series of 100 carotid endarterectomies, 2 intraoperative minor strokes occurred. One had massive embolization during several minutes at release of the clamp, the other showed a 75 per cent reduction of blood-flow velocity upon cross-clamping and developed a watershed infarct. In this patient the EEG revealed asymmetry of 10 to 15 per cent during test clamping and, therefore, a shunt was not used. Finally, one patient developed a hematoma in the territory of an old infarct 5 days after surgery. Intraoperative morbidity has declined in our institution after the introduction of TCD monitoring during carotid endarterectomy. It shows that careful intraoperative monitoring and the continuous auditive feedback from the TCD unit may help to reduce the number of intraoperative strokes.

REFERENCES

1. Aaslid R, Markwalder TM, Nornes H: Non-invasive Doppler ultrasound recording of flow velocity in basal cerebral arteries. Neurosurgery 1982;57:769–774.
2. Bogousslavsky J, Barnett HJM, Fox AJ, Hachinski VC, Taylor W: Atherosclerotic disease of the middle cerebral artery. Stroke 1986;17:1112–1120.
3. Grolimund P, Seiler RW: Age dependency of the flow velocity in the basal cerebral arteries— a transcranial Doppler ultrasound study. Ultrasound Biol 1988;14:191–198.
4. Vriens EM, Kraaier V, Musbach M, Wieneke G, van Huffelen AC: Transcranial pulsed Doppler measurements of blood velocity in the middle cerebral artery: Reference values at rest and during hyperventilation in healthy volunteers in relation to age and sex. Ultrasound Med Biol 1989;15:1–18.

5. Ackerstaff RGA, Keunen RWM, van Pelt W, Montauban van Swijndregt AD, Stijnen T: Influence of biological factors on changes in mean cerebral blood flow velocity in normal ageing: A transcranial Doppler study. Neurol Res 1990;*12*:187–192.

6. Lindegaard K-F, Bakke SJ, Aaslid R, Nornes H: Doppler diagnosis of intracranial occlusive disorders. J Neurol Neurosurg Psychiatr 1986;*49*:510–518.

7. Arnolds B, Oehme A, Schumacher M, Reutern C-M von: Detection of intracranial stenosis and occlusion with transcranial Doppler sonography. J Cardiovasc Ultrasonogr 1986;*5*:Abstract 22.

8. Mattle H, Grolimund P, Huber P, Strurzenegger M, Zurbrügg HR: Transcranial Doppler sonographic findings in middle cerebral artery disease. Arch Neurol 1988;*45*:289–295.

9. Ley-Pezo J, Ringelstein EB: Noninvasive detection of occlusive disease of the carotid siphon and middle cerebral artery. Ann Neurol 1990;*28*:640–647.

10. Aaslid R, Huber P, Nornes H: A transcranial Doppler method in the evaluation of cerebrovascular spasm. Neuroradiology 1986;*26*:11–16.

11. Grolimund P, Seiler RW, Aaslid R: Evaluation of cerebrovascular disease by combined extracranial and transcranial Doppler sonography. Experience in 1039 patients. Stroke 1987;*18*:1018–1024.

12. Dyken M, Pokras R: The performance of endarterectomy for disease of the extracranial arteries of the head. Stroke 1984;*15*:948–950.

13. Warlow C: Carotid endarterectomy, does it work? Stroke 1984;*15*:1068–1076.

14. Toronto Cerebrovascular Study Group: Risks of carotid endarterectomy. Stroke 1986;*17*:848–852.

15. North American Symptomatic Carotid Endarterectomy Study Group: Carotid endarterectomy: Three critical evaluations. Stroke 1987;*18*:987–989.

16. Warlow CH: MRC European carotid surgery trial: Interim results for symptomatic patients with severe carotid stenosis and with mild carotid stenosis. Lancet 1991 accepted for publication.

17. Rocderer GO, Langlois YE, Jager KA, et al: The natural history of carotid arterial disease in asymptomatic patients with cervical bruits. Stroke 1984;*15*:605–613.

18. Chambers BR, Norris JW: Outcome in patients with asymptomatic neck bruits. Engl Med 1986;*315*:860–865.

19. Barnes RW, Nix ML, Sansonetti D, Tuley DG, Goldman MR: Late outcome of untreated asymptomatic carotid disease following cardiovascular operations. J Vasc Surg 1985;*2*:843–849.

20. Bogousslavsky J, Despland P-A, Regli F: Asymptomatic tight stenosis of the internal carotid artery: Long-term prognosis. Neurology 1986;*36*:861–863.

21. Hennerici M, Hulsbomer H-B, Hefter H, Lammerts D, Rautenberg W: Natural history of asymptomatic extracranial arterial disease: Results of a long-term prospective study. Brain 1987;*110*:777–791.

22. Moneta GL, Taylor DC, Nicholls SC, et al: Operative versus nonoperative management of asymptomatic high-grade internal carotid artery stenosis: Improved results with endarterectomy. Stroke 1987;*18*:1005–1010.

23. Moll FL, Eikelboom BC, Vermeulen FEE, van Lier HJJ: Dynamics of collateral circulation in progressive asymptomatic carotid disease. J Vasc Surg 1986;*3*:470–474.

24. Eikelboom BC, Vermeulen FEE: The value of ocular pneumoplethysmography versus angiography in the determination of the potential collateral hemispheric circulation. *In* Diethrich G, ed: Noninvasive Cardiovascular Diagnosis, 2nd ed. Littleton, MA, PSG Publishing, 1981.

25. Eikelboom BC, Welten RJTH, Ackerstaff RGA, Vermeulen FEE: Recognizing stroke prone patients with a poor collateral circulation. Eur J Vasc Surg 1987;*1*:381–384.

26. Schneider PA, Rossman ME, Bernstein EF, Ringelstein EB, Otis SM: Noninvasive assessment of cerebral collateral blood supply through ophthalmic artery. Stroke 1991;*22*:31–36.

27. Schneider PA, Rossman ME, Bernstein EF, Torem S, Ringelstein EB, Otis SM: Effect of internal carotid artery occlusion on intracranial haemodynamics. Transcranial Doppler evaluation and clinical correlation. Stroke 1988;*19*:589–593.

28. Norris JW, Krajewski A, Bornstein NM: The clinical role of the cerebral collateral circulation in carotid occlusion. J Vasc Surg 1990;*12*:113–118.

29. Bishop CCR, Powell S, Rutt D, Browse NL: The effect of internal carotid artery occlusion on middle cerebral artery blood flow, at rest and response to hypercapnia. Lancet 1986;*1*:710–712.

30. Brown MM, Wade JPH, Bishop CCR, Ross Russell RW: Reactivity of the cerebral circulation in patients with carotid occlusion. J Neurol Neurosurg Psychiatry 1986;*49*:899–904.

31. Schroeder T: Cerebrovascular reactivity to azetazolamide in carotid artery disease. Echancement of side-to-side asymmetry indicates critically reduced perfusion pressure. Neurol Res 1986;*8*:231–236.

32. Keunen RWM: Transcranial Doppler sonography of the cerebral circulation in occlusive cerebrovascular disease. Thesis, Benda BV, Nijmegen, 1991.

33. Barnett HJM: A critique of surgical treatment in cerebrovascular ischemia. *In* McDowell F, Caplan LR, eds: Cerebrovascular Survey Report, 1985;189–209.

34. Lusby RJ, Wylie EJ: Complications of carotid endarterectomy. Surg Clin North Am 1983;*63*:1293–1302.
35. Krul JMJ, van Gijn J, Ackerstaff RGA, et al: Site and Pathogenesis of Infarcts Associated With Carotid Endarterectomy. Stroke 1989;*20*:324–328.
36. Ferguson GG: Intraoperative monitoring and internal shunts: Are they necessary in carotid endarterectomy? Stroke 1982;*13*:287–289.
37. Sundt TM: The ischemic tolerance of neural tissue and the need for monitoring and selective shunting carotid endarterectomy. Stroke 1983;*14*:93–98.
38. Hallenbeck JM, Dutka AJ: Background review and current concepts of reperfusion injury. Arch Neurol 1990;*47*:1245–1254.
39. Schroeder T, Sillesen H, Sorensen O, Engell HCh: Cerebral hyperperfusion following carotid endarterectomy. J Neurosurg 1987;*66*:824–829.
40. Powers AD, Smith RR: Hyperperfusion syndrome after carotid endarterectomy. A transcranial Doppler evaluation. Neurosurgery 1990;*26*:56–60.
41. Pronk RAF, Simons AJR: Automatic EEG monitoring during anesthesia. *In* Prakash O, ed: Computing in Anesthesia and Intensive Care. Boston, Martinus Nijhof Publishers, 1983;227–257.
42. Padayachee TS, Gosling RG, Bishop CC, et al: Monitoring middle cerebral artery blood velocity during carotid endarterectomy. Br J Surg 1986;*73*:98–100.
43. Schneider PA, Bernstein EF: The use of transcranial doppler in carotid surgery. *In* Bergan JJ, Yao JST, eds: Arterial Surgery: New Diagnostic and Operative Techniques. London, Grune and Stratton, 1988;147–159.
44. Pugsley W: The use of Doppler ultrasound in the assessment of microemboli during cardiac surgery. Perfusion 1989;*4*:115–122.
45. Russell D, Madden KP, Clark WM, et al: Detection of Arterial Emboli Using Doppler Ultrasound in Rabbits. Stroke 1991;*22*:253–258.
46. Spencer MP: Decompression limits for compressed air determined by ultrasonically deteted blood bubbles. J Appl Physiol 1976;*40*:229–235.
47. Padayachee TS, Parsons S, Theobold R, et al: The detection of microemboli in the middle cerebral artery during cardiopulmonary bypass: A transcranial Doppler ultrasound investigation using membrane and bubble oxygenators. Ann Thorac Surg 1987;*44*:298–302.
48. Spencer MP, Thomas GI, Nicholls SC, Sauvage LR: Detection of middle cerebral artery emboli during carotid endarterectomy using transcranial Doppler ultrasonography. Stroke 1990;*21*:415–423.

14

TRANSCRANIAL DOPPLER: A New Test for Cerebral Embolism?

JOHN W. NORRIS and C.Z. ZHU

The diagnosis of cerebral embolism is notoriously difficult, yet critical in managing stroke patients, since anticoagulant therapy is a valuable prophylactic against further strokes in cardioembolic strokes, but not in those due to carotid stenosis.[1]

Diagnostic criteria of embolic stroke are so far entirely clinical. Textbooks on stroke indicate the embolic stroke profile as of sudden and dramatic onset, but often with rapid recovery (presumably as the embolus is rapidly lysed). Sometimes there are major seizures at onset, and usually there is an embolic source such as atrial fibrillation, valvular heart disease, or recent myocardial infarction.[2,3] Dissolution of emboli may cause a severe initial hemiplegia, with rapid recovery but with residual cortical deficits such as aphasia, as the embolus lodges distally.[3]

The advent of single-photon emission computerized tomography (SPECT) scanning in recent years allows an evaluation of cerebral perfusion by producing a color-coded image of cerebral perfusion.[4] Recent data of SPECT in stroke indicate that severe perfusion deficits indicate a poor prognosis[5] and that patients with "luxury" perfusion (high flow in the ischemic area) do well and may have embolic stroke.[6]

Transcranial Doppler (TCD) has now been subjected to a variety of evaluations in patients with acute cerebrovascular disorders, and blood-flow velocities (BFV) have been found to be normal, higher, or lower than normal.[6] Because of these preliminary data, we decided to compare clinical features of acute stroke to the findings of TCD and SPECT to determine if a definite relationship could be established in the diagnosis of cardioembolic stroke.

MATERIALS AND METHODS

All patients admitted over a 2-year period to the Acute Stroke Unit in Toronto with hemispheric cerebral infarction and evaluated by TCD were included. They were not consecutive, since not all patients had TCD. Some were too ill for the procedure, or the TCD was not performed for technical reasons, and patients with vertebrobasilar stroke were excluded.

Clinical stroke scores were measured on each patient twice in the first week and thereafter for 3 weeks, weekly, using the Toronto Stroke Scale.[7]

TABLE 14–1. CLINICAL CRITERIA FOR CEREBRAL EMBOLISM[a]

Major criteria
    Simultaneous multiple neurologic events; e.g., bihemispheric infarcts
    Evidence of systemic embolic; e.g., femoral artery occlusion
    Presence of cardiac source; e.g., cardiomyopathy, <3 months MI, atrial fibrillation
    Seizure at onset
Minor criteria
    Sudden and abrupt onset of neurological deficit, often with transient loss of consciousness
    Prominent vascular headache
    Emphasis on cortical events; e.g., aphasia without hemiplegia in hemispheric infarcts
    CT—hemorrhagic infarction or infarcts in more than one vascular territory.

[a] High risk, 1 major criteria; medium risk, 3 minor criteria; low risk, 1 or 2 minor criteria.

An empirical Toronto Embolic Score was created (Table 14–1) with three grades of probability—high, medium, none. Since there is no "gold standard" for cardioembolic stroke, this score could not be objectively evaluated. Points were allotted for major criteria (3), minor criteria (2), and no criteria for cerebral embolism (1).

Single-photon emission computerized tomography scanning was performed using twenty mC of ^{99m}Tc HmPAO (Ceretec) injected intravenously and tomoscintography begun 15 to 30 minutes later. Scans were performed parallel to the orbitomeatal line using a laser positioning system to allow comparison to computed tomographic (CT) scans. Computerized reconstructions were in the axial, coronal, and sagittal planes, correcting for small degrees of head tilt or movement. Color-coded images were displayed using the highest count and the lowest count to determine the color range. Three patterns of flow were recognized: normal, focal low flow, and focal high flow. Two-dimensional echocardiography was performed when clinically indicated.

The transcranial Doppler was an EME-2-64 (Uberlingen, FRG). This is a 2-MHz pulsed-wave, range-gated transcranial Doppler. The probe was placed in each of the three standard insonation windows: orbital, temporal, and foramen magnum. Both anterior and posterior circulations were assessed whenever possible, and a flow-diagram constructed for each patient, noting direction of flow and BFV. Peak values were used in all cases. Transcranial Doppler values were divided into high, normal, and low, using the side ratio:

$$\frac{MCA - \text{blood flow velocity } (s)}{MCA - \text{blood flow velocity } (n)}$$

where (s) is the stroke side and (n) is the nonstroke side.

For example, with a BFV stroke side of 150 cm/sec, and BFV normal side of 100 cm/sec, the side ratio would be $150/100 = 1.5$.

We have previously estimated the mean side ratio (± 2 SD) as varying from 0.7 to 1.3 in 20 normal subjects. All patients with TCD had duplex scanning of the carotid arteries when possible.

RESULTS

There were 160 patients included in the study, but 21 (13 per cent) could not be evaluated because the density of the temporal bone made insonation of the middle cerebral artery impossible. All TCDs were assessed within 1 day of admission. Of the 139 patients evaluated, 32 had SPECT examinations within

TABLE 14–2. RELATIONSHIP OF TCD RESULTS TO CLINICAL AND OTHER LABORATORY RESULTS

	MCA-BFV Side Ratios		
	High	*Normal*	*Low*
	17	94	28
TSS[a]	2.29 ± 0.2 (SEM)[c]	1.79 ± 0.1	2.71 ± 0.11[d]
TES[b]	2.47 ± 0.24 (SEM)	1.96 ± 0.12	1.83 ± 0.2
SPECT	2 low	8 low	11 low
(32)	1 high	1 high	7 high
			2 normal
Echo	1 normal	18 normal	6 normal
(48)	3 abnormal	12 abnormal	12 abnormal

[a] TSS, stroke score.
[b] TES, embolic score.
[c] $p < 0.001$, low-flow group differs from normal-flow group in score severity.
[d] $p < 0.04$, high-flow group differs from normal-flow group in score severity.

the first 3 days, and 48 had two-dimensional echocardiography within the first week. The comparative results are tabulated in Table 14–2.

In patients with middle cerebral artery (MCA) occlusion, two patterns of compensatory flow were seen (Fig. 14–1). In the first, anterior cerebral artery (ACA), flow was markedly augmented on the contralateral side, and reversed (with or without increased BFV) on the ipsilateral side. In the second, there was increased BFV in the ipsilateral posterior cerebral artery (PCA), but often without alteration in other vessels in the vertebrobasilar circulation; sometimes flow as at the upper limit in the basilar artery, reflecting the increased collateral flow from the posterior circulation to the anterior circulation. Why one flow pattern is favored over another is uncertain. Presumably the pattern of collateral flow is largely determined by the size and fit of existing vascular anatomy.

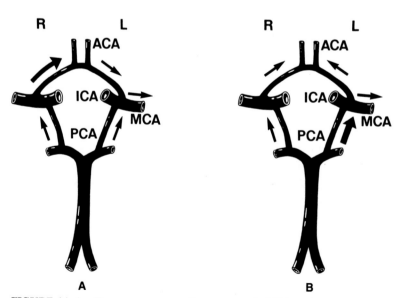

FIGURE 14–1. Two most common flow patterns in MCA occlusion *A,* Reversal of ipsilateral ACA flow with increased flow in contralateral ACA. *B,* Increased in flow in ipsilateral PCA.

Patients were subdivided into three categories according to their TCD side-ratio results: High, normal, and low flow. The only differences in the three TCD groups were in score severity; only patients with severe neurological deficits showed changes in MCA-BFV. Although the clinical embolic scores were higher in the TCD high-velocity groups, this was not statistically significant. Unfortunately, only three patients in the high-flow group had SPECT, so these results are unassessable. Echocardiography was abnormal in 22 of the 48 patients assessed. These included valvular abnormalities such as mitral valve prolapse and ventricular dyskinesia, and were all assumed to have embolic potential. However, the incidence of these abnormalities was random in the three TCD groups, and showed no association with the high-flow TCD group (Table 14–2).

DISCUSSION

The most striking finding was that MCA blood-flow velocities were only altered in patients with severe strokes. Patients with mild strokes, in whom management might be most beneficial, showed no changes on TCD. This, in conjunction with the 13 per cent failure to insonate adequately the intracranial circulation, indicates that this technique is of limited value in assessing patients with acute ischemic stroke. The low SPECT rate in the high-flow group leaves the interpretation of this test difficult, but as we recruit more patients and have a higher yield of SPECT procedures we may be able to draw more definite conclusions.

There have been surprisingly few evaluations of TCD in patients with acute ischemic stroke. Most published series are concerned with evaluating intracranial arterial blood velocities for collateral flow. This topic was reviewed in detail by Ringelstein.[8] However, we disagree with his statement that normal TCD findings in an acute stroke patient focus clinical interest on the heart, since we found that MCA-BFV changes are more likely to reflect the disordered metabolism of infarcted brain. Also in our series, half the patients with normal TCD values had abnormal (potentially cardioembolic) echocardiographic findings.

We also did not confirm his finding that TCD can differentiate "small-vessel" strokes from those with large-vessel occlusive disease, since failure of insonation may occur in patients with a normal complement of vessels angiographically. Ringelstein found a specificity and sensitivity of 90 per cent, indicating 10 per cent false-negative and 10 per cent false-positive values when compared to angiography.[8] These figures are even less accurate in the vertebrobasilar system. For instance, in the study of Mull et al., TCD findings were compared to angiographic findings in 58 patients. They found serious technical limitations owing to failure to insonate thick tissues. Only five patients had insonation of the length of the basilar artery in their series. They concluded that TCD examination alone (without angiography) leads to "ambiguous" results.[9]

In a small series of 15 patients with acute ischemic hemiplegia, Halsey found that if the TCD is performed within 12 hours, and MCA-BFV was greater than 30 cm/sec, prognosis was relatively favorable; if it was below this value, and remained so, recovery was invariably poor[10] (Fig. 14–2). In his study, three patients could not be assessed because of impenetrable temporal "windows," a failure rate of 20 per cent (even higher than ours).

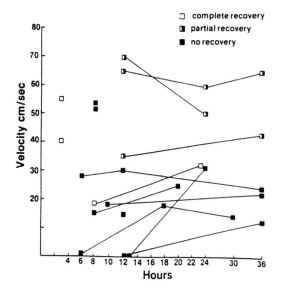

FIGURE 14–2. Plot of middle cerebral artery blood velocity and time of transcranial Doppler ultrasonography after hemiplegia. (Reproduced with permission from Halsey JH: Prognosis of acute hemiplegia estimated by transcranial Doppler ultrasonography. Stroke 1988;*19*:648–649.)

During the course of a multicenter study in acute stroke where patients were recruited within 4 hours of the ictus, TCDs were performed on 42 patients within 6 hours.[11] Unobtainable or low MCA signals were associated with MCA occlusions on angiography, and large infarcts on CT. There was no mention of increased MCA-BFV. The authors concluded that normal or "near normal" MCA-BFV values were associated with a good prognosis.

It appears from these studies that MCA occlusion (which is nearly always embolic) with permanently low MCA-BFV implies a bad prognosis and extensive brain damage. However, there is no mention of the state of "luxury perfusion," as indicated by initially high MCA-BFV values.

A major problem with TCD in stroke patients is deciding whether high MCA-BFV values represent local arterial stenosis or reflect the metabolic state of the infarcted hemisphere. Also, as indicated by Wechsler et al. in 1986, ipsilateral hemodynamic carotid stenosis often produces low MCA-BFV, with blunted systolic peaks on spectral analysis and reduced peak-systolic and end-diastolic differences.[12] These abnormalities spring back to normal after carotid surgery has restored normal flow (Fig. 14–3).

In a study of 48 patients, all examined within 6 hours of acute ischemic stroke, TCD, angiography, and CT scan were performed.[13] In nine (19 per cent) cases, impenetrable temporal windows made evaluation by TCD impossible. When there was occlusion of the carotid siphon or origin of the MCA on angiography, MCA-BFV were not detected, and velocities were reduced when the terminal branches of the MCA were occluded[13]; even more significant, six of eight patients with terminal branch MCA occlusions had normal TCD findings.

In addition, there are a number of other technical limitations to TCD interpretation in cerebrovascular disease.[14] First, there are large variations of normal values, and often, normal vessels cannot be separated using a hand-held probe. Some of these problems arise from the large sampling volume, which may be overcome by future developments in technology.

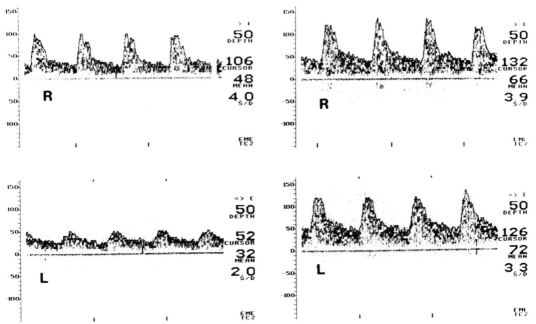

FIGURE 14–3. Transcranial Doppler studies of middle cerebral arteries before and after left carotid endarterectomy. Before surgery, peak systolic velocity was reduced on the left. Left/right middle cerebral artery peak velocity ratio (0.49) was reduced. Following left endarterectomy ipsilateral middle cerebral artery peak velocity more than doubled (126 cm/sec) and left/right ratio became normal (0.95). Cursor indicates peak systolic velocity for each trace. (Reproduced with permission from Wechsler LR, Ropper AH, Kistler JP: Transcranial Doppler in cerebrovascular disease. Stroke 1986;*17*:905–912.)

Second, physiological variations of the circle of Willis, such as absent or atrophic posterior communicating arteries, produce apparent abnormalities in TCD findings where flow is normal, just as emboli producing branch occlusions are often undetected.

Third, increased MCA-BFVs may be due to local stenoses or an overall increase in metabolic demand. This problem is partly overcome by reversal to normal values during the subsequent course of the stroke, though this might equally apply to lysis of thrombus with recanalization.

Fourth, reversal of flow in the anterior cerebral circulation, in response to MCA occlusion, may simulate high flow in the MCA, when in fact there is no flow.

In conclusion, we have failed to demonstrate a consistent and clinically useful method of determining whether an ischemic stroke is of cardioembolic origin. Clearly, even if our results were more convincing, the 15 to 19 per cent rate of insonation of the intracranial circulation is a major limitation. However, our numbers with laboratory confirmation are small. It may be that a "hot spot" of high perfusion on SPECT scanning associated with high blood-flow velocities may represent an embolic infarct, but in that case the TCD findings may be irrelevant (Fig. 14–4). It certainly seems to imply a better prognosis.

Many of these problems may be resolved as we continue to evaluate more patients and can make a more valid comparison of the laboratory data. However, we have not been able to draw any definitive conclusions in 160 patients, so whatever associations we ultimately discover cannot be very striking.

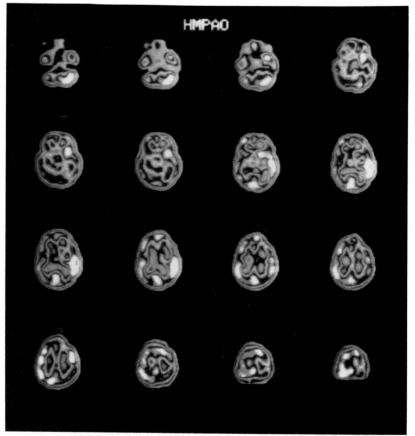

FIGURE 14–4. SPECT-HmPAO scan performed on Day 3 in a 27-year-old female with a right hemiplegia and severe aphasia following an acute left cerebral hemisphere embolic infarction. Note the focal area of high flow in the left cerebral hemisphere. Left MCA blood velocities were consistently high for 2 weeks following the infarction.

REFERENCES

1. Easton JD: Present status of anticoagulant prophylaxis. *In* Norris JW, Hachinski VC, eds: Prevention of Stroke. New York, Springer Verlag, 1990;139–147.
2. Mohr JP, Gautier JC, Hier DB, Stein RW: Middle cerebral artery. *In* HJM Barnette, BM Stein, JP Mohr, FM Yatsu, eds: Stroke. New York, Churchill Livingstone, 1986;387.
3. Toole JF: Cerebrovascular Disorders. New York, Raven Press, 1984;193.
4. Holman BL, Moretti JL, Hill TC: SPECT perfusion imaging in cerebrovascular disease. *In* Wwinberger J, ed: Noninvasive Imaging of Cerebrovascular Disease. New York, Alan R. Liss, 1989;147–162.
5. Limburg M, van Royen EA, Hijdra A, de Bruine JF, Verbeeten BWJ Jr: Single-photon emission computed tomography and early death in acute ischemic stroke. Stroke 1990;*21*:1150–1155.
6. Luo YM, Bondar RL, Norris JW: Clinical value of transcranial Doppler in stroke (abstract). J Cardiovasc Tech 1989;*8*:2.
7. Norris JW: Comment on "Study design of stroke treatments" (letter). Stroke 1982;*13*:527–528.
8. Ringelstein EB: Continuous-wave Doppler sonography of the extracranial brain-supplying arteries. *In* Weinberger J, ed: Noninvasive Imaging of Cerebrovascular Disease. New York, Alan R. Liss, 1989;94.
9. Mull M, Aulich A, Hennerici M: Trancranial Doppler ultrasonography versus arteriography for assessment of the vertebrovasilar circulation. J Clin Ultrasound 1990;*18*:539–549.
10. Halsey JH: Prognosis of acute hemiplegia estimated by transcranial Doppler ultrasonography. Stroke 1988;*19*:648–649.

11. Kushner MJ, Zanette EM, Bastianello S, et al: Transcranial Doppler in acute hemispheric brain infarction. Neurology 1991;*41*:109–113.
12. Wechsler LR, Ropper AH, Kistler JP: Transcranial Doppler in cerebrovascular disease. Stroke 1986;*17*:905–912.
13. Zanetta EM, Fieschi C, Bozzao L, et al: Comparison of cerebral angiography and transcranial Doppler sonography in acute stroke. Stroke 1989;*20*:899–903.
14. Hennerici M: New technical and clinical aspects for cerebrovascular applications of ultrasound methods. J Neurosci Meth 1990;*34*:169–177.

15

USE OF DUPLEX SCANNING IN RENOVASCULAR HYPERTENSION

KIMBERLEY J. HANSEN, SCOTT W. REAVIS, and
RICHARD H. DEAN

Historically, evaluation of patients for renovascular occlusive disease has evolved through several screening methods. During respective eras, rapid sequence intravenous pyelography, peripheral plasma renin activity, infusion of angiotensin-II antagonists, and radionuclide renography have been suggested as valuable screening tests to detect functionally significant renovascular disease. Nevertheless, none of these methods have survived close scrutiny or sustained use owing to a lack of sensitivity, specificity, or both.

Although standard "cut-film" renal arteriography has continued to be the most reliable method to identify renovascular lesions potentially causing renovascular hypertension (RVH), its cost and invasiveness have limited its widespread use for this purpose. This reluctance is augmented when renal insufficiency coexists due to the potential nephrotoxicity of contrast material in such patients. These limitations of arteriography as a screening tool have led us to continue our search for an accurate noninvasive technique on which to base decisions regarding more-invasive angiographic evaluation.

Through continued improvements in probe design and duplex sonographic technology, imaging and Doppler-shift interrogation of deep abdominal vasculature has been introduced as a potentially accurate screening method to identify and quantify visceral and renal artery occlusive disease. Our clinical experience with its use has centered on evaluation of renovascular disease. We have evaluated the role of duplex sonography as an initial surface screening test, an intraoperative study to confirm technical success of reconstructive procedures, and as a postoperative surveillance method to follow progression of disease and stability of reconstructions. This discussion will summarize the methods we use for these studies and our results to date.

SCREENING IN RENOVASCULAR DISEASE

During the past 22 months, we have performed over 680 surface renal duplex sonography (RDS) studies to screen patients ranging from 2 to 90 years of age. Technically satisfactory studies defined as complete main renal artery Doppler interrogation from aortic origin to renal hilum were obtained in 94.4 per cent of patients studied. These results were ensured by proper patient preparation and method of examination.[1]

Patients for elective examination are fasted overnight and receive 10 mg bisacodyl by mouth to minimize bowel gas interference. The B-scan images and Doppler-shifted signals from the aorta, visceral, and renal arteries are first obtained in the supine position with either a 3-MHz mechanical long-focus probe or a 2.25-MHz phase array probe with Doppler color flow capability. Positioned in the abdominal midline just below the xiphoid process, the sagittal B-scan image of the upper abdominal aorta defines the origins of the celiac and superior mesenteric arteries. At this level, a centerstream aortic peak systolic velocity may be obtained for a future calculation of renal artery to aortic peak systolic velocity ratio. Using the origin of the superior mesenteric artery and the left renal vein as visual references, the origin of each main renal artery can usually be defined in transverse projection during peak inspiration (Fig. 15–1). We require that sequential renal artery Doppler-shifted signals and calculated peak systolic velocities are obtained throughout the renal artery in continuity from aorta to renal hilum. Doppler color flow capability permits a more rapid identification of renal artery origins and anatomic course to the kidney (Fig. 15–2). In kidneys with normal parenchymal renovascular resistance, demonstration of forward flow throughout diastole is consistent, but not uniquely characteristics of the renal artery color flow signal—the celiac axis and its branches also demonstrate a forward flow during diastole and may occasionally be confused with a renal artery signal. B-scan identification and Doppler

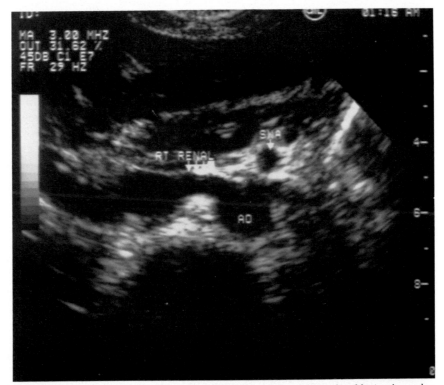

FIGURE 15–1. Transverse projection of aorta (red) and renal arteries (blue) using color flow Doppler.

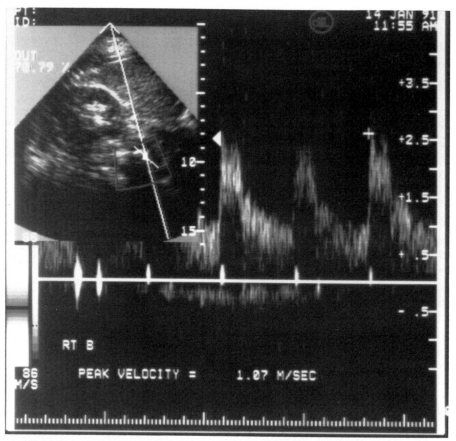

FIGURE 15–2. Normal Doppler spectral analysis during surface RDS from undiseased right renal artery.

interrogation is then repeated using a flank approach with the patient in a decubitus position. This flank approach improves B-scan image quality and Doppler signal. From the flank, the liver (right) and kidney (left) provide solid organ acoustic windows free of bowel gas interference, and the surface transducer can be placed closer to the areas of renal artery interrogation, improving image quality. Inherent errors in estimation of renal artery peak systolic velocity (RA-PSV) are reduced by decreasing the angle of insonation. Finally, the kidney length, width, and thickness are determined. Doppler shifted signals are obtained from regions of arcuate and interlobar arteries, and color flow parenchymal mapping performed. Color flow Doppler from the flank approach helps to identify the intraparenchymal vascular anatomy. Other investigators have suggested that Doppler spectral analysis from these parenchymal vessels alone may be sufficient to detect the renal artery stenosis (RAS). We have examined Doppler spectra from the arcuate and interlobar arteries, but only consider this information a qualitative expression of renal parenchymal disease.

Renal duplex sonography criteria for critical renal artery stenosis are depicted in Table 15–1. Assuming that RA-PSV varied with the degree of renal artery stenosis and aortic PSV (i.e., inflow), most authors[2-5] have advocated the ratio of RA-PSV to aortic PSV (the renal-aortic ratio) to define critical renal artery stenosis. In contrast, we have found no relationship between RA-PSV

TABLE 15–1. DOPPLER VELOCITY CRITERIA FOR B-SCAN DEFECTS

Defect	Criteria
<60% diameter-reducing RA defect	RA-PSV from entire RA <2.0 m/sec
≥60% diameter-reducing RA defect	Focal RA-PSV ≥2.0 m/sec and distal turbulent velocity waveform
Occlusion	No Doppler-shifted signal from renal artery B-scan image
Inadequate study for interpretation	Failure to obtain Doppler samples from entire main renal artery

and aortic PSV in the presence or absence of disease (Fig. 15–3). Focal RA-PSV 2 m/sec or more in combination with distal poststenotic turbulence has proved to correlate highly with the angiographic presence of 60 per cent or greater diameter reducing stenosis of the renal artery.[1] In 122 kidneys with single renal arteries with renal angiography for comparison, RDS correctly identified 67 of 68 kidneys with normal and less than 60 per cent renal artery stenosis, and 35 of 39 kidneys with 60 to 99 per cent renal artery stenosis (Table 15–2). All 15 renal artery occlusions were correctly identified by failure to obtain a Doppler-shifted signal from an imaged renal artery. Using this methodology and criteria for interpretation, renal duplex was 93 per cent sensitive and 98 per cent specific, with a positive predictive value of 98 per cent and a negative predictive value of 94 per cent. Overall accuracy was 96 per cent when compared prospectively with cut-film angiography.

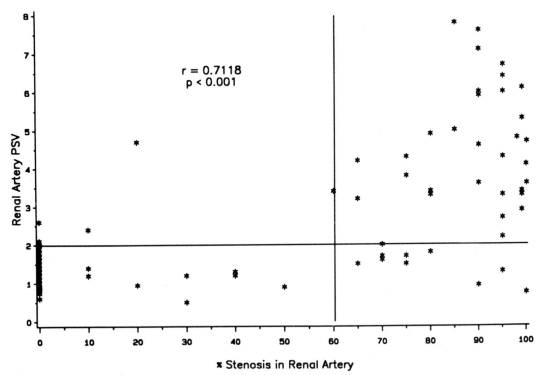

FIGURE 15–3. Scatter plot and Pearson correlation coefficient for renal artery peak systolic velocity (PSV) versus per cent renal artery stenosis. A 60 per cent or greater diameter reducing stenosis is indicated by a renal artery PSV 2.0 m/sec or more. (Reproduced with permission from Hansen KJ, et al. Renal duplex sonography: Evaluation of clinical utility. J Vasc Surg 1990;*12*:227–236.)

TABLE 15–2. COMPARATIVE ANALYSIS PARAMETER ESTIMATES AND THEIR 95 PERCENT CONFIDENCE INTERVALS

Group	N	Measure	Estimate	95 Percent Confidence Interval
All kidneys	142 (kidneys)	Sensitivity	.88	(.84, .92)
		Specificity	.99	(.97, 1.00)
		PPV	.98[b]	(.96, .99)
		NPV	.92[c]	(.89, .95)
	148 (kidneys)	Accuracy	.91	(.87, .95)
Kidneys with single renal artery	122 (kidneys)	Sensitivity	.93	(.90, .96)
		Specificity	.98[b]	(.96, 1.00)
		PPV	.98[c]	(.96, 1.00)
		NPV	.94	(.91, .97)
	148 (kidneys)	Accuracy	.91	(.87, .95)
Kidneys with multiple renal arteries	21 (arteries)	Sensitivity	.67	(.53, .81)
		Specificity	1.00[a]	—
		PPV	1.00[ab]	—
		NPV	.79[c]	(.68, .90)
		Accuracy	.86	(.76, .96)
All patients	74 (subjects)	Sensitivity	.93	(.87, .99)
		Specificity	1.00[a]	—
		PPV	1.00[ab]	—
		NPV	.91[c]	(.84, .98)
		Accuracy	.96	(.91, 1.00)

[a] Estimated standard error is zero, confidence level is inestimable.
[b] PPV, positive predictive value.
[c] NPV, negative predictive value.

These results are superior to all other alternative screening tests for renovascular disease; however, strict attention to patient preparation, skilled performance of the scan, and adherence to criteria are prerequisites for this level of success. We feel that interrogation of the entire renal artery is necessary to ensure these results, since accelerated flow velocity secondary to stenosis may normalize two vessel diameters distal to the lesion.[6] Furthermore, the increase in RA-PSV must be focal *and* accompanied by "turbulent" distal spectral waveforms (Fig. 15–4). Turbulent waveforms are characterized by delayed acceleration in early systole with mosaic Doppler color flow patterns. Four per cent of our patients screened for significant renovascular disease will demonstrate more than 2.0 m/sec RA-PSV uniformly throughout the renal artery. In general, these patients are less than 50 years of age, fail to demonstrate distal turbulent spectral waveforms, and invariably fail to demonstrate anatomic disease by conventional cut-film angiography. The lack of focality and distal turbulence distinguishes this subgroup from those patients with anatomic disease. Although not confirmed by prospective study, our experience with color flow mapping suggests that a mosaic parenchymal pattern coincides with grossly disturbed, poststenotic turbulence.

Multiple or polar renal arteries pose a potentially serious limitation of surface RDS. Nineteen per cent of the patients presenting to our institution for evaluation of renovascular hypertension have had polar renal arteries by angiography. Among these patients, 43 per cent have had multiple vessels to both kidneys and 40 per cent of all the multiple vessels have demonstrated 60 per cent or greater diameter reducing stenosis or occlusion. Because of variable polar vessel origin, small vessel size, and compromised image quality associated with low-frequency probes, identification of polar vessels and their associated disease is difficult. In our validity analysis of surface RDS, we identified only

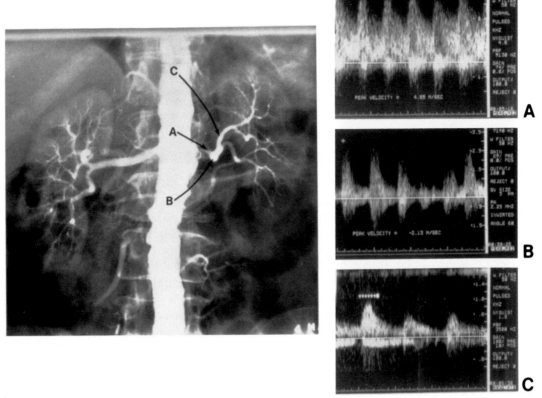

FIGURE 15–4. Radiograph cut-film angiogram demonstrating high-grade left renal artery stenosis. *A,* Doppler spectral analysis at the site of stenosis demonstrating focal increase in RA-PSV (4.6 m/sec). *B,* Distal spectral analysis demonstrating turbulent waveform—decreased RA-PSV with ragged spectral envelope and spontaneous bidirectional signals. *C,* Spectral analysis several vessel diameters distal to stenosis demonstrating return of near-normal waveform.

1 of 43 polar arteries. Although Doppler color flow has enhanced recognition of multiple renal arteries, failure to identify these polar vessels and their associated disease constituted the largest single source of false-negative studies.

The pertinence of RDS insensitivity to polar vessel disease relates to the prevalence of such disease within the patient population examined and the clinical indication for surface RDS. Fourteen per cent of our patients who submitted to repair for unilateral renovascular disease and presumed renovascular hypertension have had only polar branch disease. We believe this group constitutes a significant minority of patients. Therefore, we proceed with conventional angiography in patients less than 60 years of age with poorly controlled hypertension despite multidrug therapy, even in the presence of a negative surface RDS. When RDS is used to screen for ischemic nephropathy and renal insufficiency, however, a negative RDS study effectively excludes significant RVD, since polar vessel disease alone does not account for renal insufficiency.[7]

Finally, the suggestion that diastolic features of the renal artery Doppler spectra might predict the clinical success of renovascular reconstruction has not proved valid in our experience (Table 15–3). A screening test which simultaneously determined the presence of anatomic renal artery disease *and* the

TABLE 15–3. ANOVA FOR RA-EDR VERSUS HYPERTENSION AND FUNCTION RESPONSE AFTER RENAL REVASCULARIZATION

	N	Mean RA-EDR (± SD)	p-Value
Hypertension response*			
Cured	8	0.25 ± 0.04	
Improved	22	0.29 ± 0.02	0.225
No change	5	0.22 ± 0.04	
Total	35		
Functional response†			
Improved	9	0.26 ± 0.04	
No change	10	0.29 ± 0.03	0.278
Worse	3	0.20 ± 0.05	
Total	22		

clinical response to repair would have wide applicability. Although we have observed the inverse correlation between renal artery end-diastolic velocity (RA-EDV) and estimated creatinine clearance reported by others, RA-EDV has not correlated with hypertension response or change in serum creatinine following renovascular repair in 35 patients (*p* - 0.225).[1] Even though low RA-EDV is consistent with high intrarenal vascular resistance and intrinsic renal parenchymal disease, a low RA-EDV does not preclude a favorable clinical response after renovascular repair and should not be used to support any particular plan of management.

INTRAOPERATIVE RDS AS A COMPLETION STUDY

In comparison to vascular reconstruction at other anatomic locations, intraoperative assessment of renovascular reconstructions has proved difficult by traditional angiographic methods. Intraoperative angiography provides anatomic evaluation in only one projection. Frequent branch renal artery and intraparenchymal arteriolar vasospasm in response to high-concentration contrast injection may provide an inaccurate impression of an intrarenal vascular catastrophe. Finally, one half of our hypertensive patients subjected to renovascular reconstruction have associated renal insufficiency (ischemic nephropathy), increasing the potential risk of contrast nephropathy superimposed upon the changes associated with reperfusion of chronic renal ischemia.[8,9] By comparison, intraoperative renal duplex is theoretically free of these limitations and potential complications. B-scan images are generated by 10-MHz mechanical or 5.0-MHz linear array probes providing excellent anatomic detail, sensitive to small (less than 1 mm) anatomic defects.[10,11] Real-time imaged defects can be viewed in a variety of longitudinal and transverse projections with no adverse consequence on renal function. Addition of pulsed Doppler sampling (5.0 MHz) proximal and distal to imaged postreconstruction defect provides potentially important physiologic information regarding associated flow significance. Freedom from limited anatomic projections, absence of potential renal toxicity, and the addition of hemodynamic data provided by Doppler interrogation make RDS the preferred method of objective assessment of renovascular reconstructions.[12]

Intraoperative studies are performed with either a 10-MHz mechanical probe with 5.0-MHz Doppler, or a 5.0-MHz linear array probe with Doppler color flow. The probe head is placed in a sterile plastic sheath containing acoustic gel. Although plastic caps are available and designed to increase gel coupling to the mechanical scan head, we have found that these add undesirable acoustic artifact. The operative field is flooded with warm saline and B-scan images are obtained first in the longitudinal projection. Care is taken to image the perirenal aorta, renal artery origin, and entire renal artery from origin to hilum. All defects seen in longitudinal projection are imaged in transverse projection to confirm their anatomic presence and contribution to luminal narrowing. Doppler samples are then obtained just proximal and distal to the imaged lesions in longitudinal projection to determine their potential contribution to flow disturbance.

Our criteria for hemodynamic defects (60 per cent or more diameter reduction) are similar to the surface RDS studies (Table 15–1).[1] These criteria have been found valid in our laboratory using a canine model of graded RAS and valid compared with preoperative cut-film angiography in 19 patients and 34 renal arteries when radiographic studies were compared with the intraoperative prerepair RDS. Unlike surface RDS in which the Doppler sample volume is large relative to the renal artery diameter, the Doppler sample volume can be accurately positioned within midcenter streamflow. At this midcenter stream location, our laboratory experience suggests that spectral broadening, increased peak systolic, and end-diastolic velocities relate to luminal narrowing in a fashion similar to that recognized in the carotid system. However, after renal artery repair, at least moderate spectral broadening seems inherent to the Doppler signal and unassociated with anatomic defects.

We have used RDS to assess 57 renovascular reconstructions in 35 patients who underwent unilateral (13 patients) or bilateral (22 patients) repair. Methods of reconstruction included aortorenal bypass (RAB) in 29 repairs (20 saphenous vein, Polytetrafluoroethylene [PTFE], 4 Dacron), reimplantation in 7 repairs, transrenal thromboendarterectomy (TEA) with PTFE-patch angioplasty in 13 repairs, and transaortic extraction TEA in 8 repairs. The group included branch renal artery repair in 6 cases (5 in vivo, 1 ex vivo), while 14 had combined aortic replacement (11 patients: 8 AAA, 3 occlusive disease) or visceral artery reconstruction (3 patients: 3 SMA-TEA, 1 IMA-TEA).

Average time for intraoperative RDS was 4.5 minutes, and studies provided complete B-scan and Doppler information in 56 of 57 repairs (98 per cent). Renal duplex sonography was considered normal in 44 repairs (77 per cent), while B-scan defects were present in 13 (23 per cent) (Fig. 15–5). Six of these B-scan defects (11 per cent) had Doppler spectra with focal increases in peak systolic velocity of 2.0 m/sec or more with poststenotic turbulence, and were defined as major. These major defects prompted immediate operative revision. In each of these revision, a significant defect was discovered and corrected. Seven B-scan defects without Doppler spectral abnormality were defined as minor and were not repaired. At mean follow-up of 12.4 months, the status of 55 renal artery reconstructions in 34 patients was determined by either surface RDS or renal angiography. Forty-two of forty-three renal artery repairs with normal intraoperative RDS, and six of six repairs with minor B-scan defects were patent and free of critical stenosis. Of the six revisions prompted by abnormal B-scan, with Doppler criteria for significant stenosis (i.e., major defects), four were patent without stenosis, one re-stenosed, and one occluded. Intraoperative RDS was 86 per cent sensitive and 100 per cent specific for technical defects associated with postoperative stenosis and occlusion of renovascular repair. These anatomic results were supported by the clinical response to operation. Ninety-six per cent of hypertensive patients demonstrated a

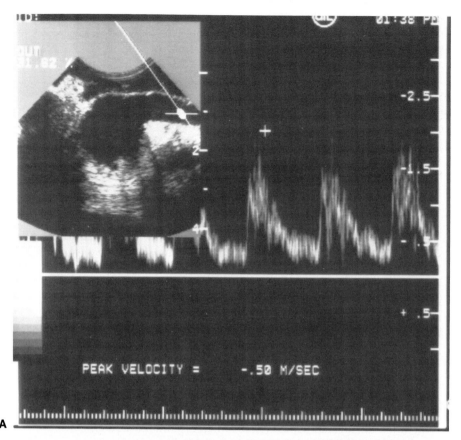

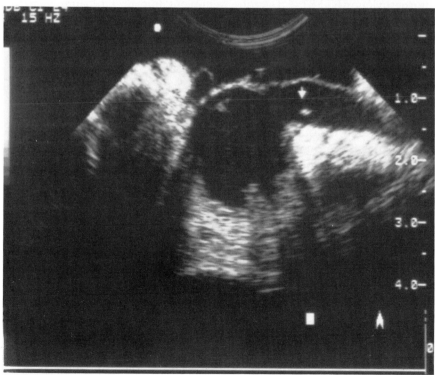

PEAK VELOCITY =   -.50 M/SEC

A

B

FIGURE 15–5. *A*, B-scan image with defect (proximal flap) within a left renal artery reimplantation. *B*, Doppler spectral analysis demonstrates normal RA-PSV (0.5 m/sec) characteristic of a minor B-scan defect.

favorable blood pressure response, while 80 per cent of patients with renal insufficiency demonstrated a favorable functional response after surgery.

We believe our experience with intraoperative RDS as a completion study following renovascular reconstruction supports RDS as the method of choice to objectively assess for technical error after repair. Ninety-seven per cent of reconstructions with normal intraoperative RDS remained patent and free of stenosis on follow-up. B-scan image defects which are not associated with significant pressure-flow disturbance by Doppler velocity spectra do not seem to predispose to restenosis or renal artery occlusion and do not require operative treatment. However, B-scan defects associated with focal increases in RA-PSV 2.0 m/sec or more with distal turbulent waveforms should be considered for immediate revision.

FOLLOW-UP STUDY OF RENOVASCULAR REPAIR

Over the past 19 months, we have performed 67 surface RDS studies in 50 patients following renovascular repair, defining renal artery anatomy to 129 kidneys. In this patient group, seven patients had undergone prior percutaneous balloon angioplasty of nine critical renal artery stenoses. Over a follow-up period ranging from 1 week to 9 years (mean follow-up: 3.2 years), three of nine balloon angioplasties demonstrated critical restenosis, while two contralateral renal arteries developed new stenoses with 60 per cent or greater diameter reduction. In addition, 59 patients were submitted to a total of 77 surface RDS follow-up studies for postoperative evaluation of 84 renal artery reconstructions. Thirty-four patients had undergone unilateral renal artery repair, while 25 patients underwent simultaneous bilateral renal artery reconstruction. Forty-one repairs (49 per cent) were aortorenal bypass, 9 (11 per cent) were renal artery reimplantation, while 26 (31 per cent) were either transaortic or transrenal thromboendarterectomy. In 14 patients, renovascular repair was combined with aortic reconstruction (11 abdominal aortic aneurysms; 3 occlusive disease). The period of follow-up ranged from 3 weeks to 6 years, with a mean of 2.2 years. Renal duplex sonography studies of four renal artery bypasses (5 per cent) were technically inadequate for interpretation (two combined with aortic reconstruction). In each case, bowel gas interference prohibited complete Doppler interrogation of the bypass. Of the 73 interpretable studies in 55 patients to 80 renal artery reconstructions, critical restenosis was present in four saphenous vein aortorenal grafts. In each case, the stenosis was apparently located within the proximal graft. Three of thirty-one contralateral unrepaired kidneys (10 per cent) demonstrated new critical stenosis (contralateral unrepaired renal arteries) which was not present at the time of the initial reconstruction. Medical history and follow-up is adequate in 34 of these patients for assessment of their hypertension and renal function response. In those patients demonstrating patent renal artery reconstruction and freedom of significant renovascular disease, 31 patients (91 per cent) have enjoyed a favorable hypertension response and 9 of 19 patients (47 per cent) have had improved renal function.

Although angiographic correlation is available postoperatively in only nine patients providing anatomy to ten renal artery repairs, there is perfect correlation in this small patient population between postoperative surface RDS and follow-up angiography. Because of the limitations of surface RDS relative to small polar vessels discussed earlier, we recommend angiographic follow-up of branch renal artery repairs.

In contrast to the prior reports from other investigators,[13] we have had few technically inadequate postoperative studies despite our stringent criteria for complete renal artery interrogation. We have not noted an increase in technical inadequacy in evaluation of renal artery repair in combination with aortic reconstruction when studies are performed at least 3 weeks postoperatively. However, when attempts were made at study in the very early postoperative period, acute postoperative changes do contribute significantly to an increase in incomplete studies.

We believe our experience with RDS supports its use as a surface screening study for main renal artery stenosis, as an intraoperative completion study to confirm the technical adequacy of renal reconstruction, and as a surface follow-up study to confirm continued patency of such repairs. The greatest limitations occur in the evaluation of small polar vessels and segmental renal arteries while screening for RVH or the postoperative study of branch renal artery repairs.

REFERENCES

1. Hansen KJ, Tribble RW, Reavis S, et al: Renal duplex sonography: Evaluation of clinical utility. J Vasc Surg 1990;*12*:227–236.
2. Norris CS, Pfeiffer JS, Rittgers SE, Barnes RW: Noninvasive evaluation of renal artery stenosis and renovascular disease. J Vasc Surg 1984;*1*:192–201.
3. Kohler TR, Zierler RE, Martin RL, et al: Noninvasive diagnosis of renal artery stenosis by ultrasonic duplex scanning. J Vasc Surg 1986;*4*:450–456.
4. Taylor DC, Kettler MD, Moneta GL, et al: Duplex ultrasound scanning in the diagnosis of renal artery stenosis: A prospective evaluation. J Vasc Surg 1988;*7*:363–369.
5. Barnes RW: Utility of duplex scanning of the renal artery. *In* Bergan JJ, Yao JST, eds: Arterial Surgery: New Diagnostic and Operative Techniques. 1st ed. Orlando, Grune & Stratton, 1988;351–366.
6. Burns PN: The physical principles of Doppler and spectral analysis. J Clin Ultrasound 1987;*15*:567–590.
7. Dean RH: Renovascular hypertension. Curr Prob Surg 1985;*22*:6–67.
8. Hansen KJ, Ditesheim JA, Metropol SH, et al: Management of renovascular hypertension in the elderly population. J Vasc Surg 1989;*10*:266–273.
9. Metropol SH, Hansen KJ, Holmes RP, Iskandar SS, Strandhoy JW, Dean RH: Reperfusion changes after relief of sustained renal ischemia. Surg Forum 1989;*XL*:300–301.
10. Coelho JC, Sigel B, Flanigan DP, Schuler JJ, Spigos DG, Nyhus LM: Detection of arterial defects by real-time ultrasound scanning during vascular surgery: An experimental study. J Surg Res 1981;*30*:535–543.
11. Coelho JC, Sigel B, Flanigan DP, et al: An experimental evaluation of arteriography and imaging ultrasonography in detecting arterial defects at operation. J Surg Res 1982;*32*:130–137.
12. Okuhn SP, Reilly LM, Bennett JB, et al: Intraoperative assessment of renal and visceral artery reconstruction: The role of duplex scanning and spectral analysis. J Vasc Surg 1987;*5*:137–147.
13. Eidt JF, Fry RE, Clagett GP, Fisher DF, Alway C, Fry WJ: Postoperative follow-up of renal artery reconstruction with duplex ultrasound. J Vasc Surg 1988;*8*:667–673.

16

CLINICAL APPLICATION OF COLOR DOPPLER IN VENOUS PROBLEMS

DAVID S. SUMNER, MARK A. MATTOS, GREGG L. LONDREY,
KIM J. HODGSON, LYNNE D. BARKMEIER, and DON E. RAMSEY

It has been almost a quarter of a century since ultrasound was first applied to the diagnosis of venous disease. Shortly after the first instruments using the Doppler principle to detect blood flow transcutaneously became available, clinicians began exploring the possible role of this remarkable device in the evaluation of venous problems.[1] Quick recognition of its value in diagnosing venous obstruction and venous valvular insufficiency followed these early investigations. Guidelines for interpreting the studies were established by the early 1970s and have remained virtually unchanged since that time.[2] Although the Doppler proved quite accurate for detecting occlusive thrombi in veins above the knee, it was limited in its ability to detect clots below the knee, and frequently failed to detect early nonocclusive thrombi or thrombi in duplicated veins. Moreover, because the veins being examined could only be identified by their proximity to arterial signals, there was always some uncertainty regarding the precise location and extent of thrombosis or valvular incompetence.

A major breakthrough occurred in 1983 when Talbut demonstrated that B-mode ultrasonic scanning could be used to diagnose deep venous thrombosis (DVT).[3] Among others, Cranley and associates quickly recognized the significance of Talbut's observations, conducted exhaustive studies, and formulated the essential diagnostic criteria.[4] With this technique, veins could be individually visualized and identified, clots both occlusive and nonocclusive could be seen and their extent determined, below-knee thrombi could be detected, and valvular function could be examined directly. It was but a small step to the more versatile duplex imagers, which supplemented the B-mode image with Doppler signal information. These two modalities complemented one another. The presence of hypoechogenic thrombi seen with the B-mode scan, thrombi in poorly visualized veins, or thrombi in areas beyond the scope of the scan could be verified by the absence or distortion of the Doppler signal; and, in turn, the scan assisted in the selection and identification of the vein to be interrogated with the Doppler. Because of these advantages, duplex scanning was rapidly adopted by many laboratories as the method of choice for diagnosing DVT.[5-7] Yet, there were some drawbacks. Examination of the entire limb remained a time-consuming, tedious exercise, requiring evaluation of venous compressibility or multiple sampling of venous flow patterns along the course of each of the many veins potentially subject to thrombosis. The problem is most acute in the relatively small paired infrapopliteal veins, where clots are frequently nonocclusive, may be isolated, and often involve only a short segment of vein.[8,9] Because below-knee veins are so difficult to survey in their entirety and because their clinical significance has been questioned, many laboratories restrict duplex scanning to the popliteal and more proximal veins.

Technological advances in the late 1980s led to the development of color flow duplex imaging. These devices superimpose a real-time color-coded Doppler flow map on the conventional B-mode image, thereby providing instantaneous flow information over an extended length of vessel. Advantages include immediate identification of vascular structures, and unequivocal differentiation of veins from arteries. Absence of flow and distorted flow patterns are visually evident. Visualization of flow over a wide area reduces the need to assess flow patterns by direct Doppler interrogation, and facilitates longitudinal scanning of veins. A change in color signifying a reversal of blood flow not only discloses the presence of valvular incompetence, but also identifies the incompetent vein. Despite these apparent advantages, there have been no reports comparing the accuracy of color flow imaging and conventional duplex scanning. In fact, because color flow imaging has only recently been applied to the study of venous disease, there are few reports concerning its accuracy.

This chapter summarizes the experience of the authors and that of other investigators with color Doppler in the diagnosis of deep venous thrombosis and compares the results with those obtained with conventional duplex scanning, both in patients with clinically suspected disease and in asymptomatic patients undergoing orthopedic procedures associated with a high incidence of postoperative venous thrombosis. The latter poses a far greater challenge than the former, since surveillance of postoperative patients requires recognition of clots in their formative stage, when they are isolated, nonocclusive, and usually confined to infrapopliteal veins.[7,10,11]

COLOR FLOW INSTRUMENTS

Currently, a number of high-quality color flow scanners are commercially available. Each instrument has its own peculiar advantages and drawbacks. Our experience is confined to the use of the Quad I and Quad 2000 machines (Quantum Medical Systems, Issaquah, WA). All employ linear array transducers, in which crystals aligned along the axis of the transducer are serially activated to produce a rectangular field of view. Sector scanners are also available and can be used when increased maneuverability is required to survey regions that are difficult to visualize with linear array. Stationary reflectors are displayed by varying intensities of a gray scale, producing a conventional B-mode image of the vessels and other structures underlying the skin. Moving particles shift the ultrasound frequencies according to the Doppler effect, creating a colored "flow map" that is superimposed on the static image. Direction of flow relative to the transducer is indicated by color, red or blue. Color is assigned by the operator so that centrally directed flow is blue to coincide with predominantly venous flow, and peripherally directed flow is red to coincide with predominantly arterial flow. The magnitude of the frequency shift, which depends on the velocity of the flow vectors relative to the sound beam, is indicated by color saturation. Provided the angle of insonation is acute and remains constant, a more intense or deeper color represents a low velocity, while a lighter, whiter color signifies a high velocity. When flow is absent, too slow to be detected, or when the flow vectors are at a right angle to the sound beam, there is no color and the image appears black. "Slow flow" software, which permits velocities as low as 0.3 cm/sec to be detected, is of great help in studying veins. By placing the pulsed-Doppler sample volume in the flow stream, the operator can also evaluate flow patterns audibly or by means of real-time spectral analysis, precisely as is done with conventional duplex scanning. Hard-copy images can be made and critical portions of the study can be recorded on videotape for later review and analysis.

Although a 7.5-MHz probe can be used to examine the more superficial veins, a 5-MHz probe is better suited for the deeper veins of the thigh and calf. One problem with the older instruments was the size of the probe, which made them somewhat difficult to use in tight spots. Newer probes have much smaller footprints, permitting better maneuverability.

SCANNING METHODS

The procedure is similar to that used with conventional duplex or B-mode scanning.[11-13] To optimize venous filling, patients lie supine on a bed or examination table tilted to a 20- to 30-degree reversed Trendelenburg position. The legs are slightly separated and externally rotated. It is most important that the patient be comfortable and relaxed to avoid venous compression. Scanning begins at the groin with the common femoral vein and its tributaries and then proceeds distally along the anterior medial thigh, just posterior to the quadriceps muscle, to the adductor canal region where the superficial femoral vein emerges from deep in the popliteal space. At this point, the patient is requested to assume a lateral decubitus position to facilitate access to the above- and below-knee popliteal space of the uppermost limb. Alternatively, the popliteal vein may be examined with the patient prone, the feet being supported on a pillow to flex the knee about 30 degrees. Flexion of the knee relaxes the popliteal space, avoids venous compression, and makes application of the probe easier. Although the tibioperoneal veins are best studied with the patient sitting with the foot on the examiners knee or resting on a low stool, many patients—owing to recent operations, serious illness, or orthopedic problems—are unable to assume this position. In these patients, the infrapopliteal veins are surveyed with the patient supine and with the knees slightly flexed to relax the calf muscles. Studies are begun at the ankle and the veins traced up the leg to the popliteal fossa. To visualize the posterior tibial vein, the probe is placed along the medial calf just behind the tibia and is directed laterally and slightly anteriorly. The anterior tibial veins are examined with the probe placed over the anterior compartment, oriented to direct the sound beam posteriorly and medially. Peroneal veins can be seen through both views, lying deep to the posterior tibial vein or deep to the anterior tibial vein just beyond the interosseous membrane. The probe angle will usually need to be readjusted to see the peroneal veins and both venae comitantes of the anterior tibial or posterior tibial veins, since these vessels may lie in different planes.

Longitudinal tracking of veins, which is often difficult with conventional duplex scanning, is greatly facilitated by color, allowing the technologist to use the long-axis view for most of the examination—thus decreasing the time required to complete the study. At selected sites, cross-sectional views are also obtained. Cross-sectional views are especially important to avoid overlooking a parallel vein in regions where veins are frequently duplicated (e.g., veins in the mid thigh, popliteal fossa, and calf).

Color expedites the identification of vessels and affords a rapid method of distinguishing veins from arteries. Unless there is arterial obstruction, flow in all named arteries of the extremities is almost always spontaneously visible. Locating the corresponding artery, which helps identify the anatomically associated venous structures, should be the initial step at each level. This is especially important below the knee, where there is a large number of small vessels and the anatomy is relatively complex. After the artery is visualized, the probe can then be tilted slightly and its longitudinal orientation shifted to optimize the venous image. Although the velocity of blood flow in femoral and popliteal veins is usually sufficiently high to insure a "spontaneous" color image, that in the infrapopliteal veins may not be visible without augmentation. Gentle manual compression of the foot or calf below the site of the probe or compression and release of the calf proximal to the probe is usually sufficient to produce a color image in patent tibioperoneal veins. At selected points, the cursor of the pulsed Doppler may be placed in the vessel lumen to sample the audible signal or record a frequency spectrum. Audible signals or recordings are necessary for estimating the velocity of flow and may be quite helpful for evaluating flow patterns when access to the entire venous segment is restricted by surgical incisions, casts, braces, or external orthopedic fixation devices.

INTERPRETATION

The B-mode image outlines blood vessel walls, and the color flow map defines their lumen. With color "off," the gain control is adjusted so that the arterial lumen is devoid of echoes and appears black. Even at this setting, slowly flowing blood in large veins often produces echoes that appear to move with the flow stream and may be confused with a free-floating thrombus. The mechanism by which these echoes are produced remains poorly understood.[14] With color "on," the lumen of large veins, such as the common femoral, superficial femoral, and popliteal, is completely filled with blue pixels, signifying antegrade flow. Phasic variations in flow velocity coinciding with respiration are clearly evident. Augmentation of flow produced by compressing the limb below the site of the probe causes the lumen to distend and the color to assume a lighter shade of blue. When venous valves are incompetent, color shifts from blue to red in response to a Valsalva maneuver or proximal limb compression. Normal veins collapse when the probe is used to apply moderate pressure to the skin. The effect of probe pressure is best observed in transverse views (with color off), since pressure applied when the probe is oriented longitudinally with respect to the vein may shift the vein from the field of view.

The common femoral vein is easily seen lying just medial to the common femoral artery. Manipulation of the probe reveals the saphenous, superficial femoral, and profunda femoris veins, and demonstrates their junction with the common femoral vein. All four veins may be simultaneously visible when the proper plane is selected. As the superficial femoral vein is traced down the leg, tissues on both sides of the superficial femoral artery should be interrogated to avoid overlooking a duplicate channel. Behind the knee, the junction of the lesser saphenous and popliteal vein is usually seen without difficulty. As mentioned earlier, transverse views, which identify all parallel structures, are helpful in the superficial femoral and popliteal areas.

Examination of infrapopliteal veins is much more challenging. Although tibioperoneal veins can be visualized on the gray-scale image, they may be confused with the arteries to which they are closely applied, and their patency is difficult to determine owing to their relatively small diameters. The presence of spontaneous flow, indicated by a blue color, confirms venous patency. It is usually necessary, however, to augment flow to obtain satisfactory visualization of the venous lumen. Because clots may be limited to only one of the two venae comitantes, flow in both must be visualized for the full extent of the vein. Pollak and coworkers, in a study focusing on deep veins of the calf, reported that augmentation produced color flow images in all normal posterior tibial and peroneal veins, but that 45 per cent of normal anterior tibial veins were not imaged.[15] Failure to image these veins, however, may not be a serious indictment of the test, since involvement of these veins is usually associated with concomitant thrombi in other veins of the calf or thigh.[16] On the other hand, van Bemmelen and colleagues studied 30 normal subjects and found that all paired calf veins could be visualized throughout their entire length from the ankle to the popliteal fossa.[17]

Fresh thrombi are hypoechoic and may not be visible on the gray-scale image. With conventional duplex scanning, lack of or incomplete venous compressibility provides indirect evidence of the presence of such clots.[4] Expansion of the venous lumen is also suggestive of venous thrombosis. In doubtful cases, the diagnosis must be confirmed by demonstrating the absence of Doppler signals in the venous lumen—a time-consuming process requiring an additional step.[8] In contrast, absence of spontaneous color immediately suggests the presence of an occlusive clot; and when no color appears with augmentation, the diagnosis of thrombosis is virtually assured (Fig. 16–1).[11–13] Compression studies are rarely necessary. With maturation, clots become more echogenic and may be clearly visible on the B-mode image. Problems still arise, particularly in the small infrapopliteal veins, where it may be difficult to

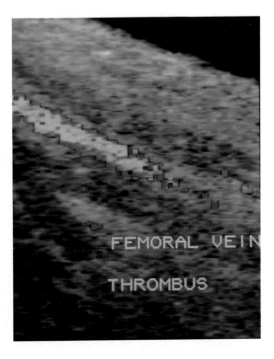

FIGURE 16–1. Thrombus totally occluding common femoral, superficial femoral, and profunda femoris veins. Femoral artery is indicated by red flow image.

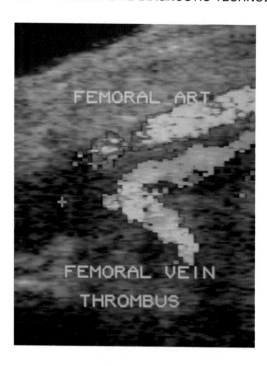

FIGURE 16–2. Thrombus occluding common femoral vein. Residual flow (blue) is shown in partially occluded superficial femoral and profunda femoris veins.

differentiate wall echoes from those emanating from the venous lumen. Compression studies of tibioperoneal veins are exceedingly hard to interpret owing to their small diameters. Again, failure to detect the blue color of venous flow in the tissues surrounding the tibial or peroneal arteries during augmentation is diagnostic of venous thrombosis.[11]

Partially occluding thrombi produce a filling defect in the color flow image (Fig. 16–2). Depending on their echogenicity, these clots may or may not be visible on the B-mode scan. "Free-floating clot," those with tails that are unattached to the venous wall, may be observed to wave about in the flow stream on the B-mode image and to distort the color flow pattern.[18] Recanalization is evident when flashes of color are seen within the echogenic substance of an old thrombus.

Sources of Error

Some anatomic areas prove difficult or impossible to scan. Visualization of the external iliac vein may be inadequate in overweight patients or in the presence of bowel gas. In such cases, the status of the iliac system can be inferred from characteristics of the flow pattern in the common femoral vein. Spontaneous phasic flow implies patency, whereas sluggish or continuous flow suggests proximal venous occlusion.[2,13] The diagnosis of occlusion is supported by finding multiple collateral channels carrying blood at an increased velocity. Although observation of the color flow image may suffice, it is usually necessary to study the audible flow pattern or the recorded spectral wave form. At the adductor canal, where the superficial femoral vein angles away from the skin and is deeply imbedded in muscle, a clear view is often difficult to obtain. Patency or occlusion of the intervening venous segment can be confirmed indirectly by observing flow patterns in the superficial femoral vein just above the hiatus and in the popliteal vein below. Compression maneuvers are not helpful, since the normal vein in this region is deeply situated and resists compression.[8,9] The point in the upper calf where the proximal tibial and peroneal veins coalesce to form the popliteal vein may also present a problem, owing not only to the large number of veins and their complex anatomy, but also to their depth.[11]

Although in normal limbs the six tibial and peroneal veins are ordinarily easy to trace throughout much of their length,[17] it may be difficult to exclude clots isolated to one or more of the venae comitantes. Uncertainties arise because there are a large number of deeply situated, relatively long veins with small diameters that carry blood at low velocities. The problem is further compounded by the presence of numerous perforating veins, some of which may contain small thrombi, and by the potential involvement of the soleal and gastrocnemial sinusoids. Thus, of all regions of the lower extremity, the below-knee veins are the most challenging for the sonographer.[9]

Accuracy, of course, is highly influenced by the adequacy of the color flow examination.[16] Technically limiting factors include obesity, swelling, small veins, collateral channels that obscure visualization, pain, and the inability to relax or combativeness on the part of the patient. In addition to those factors that negatively influence the accuracy of color flow scans in symptomatic patients, other limitations such as the presence of surgical wounds, casts, and braces also frequently interfere with surveillance studies conducted on postoperative patients. Moreover, positioning these patients for optimum access to the underlying veins is often restricted by pain or concern that movement may result in joint dislocation.

Diagnostic Criteria

Color flow scan results can be classified into one of three categories.

Normal. No thrombus is visualized; flow is either spontaneous and phasic or easily augmented; and the color image fills the entire venous lumen. Most normal veins are also easily compressed by probe pressure.

Positive for Thrombi. Flow is absent with augmentation or there is definite encroachment on the flow image. Clots, depending on their echogenicity, may or may not be visualized, and venous compressibility is usually absent or incomplete.

Equivocal. No thrombus is seen, but spontaneous or augmented flow patterns are abnormal. The flow image may be nonconfluent in that there are time- and spatially-dependent irregularities of the image without consistent areas of encroachment being observed. (In our experience, most of equivocal scans have turned out to be positive for small, isolated, nonocclusive thrombi.)

In arriving at an overall assessment, the technologist should also incorporate audible Doppler flow information (or recorded information) using the criteria developed for evaluating hand-held Doppler venous surveys.[2] As mentioned above, this information is especially valuable when clots may be hidden in inaccessible areas. The demonstration of increased flow velocities in superficial veins that act as collateral channels is highly suggestive of deep venous thrombosis, even when no definite clots have been identified on the color image. The presence or absence of this finding may resolve the question when clots are suspected in the iliac or below-knee veins.

ANALYSIS OF CLINICAL RESULTS

Although the deficiencies of phlebography are universally acknowledged, phlebography remains the most appropriate "gold standard" for determining the diagnostic accuracy of noninvasive tests designed to detect deep venous thrombosis. In comparing color flow scans with phlebographic images, one must remember that ascending phlebography seldom reveals the profunda femoris vein, often opacifies the iliac system inadequately, and may fail to opacify many veins of the calf or thigh, especially in the presence of thrombus. Therefore, some of the false-positive studies observed with color flow imaging may in fact represent phlebographic errors. Because of a low but real incidence of associated complications and because the procedure is frequently uncomfortable, physicians are reluctant to order phlebograms when noninvasive tests have been performed, especially when the diagnosis of deep venous thrombosis seems doubtful. This attitude restricts the number of phlebograms available for comparison with noninvasive tests and tends to increase the proportion of positive results in those patients undergoing phlebography. As a result, it has proved to be difficult to obtain an accurate assessment of noninvasive test accuracy in a true cross-section of symptomatic patients.

Unlike physiologically based tests (Doppler surveys, impedance plethysmography, phleborheography), which are limited to assessing above-knee veins and are ordinarily interpreted as being positive or negative for the entire limb, color flow provides anatomic information throughout the limb, permitting the extent and location of clots to be determined. Thus, it is appropriate to evaluate the accuracy of color flow scanning in individual segments, such as the common femoral, superficial femoral, popliteal, and tibioperoneal veins. It is also informative to analyze accuracy in the larger above-knee and below-knee segments of the limb, in the entire limb, and in the patient as a whole. The latter information is particularly important as regards therapeutic decisions.

Although most noninvasive tests tend to overlook nonocclusive thrombi that do not interfere with blood flow and are relatively insensitive to thrombi isolated to a single short segment of vein (especially below the knee), color flow is at least theoretically capable of detecting these clots. Thus, color flow must be held to a higher standard of excellence than most other noninvasive tests. Finally, it is well known that all tests for deep venous thrombosis are more sensitive in limbs with clinically suspected disease than they are when used for surveillance of asymptomatic patients at high risk for developing venous thrombi.

Clinically Suspected Deep Venous Thrombosis

In our laboratory, color flow scans have been positive in all patients with deep venous thrombosis who have undergone phlebography (sensitivity of 100 per cent).[19] No superficial femoral thrombi and only 6 per cent of those below the knee have escaped detection (Table 16–1). We attribute the high sensitivity to the extensive nature of the thrombotic process in these symptomatic patients. (Over half of these clots proved to be totally occlusive and almost three quarters involved both above-knee and below-knee veins.) Negative predictive values approach 100 per cent for the patient as a whole, and exceed 92 per cent for all individual venous segments.

Although specificity, in our experience, exceeds 95 per cent above the knee, it hovers around 75 per cent below the knee, probably due to our practice

TABLE 16–1. ACCURACY: SYMPTOMATIC DVT

	Limbs (N)	Above-Knee		Below-Knee	
		Sensitivity (%)	Specificity (%)	Sensitivity (%)	Specificity (%)
Color flow					
Mattos et al.[19]	77	100	98	94	75
Persson et al.[20]	24	100	100	—	—
Schindler et al.[18]	94	98	100	—	—
Duplex or B-mode					
Elias et al.[5]	430	100	98	91	96
Semrow et al.[23]	36	—	—	98	92
Comerota et al.[7]	72	100	86	86	86

of classifying equivocal studies as positive.[19] Above the knee, positive predictive values have been 95 per cent or better, but approximately 20 per cent of our positive scans in the tibioperoneal veins have not been verified phlebographically. For the patient as a whole, positive predictive values are about 80 per cent—reflecting the relatively high false-positive rate in the below-knee segments.

Literature Review

There are few reports in the literature concerning the accuracy of color flow scanning for the detection of clinically suspected deep venous thrombosis (Tables 16–1 and 16–2). Among the first studies was that of Persson and associates, who compared the results of color flow scanning with phlebography in 24 symptomatic legs.[20] All 16 positive studies were correct, for a sensitivity of 100 per cent; but only one thrombus was isolated to the calf veins—the remainder were located in the popliteal or more proximal veins. Specificity was 100 per cent. Foley and colleagues reported complete agreement between color flow and phlebography in 12 positive and 35 negative studies at the femoral level and in 4 positive and 12 negative studies of the tibioperoneal veins, but none of the tibioperoneal thrombi were isolated to the calf veins.[12] Two of seven isolated popliteal thrombi were not detected. In a prospective study of 94 symptomatic limbs (55 of which were positive for thrombi), Schindler and associates reported a 98 per cent sensitivity and 100 per cent specificity for color coded duplex scanning.[18] Below-knee veins were not examined.

TABLE 16–2. ACCURACY OF COLOR FLOW SCANNING IN 75 SYMPTOMATIC LIMBS[a]

	Limbs (N)	Thrombi (N)	Sensitivity (%)	Specificity (%)	PPV (%)	NPV (%)
Limbs	75	34	79	88	84	84
Above-Knee	75	25	92	100	100	96
Tibio-peroneal	74	30	73	86	79	83
Adequate	44	20	95	100	100	96
Inadequate	30	10	30	70	33	67
Isolated tibio-peroneal	49	9	44	88	44	88
Adequate	28	5	80	100	100	96
Inadequate	21	4	0	71	0	75

[a] Data derived from Rose SC, et al: Symptomatic lower extremity deep venous thrombosis: Accuracy, limitations, and role of color duplex flow imaging in diagnosis. Radiology 1990;*175*:639–644.

Results of the comprehensive report of Rose and colleagues, who compared color flow scanning and phlebography in 75 limbs of 69 symptomatic patients, were similar to ours (Table 16–2).[16] Accuracy for detecting or excluding thrombi in above-knee veins was excellent. Although accuracy was also reasonably good below the knee, only 8 of 30 tibioperoneal clots were isolated to that region; the remainder occurred in conjunction with above-knee thrombi. The sensitivity below the knee was greatly influenced by whether the study was considered adequate (visualization of all portions of the tibioperoneal veins) or inadequate (visualization limited by technical factors) and by whether the clots were isolated to the tibioperoneal segment. They also noted that nonocclusive small thrombi (less than 3 cm in length) were difficult to detect, only one of four being correctly identified on color flow scanning.

Diagnosis of Symptomatic DVT with a B-Mode or Duplex Scans

Pooled data from 12 reports in which conventional B-mode or duplex scans were compared to phlebography in 1835 patients with clinically suspected DVT yield a cumulative sensitivity and specificity of 96 per cent.[21] Five of these studies were confined to veins above the knee and few of the others singled out below-knee thrombi for consideration (many papers mention calf veins only in passing). Thus, these figures probably represent the accuracy of duplex scanning above the knee relatively accurately, but are unlikely to reflect the accuracy of duplex scanning below the knee. It is generally acknowledged that most errors with duplex scanning are made in surveys of the infrapopliteal veins.[8,9]

Several papers, however, report excellent accuracy for detecting calf vein thrombosis in symptomatic patients (Table 16–1). In a prospective study of 430 patients with suspected DVT, Elias and colleagues obtained positive duplex scans in 84 of 92 limbs with isolated calf vein thrombi (sensitivity, 91 per cent).[5] The specificity was 96 per cent. Rollins and co-workers investigated 319 individual veins in 46 limbs with suspected DVT and found that the location and anatomic extent of thrombi detected with B-mode scans corresponded within ±1.5 cm with that disclosed by phlebography in 84 per cent of anterior tibial, 86 per cent of posterior tibial, and 93 per cent of peroneal veins.[22] In another study by this same group, Semrow examined 203 individual calf veins in 36 limbs with symptoms suggesting acute DVT.[23] Thrombi were detected by B-mode scanning in 127 of 130 venous segments in which the phlebogram was positive for acute or chronic DVT (sensitivity, 98 per cent); and negative results were obtained in 67 of 73 phlebographically normal veins (specificity, 92 per cent). These remarkable results are more likely to be the exception rather than the rule; but they do confirm that a high degree of accuracy is possible. Somewhat less favorable results with duplex scanning were reported by Comerota and associates.[7] In their prospective study of 72 legs with suspected DVT, the sensitivity (6 of 7) and specificity (24 of 28) for detecting or ruling out calf vein thrombi were both 86 per cent.

Surveillance of High-Risk Patients

In our early surveillance studies of asymptomatic high-risk patients undergoing total hip or knee arthroplasty, less than 30 per cent of clots developing during the postoperative period were detected with color flow scanning.[11,19] Increasing experience on the part of technologists, more skillful interpretation of the scans, and the acquisition of more sophisticated instruments with "slow flow" capabilities and an enhanced gray scale have resulted in an improved sensitivity, which now (in the last 50 patients) approaches 80 per cent.[19] Over 90 per cent of these developing thrombi were nonocclusive, were only a few centimeters long, and were isolated to the below-knee veins. Therefore, the relative lack of sensitivity was not unanticipated. Specificity, however, was quite good, exceeding 97 per cent for all venous segments—both above and below the knee (Table 16–3).

Although a positive result in a surveillance study provides reasonable assurance that a clot is present (positive predictive value of 90 per cent), a negative result cannot be relied upon to exclude the presence of a postoperative thrombosis developing in the infrapopliteal veins (negative predictive value of 75 per cent). Above the knee, however, the negative predictive value approximates 100 per cent.

Surveillance of High-Risk Patients with Conventional Duplex Scans

Except for our preliminary study, there are no reports in the literature concerning surveillance of high-risk patients with color flow scanning.[11] Although the results of a number of surveillance studies with conventional duplex scanning have been reported, there is little information concerning the accuracy of this modality for detecting asymptomatic thrombi originating in veins below the knee (Table 16–3).

Positive duplex scans were obtained by Flinn and associates in 17 (4.7 per cent) of 361 consecutive patients following major neurosurgical procedures.[24] All clots were detected in veins proximal to the tibioperoneal level. Calf veins were not scanned routinely, and therefore the accuracy in this area was not determined. Phlebograms were obtained in 14 patients, 10 with positive scans and 4 with negative scans. In this small sample of the entire series, the positive predictive value of B-mode scanning was 80 per cent (8 of 10) for proximal DVT, and the negative predictive value was 100 per cent (4 of 4).

Barnes and coauthors compared the results of duplex scanning and phlebography in 78 patients undergoing total hip or knee arthroplasty.[25] Again, scans were confined to the popliteal and more proximal veins. The sensitivity of conventional duplex scans for proximal deep venous thrombosis was 83 per cent (10 of 12 limbs), and the specificity was 96 per cent (135 of 141 limbs). In

TABLE 16–3. ACCURACY: SURVEILLANCE DVT

	Limbs (N)	Above-Knee		Below-Knee	
		Sensitivity (%)	Specificity (%)	Sensitivity (%)	Specificity (%)
Color flow					
Mattos et al.[19]	190	67	100	56	98
Duplex or B-mode					
Barnes et al.[25]	153	83	96	—	—
Woolson et al.[26]	150	89	100	—	—
Comerota et al.[7]	38	100	100	50	100
Borris et al.[27]	60	59	91	29	91
Borris et al.[28]	61	73	96	67	—

13 (52 per cent) of 25 patients with postoperative DVT, clots were confined to the infrapopliteal veins and therefore escaped detection.

A third study of postoperative DVT in which duplex scanning was confined to the proximal veins was reported by Woolson and colleagues.[26] All patients underwent phlebography 4 to 23 days following total hip replacement. Seventeen of nineteen above-knee thrombi were detected, representing a sensitivity of 89 per cent. Eight limbs, however, had isolated calf thrombi; and since none of these were detected, the overall sensitivity was only 63 per cent. There were no false-positive studies in the 131 patients with negative phlebograms.

Three reports include data concerning the detection of below-knee thrombi.

1. Comerota and associates evaluated the accuracy of duplex scanning for detecting postoperative DVT in 38 legs of patients undergoing total joint replacement.[7] All seven proximal thrombi were detected by duplex scanning (sensitivity, 100 per cent), but only one of two clots confined to the infrapopliteal veins were identified (sensitivity, 50 per cent). The overall specificity was 100 per cent.

2. Borris and colleagues compared the results of postoperative B-mode scanning (without Doppler) to phlebography in a prospective study of 60 patients undergoing total hip replacement.[27] B-mode scanning was positive in 15 of 28 patients with positive phlebograms, for a sensitivity of 54 per cent. All clots were nonocclusive. The specificity was 91 per cent (29 of 32). Sixteen (59 per cent) of 27 proximal thrombi were identified, but only 4 (29 per cent) of 14 calf vein thrombi were detected. The length of the thrombus also influenced accuracy. Whereas the sensitivity was 64 per cent (18 of 28) for clots longer than 1 centimeter, it was only 15 per cent (2 of 13) for those shorter than 1 centimeter.

3. In a subsequent similar study, the same authors found the sensitivity and specificity of B-mode scanning to be 73 per cent and 96 per cent for proximal venous thrombosis, respectively; but no clot less than 1 centimeter was detected.[28] There were three isolated calf vein thrombi, one of which was missed.

APPLICATION

Symptomatic Patients

The diagnosis of DVT in symptomatic patients constitutes the major role of color flow imaging in the clinical assessment of venous disease. In recent years, duplex scanning has become the standard noninvasive diagnostic test. Our results and those of others with color flow compare favorably with the best results reported with conventional duplex scanning. For detecting and ruling out thrombi in the large veins above the knee, color flow imaging has proved to be highly accurate, with sensitivities and specificities approaching 100 per cent. Even below the knee, most clots in the tibioperoneal veins can be detected, albeit at the expense of a reduced specificity. Again, results with color flow imaging below the knee approximate the best of those achieved with conventional duplex scanning and far exceed the experience of most investigators with this modality.

Whether to treat or not to treat a symptomatic patient is a decision that rests on the accuracy of the diagnostic test as it applies to the patient as a whole. If the decision is made to treat only proximal DVT, color flow may be relied upon to reach the proper conclusion (Fig. 16–3). This is the approach championed by those who advocate physiological testing and by many of the proponents of B-mode or duplex imaging.[29] If, however, calf vein thrombosis is not assumed to be innocuous and the decision is made to treat DVT regardless of location, it would seem prudent to confirm the diagnosis of isolated calf vein DVT with phlebography—a conclusion based on the relatively low positive predictive value (~80 per cent) of color flow imaging below the knee. On the other hand, a totally negative study below the knee in symptomatic patients can usually be relied upon.

Surveillance

In our experience, less than 60 per cent of the thrombi developing during the early postoperative period in patients undergoing joint arthroplasty were detected.[19] These clots were almost exclusively located below the knee; most were isolated, nonocclusive, and of limited extent. Some involved perforating veins or venous sinusoids, and therefore were not along the main track of interrogation. Although results improved with experience, it is doubtful that the accuracies achieved in symptomatic patients will ever be matched. If one considers all segments of both limbs (i.e., the patient as a whole), the negative predictive value of 75 per cent suggests that clots will actually be present in about one fourth of all patients with negative surveillance studies (Fig. 16–4). On the other hand, specificity and the positive predictive value is good. In other words, if the scan results are positive, the clinician can be about 90 per cent certain that a thrombus is present and can institute appropriate treatment.

From these preliminary studies, it is not clear what role surveillance with color flow Doppler should play. Surveillance studies are not only expensive, time consuming, and labor intensive, but also miss an appreciable number of clots, especially below the knee. Although repeating the scan at intervals of several days in patients with negative studies is likely to detect significant proximal propagation, this program, if adopted, would greatly increase the expense (Fig. 16–4). To arrive at a conclusion, it is necessary to balance the expense and efficacy of color Doppler scanning against that of routine prophylaxis. Clearly, prophylaxis in not the complete answer, since 40 per cent of

FIGURE 16–3. Algorithm showing approach to diagnosis and management of DVT in symptomatic patients based on results of color flow scanning. (Positive (PPV) and negative (NPV) predictive values are derived from the data of Mattos MA, et al: Color flow duplex scanning for the surveillance and diagnosis of acute deep venous thrombosis. Derived from data presented at the 45th annual meeting of the Society for Vascular Surgery, Boston, MA, June 5, 1991.)

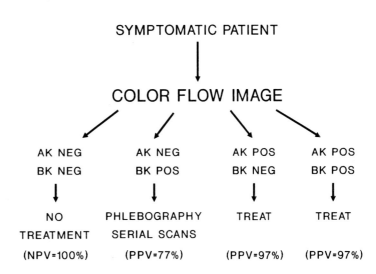

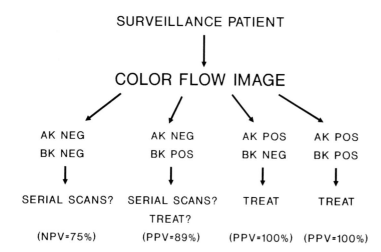

SURVEILLANCE PATIENT

COLOR FLOW IMAGE

| AK NEG | AK NEG | AK POS | AK POS |
| BK NEG | BK POS | BK NEG | BK POS |

| SERIAL SCANS? | SERIAL SCANS? | TREAT | TREAT |
| | TREAT? | | |

| (NPV=75%) | (PPV=89%) | (PPV=100%) | (PPV=100%) |

FIGURE 16–4. Algorithm showing approach to diagnosis and management of DVT in high-risk patients based on surveillance with color flow scanning. (Positive (PPV) and negative (NPV) predictive values are derived from the data of Mattos MA, et al: Color flow duplex scanning for the surveillance and diagnosis of acute deep venous thrombosis. Derived from data presented at the 45th annual meeting of the Society for Vascular Surgery, Boston, MA, June 5, 1991.)

the patients in our study developed thrombi despite all having received some form of perioperative prophylaxis.[19]

Below-Knee Thrombi

Color flow imaging detects most below-knee thrombi in symptomatic patients even when they are isolated or nonocclusive; and, as our most recent experience shows, almost 80 per cent of below-knee thrombi are identified in surveillance patients. Because one of the potential advantages that color imaging has over other noninvasive techniques is its ability to detect below-knee thrombi, it is fair to ask: What is the importance of thrombi in this location—is it really necessary to expend the extra effort required to identify them?

Most investigators agree that thrombi isolated to the tibioperoneal veins are seldom responsible for pulmonary emboli.[30] Moreno-Cabal and colleagues, however, found positive ventilation-perfusion lung scans in 66 per cent of patients with popliteal thrombi and in 33 per cent of patients with tibioperoneal thrombosis.[31] None of these patients had extension of the clot into proximal veins. About half of the patients with positive scans had "silent" emboli that would not have been detected had the scans not been performed. Moreover, in the surveillance study of Flinn and associates,[24] the only three pulmonary emboli that occurred were in patients with negative duplex scans of the proximal veins; and in a similar study of Barnes and colleagues,[25] the only two patients to develop pulmonary emboli had clots isolated to the infrapopliteal veins. Therefore, it is likely that at least some calf vein clots have the potential to embolize.

Undoubtedly, many below-knee thrombi are missed in symptomatic patients when the examination is limited to above-knee veins by the nature of the study (plethysmography) or by the practice of the laboratory (B-mode or duplex scanning).[29,32] A number of investigators have shown that this poses little hazard for the patient, provided serial plethysmographic, Doppler, or duplex studies are performed on all patients with negative studies to detect potentially dangerous propagation into more proximal veins.[30,32] Because only a fraction of patients with negative above-knee studies have undetected infrapopliteal thrombi and because only 20 per cent of these thrombi propagate into the popliteal or more proximal veins, serial testing yields few positive results and is unlikely to be cost-effective. Even if it were elected not to treat isolated below-knee thrombi in symptomatic patients, color flow imaging of calf veins has the advantage of permitting serial testing to be restricted to those patients with positive findings (Fig. 16–3). Unlike the requirements posed by the limitations of other testing methods, there is no need to follow symptomatic patients with negative color flow studies.

Of equal interest is the accumulating evidence that tibio-peroneal DVT may be responsible for chronic venous insufficiency.[33–35] This by itself may put a different complexion on the issue of the importance of calf vein thrombosis and the role of color flow scanning in its detection.

CONCLUSION

We believe that color flow imaging is the current noninvasive method of choice for diagnosing deep venous thrombosis in symptomatic patients, that it holds promise as a method for detecting clots forming in the perioperative period, and that it is the best noninvasive method for identifying calf vein thrombosis. Even if it were proved to be no more accurate than conventional duplex scanning, color flow scanning has the advantages of facilitating the identification of veins and of decreasing the time and effort spent on each examination.

REFERENCES

1. Sumner DS, Baker DW, Strandness DE Jr: The ultrasonic velocity detector in a clinical study of venous disease. Arch Surg 1968;97:75–80.
2. Sumner DS: Diagnosis of venous thrombosis by Doppler ultrasound. *In* Bergan JJ, Yao JST, eds: Venous Problems. Chicago, Year Book Medical Publishers, 1978;159–185.
3. Talbut SR: Use of real-time imaging in identifying deep venous obstruction: A preliminary report. Bruit (June) 1982;6:41–42.
4. Flanagan LD, Sullivan ED, Cranley JJ: Venous imaging of the extremities using real-time B-mode ultrasound. *In* Bergan JJ, Yao JST, eds: Surgery of the Veins. Orlando, Grune & Stratton, 1985;89–98.
5. Elias A, Le Corff G, Bouvier JL, Benichou M, Serradimigni A: Value of real-time B-mode ultrasound imaging in the diagnosis of deep vein thrombosis of the lower limbs. Int Angio 1987;6:175–182.
6. Becker DM, Philbrick JT, Abbitt PL: Real-time ultrasonography for the diagnosis of lower extremity deep venous thrombosis. The wave of the future? Arch Intern Med 1989;149:1731–1734.
7. Comerota AJ, Katz ML, Greenwald LL, Leefmans E, Czeredarczuk M, White JV: Venous duplex imaging: Should it replace hemodynamic tests for deep venous thrombosis? J Vasc Surg 1990;11:53–61.
8. Killewich LA, Bedford GR, Beach KW, Strandness DE: Diagnosis of deep venous thrombosis: A prospective study comparing duplex scanning to contrast venography. Circulation 1989;79:810–814.
9. Wright DJ, Shepard AD, McPharlin M, Ernst CB: Pitfalls in lower extremity venous duplex scanning. J Vasc Surg 1990;11:675–679.
10. Comerota AJ, Katz ML, Grossi RJ, et al: The comparative value of noninvasive testing for diagnosis and surveillance of deep vein thrombosis. J Vasc Surg 1988;7:40–49.
11. Sumner DS, Londrey GL, Spadone DP, Hodgson KJ, Leutz DW, Stauffer ES: Study of deep venous thrombosis in high-risk patients using color flow Doppler. *In* Bergan JJ, Yao JST, eds: Venous Disorders. Philadelphia, WB Saunders Co, 1991;63–76.
12. Foley WD, Middleton WD, Lawson TL, Erickson S, Quiroz FA, Macrander S: Color Doppler ultrasound imaging of lower-extremity venous disease. AJR 1989;152:371–376.
13. Knighton RA, Priest DL, Zwiebel WJ, Lawrence PF, Miller FJ, Rose SC: Techniques for color flow sonography of the lower extremity. Radiographics 1990;10:775–786.
14. Sigel B, Machi J, Beitler JC, Justin JR: Red cell aggregation as a cause of blood flow echogenicity. Radiology 1983;148:799–802.

15. Polak JF, Culter SS, O'Leary DH: Deep veins of the calf: Assessment with color Doppler flow imaging. Radiology 1989;*171*:481–485.
16. Rose SC, Zwiebel WJ, Nelson BD, et al: Symptomatic lower extremity deep venous thrombosis: Accuracy, limitations, and role of color duplex flow imaging in diagnosis. Radiology 1990; *175*:639–644.
17. van Bemmelen PS, Bedford G, Strandness DE: Visualization of calf veins by color flow imaging. Ultrasound Med Biol 1990;*16*:15–17.
18. Schindler JM, Kaiser M, Gerber A, Vuilliomenet A, Popovic A, Bertel O: Colour coded duplex sonography in suspected deep vein thrombosis of the leg. Br Med J 1990;*301*:1369–1370.
19. Mattos MA, Londrey GL, Leutz DW, et al: Color flow duplex scanning for the surveillance and diagnosis of acute deep venous thrombosis. Presented at the 45th annual meeting of the Society for Vascular Surgery, Boston, MA, June 5, 1991.
20. Persson AV, Jones C, Zide R, Jewell ER: Use of triplex scanner in diagnosis of deep venous thrombosis. Arch Surg 1989;*124*:593–596.
21. Sumner DS: Diagnosis of deep venous thrombosis. *In* Rutherford RB, ed: Vascular Surgery, 3rd ed. Philadelphia, WB Saunders Co, 1989;1520–1560.
22. Rollins DL, Semrow CM, Friedell ML, Calligaro KD, Buchbinder D: Progress in the diagnosis of deep venous thrombosis: The efficacy of real-time B-mode ultrasonic scanning. J Vasc Surg 1988;*7*:638–641.
23. Semrow CM, Friedell ML, Buchbinder D, Rollins DL: The efficacy of ultrasonic venography in the detection of calf vein thrombosis. J Vasc Technol 1988;*12*:240–244.
24. Flinn WR, Sandager GP, Cerullo LJ, Havey RJ, Yao JST: Duplex venous scanning for the prospective surveillance of perioperative venous thrombosis. Arch Surg 1989;*124*:901–905.
25. Barnes RW, Nix ML, Barnes CL, et al: Perioperative asymptomatic venous thrombosis: Role of duplex scanning versus venography. J Vasc Surg 1989;*9*:251–260.
26. Woolson ST, McCrory DW, Walter JF, Maloney WI, Watt JM, Cahill PD: B-mode ultrasound scanning in the detection of proximal venous thrombosis after total hip replacement. J Bone Joint Surg 1990;*72-A*:983–987.
27. Borris LC, Christiansen HM, Lassen MR, Olsen AD, Schøtt P: Comparison of real-time B-mode ultrasonography and bilateral ascending phlebography for detection of post operative deep vein thrombosis following elective hip surgery. Thromb Haemost 1989;*61*:363–365.
28. Borris LC, Christiansen HM, Lassen MR, Olsen AD, Schøtt P: Real-time B-mode ultrasonography in the diagnosis of postoperative deep vein thrombosis in non-symptomatic high-risk patients. Eur J Vasc Surg 1990;*4*:473–475.
29. Lensing AWA, Prandoni P, Brandjes D, et al: Detection of deep-vein thrombosis by real-time B-mode ultrasonography. N Engl J Med 1989;*320*:342–345.
30. Philbrick JT, Becker DM: Calf deep venous thrombosis: A wolf in sheep's clothing? Arch Intern Med 1988;*148*:2131–2138.
31. Moreno-Cabral R, Kistner RL, Nordyke RA: Importance of calf vein thrombophlebitis. Surgery 1976;*80*:735–742.
32. Hull RD, Hirsh J, Carter CJ, et al: Diagnostic efficacy of impedance plethysmography for clinically suspected deep-vein thrombosis. A randomized trial. Ann Intern Med 1985; *102*:21–28.
33. Strandness DE, Langlois Y, Cramer M, Randlett A, Thiele BL: Long-term sequelae of acute venous thrombosis. JAMA 1983;*250*:1289–1292.
34. Moore DJ, Himmel PD, Sumner DS: Distribution of venous valvular incompetence in patients with the postphlebitic syndrome. J Vasc Surg 1986;*3*:49–57.
35. Schulman S, Granqvist S, Juhlin-Dannfelt J, Lockner D: Long-term sequelae of calf vein thrombosis treated with heparin or low-dose streptokinase. Acta Med Scand 1986;*219*:349–357.

17

INTRAOPERATIVE USE OF B-MODE AND COLOR DOPPLER IMAGING

JUNJI MACHI, BERNARD SIGEL, and ANDREW B. ROBERTS

A variety of diagnostic technologies have been introduced for diagnosis of vascular problems. Particularly, the use of noninvasive techniques has increased dramatically both preoperatively and postoperatively. Diagnostic procedures are also important during vascular operations. Vascular defects such as intimal flaps, strictures, and thrombi may occur during vascular reconstructive operations. These defects may result in early graft occlusion. Therefore, the detection and correction of significant vascular defects at the time of the initial operative procedure is a major concern for vascular surgeons. The imaging method that has been used most frequently and generally is regarded as the standard intraoperative procedure to detect vascular defects is radiographic arteriography. Although highly accurate in diagnosing vascular problems, operative arteriography has certain inherent risks and disadvantages.[1-3] For this reason, we have applied high-resolution ultrasound imaging during vascular operations as a safer and simpler method.

Over the past 10 years, intraoperative B-mode imaging was performed during more than 500 vascular operations, and the accuracy and the benefits of this new method was compared to operative arteriography.[4-11] More recently, color Doppler imaging was introduced in addition to B-mode imaging.[12-14] In this report, we summarize our experience with B-mode and color Doppler imaging by reviewing the indications, technique, clinical results, benefits, and limitations of operative imaging ultrasonography during vascular surgery.

INDICATIONS

There are two principal indications for the use of intraoperative ultrasonography for vascular surgery: (1) preconstruction evaluation of vascular abnormalities, and (2) postreconstruction detection and assessment of vascular defects. Preconstruction evaluation is usually complimentary to preoperative imaging studies. In the majority of operations, preoperative arteriography provides detailed information about the location and the extent of vascular diseases, which is sufficient for surgeons to approach, expose, and open vessels. Therefore, preconstruction ultrasonography is not often indicated. However, there are situations in which preoperative arteriography may not adequately demonstrate the exact vascular anatomy beyond a proximal occlusion or stenosis. Even when preoperative arteriography is complete, the localization of a particular vascular lesion or a blood vessel itself in the operative field may be difficult due to distorted anatomy resulting from diseases or previous operations. In such circumstances, prereconstruction operative ultrasonography may accurately identify the location and the extent of vascular diseases not adequately visualized by arteriography, thus facilitating the approach and exposure of vessels. Color Doppler imaging may be more advantageous than B-mode imaging in localizing small vascular abnormalities or detecting preoperatively unclear vascular diseases prior to reconstruction.

Postreconstruction operative ultrasonography is generally indicated in all vascular procedures as a completion examination prior to closure of the operative site. This is apparently the more common and important indication for the use of ultrasound imaging during vascular operations. Significant vascular defects that result from technical problems during vascular procedures should not be inadvertently left behind. Many vascular defects such as intimal flaps and thrombi may be too small to produce discernible hemodynamic changes, and thus may not be identifiable by conventional Doppler or other flow studies. Consequently, intraoperative imaging studies are required. Operative arteriography, a traditional method, and intraoperative ultrasonography, a newer method, are currently available intraoperative imaging studies. These two methods should be used in a complementary fashion, on the basis of advantages and disadvantages of each method. In general, because of its safety and simplicity, intraoperative ultrasonography can be used as a first-choice screening procedure to evaluate all reconstructive sites including anastomotic and endarterectomized segments. Once a vascular defect is found, its potential as a problem should be assessed in order to determine whether or not the vessel should be reopened and the defect repaired. This determination is based on the type, size (or magnitude), and location of each vascular defect. Real-time B-mode ultrasonography, which provides multiple image views of vascular defects, is particularly useful in assessing the identified defects, and thereby helps determine their clinical significance. Intraoperative color Doppler imaging may be more helpful in some instances because it is able to provide supplemental blood flow information in addition to anatomic information.

INSTRUMENTATION AND TECHNIQUE

The high-resolution real-time B-mode ultrasound system is the equipment employed for intraoperative use during vascular surgery. The color Doppler imaging system also may be used during operation and should be high-resolution with a capability of detecting small vascular abnormalities. Transducer frequencies of 7.5 to 10-MHz are required. With such frequency instruments, vascular defects (i.e., intimal flaps, thrombi) as small as 1 mm can be delineated. The size and the shape of the ultrasound probe is important. Scanning of deeply seated or small peripheral vessels requires a probe with a small head. A pencil-like, cylindric probe with a small end-viewing head is the best instrument for manipulating in the operative fields of vascular surgery.

Prereconstruction scanning can be performed whenever necessary before arteriotomy, while postreconstruction scanning is performed immediately after closure of vessels and restoration of blood flow. The most important maneuver to scan blood vessels is the "probe stand-off technique," in which the probe is held about 1.0 to 2.0 cm away from the surface of the vessel. This method permits clear visualization of vascular structures, particularly the superficial wall of the vessel, and prevents the compression of the vessel by the probe. Saline solution is introduced into the operative fields for acoustic coupling. Frequently, it is necessary to retract the edges of the operative wound or the skin flap upward to fill saline in the operative fields. The blood vessels are imaged routinely along their longitudinal axis. During this longitudinal scanning, the vessels should be examined in multiple planes. Transverse scanning is also performed at locations of interest. When a vascular defect is detected by longitudinal scanning, transverse scanning should always be added to confirm its presence and to better evaluate its extent. It is important to scan all segments of the vessels that are manipulated at operation. These include not only all arteriotomy closures, anastomoses, and endarterectomized segments, but also sites at which vascular clamps or occlusion tapes are placed. In addition, bypass grafts, particularly saphenous vein grafts, can be examined intraoperatively. Color Doppler imaging has been particularly useful in detecting arteriovenous fistulas of in situ vein-graft bypasses.

CLINICAL RESULTS

Intraoperative B-mode Imaging

B-mode imaging ultrasonography using 7.5- or 10-MHz systems was performed during 519 vascular operations[4,5] (Table 17–1). The majority of operations were lower extremity bypasses and carotid endarterectomies. Pre-reconstruction ultrasonography was selectively used only in 23 operations (4.4 per cent). On the other hand, postreconstruction ultrasonography was performed routinely in all operations, and a total of 960 operative sites (e.g., anastomotic sites, endarterectomized areas) were examined (Table 17–1).

In 364 of 519 operations (70.1 per cent), no vascular defects were detected by intraoperative postreconstruction B-mode imaging. In the remaining 155 operations (29.9 per cent), a total of 194 vascular defects were diagnosed. The vascular surgeon assessed those vascular defects to determine their clinical significance in terms of the need for reexploration and repair.

Of the 194 discovered vascular defects, 134 defects that were found in 107 operations (20.6 per cent of total operations) were judged not to need repair because they were too small or located in a noncritical position. Most of these defects designated as insignificant (not repaired) were small intimal flaps (3

TABLE 17–1. INTRAOPERATIVE B-MODE IMAGING DURING VASCULAR OPERATIONS

Type of Operations	Number of Operations (%)	Number of Sites Examined
Carotid endarterectomy	153 (29.5)	154
Carotid bypass	6 (1.2)	10
Axillo-femoral bypass	11 (2.1)	30
Aorto-femoral bypass	82 (15.8)	237
Lower extremity bypass	218 (42.0)	459
Porto-systemic shunt	12 (2.3)	14
Others	37 (7.1)	56
Totals	519 (100%)	960

mm or less in size) and mild strictures (less than 30 per cent), and were situated in relatively large vessels (Table 17–2). The remaining 60 vascular defects that were found in 48 operations (9.3 per cent of total operations) were judged to require repair because they were of such a large size or located in such a position that they would endanger the patency of the vascular reconstruction. The majority of these significant defects (repaired) were large intimal flaps (3 mm or greater in size), thrombi causing significant or total occlusion, and moderate to severe strictures (greater than 30 per cent), which were situated in relatively smaller or critical vessels or grafts themselves (Table 17–3). Figure 17–1 shows a vascular defect not repaired, and Figures 17–2 and 17–3, show vascular defects repaired.

The outcome of operations was basically the same whether vascular defects were present or absent, repaired or not repaired. The early postoperative patency rate (1 to 2 months after operation) of the vascular reconstruction (excluding carotid endarterectomy) was 91.5 per cent in operations without vascular defects, 90.2 per cent in operations with significant defects which were repaired, and 95.8 per cent in operations with insignificant defects which were not repaired. No statistical differences were noted among these patency rates. This suggests that our judgment of not repairing insignificant defects was probably justified. The evidence that the results of the operations with defects repaired were comparable to the operations without defects suggest that the repair of significant defects was successful.

The accuracy of intraoperative B-mode imaging was also evaluated by comparison with operative arteriography. Of 960 ultrasonically examined sites, a total of 211 sites (in 168 operations) were also examined by postreconstruction operative arteriography. Usually, the distal anastomoses in relatively small vessels such as popliteal or more distal arteries were examined by arteriography as well as ultrasonography. The results of intraoperative ultrasonography and arteriography in diagnosing vascular defects are shown in Table 17–4. When both tests were negative, these were considered to be true-negative examinations. When both or either test was positive, the result, either true or false, was established on the basis of the operative findings at reexploration. The results

TABLE 17–2. VASCULAR DEFECTS DETECTED BY B-MODE IMAGING: NOT REPAIRED

Vascular Defects	Size (Magnitude)	Number	Location[a]
Intimal flap	1 mm	16	CC, IC(4), EC, F(7), P(2), T
	2 mm	65	CC(5), IC(3), EC(9), A, F(37), P(8), T, S
	3 mm	17	CC(6), EC(4), A(3), F(3), P
	4 mm	10	A(2), F(5), P(3)
	5 mm	3	EC, A, F
	6 mm	2	A(2)
Thrombus	2 × 2 mm	2	F, SR
	3 × 3 mm	1	SR
	3 × 5 mm	1	F
Stricture	20–30%	16	IC, EC(2), F(7), P(2), T, VG, SR, PC
	40%	1	P
Total		134 (107 operations)	

A, aorta; B, brachial artery; CC, common carotid; IC, internal carotid; EC, external carotid; F, femoral artery; P, popliteal artery; T, tibial or peroneal artery; S, subclavian artery; SR, splenorenal shunt; PC, portocaval shunt; VG, vein graft; P-T, popliteal-tibial bypass.

TABLE 17–3. VASCULAR DEFECTS DETECTED BY B-MODE IMAGING: REPAIRED

Vascular Defects	Size (Magnitude)	Number	Location[a]
Intimal flap	1 mm	1	T
	2 mm	2	P, T
	3 mm	7	IC(2), F(2), P(2), T
	4 mm	4	F(3), T
	5 mm	6	IC, F(2), P(3)
	6 mm	1	F
	7 mm	2	CC, F
	8 mm	1	A
Plaque	4 × 3 mm	1	EC
Thrombus	4 × 2 mm	2	VG(2)
	3 × 3 mm	2	F, VG
	5 × 4 mm	1	IC
	5 × 5 mm	3	F(2), PC
	6 × 3 mm	2	A, F
	Total thrombosis	4	P, T(2), SR
Stricture	20–30%	5	F, T(3), B
	40%	5	IC, F, VG(2), PC
	50–60%	7	IC(3), F(2), T(2)
	75%	1	IC
	90%	1	F
Air bubble		1	P
Inverted graft		1	P-T
Total		60 (48 operations)	

[a] A, aorta; B, brachial artery; CC, common carotid; IC, internal carotid; EC, external carotid; F, femoral artery; P, popliteal artery; T, tibial or peroneal artery; S, subclavian artery; SR, splenorenal shunt; PC, portocaval shunt; VG, vein graft; P-T, popliteal-tibial bypass.

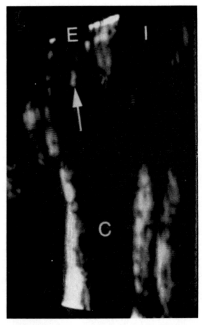 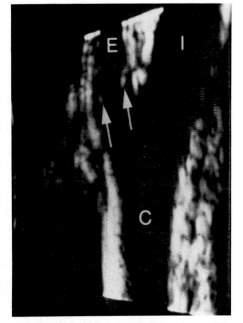

FIGURE 17–1. Three intimal flaps (arrows), 5-mm, 2-mm, and 1-mm in size, detected in an external carotid artery (E) after carotid endarterectomy. Because of their noncritical locations and sizes, these flaps were not repaired. I, internal carotid artery; C, common carotid artery. (Reprinted with permission from Sigel B: Ultrasonography during vascular surgery. *In* Sigel B, ed: Operative Ultrasonography. 2nd ed. New York, Raven Press, 1988;163.)

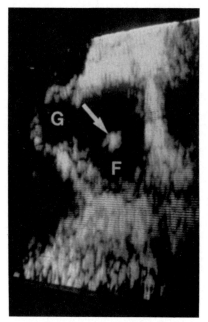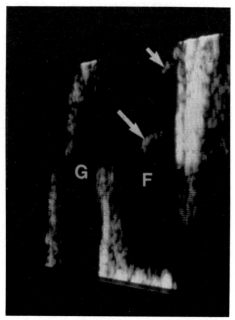

FIGURE 17–2. Two intimal flaps (arrows), 4-mm and 2-mm in length, detected in a femoral artery (F) at the proximal anastomosis after femoral-popliteal bypass. G, bypass graft. *Right,* Longitudinal scanning showing these two flaps simultaneously. *Left,* Transverse scanning demonstrating that the larger flap was 3 mm wide. These intimal flaps were excised after reexploration. (Reprinted with permission from Machi J: Operative ultrasonography during cardiac and vascular surgery. *In* Machi J, ed: Operative Ultrasonography—Fundamentals and Clinical Applications. 1st ed. Tokyo, Life Science Co Ltd, 1987;287.)

revealed that intraoperative ultrasonography had fewer false-positive examinations. Figure 17–4 is an example of false-positive operative arteriography. The accuracy indices of both tests were calculated from the results (Table 17–4). Both imaging methods were comparable in terms of sensitivity, specificity, and predictability of a negative test. Intraoperative ultrasonography provided better predictability of a positive test than arteriography.

Intraoperative Color Doppler Imaging

Color Doppler imaging using high-frequency (7.5-MHz) system has been more recently performed during 57 vascular operations,[14] and the benefits of this imaging method were assessed in comparison to intraoperative B-mode imaging. Most of the operations were carotid endarterectomies and lower extremity bypasses. Six renal artery stenosis correction procedures were included (Table 17–5). In situ saphenous vein-graft bypasses were performed in nine operations. Prereconstruction color Doppler imaging was selectively used in 18 operations (31.6 per cent). Particularly in four operations, intraoperative color Doppler imaging was valuable. In two femoral vascular operations, color Doppler imaging precisely localized a small traumatic arteriovenous fistula and the origin of a pseudoaneurysm, thus facilitating the surgical tissue dissection to gain access to the lesions. In two operations for renovascular hypertension, the presence or the extent of renal artery stenosis that was unclear preoperatively was distinctly demonstrated by intraoperative color Doppler imaging (Fig. 17–5), and this was useful for surgical decision-making before abdominal tissue

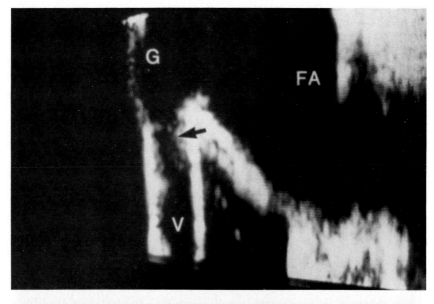

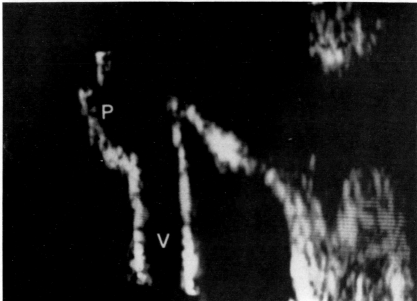

FIGURE 17–3. *Top,* Anastomotic stricture (arrow) detected at the proximal anastomosis between a femoral artery (FA) and a saphenous vein graft (V) after femoral-femoral-popliteal bypass. G, graft of femoral-femoral bypass. This was a 50 per cent stricture and required reexploration and repair. *Bottom,* The stricture was corrected by a saphenous vein patch angioplasty (P) over the stenotic portion (Reprinted with permission from Sigel B: Ultrasonography during vascular surgery. *In* Sigel B, ed: Operative Ultrasonography. 2nd ed. New York, Raven Press. 1988;165.)

dissection. In the remaining 14 operations, prereconstruction color Doppler imaging did not provide significant additional information regarding structural abnormalities; however, abnormal blood flow patterns observed on prereconstruction imaging were helpful for comparison to flow patterns at the time of postreconstruction imaging (Fig. 17–6).

TABLE 17–4. RESULTS AND ACCURACIES OF INTRAOPERATIVE ULTRASONOGRAPHY AND ARTERIOGRAPHY

	Ultrasonography (B-mode Imaging)	Arteriography
True-Positive	27	27
True-Negative	178	172
False-Positive	4	10
False-Negative	2	2
Total	211	211
Sensitivity	93.1%	93.1%
Specificity	97.8%	94.5%
Predictability of a negative test	98.9%	98.9%
Predictability of a positive test	87.1%	73.0%
Overall Accuracy	97.2%	94.3%

Postreconstruction color Doppler imaging was performed routinely in all operations except one operation in which nephrectomy was done for treatment of renovascular hypertension. A total of 99 reconstruction sites were examined (Table 17–5). Vascular defects were not detected in 40 of 56 operations (71.4 per cent). However, mild blood flow disturbances were occasionally observed, mainly at the anastomotic sites. In the saphenous vein grafts, the venous valve remnants frequently produced blood flow disturbances (Fig. 17–7).

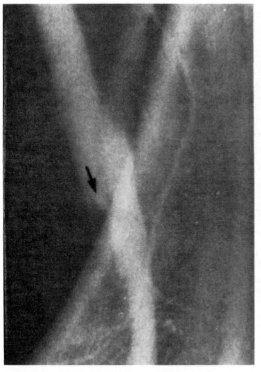 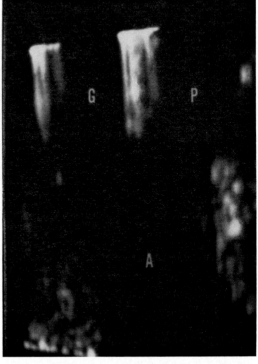

FIGURE 17–4. False-positive operative arteriography. A 3-mm filling defect (arrow) was demonstrated at the distal anastomosis by arteriography after femoral-popliteal bypass. On the other hand, the corresponding intraoperative ultrasonography appeared normal. G, graft; P, popliteal artery; A, anastomosis. Upon reexploration, no vascular defects were found. (Reprinted with permission from Sigel B, Coelho JCU, Flanigan DP, et al: Comparison of B-mode real-time ultrasound scanning with arteriography in detecting vascular defects during surgery. Radiology, 1982;*145*:778.)

TABLE 17–5. INTRAOPERATIVE COLOR DOPPLER IMAGING DURING VASCULAR OPERATIONS

Type of Operations	Number of Operations (%)	Number of Sites Examined (Postreconstruction)
Carotid endarterectomy	22 (38.6)	23
Other carotid operations	2 (3.5)	4
Lower extremity bypass	20 (35.1)	52
Renal artery stenosis correction	6 (10.5)	10
Others	7 (12.3)	10
Totals	57 (100%)	99

In 16 operations (28.6 per cent), vascular defects were identified by color Doppler imaging (Table 17–6). The vascular defects in eight operations required immediate repair, whereas the defects in eight operations were left alone. Intimal flaps were present in four operations. Three of four flaps were 1 to 2 mm in size, situated in the femoral and external carotid artery, and thus were not repaired. These three flaps did not cause any blood flow disturbances on color Doppler imaging. One intimal flap which required repair was 4 mm, located in the common carotid artery and was associated with blood flow reversal (Fig. 17–8). Anastomotic strictures were detected in seven operations. Mild (15 to 30 per cent) anastomotic strictures in four operations, which were associated with only minimal flow disturbances, were not repaired. More severe (30 to 50 per cent) strictures at the distal anastomoses in three operations demonstrated marked poststenotic flow turbulences (Fig. 17–9) and were repaired. Intra-

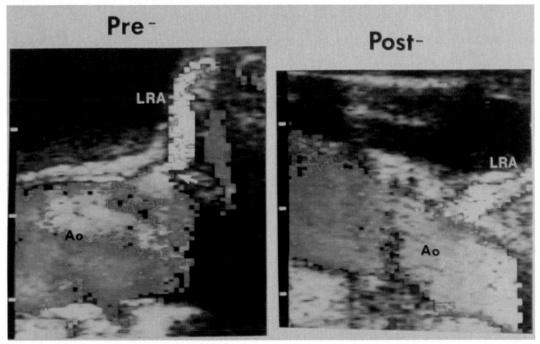

FIGURE 17–5. *Left,* Prereconstruction intraoperative color Doppler imaging demonstrating a renal artery stenosis (arrow) which was unrecognized by preoperative arteriography. A 75 per cent stenosis was present at the origin of the aberrant left renal artery (LRA) originating from the ventral surface of the aorta (Ao). *Right,* Post-reconstruction imaging after correction of the renal artery stenosis. (Reprinted with permission from Machi J. Sigel B, Roberts A, et al: Operative color Doppler imaging for vascular surgery. J Ultrasound Med, in press).

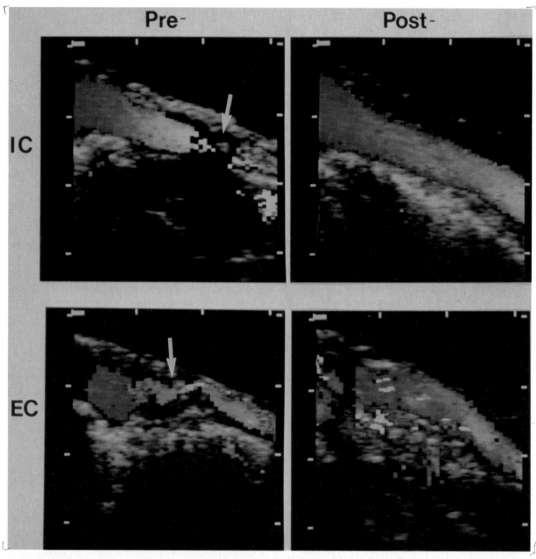

FIGURE 17–6. Prereconstruction (*left*) and postreconstruction (*right*) intraoperative color Doppler imaging during carotid endarterectomy. Prereconstruction scanning showed severe stenoses (arrows) in the internal carotid artery (IC: *upper*) and the external carotid artery (EC: *lower*). Abnormal turbulent blood flow was seen at the poststenotic segments of each artery. Postreconstruction scanning demonstrated wide open lumens of both arteries without significant flow disturbance. (Reprinted with permission from Machi J, Sigel B, Roberts A, et al: Operative color Doppler imaging for vascular surgery. J Ultrasound Med, in press).

operative color Doppler imaging was particularly helpful in detecting and precisely localizing arteriovenous fistulas that resulted from arterialization of the saphenous vein during in situ saphenous vein graft bypass operations. In two operations, intraoperative color Doppler imaging diagnosed four fistulas that were not recognized with operative arteriography (Fig. 17–10). In two other operations, color Doppler imaging that was conducted prior to arteriography delineated multiple fistulas. Because the ultrasound probe was placed just above the bypass graft, these arteriovenous fistulas, whenever seen on the imaging screen, were readily localized by the surgeon in the operative field.

TABLE 17–6. VASCULAR DEFECTS DETECTED BY COLOR DOPPLER IMAGING

Vascular Defects	Size (Magnitude)	Number of Operations	Defects Not Repaired	Defects Repaired
Intimal flap	1–2 mm	3	3	
	4 mm	1		1
Stricture	15–30%	4	4	
	30–50%	3		3
Patch bulging		1	1	
Arteriovenous fistula		4	—	4
Totals		16	8	8

All the fistulas were subsequently repaired (ligated) successfully. The arteriovenous fistulas of in situ vein graft bypasses were not visualized by B-mode imaging alone, probably because of their small size (less than 2 to 3 mm). However, intraoperative color Doppler imaging readily detected these small fistulas by demonstrating intravascular blood flow in color.

From the present preliminary study, we have identified four advantages of intraoperative color Doppler imaging over B-mode imaging:

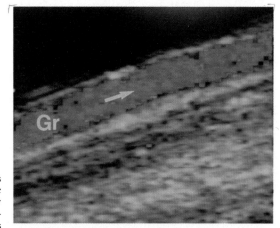

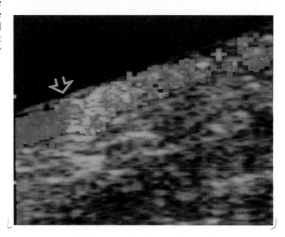

FIGURE 17–7. *Top,* In situ saphenous vein bypass graft (Gr) where no venous valve was present. The blood flow was smooth without disturbance. Arrow indicates the direction of blood flow. *Bottom,* A saphenous vein segment where a valve remnant was present. An open arrow indicates the site of the valvulotomized venous valve. A blood-flow turbulence was seen at the distal side of the valve. (Reprinted with permission from Machi J, Sigel B, Roberts A, et al: Operative color Doppler imaging for vascular surgery. J Ultrasound Med, in press).

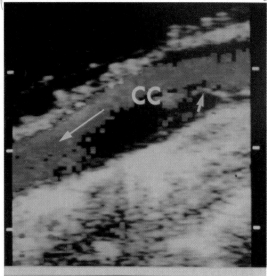

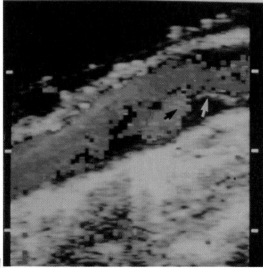

FIGURE 17–8. A 4-mm intimal flap (small white arrow) detected in a common carotid artery (CC) after carotid endarterectomy. This flap was located at the proximal end of the endarterectomized segment. Long white arrow indicates the direction of blood flow (red color). A black arrow indicates a reversed blood flow (blue color) which was observed just distal to the starting point of the endarterectomy where the intimal flap was present. (Reprinted with permission from Machi J, Sigel B, Roberts A, et al: Operative color Doppler imaging for vascular surgery. J Ultrasound Med, in press).

1. Improved localization of small vascular structural abnormalities or detection of preoperatively unknown vessel stenosis before vascular reconstruction.

2. Faster recognition of vascular defects after reconstruction.

3. Unique ability to detect vascular problems (i.e., small arteriovenous fistulas) that are not identifiable by B-mode imaging.

4. Provision of supplemental blood flow information for making decisions regarding the need to repair the vascular defects of marginal anatomic significance.

BENEFITS AND LIMITATIONS

In order to use intraoperative ultrasound imaging appropriately during vascular surgery, surgeons should be aware of its benefits (or advantages) and

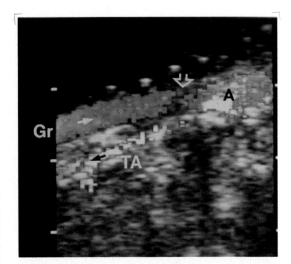

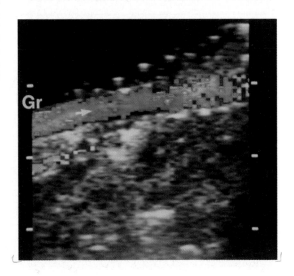

FIGURE 17–9. *Top,* Anastomotic stricture after femoral-tibial bypass. A 50 per cent stricture (open arrow) was detected at the distal anastomosis (A) between a saphenous vein graft (Gr) and a tibial artery (TA). A disturbed blood flow was seen at the poststricture area. White arrow indicates the direction of blood flow in the graft, black arrow indicates a reversed blood flow in the native tibial artery. *Bottom,* This anastomotic stricture was repaired. Color Doppler imaging after repair demonstrated a wide open anastomotic site without significant flow disturbance. (Reprinted with permission from Machi J, Sigel B, Roberts A, et al: Operative color Doppler imaging for vascular surgery. J Ultrasound Med, in press).

limitations (or disadvantages). As compared to operative arteriography, intraoperative ultrasonography has several advantages, which include:[4–17]

1. Comparable or higher accuracy than arteriography.
2. More imaging information of vascular abnormalities.
3. Safety.
4. Wider applications to reconstruction sites.
5. Ability for repeated use.
6. Low cost.

Our experimental studies[18–20] as well as clinical studies[4–11] revealed that B-mode ultrasonography was highly accurate and, in a certain aspect, more accurate than arteriography in identifying vascular defects associated with vascular reconstruction. Intraoperative ultrasonography provided the sensitivity and specificity comparable to arteriography, and provided better predictability of a positive test. This indicates that fewer unnecessary negative reexplorations will occur following a decision based on ultrasound results than arteriographic results.

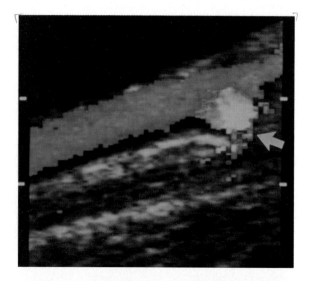

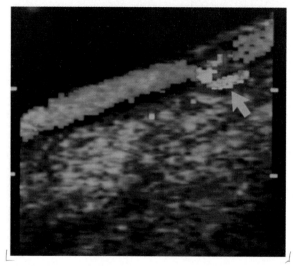

FIGURE 17–10. Arteriovenous fistulas (arrows) detected by intraoperative color Doppler imaging after in situ saphenous vein graft bypass. These fistulas were not identified by operative arteriography. (Reprinted with permission from Machi J, Sigel B, Roberts A, et al: Operative color Doppler imaging for vascular surgery. J Ultrasound Med, in press).

Intraoperative ultrasonography has an ability to present more imaging information regarding vascular defects. Operative arteriography in common use is a single exposure in one plane following a single injection. On the other hand, ultrasonography can offer multiple images (including longitudinal and transverse scanning) from various angles in different planes. The size and shape of vascular defects such as intimal flaps or thrombi and the degree of strictures can be more accurately determined. The real-time feature of ultrasonography makes the evaluation of vascular defects easier and more precise. In addition, real-time B-mode imaging allows the display of the motion of intimal flaps, thus permitting the distinction of flaps from thrombi without difficulty. Because intraoperative ultrasonography requires no contrast and demonstrates vascular defects as a positive (echogenic) images, ultrasound images are not affected by inadequate concentration of contrast media or other radiographic problems, which at times results in inappropriate arteriograms. Color Doppler imaging provides blood flow information in addition to anatomic information. The presence and extent of flow disturbances are demonstrated by color Doppler imaging, and this information may improve decision-making for operative repair if the extent of anatomic abnormalities is of borderline significance. All these characteristics of intraoperative ultrasonography are advantageous not only in detecting vascular defects but in assessing the detected defects in terms of the necessity of repair.

Safety is an important advantage of intraoperative ultrasonography during vascular surgery. Arteriography requires cannulation or puncture of the vessels, injection of contrast, and irradiation, all of which entail risks to the patient and the operative team. In particular, during carotid endarterectomy, serious complications such as a stroke have been reported due to technical problems associated with operative arteriography.[2,3] In addition, the number of arteriographic studies may be limited due to the possible side effects of contrast materials. Because of its inherent risks, operative arteriography is usually used only for selected reconstruction sites. On the other hand, because of its inherent safety, intraoperative ultrasound imaging can be used more widely and routinely for all reconstruction sites, including the carotid artery. It can be repeated whenever necessary during operation. Because of the real-time feature of B-mode or color Doppler imaging, the results of imaging are obtained immediately in the operating room, and saves operating time.

There are disadvantages or limitations of intraoperative ultrasound imaging, which include (1) a prolonged learning period, and (2) inability to provide extended views of the distal arterial bed. Surgeons are usually unfamiliar with performance and interpretation of ultrasonography. The learning curve for intraoperative ultrasound examination is slow. This problem will be solved if the surgeon is interested and patient enough to obtain the requisite experience in performing the intraoperative scanning and interpreting ultrasound images. The establishment of working relations with radiologists or ultrasonographers is helpful in learning the procedure for intraoperative ultrasonography. The use of color Doppler imaging might be useful to enhance the learning process of ultrasonography.

The major limitation of intraoperative ultrasonography is that it provides a view of the vascular system only within the operative field. Operative arteriography can demonstrate the entire arterial bed distal to the operative site. Such extended panoramic views of the arterial system is unobtainable by B-mode ultrasonography. Therefore, intraoperative B-mode ultrasonography is applicable only for gathering information about the vessels within the operative field. Our preliminary experience on color doppler imaging suggests that this new ultrasound imaging modality may also be useful for examination of vessels outside the operative field during operation. This will require further experience. At present, if detailed information regarding the distal arterial tree is needed, operative arteriography should be performed.

CONCLUSION

Our present study indicates that intraoperative ultrasonography employing high-resolution systems is a valuable, reliable, and cost-effective modality during vascular reconstruction surgery. Prereconstruction scanning, although not so frequently indicated, may help to approach the blood vessels and to make a final decision regarding the type of operation to be performed. Particularly, prereconstruction color Doppler imaging has a potential to diagnose vascular abnormalities which are unknown by preoperative studies. Postreconstruction scanning is indicated as a routine completion examination. Intraoperative ultrasonography is highly accurate and, in terms of a predictability of a positive test, more accurate than arteriography in detecting vascular defects. Important features of intraoperative ultrasonography such as multiple images, real-time, and repetitive performance contribute to such accuracy.

Intraoperative ultrasonography is so sensitive that postreconstruction vascular defects were identified by this technique in approximately 30 per cent of vascular operations in our study. This high discovery rate is consistent with the findings of other investigators.[15-17] Among these vascular defects, only about one third were considered to be clinically significant to justify reexploration of the vessels for repair. A decision to reexplore (or not) is based on the risk of attempting reexploration against the risk of leaving the vascular defects behind. The surgeon should determine the significance of the defects by evaluating such factors as the type, magnitude, and location of the defects, in addition to the clinical conditions of the patient. Intraoperative B-mode imaging is more informative in providing such factors than arteriography. Furthermore, intraoperative color Doppler imaging, which is capable of providing supplemental blood flow information, may be helpful for formulating decisions on the need to repair defects of marginal significance on the basis of anatomic features alone.

In addition to its accuracy, intraoperative ultrasonography has advantages including safety, ability for repeated use, and low cost. For this reason, we recommend the use of intraoperative ultrasound examination as a first-choice procedure for screening vascular defects. However, intraoperative ultrasonography has an inherent disadvantage; namely, inability to display extended images of the distal arterial bed. This information is obtained by operative arteriography. Therefore, intraoperative ultrasonography and arteriography should be used in a complementary fashion. Our current recommendation for applications of these imaging methods is as follows:

1. Intraoperative ultrasonography is routinely used for examination of all reconstruction sites including endarterectomized segment, proximal and distal anastomotic sites of bypass grafts, and vascular clamp and tourniquet placement sites.

2. Operative arteriography is selectively used for examination of distal anastomotic sites, particularly in popliteal or more distal arteries where vascular defects, if present, are more likely to be clinically significant.

3. Intraoperative ultrasonography is solely used during carotid operations.

4. Intra-abdominal vessels are usually examined only with intraoperative ultrasonography.

5. Evaluation of a distal arterial bed, whenever necessary, is performed by operative arteriography.

Introduction of color Doppler imaging during surgery may further widen the applications of this intraoperative imaging method. For example, arteriovenous fistulas associated with in situ saphenous vein graft bypass, which are usually impossible to detect with B-mode imaging, are now identifiable by the use of intraoperative color Doppler imaging. Although more investigation is required, color Doppler imaging has a beneficial potential for further improvement of the outcome of vascular surgery because of its unique ability to simultaneously provide anatomic and flow information in one image. Operative arteriography is an important tool to complete vascular operations. However, we believe that intraoperative ultrasonography, particularly with further experience with color Doppler imaging, will assume a more important role in vascular reconstructive surgery.

REFERENCES

1. Ansell G: Adverse reactions to contrast agents: Invest Radiol 1970;5:374–384.
2. Collins GJ Jr, Rich NM, Anderson CA, et al: Stroke associated with carotid endarterectomy. Am J Surg 1978;135:221–225.
3. Pories WJ, Plecha FR, Castele TJ, et al: Complications of arteriography and phlebography. In Beebe GH, ed: Complications in vascular surgery. Philadelphia, JB Lippincott, 1973;1–44.
4. Sigel B: Ultrasonography during vascular surgery. In Sigel B, ed: Operative Ultrasonography. 2nd ed. New York, Raven Press, 1988;151–174.
5. Machi J: Operative ultrasonography during cardiac and vascular surgery. In Machi J, ed: Operative Ultrasonography—Fundamentals and Clinical Applications. 1st ed. Tokyo, Life Science Co Ltd, 1987;255–317.
6. Sigel B, Machi J, Anderson KW III, et al: Operative ultrasonic imaging of vascular defects. Semin Ultrasound CT MR 1985;6:85–92.
7. Schuler JJ, Machi J, Ramos J, et al: The role of intraoperative ultrasonography in vascular surgery. Bruit 1984;8:234–238.
8. Sigel B, Flanigan DP, Schuler JJ, et al: Imaging ultrasound in the intraoperative diagnosis of vascular defects. J Ultrasound Med 1983;2:337–343.
9. Sigel B, Coelho JCU, Flanigan DP, et al: Detection of vascular defects during operation by imaging ultrasound. Ann Surg 1982;196:473–480.
10. Flanigan DP, Douglas DJ, Machi J, et al: Intraoperative ultrasonic imaging of the carotid artery during carotid endarterectomy. Surgery 1986;100:893–899.
11. Sawchuk AP, Flanigan DP, Machi J, et al: The fate of unrepaired minor technical defects detected by intraoperative ultrasound during carotid endarterectomy. J Vasc Surg 1989;9:671–676.
12. Roberts AB, Bakshi KR, Samhouri FA, et al: Intraoperative use of color Doppler imaging in the correction of renal artery stenosis. Dyn Cardiovasc Imaging 1989;2:43–48.
13. Samhouri FA, Bakshi KR, Roberts AB, et al: Arteriovenous fistula following cardiac catheterization: peri- and intraoperative evaluation using color Doppler imaging. Dyn Cardiovasc Imaging 1989;2:167–169.
14. Machi J, Sigel B, Roberts A, et al: Operative color Doppler imaging for vascular surgery. (J Ultrasound Med, in press).
15. Lane RJ, Ackroyd N, Appleberg M, Graham J: The application of operative ultrasound immediately following carotid endarterectomy. World J Surg 1987;11:593–597.
16. Lane RJ, Appleberg M: Real-time intraoperative angiosonography after carotid endarterectomy. Surgery 1982;92:5–9.
17. Rosenbloom MS, Flanigan DP: The use of ultrasound during reconstructive arterial surgery of the lower extremities. World J Surg 1987;11:598–603.
18. Coelho JCU, Sigel B, Flanigan DP, et al: An experimental evaluation of arteriography and imaging ultrasonography in detecting arterial defects at operation. J Surg Res 1982;32:130–137.
19. Coelho JCU, Sigel B, Flanigan DP, et al: Detection of arterial defects by real-time ultrasound scanning during vascular surgery: an experimental study. J Surg Res 1981;30:535–543.
20. Coelho JCU, Sigel B, Flanigan DP, et al: Arteriographic and ultrasonic evaluation of vascular clamp injuries using an in vitro human experimental model. Surg Gynecol Obstet 1982;155:506–512.

18

NONINVASIVE FOLLOW-UP OF ENDOVASCULAR PROCEDURES

JOHN L. GLOVER and PHILLIP J. BENDICK

One of the most important contributions of noninvasive tests for arterial function is the ability to provide objective evidence of the degree of relative ischemia and of any improvement gained by surgical treatment. These tests are now routinely used by vascular surgeons.[1] Predictions that regular testing would also allow surgeons to detect impending failure of grafts have not been borne out with standard tests, however, which is unfortunate because so few vein grafts can be reopened successfully once thrombosis has occurred, even using thrombolytic therapy.[2-4] More recently, Bandyk and associates have been able to detect certain changes in vein grafts that would most likely have caused occlusion if left alone, such as stenosis at valve sites; they have obtained good long-term patency after repair of these lesions, indicating a role for regular surveillance, at least of vein grafts.[5]

If detection of failure is important for bypass grafting, it is equally important for endovascular interventions for at least three reasons. First, since these procedures are often used in high-risk patients with ischemia at rest, it is likely that ischemia will return when restenosis occurs; and theoretically at least, one could repeat the dilation and maintain improved flow. Second, one might detect different patterns of scarring and its resulting stenosis after interventions, which would negate the possibility of repeat dilatation and require surgical treatment if ischemia returned. Third, unless good objective data are provided to show the natural history of interventions, we will continue to have entrepreneurial publicity, which will delay our understanding of the appropriate place for these procedures. In some general respects, the surveillance of endovascular procedures is more important than that of grafts because of the potential risk of delay of treating recurrent ischemia when the procedure and the follow-up care are done by different physicians, neither of whom are surgeons, as is often the case.

Conventional vascular laboratory testing has traditionally incorporated flow waveforms, using either the ultrasound Doppler flowmeter or some type of plethysmographic device, and the ankle brachial pressure index.[6] While suited for certain screening procedures, these indirect techniques have significant limitations in maintaining a follow-up surveillance program to assess the hemodynamics of limbs that have had some type of endovascular intervention. The major limitation is that the conventional techniques provide only indirect measures of overall hemodynamic changes throughout a limb. In addition, there is significant scatter and overlap of ankle brachial pressure index data, when attempting to objectively categorize a patient's clinical condition.[7] These techniques do not appear to be sensitive enough to detect the early changes associated with restenosis following angioplasty. Although angiography is routinely performed immediately following endovascular intervention and provides anatomic information as to the patency of the angioplasty site, it clearly is unsuited for routine follow-up and, furthermore, provides very little or no hemodynamic data necessary for the evaluation of intervention.

In the noninvasive assessment of peripheral arterial disease, it is desirable to have objective data regarding the location and extent of any atherosclerotic occlusive lesions that may be present, the anatomic severity of these lesions, and their hemodynamic significance, both locally and as they affect flow throughout the entire limb. Two new technologies in noninvasive testing that help provide this data in a quantitative fashion are duplex ultrasound with color Doppler imaging (CDI) and magnetic resonance blood flow measurements. Both of these techniques provide direct measurements that quantify the local and global hemodynamic effects of endovascular intervention.

Duplex ultrasound has been a primary evaluation technique in the peripheral vascular laboratory for nearly 10 years, but its principal site of application has been the carotid arterial system. Only recently has its value in the lower extremity circulation been appreciated, corresponding to the development of color displays of Doppler information.[8] Both conventional and color duplex systems provide real-time high-resolution B-mode images. But while conventional systems rely on a gray-scale image presentation to differentiate tissue types and vascular structures, the color duplex systems simultaneously process the returned echoes for this tissue information as well as Doppler flow information. The frequency-shift data derived from Doppler signal processing is then presented in a color display, which is superimposed on the gray-scale tissue information. By coding specific colors as to flow direction and the magnitude of the frequency shift, a vascular "road map" is provided in real time. This vascular map speeds up the process of vessel identification, and helps to differentiate sites with normal flow from those with disturbed flow, making it easier to localize areas of stenosis.

It must be pointed out, however, that while color duplex imaging simplifies the task of identifying stenotic regions of interest, *it is not a quantitative technique.* It does allow one to quickly focus a follow-up examination on a few specific sites, but *objective data* regarding stenosis is obtained from *conventional gray-scale images and Doppler spectrum analysis.* High-resolution imaging allows a precise measure of the anatomic degree of restenosis, particularly in cross-sectional views where per cent area reduction can also be calculated. With the pulsed Doppler sample volume placed in the center of the patent lumen, the entire region of interest can be scanned to acquire quantitative flow-velocity data and evaluate hemodynamic disturbances associated with restenosis.

The second technology utilizes the magnetic resonance properties of whole blood to quantify limb volume flows. The flow cylinder contains a 0.1 tesla permanent magnet, which is used to magnetize the blood passing through a selected cross-sectional slice of the extremity. A high-frequency RF signal then perturbs this nuclear magnetization and a sensitive receiver coil is used to detect the magnetic resonance relaxation as the flowing blood passes through this coil.

The magnitude of this output signal is proportional to the volume of blood crossing the detecting plane, with the factor of proportionality having been determined in a flow calibration model.[9] For a given measurement site, data over 15 to 20 successive cardiac cycles are averaged to produce a volume flow ml/min. Multiple cross-sectional slices can be selected for each limb providing a complete set of volumetric flow data from mid-thigh to the ankle. The entire procedure is noninvasive, involves no ionizing radiation, and requires only approximately 15 minutes to complete both lower extremities.

An example of magnetic resonance flowmeter data is shown in Figure 18–1. Throughout both extremities, each cross-sectional site of measurement is identified as to its location (in cm) proximal to the anatomic landmark of the medial malleolus, the number of cardiac cycles averaged to obtain the displayed analog flow waveform, and the measured volume flow in ml/min at that site. In this example, the right lower extremity is hemodynamically normal. Qualitatively, the analog flow waveforms resemble those of normal limb plethysmography, with a well-defined systolic peak and evidence of the dicrotic notch during mid-diastole. Volume flows are seen to progressively decrease as the measurement site becomes more distal. Proximally on the left lower extremity, the flow waveforms also appear normal, though volume flows are significantly diminished compared to those on the right at all measurement sites, and flow waveforms in the lower leg are dampened without a sharply defined systolic peak. This patient was noted to have significant chronic left lower leg trifurcation

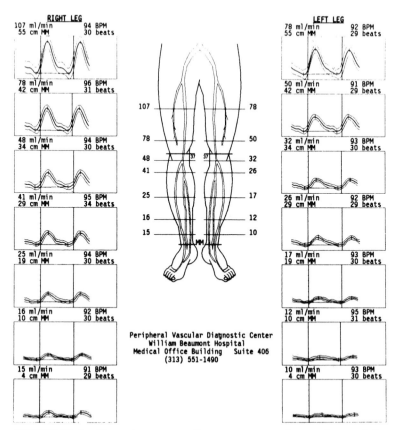

FIGURE 18–1. Magnetic resonance flow measurement data at characteristic cross-sectional sites in a patient with normal right lower extremity arterial hemodynamics and chronic left lower leg trifurcation vessel occlusive disease.

vessel thromboembolic occlusive disease; the hemodynamic effects are seen to be not only local, but also limiting to inflow and distal runoff.

In addition, as flow is measured at each cross-sectional site, the limb circumference at this site is also measured. These data are entered into the computer, which uses a finite element algorithm to calculate segmental limb volumes. The volume-flow data and the data regarding volume of tissue in the limb are combined to express limb perfusion in ml/min/100 cc of tissue. Figure 18–2 shows this perfusion data for the patient above. Each measurement site is labeled as before as to site of data acquisition (cm MM) and volume flow (Q). In addition, the measured limb circumference data is shown (Circ) along with the calculated segmental volumes (S.V.). These data are combined to give a derived limb perfusion value (L.P.) in ml/min/100 cc tissue by dividing volume flow at a given site by the total limb volume distal to that site. Just below the knee on the right side (site 29 cm) a normal perfusion value of 1.72 is shown. The effects of the lower leg trifurcation vessel occlusive disease on the left are seen at its corresponding site where distal limb perfusion is only 1.09.

The accuracy and repeatability of magnetic resonance flow measurements have been tested both in vitro and in vivo. In vitro studies in a pulsatile flow system using a copper sulfate solution to mimic the magnetic resonance relaxation properties of whole blood compared magnetic resonance flow values to those of an electromagnetic flowmeter.[10] There is a linear relationship between these two over a range of 5 to 300 ml/min with an absolute accuracy and repeatability within ± 5 per cent. In vivo studies have compared magnetic resonance blood-flow measurement with those of venous occlusion strain-gauge plethysmography.[11] Mean flows with the strain-gauge technique were 100 ml/min; those with the magnetic resonance flowmeter 93 ml/min. Repetitive studies on the same limb showed a coefficient of variance of 15 per cent for the magnetic resonance flowmeter, data comparable to the variance seen in clinical studies of the measurement of segmental systolic blood pressures and signifi-

PERFUSION ANALYSIS

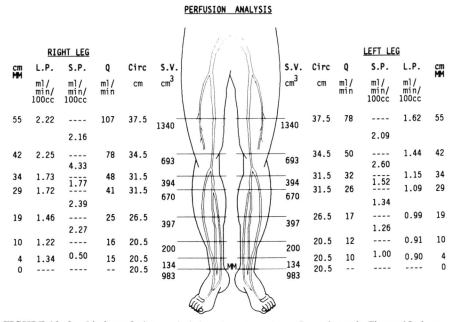

	RIGHT LEG						LEFT LEG				
cm MM	L.P. ml/min/100cc	S.P. ml/min/100cc	Q ml/min	Circ cm	S.V. cm³		S.V. cm³	Circ cm	Q ml/min	S.P. ml/min/100cc	L.P. ml/min/100cc	cm MM
55	2.22	----	107	37.5	1340		1340	37.5	78	----	1.62	55
		2.16								2.09		
42	2.25	----	78	34.5	693		693	34.5	50	----	1.44	42
		4.33								2.60		
34	1.73	---- 1.77	48	31.5	394		394	31.5	32	---- 1.52	1.15	34
29	1.72	----	41	31.5	670		670	31.5	26	----	1.09	29
		2.39								1.34		
19	1.46	----	25	26.5	397		397	26.5	17	----	0.99	19
		2.27								1.26		
10	1.22	----	16	20.5	200		200	20.5	12	----	0.91	10
4	1.34	0.50	15	20.5	134		134	20.5	10	1.00	0.90	4
0	----	----	--	20.5	983		983	20.5	--	----	----	0

FIGURE 18–2. Limb perfusion analysis based on the volume flows shown in Figure 18–1. cm MM, site of measurement; L.P., distal limb perfusion beyond that site; Q, measured volume volume flow; Circ, measured limb circumference; S.V., calculated limb segmental tissue volume.

cantly better than the coefficient of variation of 26 per cent found for strain-gauge plethysmography.

Both of these new techniques provide direct measurements that quantify both the physical and hemodynamic effects of endovascular intervention. The combination of duplex ultrasound (with or without color imaging) plus magnetic resonance flow measurements allows a direct, quantitative anatomic and functional evaluation. The patient shown in Figure 18–3 and succeeding illustrations presented with bilateral calf claudication of increasing severity with onset at approximately one half block and a small area of ulceration on the lateral left ankle. Baseline magnetic resonance flow studies (Fig. 18–3) showed the hemodynamic effects of bilateral superficial femoral artery occlusions with diminished, damped runoff in both lower legs. Distal limb perfusions were calculated to be 0.73 and 0.61 for the right and left sides, respectively. A balloon angioplasty of the left superficial femoral artery successfully restored patency, and the follow-up study done at 3 months is shown in Figure 18–4. There have been no changes on the right (limb perfusion = 0.76) while perfusion on the left has increased to 1.22 with qualitatively improved, though not completely normal, flow waveforms. Color Doppler imaging through the angioplasty site (Fig. 18–5) shows diffuse residual wall irregularity with areas of mild localized flow-velocity acceleration, but no hemodynamically significant stenoses. The left ankle ulcer at that time was noted to be nearly completely healed. The ulcer had become worse, however, when the patient returned for a 6-month follow-

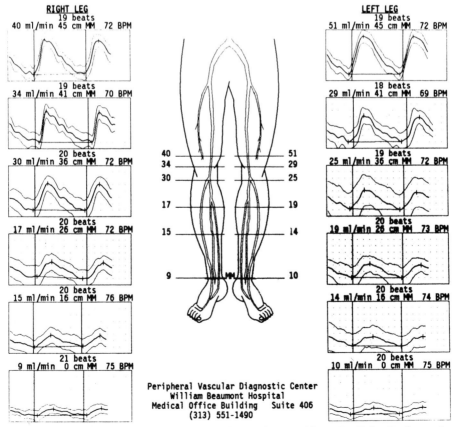

FIGURE 18–3. Baseline flow studies in a patient with severe bilateral calf claudication and a nonhealing left foot ulcer.

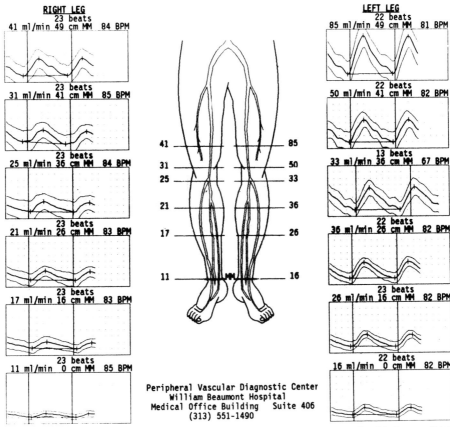

FIGURE 18–4. Flow measurements taken 3 months following a laser-assisted left superficial femoral artery angioplasty.

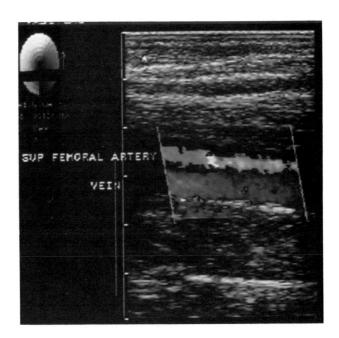

FIGURE 18–5. Color Doppler image at the angioplasty site (3-month follow-up) showing diffuse residual wall irregularity without any significant stenosis.

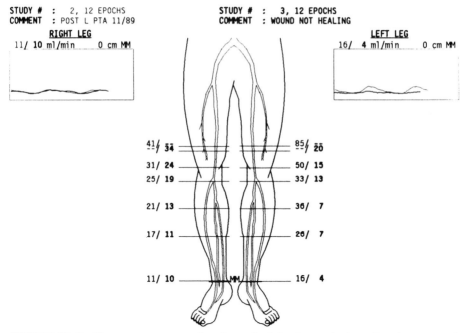

STUDY # : 2, 12 EPOCHS
COMMENT : POST L PTA 11/89

RIGHT LEG

11/ 10 ml/min   0 cm MM

STUDY # : 3, 12 EPOCHS
COMMENT : WOUND NOT HEALING

LEFT LEG

16/ 4 ml/min   0 cm MM

41/ 34   85/ 20
31/ 24   50/ 15
25/ 19   33/ 13
21/ 13   36/ 7
17/ 11   26/ 7
11/ 10   16/ 4

FIGURE 18–6. Flow measurements taken 6 months following angioplasty directly compared to those at 3 months.

up. Magnetic resonance flow measurements at that time are shown in Figure 18–6, where they are compared to those at 3 months postangioplasty. The significant decreases in flow throughout the left leg gave a limb perfusion value of only 0.31, indicative of the degree of resting ischemia in the left lower leg and foot. Color Doppler imaging (Fig. 18–7) confirmed complete reocclusion of the left superficial femoral artery and the absence of any identifiable major collateral vessels.

A number of studies are underway evaluating duplex ultrasound in the role of primary technique for the follow-up evaluation of angioplasty.[12,13] Anecdotally, these have provided reliable information on the site and extent of occlusions in the lower extremities, patency of the major vessels, sites of flow

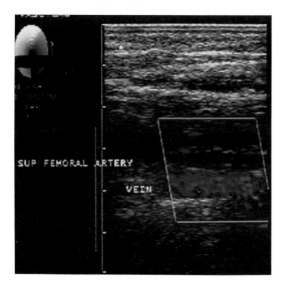

SUP FEMORAL ARTERY

VEIN

FIGURE 18–7. Corresponding color Doppler image showing reocclusion of the superficial artery at the previous angioplasty site.

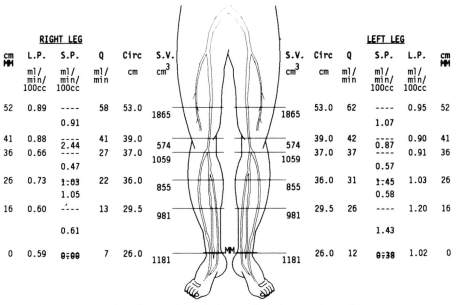

FIGURE 18–8. Baseline flow and perfusion analysis in a patient with severe right calf claudication.

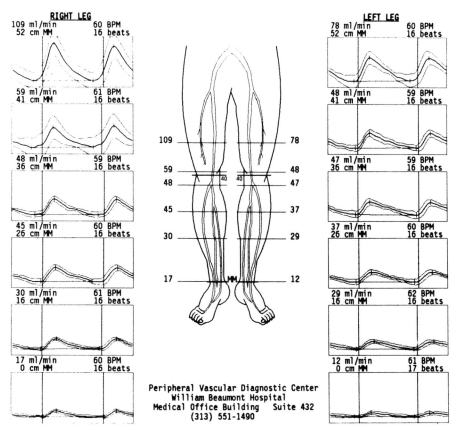

FIGURE 18–9. Flow measurements taken 1 month following excimer laser-assisted right superficial artery angioplasty showing a marked increase in right lower leg flows and perfusion.

disturbance, and in some cases, the adequacy of collateral circulation. Objective criteria for evaluating sites of intervention are just now becoming available. Bandyk et al. have investigated a series of femoral-popliteal percutaneous transluminal angioplasties using color duplex ultrasound and grading the degree of residual or recurrent stenosis based on hemodynamic criteria.[13] Diameter stenoses up to 25 per cent produced no measurable hemodynamic disturbances. Stenoses ranging from 25 to 50 per cent produced some late systolic or early diastolic spectral broadening, occasionally with minor acceleration of peak systolic flow velocities. Diameter reductions from 50 to 70 per cent had pronounced effects on peak systolic velocity, elevating it to greater than 125 to 150 cm/sec and causing marked spectral broadening. Stenoses greater than 75 per cent caused very disturbed, turbulent flow throughout the cardiac cycle with an elevation of end-diastolic velocity typically greater than 100 cm/sec. They have found these hemodynamic criteria to correlate quite well with duplex ultrasound images as well as angiography when available. High-resolution duplex imaging has the further advantage of being able to characterize residual plaque or the nature of reocclusive lesions, and with the help of color flow imaging, to define the true vessel lumen and identify sites of plaque dissection or intimal disruption.

Very little data is available at this time regarding clinical magnetic resonance flow measurements.[14,15] Absolute flow values have not been helpful in distinguishing normal from stenosed vessels because of the wide scatter among patients. In our experience, lower leg limb perfusion appears to be a much more reliable index of hemodynamic function. An initial series of normal patients had lower leg limb perfusion values ranging from 1.3 to 1.9 with a mean of 1.63 ± 0.10 ml/min/100 cc of tissue, consistent with other reports in the literature. A series of 39 patients undergoing conventional or laser assisted femoropopliteal endovascular intervention have been studied at intervals, up to a minimum of 6 months, using limb perfusion measurements. Baseline limb

PERFUSION ANALYSIS

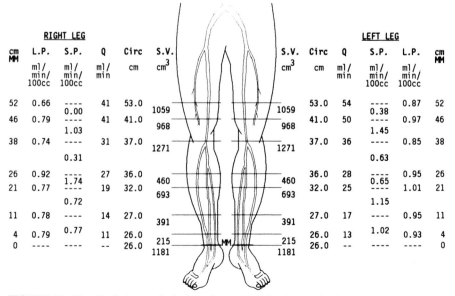

RIGHT LEG

cm MM	L.P. ml/min/100cc	S.P. ml/min/100cc	Q ml/min	Circ cm	S.V. cm³
52	0.66	----	41	53.0	
		0.00			1059
46	0.79	----	41	41.0	
		1.03			968
38	0.74	----	31	37.0	
		0.31			1271
26	0.92	----	27	36.0	
		1.74			460
21	0.77	----	19	32.0	
		0.72			693
11	0.78	----	14	27.0	
		0.77			391
4	0.79	----	11	26.0	
					215
0	----	----	--	26.0	
					1181

LEFT LEG

S.V. cm³	Circ cm	Q ml/min	S.P. ml/min/100cc	L.P. ml/min/100cc	cm MM
	53.0	54	----	0.87	52
1059			0.38		
	41.0	50	----	0.97	46
968			1.45		
	37.0	36	----	0.85	38
1271			0.63		
	36.0	28	----	0.95	26
460			0.65		
	32.0	25	----	1.01	21
693			1.15		
	27.0	17	----	0.95	11
391			1.02		
	26.0	13	----	0.93	4
215					
	26.0	--	----	----	0
1181					

FIGURE 18–10. Perfusion analysis done 6 months following angioplasty, showing a decrease in right leg perfusion from 1.18 at 1 month to 0.74 at 6 months.

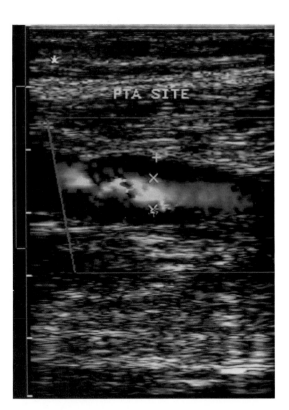

FIGURE 18–11. Longitudinal color Doppler image of the angioplasty site at 6-months follow-up showing recurrent disease with significant flow velocity acceleration and some degree of flow turbulence.

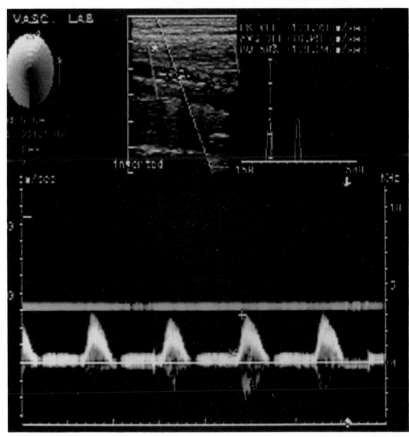

FIGURE 18–12. Doppler spectrum at the point of maximum flow disturbance in the angioplasty site showing increased peak systolic velocity (140 cm/sec) and spectral broadening.

perfusion averaged 0.53 ± 0.14 for the group with a range of 0.30 to 0.71. No changes in lower leg limb perfusion were noted in the four patients in which the endovascular intervention could not be technically completed. For those successful angioplasties, perfusion values rose within 48 hours to a mean of 1.37 ± 0.31, comparable to a similar group of patients who had femoropopliteal bypass procedures. In those patients in whom the angioplasty ultimately failed (4 early failures, less than 30 days; and 11 late failures, within 6 months) lower leg limb perfusion values fell to 0.66 ± 0.16, slightly greater than but not significantly different from baseline values.

At 6 months, three additional limbs were noted to have a decrease in lower leg limb perfusion to 0.7 to 1.0, representing a mean decrease of 0.52 from immediate postangioplasty levels. Duplex imaging in these three limbs has shown restenosis at the angioplasty site ranging from 45 to 75 per cent. Typical of this group is the patient shown in Figures 18–8 through 18–14. Presenting with severe calf claudication from a right superficial femoral artery occlusion, baseline flow measurements are shown in Figure 18–8, where the right lower leg limb perfusion can be seen to be 0.66 ml/min/100 cc tissue. Following an excimer laser assisted balloon angioplasty, repeat flow studies at 1 month (Fig. 18–9) show markedly increased volume flows with restoration of nearly normal flow waveforms throughout the right leg. Right lower leg limb perfusion was calculated to be 1.18 at this time, with no remarkable findings by color Doppler

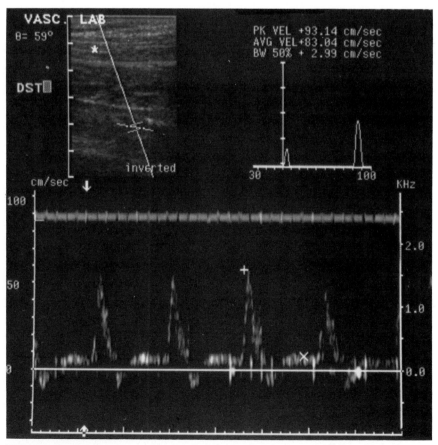

FIGURE 18–13. Doppler spectrum taken distally in the right superficial artery showing a normal triphasic velocity waveform and normal peak systolic velocity (59 cm/sec), indicating that the hemodynamic effects of the proximal stenosis are localized only.

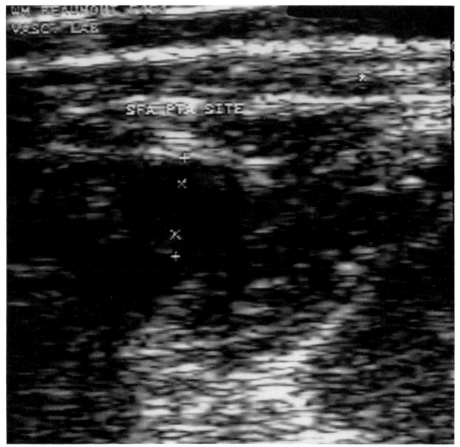

FIGURE 18–14. Gray-scale cross-sectional image of the angioplasty showing recurrent disease causing a 49 per cent diameter stenosis.

imaging. Figure 18–10 shows the flow data measured at 6 months postangioplasty; the flow waveforms had shown no significant change, but right lower leg limb perfusion had decreased to 0.74, though the patient reported no symptoms. Color Doppler imaging showed a short segmental region of possible restenosis at the angioplasty site with accelerated flow velocities and mild flow turbulence, as seen in Figure 18–11. Doppler spectrum analysis at this site showed a peak systolic velocity of 140 cm/sec, with evidence of spectral broadening; distal to this site the Doppler spectrum exhibited a normal triphasic waveform, with a peak systolic velocity of 59 cm/sec, shown in Figures 18–12 and 18–13, respectively. High-resolution gray-scale imaging at the angioplasty site in cross-section (Fig. 18–14) showed a nearly concentric, acoustically homogeneous lesion consistent with intimal hyperplasia leaving a residual lumen of 3.6-mm and causing a localized 49 per cent diameter stenosis. Careful surveillance of this site at 3-month intervals to evaluate for further restenosis has been recommended.

In summary, both of these new technologies provide a mechanism for direct evaluation of the anatomic and hemodynamic changes associated with endovascular intervention. Preintervention baseline studies using these techniques provide helpful clinical guidance for the selection of appropriate sites and types of intervention. Since both duplex ultrasound and magnetic resonance flow measurements are noninvasive, they are ideal techniques for objective, quantitative serial follow-up to evaluate the efficacy of interventional procedures. In addition, as objective parameters and indices are verified, either or both of these techniques in combination may provide the means for the early prediction of impending angioplasty failure, allowing treatment at a less severe stage of the disease process.

REFERENCES

1. Glover JL: Presidential address: Vascular surgery—the third generation. J Vasc Surg 1990;*11*:615–623.
2. Whittemore AD, Clowes AW, Couch NP, et al: Secondary femoropopliteal reconstruction. Ann Surg 1981;*193*:35–42.
3. Bandyk DF, Towne JB, Schmitt DD, et al: Therapeutic options for acute thrombosed in situ saphenous vein arterial bypass grafts. J Vasc Surg 1990;*11*:680–687.
4. Belkin M, Donaldson MC, Whittemore AD, et al: Observations on the use of thrombolytic agents for thrombotic occlusion of infrainguinal vein grafts. J Vasc Surg 1990;*11*:289–296.
5. Bandyk DF, Schmitt DD, Seabrook GR, et al: Monitoring functional patency of in situ saphenous vein bypasses: The impact of a surveillance protocol and elective revision. J Vasc Surg 1989;*9*:286–296.
6. Sumner DS: Noninvasive assessment of peripheral arterial occlusive disease. *In* Rutherford RB, ed: Vascular Surgery. 3rd ed Philadelphia, WB Saunders Co, 1989;61–111.
7. Yao JST: Hemodynamic studies in peripheral arterial disease. Br J Surg 1970;*57*:761–766.
8. Green RM, McNamara J, Ouriel K, DeWeese JA: Comparison of infrainguinal graft surveillance techniques. J Vasc Surg 1990;*11*:207–215.
9. Battocletti JH, Halbach RE, Salles-Cunha SX, Sances A: The NMR blood flowmeter: Theory and history. Med Phys 1981;*8*:435–443.
10. Salles-Cunha SX, Halbach RE, Battocletti JH, Sances A: Nuclear magnetic resonance (NMR) cylindrical blood flowmeter: In vitro evaluation. J Clin Eng 1980;*5*:205–213.
11. Salles-Cunha SX, Tolan D: Evaluation of a magnetic resonance arterial blood flowmeter: Comparison with venous occlusion strain-gauge plethysmography. J Vasc Tech 1989;*13*:155–157.
12. Bendick PJ, Glover JL: Noninvasive evaluation and follow-up of results of peripheral laser angioplasty and atherectomy. Proceedings of the International Congress IV; endovascular therapies in vascular disease. Scottsdale, AZ, February 10, 1991; III–5.
13. Bandyk DF: Applications of colorflow duplex imaging in peripheral vascular disease. Presented to the Michigan Ultrasound Society, Pontiac, MI, March, 1991.
14. Salles-Cunha SX, Andros G, Dulawa LB, et al: Changes in peripheral hemodynamics after percutaneous transluminal angioplasty. J Vasc Surg 1989;*10*:338–342.
15. Kerr TM, Cranley JJ, Johnson JR, et al: Magnetic resonance blood flow scanning—Is it reliable? Proceedings of the Forty-third Annual Meeting of the Society for Vascular Surgery, New York, June 20, 1989; 24.

IV

NEW INTRAVASCULAR DIAGNOSTIC TECHNOLOGY

19

INTRAVASCULAR ULTRASOUND: Principles and Techniques

DAVID D. McPHERSON and ROGER DAMLE

For the past 3 decades, arteriography has been widely used as one of the primary means of assessing the severity of atherosclerosis. This technique has been the basis for diagnosing the presence of atherosclerosis and, more importantly, for guiding therapy, including bypass grafting, angioplasty, and atherectomy. It has become increasingly apparent that, in spite of its clinical utility, there remain several problems with angiography. One problem is that in cases of disease of intermediate severity, there is significant interobserver and intraobserver variability in the visual interpretation of angiograms.[1,2] Another problem is that atherosclerosis is a diffuse process.[3] Since the assessment of the severity of the stenosis depends on identification of a "normal" proximal segment angiographically, this may significantly underestimate lesion severity, since it cannot identify diffuse disease. Angiography evaluates the edges of the lumen. It does not provide information concerning the vessel wall, which may be of importance when using currently available interventional devices. Finally, the presence of eccentric lesions may interfere with the accurate assessment of stenosis severity. High-frequency epicardial ultrasound probes were developed in the early 1980s to visualize coronary arteries at the time of coronary bypass surgery.[4,5] The epicardially placed probes enable an accurate assessment of the coronary arterial wall and luminal morphology as well as the extent of atherosclerosis at the time of operation. Using this technique, it was demonstrated that many segments identified as being angiographically normal actually had evidence of diffuse atherosclerosis.[5] Similar high-frequency ultrasonic probes are available for intravascular transcutaneous imaging; however, these probes are primarily employed in an intraoperative setting and often the images cannot be obtained percutaneously. Other techniques have been utilized, including fiberoptic angioscopy, which offers the advantage of direct visualization of the intraluminal surface of vascular beds.[6,7] Atheroma, thrombus, and plaque ulceration can be clearly identified under optimal conditions. However, the clinical applicability of angioscopy has been limited by the lack of appropriate delivery systems and the necessity of requiring continuous irrigation of the angioscopy field or inflation of a balloon in a proximal segment to allow visualization of the surface of the vascular walls. In addition, angioscopy is unable to yield information on the architecture of the atheroma and the surrounding vessel wall.

Intravascular ultrasound imaging uses high-resolution ultrasound imaging transducers attached to catheters to identify the arterial wall and luminal structure at the time of angiography or intervention. In this review, we will discuss the current status of intravascular ultrasound imaging, instrumentation and principles, techniques, and potential clinical applications.

PRINCIPLES AND INSTRUMENTATION

Advances in catheter and ultrasound technology have spurred the development of catheter-based ultrasound imaging systems. Two basic approaches are utilized for intravascular ultrasound transducers, both employing 20- to 40-MHz ultrasound transducers, which are small and placed near the tip of the catheter.

The basic principle underlying the development of intravascular ultrasound imaging catheters is that of all small-structure ultrasound. This is that as the frequency of ultrasound transducers increases, structural resolution increases at the expense of a decreasing imaging depth of field. Standard 2.25- to 3.50-MHz transducers have a 2-point structural resolution of 0.5 to 1.0 cm with an imaging depth of up to 30 cm. As ultrasound transducers are increased to the range of 20- to 40-MHz, the 2-point structural resolution becomes 0.1 mm, but the depth of the imaging field is limited to 3 to 10 mm. These high-frequency transducers must therefore be placed very close to the structures being imaged, but give excellent resolution of tissue components.

Generally, two types of transducers exist. Mechanical transducers have 360-degree rotating heads, and phased array transducers sequentially activate crystals through a 360-degree circular arch. With the mechanical transducers, a motor-driven rotary core inside the shaft of the catheter is attached to a mirror that reflects ultrasound transmitted from a fixed crystal at the distal end or from a ceramic ultrasound crystal at the catheter tip. Figure 19–1 illustrates a mirror-based mechanical imaging catheter. The rotary core attached

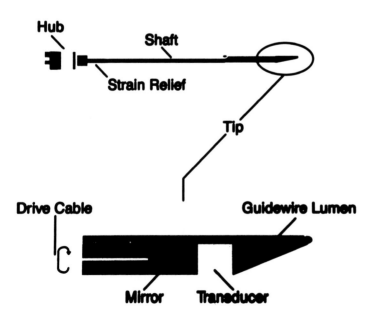

FIGURE 19–1. An illustration of the internal design of an intravascular imaging catheter. This demonstrates the rotating shaft, the fixed ultrasound crystal and the rotating mirror. (This illustration reproduced courtesy of Cardiovascular Imaging Systems, Inc., Sunnyvale, CA).

to either the crystal or the mirror rotates at rates between 700 to 1500 revolutions per minute and ultrasound is transmitted and received over the full 360-degree arch to produce an image. In the phased array imaging transducer approach, 32 or 64 transducer elements are constructed around the circumference of the catheter tip. The elements are activated in a sequence to produce a circular image. All transducers are attached near the distal end of the intravascular catheters. Catheters and transducers are sized according to the vessel to be imaged. For peripheral vascular imaging, 5-F and 8-F catheters are presently available; for coronary arteries, 3.5- to 5.0-F imaging catheters are available. Both fixed and removable guidewire catheters are available for peripheral vascular imaging and removable guidewire systems for coronary arterial imaging. The systems for intravascular ultrasound are either stand-alone or attached to multipurpose vascular ultrasound imaging machines.

TECHNIQUE AND IMAGING

The procedure for obtaining images with an ultrasound imaging catheter starts with an appropriate sized transducer sheath being placed into a femoral artery. For peripheral imaging, the catheters advance under fluoroscopic guidance either retrograde into the iliac or abdominal aorta, or antegrade into the femoral artery. For coronary imaging, the catheters are advanced through a previously placed guiding catheter. Images are then acquired and recorded onto videotape.

The images obtained by intravascular ultrasound consist first of a "blank spot" which appears as a central black area surrounded by a white ring. This represents an image processing artifact that excludes near-field echos immediately adjacent to the catheter. The arterial lumen itself is seen as a specular gray area surrounding the white catheter ring. The normal arterial wall of muscular arteries is imaged as three components. The intima is seen as a bright echogenic structure that extends circumferentially around the lumen. This echogenicity arises primarily from the internal elastic lamina. The media is an echolucent area which lies between the intima and the more peripherally placed adventitia which, like the intima, is very echogenic. In the case of elastic arteries, the interface between media and adventitia may be less distinct. In the presence of atherosclerosis pathology, the appearance of the lumen and arterial wall changes. Figure 19–2 demonstrates a normal intravascular ultrasound image of a femoral artery. The lumen, intima, media, and adventitia are well delineated and a vein is present beside the artery.

Atherosclerosis tends to demonstrate differing levels of echo intensity depending on the components of the atherosclerotic plaque. Tobis and others have demonstrated, in the coronary circulation, that calcified atherosclerotic plaques can be either brightly echogenic or echolucent; fibrous plaque is echogenic but not as brightly reflected as calcification, and has little or no shadowing; and necrotic plaques demonstrate echolucent lakes containing liquid necrotic material on gross examination.[8] Figure 19–3 demonstrates an external iliac artery following an atherectomy. The catheter and lumen are well differentiated; however, a large intimal dissection occurred with a well-defined intimal flap noted.

In addition to identifying atherosclerotic plaque and the results postintervention, saphenous vein grafts have also been imaged. Figure 19–4 demonstrates

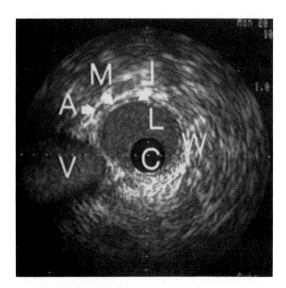

FIGURE 19–2. An intravascular ultrasound image of a femoral artery in cross-section. C, catheter; L, arterial lumen; W, arterial wall; V, femoral vein; I, intima; M, media; A, adventitia. (Reproduced with permission from Damle R, et al. and Dyn Cardiovasc Imaging 1990;*3*:165.)

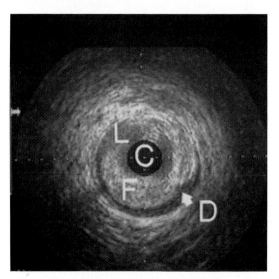

FIGURE 19–3. An intravascular ultrasound image of an iliac artery following atherectomy. A large intimal dissection with extension into the media is demonstrated. C, catheter; L, arterial lumen; F, intimal flap; D, dissection. (Reproduced with permission from Damle R, et al. and Dyn Cardiovasc Imaging 1990;*3*:166.)

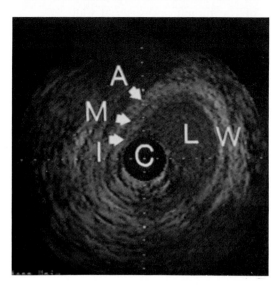

FIGURE 19–4. An intravascular ultrasound image of a saphenous vein graft. C, catheter; L, vein graft lumen; W, vein graft wall; I, intima; M, media; A, adventitia. (Reproduced with permission from Damle R, et al. and Dyn Cardiovasc Imaging 1990;*3*:167.)

images obtained from a saphenous vein graft with a large lumen and a relatively well-defined wall.

It therefore seems that intravascular ultrasound may have potential not only in identifying abnormalities of lumen and wall structural morphology, but also in identifying components within the atherosclerotic plaque.

VALIDATION AND CLINICAL UTILIZATION

Several investigators have validated data obtained using the intravascular imaging catheters by correlation with both pathologic and histologic preparations. These studies have confirmed the three-ring appearance of normal arteries.[9,10] Correlation of ultrasound images obtained in vitro with histologic analysis have demonstrated that luminal area and wall thickness can be assessed accurately in both normal and abnormal human peripheral and coronary arteries.[11,12] In vivo studies have demonstrated that intravascular imaging of peripheral and coronary arteries is feasible and that there is close correlation between ultrasound and quantitative angiography.[13-17] Investigators have demonstrated that atherosclerosis results in the appearance of a nonuniform gray area with regions of both echogenicity and echolucency.[8,18] It seems clear that one potential use for intravascular ultrasound imaging is in the accurate measurement of luminal area, wall thickness, and per cent stenosis of diseased arteries. The addition of Doppler techniques should allow for more accurate structural and physiologic information to be obtained before and after interventional procedures to assess the physiologic reactivity of vascular beds.[19]

In addition to simple assessment of luminal area, intravascular ultrasound may allow for the precise definition of plaque geometry and morphology. One aspect of plaque geometry for which it has been successfully utilized is the distinction of concentric from eccentric atherosclerotic lesions.[17] With respect to morphology, intravascular ultrasound has been used both in vitro and in vivo to identify thrombus and intimal flaps.[20-22] Thrombus appears as a mass of echogenic material attached to the vessel wall protruding into the lumen, whereas an intimal flap is seen as a linear echogenic structure with or without a free edge separating the structure from the vessel wall and protruding into the lumen. These associated morphologic features are important in guiding the type of therapy. For example, the presence of a large thrombus may indicate the need for adjunctive thrombolytic therapy. On the other hand, a large intimal flap (dissection) following angioplasty may indicate the need for an additional catheter-based procedure or bypass surgery.

Another potential use for ultrasound is in the precise determination of plaque composition. In vitro histologic studies have suggested that ultrasound can be used to distinguish plaque type.[8,18] Calcified plaques produce very bright echos, causing shadowing artifact, whereas fibrous plaques produce a less echodense and more homogenous appearance. In contrast to calcified and fibrous plaques, lipid-filled plaques appear more echolucent. This difference has potential importance in terms of research into the natural history of atherosclerosis progression, and the effects of risk-factor modification and restenosis following interventional procedures. Like plaque morphology, plaque composition may prove to be an important determinant of the type of intervention chosen.

Intravascular imaging has gained increased use in guiding decisions concerning interventional procedures. For example, the use of ultrasound before and after balloon angioplasty has been used to assess the changes in luminal area and whether or not dissection or thrombus has developed.[23,24] This information may be used to assess the need for additional balloon inflations or alternative procedures. Intravascular ultrasound has also been used to quantify tissue removal following atherectomy and laser procedures which may determine the need for further intervention.[25–27] It may be useful in localizing plaque so that atherectomy or laser devices can be used so that minimal risk of vessel damage or perforation occurs.[25] Intravascular ultrasound may be used to guide intravascular stent placement.[28] It may be important in allowing for accurate determination of long-term outcome of interventional procedures with respect to restenosis.[29] In the peripheral vascular field, intravascular ultrasound has been used to choose catheter size and assess results following renal artery angioplasty.[30]

The use of new image data processing and display stations has allowed for three-dimensional visualization of intravascular ultrasound data. Pixel data is represented in a three-dimensional "log" format and subsequently resliced so that the extent of plaque can be demonstrated during the procedure. Figure 19–5 illustrates a three-dimensional log reconstruction of intravascular ultrasound pixel data. It also demonstrates reslicing longitudinally and in cross-

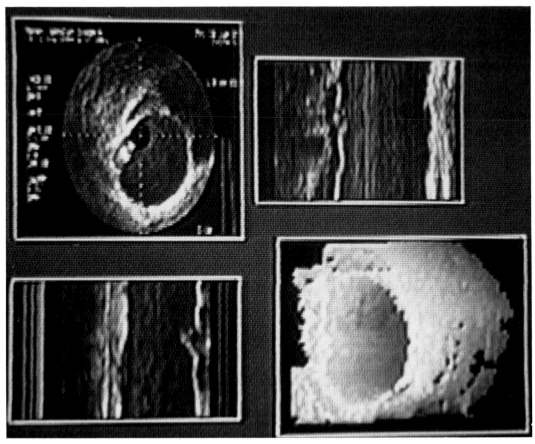

FIGURE 19–5. A three-dimensional pixel reconstruction of an arterial segment from intravascular ultrasound image data. The top left panel illustrates cross-sectional image data; the top right and lower left panels illustrate longitudinal resliced image data; and the lower right panel illustrates the three-dimensional pixel reconstruction of the intravascular ultrasound data three-dimensionally. Using reconstruction systems, the image data can be displayed three-dimensionally or cut in any axis to view internal and external geometry.

section so that the atheroma mass can be determined. Many investigators have demonstrated that these three-dimensional pixel log reconstructions aid in assessment of the need for additional procedures at the time of plaque debridement techniques.[30-33]

However, these three-dimensional representations of arterial segments assume that all images are positioned at the exact same angles and at equal intervals with respect to the other images. This is not correct, especially for arterial segments that include angles (bifurcations) or curves. In addition, the ultrasound catheter imaging varies in position inside the artery from one image to the next, adding further malalignment to the collected intravascular ultrasound images. Other factors confounding this type of three-dimensional reconstruction include the lack of cardiac cycle gating and, in the case of coronary intravascular images, the lack of respiratory gating. Our group[34] and LeFree and colleagues[35] have developed angiographic systems that identify catheter positions in space with good accuracy and thus allow true three-dimensional alignment of intravascular ultrasound data in correct three-dimensional format. We have also gated our image data to both the cardiac and respiratory cycle, and our system is designed to overcome potential data misinterpretation owing to varying speeds of catheter pullback within the arterial segment.[34] These new techniques should allow for accurate three-dimensional display of intravascular ultrasound data such that true determination of atheroma mass, extent of dissection, and physiologic reactivity can be made. All summed, these new three-dimensional display and identification techniques may rapidly improve our knowledge of atherosclerosis and our ability to treat plaque.

Intravascular ultrasound is an exciting new technique that allows the arterial wall and lumen to be visualized accurately at the time of angiography or intervention. This allows for better definition of atherosclerosis and the results following intervention to remove plaque. Intravascular ultrasound imaging allows for follow-up of atherosclerosis longitudinally to demonstrate if plaque progression or regression occurs following intervention and pharmacologic modification. With the advent of accurate three-dimensional reconstruction techniques that will allow true representation and analysis of intravascular data, and the development of forward-looking catheters that will allow imaging of the arterial segments distal to total occlusions, further uses for intravascular ultrasound data will arise. Although in its infancy, intravascular ultrasound imaging seems to provide an array of information that adds to the clinicians' and physiologists' information base, allowing for more accurate and complete diagnostic, therapeutic, and physiologic decisions to be made concerning the extent and severity of atherosclerosis in the vascular bed. These data do not replace angiography data, but add a breadth and depth of information that previously was present only in pathologic specimens.

REFERENCES

1. Detre KM, Wright E, Murphy ML, Takaro T: Observer agreement in evaluating coronary angiograms. Circulation 1975;*52*:979–986.
2. DeRouen TA, Murray JA, Owen W: Variability in the analysis of coronary arteriograms. Circulation 1975;*55*:324–328.
3. Arnet EN, Isner JM, Redwood DR, et al: Coronary artery narrowing in coronary heart disease: Comparison of cineangiographic and necropsy findings. Ann Intern Med 1979;*91*:350–356.
4. McPherson DD, Armstrong M, Rose E, et al: High frequency epicardial echocardiography for coronary artery evaluation. In vitro and in vivo validation of arterial lumen and wall thickness measurements. J Am Coll Cardiol 1986;*8*:600–606.

5. McPherson DD, Hiratzka LF, Lamberth WC, et al: Delineation of the extent of coronary atherosclerosis by high frequency epicardial echocardiography. N Engl J Med 1987;316:304–308.

6. Hickey A, Litvack F, Grundfest WS, et al: Coronary angioscopy: The spectrum of disease in the first 100 patients (abstr). J Am Coll Cardiol 1987;9:197A.

7. Grundfest WS, Litvack F, Glick D, et al: Intraoperative decisions based on angioscopy in peripheral vascular surgery (abstr). Circulation 1988;78:(suppl III):III–3.

8. Tobis JM, Mallery J, Mahon D, et al: Intravascular ultrasound imaging of human coronary arteries in vivo: Analysis of tissue characterization with comparison to in vitro histological specimens. Circulation 1991;83:913–926.

9. Siegel RJ, Fishbein MC, Chae J, et al: Origin of the 3-ringed appearance of human arteries by ultrasound: microdissection with ultrasonic and histologic correlation (abstr). J Am Coll Cardiol 1990;15:17A.

10. Webb JG, Yock PJ, Slepian MJ, et al: Intravascular ultrasound: Significance of the three-layered appearance of normal muscular arteries (abstr). J Am Coll Cardiol 1990;15:17A.

11. Potkin BN, Bartorelli AL, Gessert JM, et al: Coronary artery imaging with high-frequency ultrasound. Circulation 1990;81:1575–1585.

12. Nishimura RA, Edwards WD, Warnes CA, et al: Intravascular ultrasound imaging: In vitro validation and pathologic correlation. J Am Coll Cardiol 1990;16:145–154.

13. Gurley JC, Nissen SE, Booth DC, et al: Evaluation of peripheral vascular diameter and cross sectional area with a multi-element ultrasonic imaging catheter: Correlation with quantitative angiography (abstr). J Am Coll Cardiol 1990;15:28A.

14. Nissen SE, Gurley JC, Booth DC, et al: In vivo assessment of human coronary minimum luminal diameter with a multi-element intravascular ultrasound catheter: Comparison to quantitative cineangiography (abstr). J Am Coll Cardiol 1990;15:29A.

15. McKay CR, Hahn L, Nuno D, et al: In vivo validation of intraluminal ultrasound catheter measurements using sonomicrometers and quantitative angiography (abstr). J Am Coll Cardiol 1990;15:16A.

16. Davidson CJ, Sheikh KH, Harrison K, et al: Intravascular ultrasonography versus digital subtraction angiography: A human in vivo comparison of vessel size and morphology. J Am Coll Cardiol 1990;16:633–636.

17. Grines CL, Nissen SE, Gurley JC, et al: Quantitation of concentric and eccentric stenoses with a new phased array ultrasonic imaging catheter: correlation with angiography (abstr). Circulation 1989;80(suppl II):II–581.

18. Mallery AJ, Tobis JM, Griffith J, et al: Assessment of normal and atherosclerotic arterial wall thickness with an intravascular ultrasound imaging catheter. Am Heart J 1990;119:1392–1400.

19. Wilson RF: Assessment of the human coronary circulation using a Doppler catheter. Am J Cardiol 1991;67:44D–56D.

20. Pandian NG, Kreis A, Brockway B, et al: Intravascular high frequency two-dimensional ultrasound detection of arterial dissection and intimal flaps. Am J Cardiol 1990;65:1278–1280.

21. Pandian NG, Kreis A, Brockway B: Detection of intraarterial thrombus by intravascular high frequency two-dimensional ultrasound imaging in vitro and in vivo studies. Am J Cardiol 1990;65:1280–1283.

22. Weintraub A, Schwartz S, Pandian N: How reliable are intravascular ultrasound and fiberoptic angioscopy in the assessment of the presence and duration of intraarterial thrombosis in atheromatous vessels with complex plaques (abstr). J Am Coll Cardiol 1990;15:17A.

23. Sublett K, Nissen SE, Grines CL, et al: Application of a new phased array ultrasonic imaging catheter to assess alterations of vessel anatomy induced by balloon dilation (abstr). 1989;Circulation 80 (suppl II):II–355.

24. Tobis JM, Mallery JA, Gessert JM, et al: Intravascular ultrasound cross sectional arterial imaging before and after balloon angioplasty in vitro. Circulation 1989;80:873–882.

25. Yock PG, Fitzgerald PJ, Jang Y, et al: Initial trials of a combined ultrasound imaging/mechanical atherectomy catheter (abstr). J Am Coll Cardiol 1990;15:105A.

26. White NW, Webb JG, Rowe MH, et al: Atherectomy guidance using intravascular ultrasound: Quantitation of plaque burden (abstr). Circulation 1989;80(suppl II):II–374.

27. Linker DT, Bylock A, Amin AB, et al: Catheter ultrasound imaging demonstrates the extent of tissue disruption by excimer laser irradiation of human aorta (abstr). Circulation 1989;80(suppl II):II–580.

28. Bartorelli AL, Neville RF, Almagor Y, et al: Intravascular catheter based ultrasound in vivo imaging of artery wall and stents (abstr). Circulation 1989;80(suppl II):II–580.

29. Ip JH, Fuster V, Badimon L, et al: Syndromes of accelerated atherosclerosis: role of vascular injury and smooth muscle cell proliferation. J Am Coll Cardiol 1990;15:1667–1687.

30. Rosenfield K, Losordo DW, Harding M, et al: Intravascular ultrasound of renal arteries in patients undergoing percutaneous transluminal angioplasty: Feasibility, safety and initial findings, including 3-dimensional reconstruction of renal arteries (abstr). J Am Coll Cardiol 1991;17:204A.

31. Rosenfield K, Losordo DW, Paletski P, et al: On-line 3-D reconstruction of 2-D intravascular

ultrasound images during balloon angioplasty: Clinical applications in patients undergoing percutaneous balloon angioplasty (abstr). J Am Coll Cardiol 1991;*17*:156A.

32. Chandrasekaran K, Sehgal CM, Hsu TL, et al: Three-dimensional intravascular ultrasound imaging of arterial atherosclerosis and its complications: Improved recognition of the atheroma bulk, the span of dissection and intimal flaps, and the thrombus extent (abstr). J Am Coll Cardiol 1991;*17*:233A.

33. Rosenfield K, Harding M, Pieczek A, et al: 3-Dimensional reconstruction of balloon dilated coronary, renal and femoropopliteal arteries from 2-D intravascular ultrasound images: Analysis of longitudinal sagittal versus cylindrincal views (abstr). J Am Coll Cardiol 1991;*17*:234A.

34. Evans JL, Ng KH, Vonesh MJ, et al: Spatially correct 3-D reconstruction of intravascular ultrasound data (abstr). Circulation 1991;*82* (in press).

35. LeFree MT, Popma JJ, Manconi GBJ: Accurate 3-D reconstruction of coronary arterial segments through the combination of angiography and intravascular ultrasonographic images (abstr). J Am Coll Cardiol 1991;*17*:93A.

20

CLINICAL APPLICATIONS OF INTRAVASCULAR ULTRASOUND

RODNEY A. WHITE, MARWAN TABBARA, DOUGLAS CAVAYE, and GEORGE KOPCHOK

Intraluminal vascular ultrasound (IVUS) is developing rapidly as a method to define the transmural anatomy of vascular structures for both diagnostic and therapeutic applications (Table 20–1). Current devices use various configurations of transducers at the end of an intraluminal catheter to make real-time images of cardiac structures and vessel walls. These devices may have diagnostic applications, particularly at the time of angiography or catheterization for symptomatic cardiovascular disease. Examples of utility include observation of the progression of coronary disease in cardiac transplants,[1-2] determination of the extent of arterial wall dissection and intimal flaps,[3-4] evaluation of intravascular tumor extension,[5] and quantitation of pulmonary artery thrombosis in patients with chronic pulmonary hypertension.[6]

A thrust of current development is as an adjunct to coronary and peripheral vascular angioplasty procedures. The ultrasound technology not only has unique diagnostic capabilities by defining the distribution and character of lesions, but also provides accurate control information regarding the efficacy of current angioplasty methods. These include the monitoring of balloon angioplasty and atherectomy,[7-9] deployment of intravascular stents,[10] and ultrasound guided laser angioplasty.[11,12] This technology may offer a method of three-dimensional guidance of intraluminal instruments to provide concentric recanalizations of stenotic or occluded arteries without perforation of the vessel wall. The images may also be useful for choosing the appropriate device to remove specific types of lesions (i.e., calcified versus fibrous plaques).

INTRAVASCULAR ULTRASOUND IMAGING TECHNIQUE

General Principles

Intravascular ultrasound images are generated using 20- to 50-MHz transducers incorporated into the tip of 3.0-F to 8.0-F catheters. Although high-frequency ultrasound has limited tissue penetration, it is adequate to produce images when used in an intraluminal position. At 20-MHz, the usable depth of penetration in blood is approximately 2.0 to 4.0 cm.[13] At 50-MHz,

TABLE 20–1. APPLICATIONS OF INTRAVASCULAR ULTRASOUND

Diagnostic
    Transmural vessel wall imaging
    Differentiate normal and diseased tissue
    Determine tissue consistency (i.e., fibrous, calcified, etc.)
    Measure vessel dimensions and cross-sectional area
    Evaluate accelerated coronary syndromes (i.e., transplant arteriopathy)
    Lesion identification and quantification (i.e., flaps, dissections, coarctations)
    Assessment of chronic pulmonary thromboembolic disease
    Localize intravascular tumors
Therapeutic
    Sizing angioplasty devices (i.e., balloon, atherectomy, etc.)
    Matching lesion characteristics and interventional method
    Delineating mechanisms of angioplasty recanalizations
    Intravascular stent deployment
    Angioplasty guidance
    Assessment of preprocedure and postprocedure vessel morphology for controlled evaluation of
        lesion recurrence phenomenon

the depth of penetration is reduced to less than 2.0 cm, but the resolution of the images is finer. Tissue penetration can be improved by using lower frequency transducers or by increasing the power from longer apertures. Imaging of small vessels, such as the coronary arteries, using high-frequency transducers (50-MHz) provides visualization comparable to imaging large vessels, such as, femoral arteries, using lower frequencies (20- to 30-MHz).

Piezoelectric transducers are used to generate the ultrasound images by mechanically rotating either an echotransducer or a beam-deflecting mirror on the tip of a catheter, or by scanning using an array of stationary elements (Fig. 20–1). Each of these types of device has specific advantages and limitations that affect the design of functioning catheters, and require specialized electronics to process the signals and display the images. The rotating intraluminal devices are simpler to manufacture, but the prototypes using a rotating transducer were difficult to maneuver in tortuous vessels owing to the necessity to house rotating transducer connecting wires in the catheter shaft. This disadvantage was eliminated by fixing the transducer at the tip of the catheter and rotating a deflecting mirror just proximal to the tip. The ultrasound imaging beam is reflected at 90 degrees to the catheter axis without the need for rotating the transducer itself. Phase array configurations require an increased electronic

FIGURE 20–1. *A*, Schematic of prototype mechanical ultrasound device with (1) rotating and (2) fixed elements. Either the transducer on the mirror may be fixed with the other element in a rotating position. *B*, Schematic of a phased-array device with the elements arranged circumferentially around the tip of the catheter. (Reproduced by permission of White RA: Indications for fiberoptic angioscopy and intraluminal ultrasound. Compr Ther 1990;*16*:23–30.)

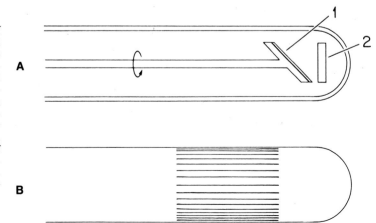

connection within the catheter, which is difficult to miniaturize, and also have the disadvantage of image loss close to the perimeter of the device ("dead zone" or "ring down" artifact). In general, with both systems, as catheter size increases, image quality improves.

Two-Dimensional Imaging Technique

Intraluminal vascular ultrasound catheters can be introduced either percutaneously or through an opening in a vessel during a surgical procedure. In either situation, blood loss and vessel trauma can be reduced by inserting the catheter through a vascular sheath that has a hemostatic introduction port. Several of the devices can be passed over a guidewire, which enhances central intravascular positioning and imaging with the catheters. A length of the vessel can be imaged by advancing and withdrawing the IVUS device up to the maximum length of the catheter. Real-time, 360-degree cross-sectional images of the vessel are displayed on a high-resolution gray-scale monitor and can be stored on both videotape or still-frame hard copy. On-line computerized morphometry allows measurement of vessel diameters, cross-sectional areas, and calculation of luminal and vessel wall volume ratios.

Three-Dimensional Imaging Technique

Three-dimensional (3D) intravascular imaging of vessels is also possible using a personal computer (PC)-based system.[14] Three-dimensional image reconstruction consists of three major computational steps: (1) segmentation and interpolation; (2) surface tracking; and (3) creation of rendered images.

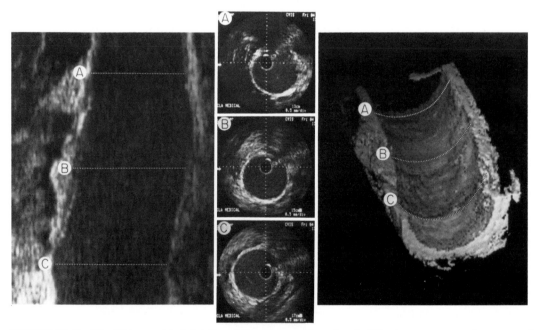

FIGURE 20–2. The 2D images labeled *A, B,* and *C* (center panel) are "stacked" by the computer, and correspond to the sites labeled with the same letter on the 3D image (*right*) and longitudinal section of the 3D image (*left*). The longitudinal section of the 3D image is displayed on the computer monitor to allow optimal adjustments of the image density threshold and viewing orientation. (Reproduced by permission of Cavaye DM, Tabbara MR, Kopchok GE, et al: Three dimensional vascular ultrasound imaging. Am Surg, in press.)

With this technology (Image Comm Systems, Inc., Santa Clara, CA), a longitudinally aligned series of consecutive two-dimensional (2D) IVUS cross-sectional images are "stacked" on top of each other (Fig. 20–2). Images may be acquired live or from videotape. The number of 2D images per 3D reconstruction is determined by the sampling rate and the total data acquisition time. Although image sampling rates of between 32 and 256 images are available in the software, we have found 90 images per 5.0-cm vascular segment optimal. To obtain the images, the IVUS catheter is positioned at the proximal end of the segment to be reconstructed. The sampling gate is opened and the catheter is manually withdrawn through the vessel segment at a rate of 1 cm per 4 seconds. A computer processing time of approximately 20 seconds is required to complete the surface tracking and creation of a coronal 2D image. The vessel segment is then viewed on a high-resolution gray-scale monitor in a longitudinal 2D view (Fig. 20–2). The image-density threshold is adjusted to optimize differentiation of structures. This is an important step, particularly when it is necessary to separate tissues of similar echodensity (e.g., soft plaque versus thrombus). The 3D image is then displayed in multiple orientations as either a complete vessel segment or in longitudinal section, depending on the viewers choice. The viewing angle is changed in real-time to allow inspection of the 3D image from all possible angles, both from within the lumen and from the adventitial surface. All data is stored on hard disk and is available for review at a later time.

PRELIMINARY STUDIES

Several studies have observed that intraluminal ultrasound determines the dimensions of the luminal diameters and wall thickness of normal or minimally diseased arteries both in vitro and in vivo and have found the method to be accurate within 0.05 mm.[15–24] Determination of outside diameter of the vessels may be less accurate, with a margin of error in some cases up to 0.5 mm.

The images produced by intravascular ultrasound catheters outline not only the luminal and adventitial surfaces of normal arterial segments, but also have the potential to discriminate between normal and diseased vessel walls (Fig. 20–3). With most IVUS devices, intraluminal thrombus can frequently be distinguished from tissue. The thrombus may produce some shadowing (loss of imaging) of tissue beyond its location. In muscular arteries, distinct layers may be visible distinguishing the vessel wall layers, with the lumen and adventitia being more echogenic than the media.[21] Smooth muscle in the media is echolucent while collagen in the adventitia and elastin in the intima are echodense (Fig. 20–3). The exact thickness of the adventitia may be difficult to determine unless the vessel is surrounded by more or less echogenic tissues (i.e., echolucent fat). Small intimal lesions are also quite well-defined in muscular arteries because of the fibrous tissue content. Large or complex plaques may compress or shadow the medial detail. The three-layer vessel image seen in muscular arteries may be lost in smaller distal arteries and larger elastic arteries, because the increased elastin content makes the media echodense. In medium-sized distal vessels, such as the femoral artery, the media is visible but is thinner than in more central vessels.

For soft tissue, the absorption coefficient for ultrasound energy is proportional to the frequency, while for hard tissue it is proportional to the square of the frequency.[13] Intraluminal ultrasound devices are thus quite sensitive for

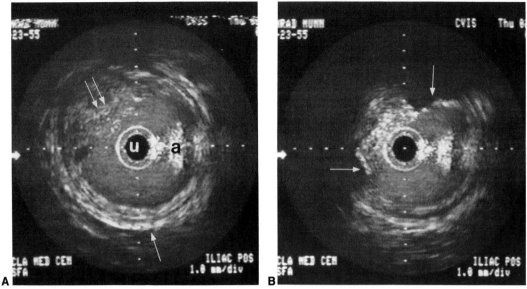

FIGURE 20–3. *A*, Intravascular ultrasound image of human iliac artery using an 8-F catheter. U, Ultrasound probe; single arrow, normal vessel wall; double arrow, soft plaque. Note the three-layer appearance of the normal arterial wall. Shadow, a, is an artifact produced by a thin metallic wire along the long axis of the catheter. This can be used to orient the catheter in the vessel by noting its location when the catheter is inserted and carefully maintaining its position throughout the exam. *B*, Intravascular ultrasound image of human iliac artery with, calcific plaque (arrow) and complete attenuation of the signal beyond the lesion. (Reproduced by permission of Tabbara MR, et al: In vivo human comparison of intravascular ultrasound and angiography. J Vasc Surg, in press.)

calcified areas. Calcium shadows adjacent structures such that medial thickness may have to be estimated by comparison to surrounding contours (Fig. 20–3).

Gussenhoven et al. have described four basic types of plaque components that can be distinguished by in vitro intravascular ultrasound imaging of human atherosclerotic arteries using a 40-MHz system.[25] Hypoechoic images denote a significant deposit of lipid. Soft echo is reflective of fibromuscular tissue (intimal proliferation) as well as lesions that consist of fibromuscular tissue and diffusely dispersed lipid. Bright echoes denote collagen-rich fibrous tissue and bright echoes with shadowing behind the lesion represent calcium.

Additional studies have compared intravascular ultrasound and uniplanar angiography for determining the luminal dimensions of normal and moderately atherosclerotic human arteries[17,26,27] (Fig. 20–4). Uniplanar angiography can be quite accurate in defining vessel luminal cross-sectional area if the vessel is circular, as it is in most normal and mildly diseased arteries. Clinically significant atherosclerotic occlusive disease is usually eccentrically positioned in the arterial lumen and the lumen may be either circular or elliptical in shape, although most are circular.[28–30] In instances where the lumen is elliptical, biplanar angiograms are needed to more-accurately define luminal cross-sectional areas and calculate a per cent area stenosis.[31]

Investigators have also shown that luminal cross-sectional areas obtained by IVUS correlate very well with those of angiography in normal and minimally diseased peripheral and coronary arteries.[26] In most studies where lumens imaged have been only mildly elliptical, cross-sectional areas evaluated from angiograms and measured using IVUS correlate significantly, while in some severely diseased arteries with elliptical lesions, the luminal cross-sectional area calculated by angiography is less accurate. In elliptical lumens, the cross-

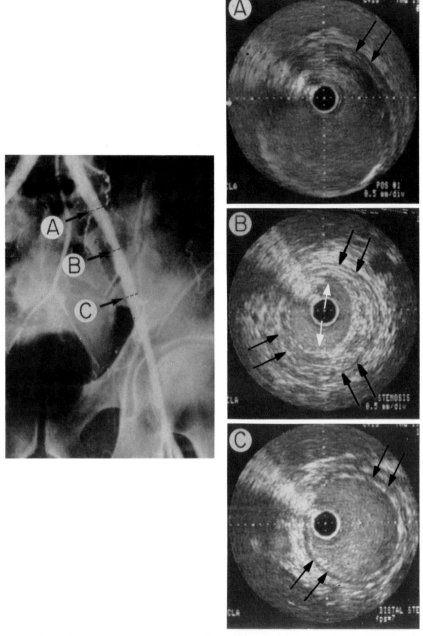

FIGURE 20–4. Comparison of angiography and intraluminal ultrasound in the common and external iliac arteries. *A*, Normal lumen; *B*, severe stenosis in the external iliac artery; and *C*, normal vessel distal to the lesion. Note the three-layer appearance of the muscular artery wall in the normal arterial segment. Single arrows delineate a 77 per cent luminal compromise in ultrasound image *B*. Double arrows identify the echolucent media in each figure. (Reproduced by permission of Tabbara et al: In vivo human comparison of intravascular ultrasound and angiography. J Vasc Surg, in press.)

sectional area calculated from angiograms is usually greater than that measured by IVUS.

In addition to the limitations of angiography in defining luminal dimensions of elliptical vessels, it gives no information about vessel wall morphology aside from calcification or aneurysms visualized on the plain radiographs. In this regard, other imaging modalities are being used to help define the extent and morphology of the atherosclerotic plaque. Angioscopy can clearly visualize the lumen of a blood vessel, but has limited ability in defining vessel wall morphology and the distribution of the atherosclerotic lesions. Intraluminal vascular ultrasound enhances the intraluminal perspective of angioscopy by defining luminal dimensions and vessel wall characteristics[32-34] (Fig. 20–5).

Comparison of angiography, angioscopy, and IVUS for determining thrombus, residual stenosis, and vessel wall dissection following percutaneous coronary angioplasty has revealed that angioscopy is more sensitive for visualizing thrombus.[33] Residual stenosis was underestimated by angiography, with IVUS being most accurate. Angioscopy did not provide a quantifiable measure of stenosis and could only be used to estimate lesion size. Angioscopy was most sensitive for determining dissection postdilatation. All three methods accurately identified atherosclerotic plaque. Angioscopy showed surface features such as pigmentation and thrombus, while IVUS was able to differentiate fibrous lesions from calcification in the arterial wall. This type of comparison emphasizes that angioscopy and IVUS provide unique information that is not available from conventional angiography.

At present, most investigators report that IVUS devices produce clear images of vessel anatomy under optimal conditions, although at times, the instruments have limited resolution in routine clinical situations. Careful positioning of catheter tips and appropriate size ratios of probe to vessel are required to optimize visualization. Image quality is best when the catheter is perpendicular to the wall, while minor angulations may affect image quality. Eccentric positioning makes the near wall appear more echogenic and thicker. Calcium at the edge of a diverging beam may project a misleading fibrotic appearance. Methods to precisely identify the location and orientation of the probes are also required. Some prototypes include an image artifact which corresponds to an external mark on the catheter to define the orientation. With

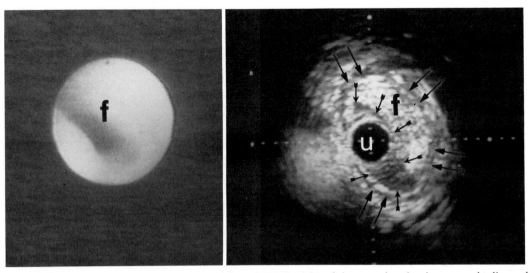

FIGURE 20–5. Comparison of angioscopy (*left*) and IVUS (*right*) of the same location in a severely diseased human superficial femoral artery. Single arrows outline the elliptical shaped lumen. Double arrows outline the echolucent media in the wall of the muscular artery as evident on the IVUS image. f, Fibrous plaque; u, ultrasound probe.

further development of these instruments, the current limitations related to image resolution and position sensitivity should be overcome. The resolution of the images is improving rapidly as clinical evaluation of the devices and the catheter-based technology progresses.

CURRENT CLINICAL APPLICATIONS

Diagnostic Applications

Intravascular ultrasound evaluations are adding a new perspective to current vascular diagnostic modalities. The benefit is apparent in two respects; for defining the distribution of disease within the arterial lumen by visualizing transmural anatomy of the vessel, and by providing control cross-sectional information regarding vessel luminal and wall morphology prior to and following interventions.

Tobis et al. compared the sensitivity of IVUS and coronary angiography for diagnosing coronary atherosclerosis.[27] In segments of arteries determined to be normal angiographically, calculations of cross-sectional area by both methods were essentially the same. In contrast, IVUS revealed a substantial amount of atheroma within the wall in either a concentric or smooth eccentric distribution involving 36.6 $\pm$ 20.8 per cent of the available area bounded by the vessel wall media, demonstrating that angiography underestimates the extent of disease in coronary arteries compared to intravascular ultrasound. Nissen et al. also confirmed a significant difference between IVUS and cine in measurements of coronary dimensions and degree of stenosis in 148 images in 46 vessels in 22 patients, particularly at sites of lesion eccentricity.[17]

Comparison of IVUS and angiography images of coronary balloon angioplasties demonstrate that IVUS is more sensitive for defining the extent of atherosclerosis and calcification.[8] Tears and dissection occurred in 80 per cent of vessels with the mean cross-sectional lumen area postdilatation of 3.7 $\pm$ 1.2 mm^2 calculated by angiography. Intraluminal vascular ultrasound documented that the mean residual atheroma area at the level of prior dilatation was 73 per cent of the available arterial cross-sectional area, and postulated that this finding may explain the high incidence of restenosis after percutaneous transluminal coronary angioplasty (PTCA).

Intraluminal vascular ultrasound is being studied as a method to evaluate accelerated coronary artery disease as a major cause of morbidity and mortality in cardiac transplant patients.[1,2] Eighty-two coronaries in twenty-one transplant recipients were imaged by angiograms and digitized IVUS. Intraluminal vascular ultrasound documented intimal thickening in all patients more than 1 year after transplant while most angiograms were normal. Intraluminal vascular ultrasound may provide a unique way to study the development of silent intimal and arterial wall thickening in these patient, and help delineate the etiology and efficacy of therapy and rejection episodes.

Intraluminal vascular ultrasound has been used to identify the location and severity of arterial dissections and intimal flaps,[3,4,34,35] and may enable treatment.[10] Cavaye et al. reported IVUS imaging of acute aortic dissections in both a canine model and in a patient[3,35] (Fig. 20–6). Intraluminal vascular ultrasound has been shown to expedite placement of intraluminal stents by accurately measuring vessel lumen dimensions and cross-sectional area[10] (Fig. 20–7). Three-dimensional computerized reconstruction of the 2D longitudinal

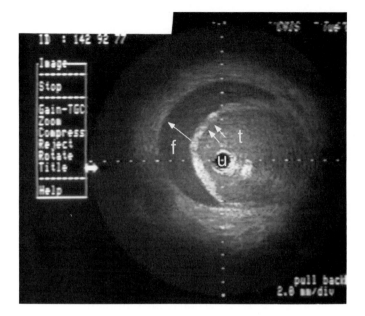

FIGURE 20–6. Intravascular ultrasound image of an abdominal aortic dissection showing aortic wall (single arrow), dissection wall (double arrows) and the true (t) and false (f) lumens. U, ultrasound probe in the true lumen. (Reproduced by permission of Cavaye D, et al: Intravascular ultrasound imaging of an acute dissecting aortic aneurysm: A case report. J Vasc Surg 1991;*13*:510–512.)

images of the aortic wall acquired by IVUS catheters imaging clearly delineated the origin, location, and length of dissections, and enabled experimental treatment using intraluminal stents deployed using IVUS imaging[35] (Fig. 20–8). Other investigators have also confirmed the utility of IVUS for detecting arterial dissection and intimal flaps.[4,8,34,36]

Sanzobrino et al. utilized IVUS to localize and treat coarctation of the aorta both experimentally and clinically.[37] In four patients (ages 5 to 17 years), IVUS crisply delineated the coarctation and accurately measured the adjacent normal aortic lumen for balloon sizing. Following dilatation, IVUS displayed the appearance of the dilation including documentation of dissections in three of four patients. They concluded that IVUS may be very useful in the diagnostic

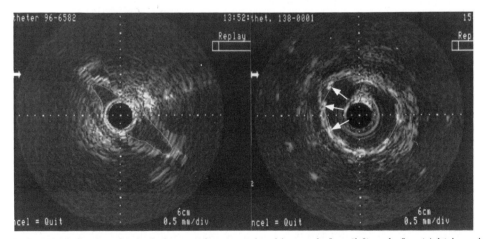

FIGURE 20–7. Intraluminal ultrasound cross-sectional images before (*left*) and after (*right*) insertion of a 5.0-mm self-expanding stent into a formalin-preserved human superficial femoral artery. A dramatic change in luminal shape is produced by the stent, resulting in an increase in cross-sectional area from 7.9 mm^2 to 16.7 mm^2, and an increase in the minimum/maximum diameter ratio from 0.26 to 0.875. Arrows identify stent struts in the vessel lumen. (Reproduced by permission of Cavaye D, et al: Intraluminal ultrasound assessment of vascular stent deployment. Ann Vasc Surg 1991;*5*:241–246.)

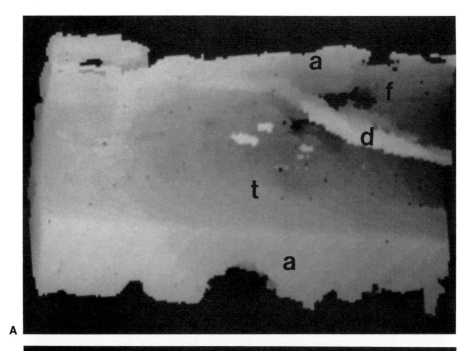

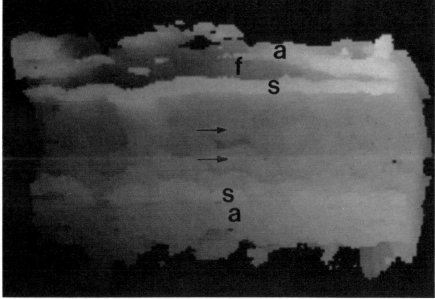

FIGURE 20–8. *A*, Three-dimensional computerized reconstruction of an experimental canine aortic dissection demonstrating the aortic wall (a), dissection wall (d), and true (t) and false (f) lumens. *B*, 3D image following intravascular stent deployment. Note residual false lumen between the aortic wall and stent(s) on the upper wall while the stent is closely apposed to the aortic wall below. Arrows identify imaging of the interwoven wire in the stent configuration at the luminal surface.

assessment and management of patients with aortic coarctation, precluding the need for excessive contrast angiography.

Ricou et al. used IVUS to determine candidacy for pulmonary thromboendarterectomy as treatment for pulmonary hypertension in patients with chronic pulmonary thromboembolic (PTE) disease.[6] In 10 patients suspected to have PTE with angiographic resistance of 667 ± 311 dynes/sec.cm^{-5}, 11 pulmonary segments determined abnormal by IVUS were confirmed at surgery. Eight of nine segments determined normal by IVUS were also confirmed, with one organized thrombus being missed in the main pulmonary artery. The investigators noted no complications and concluded that IVUS safely helped assess the location and extent of PTE in patients with pulmonary hypertension and helped identify patients most likely to benefit from surgery.

Intraluminal vascular ultrasound has also been used to localize intravascular tumors.[5] Barone et al. used IVUS preoperatively to determine vena caval extension of recurrent renal cell carcinoma and help plan successful resection[5] (Fig. 20–9). Further adaptation of this technology may enable identification of perivascular pathology similar to the uses of intraluminal ultrasound catheters in the gastrointestinal system for localizing, staging, and identifying intraluminal or periluminal lesions.[38]

Therapeutic Applications

Therapeutic applications of IVUS are rapidly developing. Several prototype instruments incorporate IVUS as the means for choosing the appropriate size and type of intraluminal device and for observing the outcome of procedures. Recent studies have indicated that PTCA balloon size is often underestimated when selection is made using quantitative angiography, and that optimal balloon size is more accurately determined by IVUS.[39] Additional findings suggest that angiographic success of balloon angioplasty is apparent when hard lesions (highly echoic components) are disrupted with dissections extending into the media of the vessel, while angiographic failure is seen in the same lesions which are nondisplacable or when circumferential dissections or intimal flaps occur.[36]

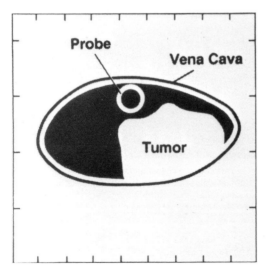
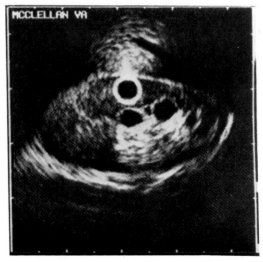

FIGURE 20–9. Intravascular ultrasonography at level of the left renal vein with adherence of tumor to caval wall. (Reproduced by permission of Barone GW, et al: Recurrent intracaval renal cell carcinoma: The role of intravascular ultrasonography. J Vasc Surg 1991;*13*:506–509.)

Angiographic success in soft lesions (mildly echoic) is associated with superficial fissures or fractures of the luminal surface, while vessel recoil and luminal disruption or thrombosis at sites of plaque rupture leads to failure. Thus, IVUS may provide information which can be used to choose lesions for balloon therapy. Many studies have noted that IVUS can be used to document lesion characteristics including eccentricity[7,17] and to quantitate residual stenosis and dissections postdilatation.[7,17,40,41]

Intraluminal vascular ultrasound is also being investigated as a method to study the mechanism of action and function of atherectomy devices, stents, and lasers.[9,10,35,42] For each type of device, the combination of the guidance and lesion assessment capabilities of IVUS with the interventional components may delineate specific benefits for a particular approach. Figures 20–7 and 20–8 highlight the potential for using IVUS to deploy intravascular stents and to assess the outcome of the procedure. An additional example of the therapeutic potential of IVUS is illustrated by preliminary studies investigating IVUS-guided laser angioplasty for recanalization of small-diameter arterial occlusions.[11,12] The combination of IVUS and lasers is particularly appealing for manufacture of cost-effective, miniature, precise ablation devices, since the fiberoptic and microchip components used for application of these modalities can be integrated in low-profile catheter systems. Initial investigations have demonstrated IVUS-guided laser recanalization of experimental arterial occlusions, followed by concentric enlargement of the recanalization by passing larger diameter multifiber laser catheters over the initial concentrically placed laser fiber (Figs. 20–10 and 20–11). Although other interventional ablation devices such as atherectomy catheters may be used to accomplish this same goal, the prerequisite of cost-effective miniaturization must be met. This factor favors laser fiberoptics, as the expense and technical difficulty for manufacturing many atherectomy devices increases with miniaturization.

Three-dimensional real-time IVUS imaging of arterial lesions and recanalizations enhances the practicality of the guided ablation concept by permitting an easily interpretable reconstruction of the vessel and recanalization procedure. This concept may be further advanced by forward-looking IVUS systems, which are currently being developed and investigated.

A particularly important aspect that IVUS adds to future endovascular device development is providing accurate control data for determining the efficacy of current devices, and for defining current failure mechanisms. As can be deduced from the preceding discussion, conventional cineangiography systems do not provide adequately sensitive data regarding either the distribution and consistency of lesions, or the outcome of current methods. Contemporary theories about recurrences (so-called restenosis) of interventional procedures are flawed by inaccurate control data regarding lesion morphology and distribution that has been measured or calculated from angiographic images. In most cases, failures that are currently attributed to smooth muscle cell restenosis are caused by inadequate removal of atherosclerotic lesions or by thrombosis and reorganization of residual intraluminal debris. The reported high-recurrence rates of almost all interventional methods, particularly balloon angioplasty, are caused primarily by inadequate removal of lesions, and by trauma to the vessel wall, which stimulates smooth muscle proliferation. The ability to accomplish long-term patency in the majority of recanalized severely diseased human arteries using improved methods of debulk lesions in a less traumatic fashion has been demonstrated.[43] Using improved methods, the 2-year patency documented by arteriography or duplex scanning approaches 70

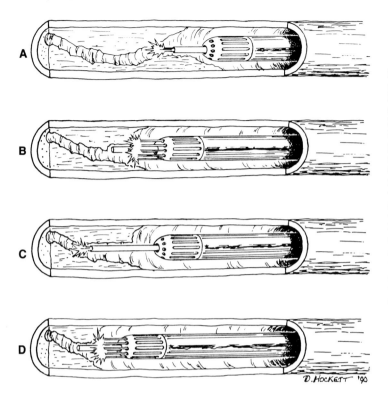

FIGURE 20–10. Schematic of a proposed ultrasound guided laser device for concentric recanalization of arterial occlusions. *A*, laser fiberoptic advanced through the center of the lumen positioned by a phase array ultrasound catheter containing a multifiber laser device; *B*, advancement of multifiber to enlarge the vessel lumen; *C* and *D*, serial, short advancements of the components to enable precise advancement of the device through the occluded lumen. (Reproduced by permission of White RA: Is laser angioplasty or atherectomy on the way out: Predictions for the future. *In* Veith F, ed: Current Critical Problems in Vascular Surgery. Vol 3. in press.)

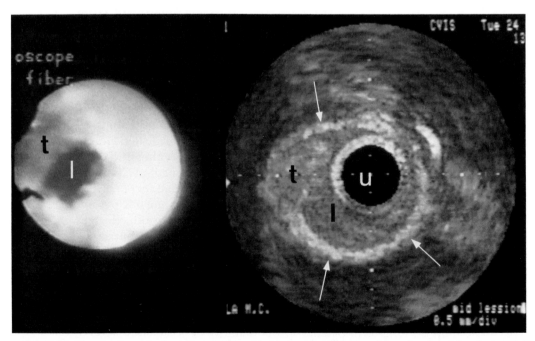

FIGURE 20–11. Angioscopic view of an IVUS-guided laser recanalization of a canine arterial occlusion (*left*), and the IVUS image of the same procedure (*right*). These images demonstrate the potential to perform precise, guided removal of lesions by combining a laser fiber with angioscopy and IVUS in a low profile catheter. 1, Vessel lumen; t, thrombus. Arrows outline the vessel wall on the IVUS image.

per cent. This degree of smooth muscle recurrence better approximates the known 10 to 15 per cent luminal narrowing that occurs following surgical endarterectomy, and negates the contemporary rapid restenosis concept. Refinement of the IVUS guided removal and debulking of lesions may further improve the long-term patency while dramatically decreasing complications from dissection and perforation of the arterial wall.

FUTURE PERSPECTIVES

Intravascular ultrasound has dramatic potential for both diagnostic and interventional application. Future angioplasty guidance devices may combine the benefits of angioscopy and intraluminal ultrasound in disposable delivery systems for various instruments, with angioscopy providing visual inspection of the lumen, and ultrasound determining the vessel wall dimensions. Improved intraluminal ultrasound devices will not only provide improved visualization of cross-sectional vessel wall anatomy, but 3D reconstruction of the vasculature from a sequence of ultrasound images. Color doppler imaging may have added applications in evaluating blood flow near vascular lesions.

Intraluminal vascular ultrasound devices are being evaluated clinically as a diagnostic aid during cardiac catheterizations in high-risk groups for coronary vascular disease such as cardiac transplant patients. Future diagnostic capabilities may enhance angioplasty device selection by delineating the distribution of tissue consituents of lesions. As an example, identification of highly calcified areas would suggest that pulsed laser energy rather than balloon angioplasty be used. Quantitative analysis of ultrasound backscatter from the vessel wall may also increase the diagnostic sensitivity.[44] These devices may help answer questions regarding the optimal level (amount of debulking) for successful angioplasty results and enable studies to determine whether medial smooth muscle exposure leads to restenosis. The technology may also be used to identify the etiology of complications (i.e., intimal flaps) leading to restenosis or to too much thinning of the vessel wall causing aneurysms.

Additional possible applications for intravascular ultrasonography include study of many exciting vascular research areas such as vascular compliance, dynamic changes in the vascular wall caused by disease or pharmacologic intervention, and further elucidation of the natural history of atherosclerosis and other arteriopathies. By combining the imaging technology with Doppler flow studies before and following interventions, the hemodynamic effect of therapy and any remaining disease can be assessed.

ACKNOWLEDGMENTS: The author recognizes the contribution of Cardiovascular Imaging Systems, Sunnyvale, CA, Immage Comm Inc., Santa Clara, CA and Endosonics, Inc., Rancho Cordova, California for the instrumentation and technical support in obtaining many of the ultrasound images used in this chapter.

REFERENCES

1. St Goar FG, Pinto FJ, Alderman EL, et al: Intracoronary ultrasound in cardiac transplant recipients: In-vivo evaluation of angiographically silent intimal thickening (abstr). J Am Coll Cardiol 1991;*17*:103A.
2. Pinto FJ, St Goar FG, Chaing M, et al: Intracoronary ultrasound evaluation of intimal thickening in cardiac transplant recipients correlation with clinical characteristics (abstr). J Am Coll Cardiol 1991;*17*:103A.

3. Cavaye DM, French WJ, White RA, et al: Intravascular ultrasound imagining of acute dissecting aortic aneurysm: A case report. J Vasc Surg 1991;13:510–512.

4. Pandian NG, Kries A, Broadway B, et al: Intravascular high frequency two-dimensional ultrasound detection of arterial dissection and intimal flaps. Am J Cardiol 1990;65:1278–1280.

5. Barone GW, Kahn MB, Cook JM, et al: Recurrent intracaval renal cell carcinoma: The role of intravascular ultrasonography. J Vasc Surg 1991;13:506–509.

6. Ricou FJ, Nicod PH, Moser KM: Intravascular ultrasound imaging of chronic pulmonary thromboembolic disease: Correlation with surgical results (abstr). Circulation 1990;82(suppl III):441.

7. Davidson CJ, Sheikh KH, Kisslo K, et al: Intracoronary ultrasound evaluation of interventional procedures (abstr). Circulation 1990;82(suppl III):440.

8. Tobis JM, Mahon D, Lehmann K, et al: Intracoronary ultrasound imaging after balloon angioplasty (abstr). Circulation 1990;82(suppl III):676.

9. Smucker ML, Scherb DE, Howard PF: Intracoronary ultrasound: How much "angioplasty effect" in atherectomy? (abstr). Circulation 1990;82(suppl III):676.

10. Cavaye DM, Tabbara MR, Kopchok GE, et al: Intravascular ultrasound assessment of vascular stent deployment. Ann Vasc Surg 1991;5:241–246.

11. White RA, Kopchok GE, Tabbara MR, et al: Intravascular ultrasound guided holmium: YAG laser recanalization of occluded arteries. Lasers Surg Med Submitted.

12. Aretz HT, Martinelli MA, LeDet EG: Intravascular ultrasound guidance of transverse laser coronary atherectomy. Intravasc J Cardiac Imaging 1989;4:153–157.

13. West AL: Endovascular ultrasound. In Moore WS, Ahs SS, eds: Endovascular Surgery. Philadelphia, WB Saunders Co, 1989;518–523.

14. Cavaye DM, Tabbara MR, Kopchok GE, et al: Three dimensional vascular ultrasound imaging, American Surgeon, in press.

15. Kopchok GE, White RA, Guthrie C, et al: Intraluminal vascular ultrasound: Preliminary report of dimensional and morphologic accuracy. Ann Vasc Surg 1990;4:291–296.

16. Kopchok G, White R, White G: Intravascular ultrasound: A new potential modality for angioplasty guidance. Angiology 1990;41:785–792.

17. Nissen SE, Gurley JC, Grines CL, et al: Comparison of intravascular ultrasound and angiography in quantitation of coronary dimensions and stenoses in man: Impact of lumen eccentricity (abstr). Circulation 1990;82(suppl III):440.

18. Tabbara M, Kopchok G, White R: In vitro and in vivo evaluation of intraluminal ultrasound in normal and atherosclerotic arteries. Am J Surg 1990;160:556–560.

19. Meyer CR, Chiang EH, Fechner KP, et al: Feasibility of high resolution intravascular ultrasonic imaging catheters. Radiology 1988;168:113–116.

20. Yock PG, Johnson EL, Linker DT: Intravascular ultrasound development and clinical potential. Am J Cardiac Imaging 1988;2:185–193.

21. Gussenhoven EJ, Essed CE, Lancee CT: Arterial wall characteristics determined by intravascular ultrasound imaging: An in-vitro study. J Am Coll Cardiol 1989;14:947–952.

22. Nissen SE, Grines CL, Gurely JC, et al: Application of new phased-array ultrasound imaging catheter in the assessment of vascular dimensions. Circulation 1990;81:660–666.

23. Neville RF, Bartorelli AL, Leon MB, et al: Validation and feasibility of in vivo intravascular ultrasound imaging with a new flexible catheter. Surg Forum ACS 1989;75:314–316.

24. Mallery JA, Tobis JM, Griffith J, et al: Assessment of normal and atherosclerotic arterial wall thickness with intravascular ultrasound imaging catheter. Am Heart J 1990;119:1392–1400.

25. Gussenhoven WJ, Essed CE, Frietman P, et al: Intravascular echographic assessment of vessel wall characteristics: A correlation with histology. Int J Cardiac Imaging 1989;4:105–116.

26. Tabbara MR, White RA, Cavaye DM, Kopchok GE: In-vivo comparison of intravascular ultrasound and angiography. J Vasc Surg in press.

27. Tobis JM, Mahon D, Lehmann K, et al: The sensitivity of ultrasound imaging compared with angiography for diagnosing coronary atherosclerosis (abstr). Circulation 1990;82(suppl III):439.

28. Zarins C, Zatura MA, Glagov S: Correlation of postmortem angiography with pathologic anatomy: Quantitation of atherosclerotic lesions. In Bond MG, Insull W, Glagov S, et al, eds: Clinical Diagnosis of Atherosclerosis. New York, Springer Verlag, 1983;283–306.

29. Roberts RW: Coronary arteries in coronary heart disease: Morphologic observations. Pathobiol Annu 1975;5:249.

30. Waller BF: The eccentric coronary atherosclerotic plaque: Morphologic observations and clinical relevance. Clin Cardiol 1989;12:14–20.

31. Sumner DS, Russell JB, Miles RD: Pulsed doppler arteriography and computer assisted imaging of carotid bifurcation. In: Bergan JJ, Yao JST, eds: Cerebrovascular Insufficiency. New York, Grune and Stratton, 1983;115–135.

32. White R: Indications for fiberoptic angioscopy and intraluminal ultrasound. Compr Ther 1990;16:23–30.

33. Ramee SR, White CJ, Jain S, et al: Percutaneous coronary angioscopy versus intravascular ultrasound in patients undergoing coronary angioplasty (abstr). J Am Coll Cardiol 1991;17:125A.

34. Neville RF, Yasuhara H, Watanabe BI, et al: Endovascular management of arterial intimal defects: An experimental comparison by arteriography, angioscopy, and intravascular ultrasonography. J Vasc Surg 1991;*13*:496–502.

35. Cavaye DM, Lerman RD, Kopchok GE, et al: Acute aortic dissection: Intraluminal ultrasound imaging and self-expanding endoluminal stenting in a canine model. Am J Cardiol, submitted for publication.

36. Leon M, Keren G, Pichard A, et al: Intravascular ultrasound assessment of plaque responses to PTCA helps to explain angiographic findings (abstr). J Am Coll Cardiol 1991;*17*:47A.

37. Sanzobrino B, Gillam L, McKay R, et al: A direct clinical role for intravascular ultrasound: utility in the assessment and treatment of coarctation of the aorta (abstr). J Am Clin Cardiol 1991;*17*:68A.

38. Tabbara M, White RA: Intraluminal ultrasound imaging. *In* White RA, Klein SR, eds: Endoscopic Surgery. Chicago, Mosby-Year Book Publishers, Inc., 1991;259–269.

39. Cacchione J, Nair R, Hodson J: Intracoronary ultrasound better than conventional methods for determining optimal PTCA balloon size (abstr). J Am Coll Cardiol 1991;*17*:112A.

40. Tobis J, Mahon D, Honye J, et al: Cross sectional morphology of balloon dilatation in vivo by intravascular ultrasound (abstr). J Am Coll Cardiol 1991;*17*:157A.

41. Gurley J, Nissen S, Grines C, et al: Comparison of intravascular ultrasound following percutaneous transluminal coronary angioplasty (abstr). Circulation 1990;*82*:90.

42. Isner JM, Rosenfield K, Losardo D, et al: Percutaneous intravascular US as adjunct to catheter-based interventions: Preliminary experience in patients with peripheral vascular disease. Radiology 1990;*175*:61–70.

43. Graor RA, Whitlow P, Bartholomew J, et al: Atherectomy of the superficial femoral and popliteal arteries: Two year patency and factors influencing patency. Presented at the Society of Vascular Surgery Meeting, Los Angeles, California, June, 1990.

44. Linker DT, Yock PG, Gronningsaether A, et al: Analysis of back scattering ultrasound from normal and diseased arterial wall. Int J Cardiac Imaging 1989;*4*:177–185.

21

PERCUTANEOUS TREATMENT OF PERIPHERAL VASCULAR DISEASE: Role of Intravascular Ultrasound

JEFFREY M. ISNER, KENNETH ROSENFIELD, DOUGLAS W. LOSORDO, ANN PIECZEK, R. EUGENE LANGEVIN, Jr., and SYED ASIF RAZVI

The short-term results of percutaneous vascular recanalization, coronary as well as peripheral, have been conventionally assessed using contrast angiography. The fact that this time-honored approach provides facile and expeditious near–on-line analysis suggests that it will remain indispensible for assessment of vascular interventions. The limitations of contrast angiography for evaluating the vascular wall as well as lumen, however, have been well documented.[1-11] Because contrast media is injected into the vascular space, alterations of the vascular wall resulting from percutaneous interventions are appreciated only indirectly. While injection of contrast media directly into the vascular space is better suited to assess luminal diameter narrowing, this examination, too, is compromised by the fact that any single site of interest is evaluated only by comparison with adjacent, less-narrowed but nevertheless diseased sites.

Previous attempts to complement conventional contrast angiography with alternative imaging modalities during percutaneous vascular interventions in human patients have included fluorescence spectroscopy[12,13] and fiberoptic angioscopy.[14-16] Intraoperative investigations of coronary physiology and anatomy[17-19] demonstrated that high-frequency, epicardial ultrasound probes could be employed to generate high-resolution images of both the vascular wall and lumen. In vitro studies[20-24] established that the ultrasound image could be further enhanced by intravascular placement of the ultrasound probe. Subsequently, intravascular ultrasound (IVUS) imaging performed by a closed-chest, percutaneous approach was used to accomplish in vivo imaging of native coronary and peripheral arteries.[25-28] More recently, intravascular ultrasound has been applied as a means of assessing the results of percutaneous vascular recanalization in vitro,[29,30] and in vivo.[27]

Recent technological developments, as well as an expanding library of clinical experience with image interpretation, have facilitated the clinical applications of intravascular ultrasound. In this chapter, we review certain of these technological modifications as well as our clinical experience using intravascular ultrasound guidance for coronary and peripheral revascularization.

CLINICAL EXPERIENCE IN PATIENTS UNDERGOING PERIPHERAL REVASCULARIZATION

Certain clinical data, including the degree of functional limitation[31] and the nature and site of the therapeutic intervention in the first 101 consecutive patients[32] in whom intravascular ultrasound examination was performed as an adjunct to percutaneous revascularization, are listed in Table 21–1. All studies were performed using a 6.2- or 4.8-F monorail-style, wire-guided IVUS catheter (Boston Scientific, Watertown, MA) with an imaging console adapted for 20-MHz operation and 360-degree scans (Diasonics, Milpitas, CA). The interventions for peripheral vascular disease included percutaneous transluminal (balloon) angioplasty (PTA) alone, PTA with implantation of an endovascular stent, directional atherectomy with or without PTA, and laser angioplasty with PTA and/or atherectomy.

As suggested by previous in vitro studies[29,30] IVUS consistently provided exquisite detail regarding alterations in the arterial wall and subjacent plaque resulting from the barotrauma of balloon inflation (Figs. 21–1 through 21–3). Intravascular ultrasound documented the presence of plaque cracks and/or dissections in most patients treated with PTA. The patterns of injury observed in these cases was remarkably similar to that which has been observed by light microscopy in patients studied at necropsy post-PTA.[8] It is not unreasonable to anticipate that improved definition of the site and extent of intraluminal flaps, cracks, and/or dissections may ultimately improve attempts to retrieve failed interventions. Long-term follow-up of a larger group of patients studied by IVUS, however, will be required to confirm the appropriate interventional response to these qualitative findings.

In contrast to IVUS findings post-PTA, IVUS images recorded post-atherectomy generally disclosed less-extensive signs of arterial wall trauma; instead, the perimeter of the neolumen was typically smooth and uninterrupted. Signs of arterial wall trauma were most completely effaced on IVUS images recorded following delivery of an endovascular stent; the fact that extensive trauma was observed at these same sites post-PTA (prestent) suggests that stent implantation acutely ameliorates arterial wall pathology.

Observations in these patients confirm previous suggestions[29,30] regarding the potential utility of IVUS for assessment of postprocedural residual narrowing. In a series of 17 patients reported previously,[27] luminal cross-sectional area at the treatment site in 5 of 17 patients was less than 69 per cent of the cross-sectional area at an apparently normal site in the same artery; in all five patients, however, conventional angiography disclosed no apparent residual luminal narrowing. The finding by IVUS of luminal narrowing at sites devoid of angiographic stenoses underscores the fact that angiographic assessment of luminal narrowing may be compromised by diffusely distributed intimal disease that allows determination of any focal stenosis only as a relative function of adjacent diseased, albeit less narrowed, sites.[1–9] On the other hand, in 6 of these 17 patients, luminal cross-sectional area postprocedure exceeded the luminal cross-sectional area of that artery arbitrarily identified as "normal." There are three possible explanations for this paradoxical outcome. In the two

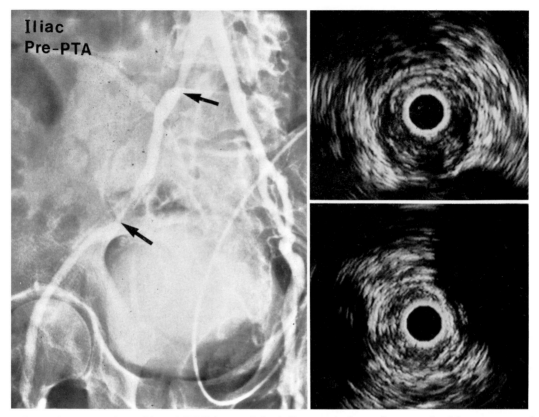

FIGURE 21–1. Angiographic and IVUS images *before* balloon angioplasty of stenoses in right common and right external iliac arteries. IVUS reveals medium density concentric plaque in both vessels (top and bottom right). (*Figure continues.*)

cases involving endovascular prostheses, it is likely that stent delivery resulted in "overstretching" of the stented segments.[33] Even without stent-implantation, overstretching of the treated arterial segment has been considered a possible mechanism for balloon angioplasty-induced augmentation of luminal patency[34]; interestingly, five of the six patients in whom there was excessive postprocedural luminal dilation had undergone balloon dilation. Finally, it is possible that attempts to identify "normal" sites on the basis of absent calcific deposits and preserved three-layered appearance of the arterial wall failed to exclude occasional cases of diffusely diseased arterial segments.

These results also suggest that IVUS may provide a superior index for gauging the diameter of balloon, stent, laser probe, and/or atherectomy catheter appropriate for a proposed intervention. There are two reasons why IVUS may constitute an improvement in this regard. First, the opportunity to image the normal segment with a coaxially positioned calibration device (i.e., the ultrasound transducer) obviates the inherent difficulty of determining radiographic magnification using a calibration instrument (catheter) which may be positioned in a plane or angle different and/or remote from the target lesion. Second, IVUS may allow more certain determination that the arterial segment judged to be normal in terms of luminal dimensions is free of important "baseline" atherosclerotic disease.

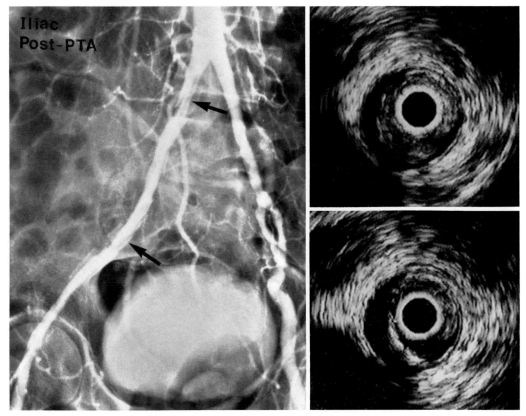

FIGURE 21–1. (*Continued.*) Angiographic and IVUS images *after* balloon angioplasty of stenoses in right common and right external iliac arteries. Angiogram reveals satisfactory result (*left*). IVUS illustrates a dissection after balloon angioplasty (top and bottom right).

Initial clinical applications of IVUS have also indicated certain limitations, some of which are generic to the technique, and others of which are related to the specific instrument employed by our group. Perhaps the most decisive limitation concerns the inability of currently available IVUS devices to consistently discriminate boundaries between the three layers of the arterial wall at sites of severe narrowing by atherosclerotic plaque. In normal arteries, or arteries mildly or moderately narrowed by atherosclerotic plaque, the media is typically observed by IVUS as an echolucent layer bounded internally by the internal elastic membrane and/or subjacent intimal deposits of plaque, and externally by the external elastic membrane and thin layer of connective tissue which constitutes the adventitia.[21–27] With more advanced degrees of atherosclerotic narrowing, however, these ultrasound patterns become blurred. This is due principally to two factors: first, emanciation of the media typically accompanies progression of the atherosclerotic process.[35] Second, extensive calcific deposits, because they are often blanketed across the intimal-medial boundary, and because they attenuate or "shadow" the ultrasound reflections from the deeper layers of the wall, further obscure the normal ultrasound depiction of the arterial wall. Ambiguity regarding the boundary between intimal thickening and media reduces the precision with which any given measurement of wall thickness can be determined to represent atherosclerotic

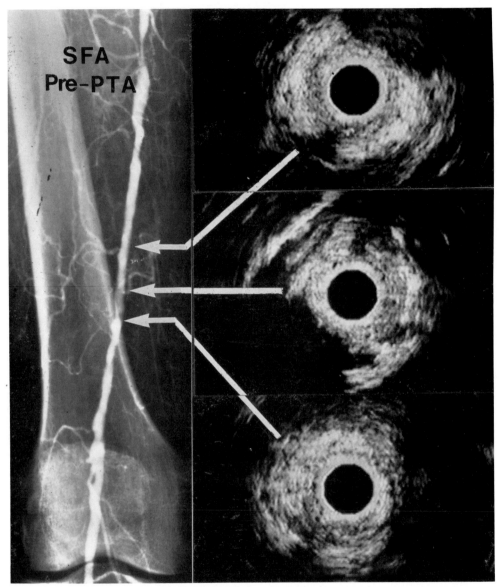

FIGURE 21–2. *Left,* Angiographic and intravascular ultrasound IVUS images taken of the SFA pre-PTA. Angiogram recorded pre-PTA suggests that distal SFA is relatively normal, compared to high-grade proximal stenosis. IVUS images recorded from the distal, relatively normal vessel, however, disclose diffuse luminal narrowing. (*Figure continues.*)

plaque versus normal wall.[36] Consequently, in those instances in which such demarcation is not possible, certain of the most potentially attractive applications of intravascular ultrasound—including precise balloon sizing and determination of cross-sectional area narrowing by atherosclerotic plaque—are seriously compromised.

A second limitation of all currently available IVUS devices in that the design of these devices allows only for side viewing. Because forward viewing is not possible, IVUS cannot be currently employed to determine the composition (e.g., thrombus versus plaque) of a total occlusion prior to recanalization.

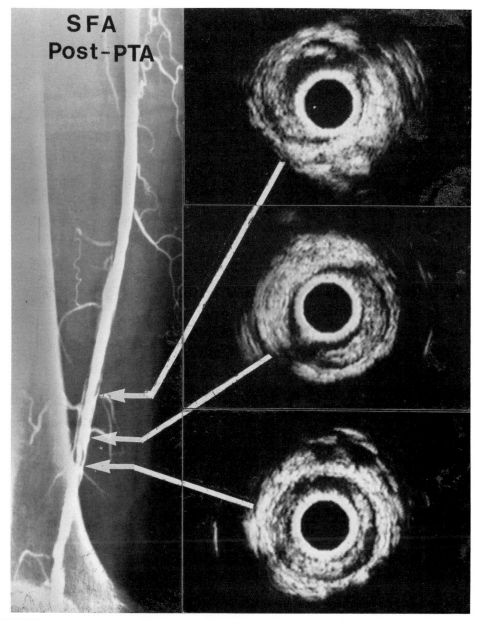

FIGURE 21–2. (*Continued.*) *Right,* Angiogram and IVUS images taken of the SFA post-PTA. Angiographic findings illustrate significant improvement in lumen, both at site of focal proximal lesion and in distal, diffusely diseased segment. IVUS images confirm post-PTA improvement in luminal cross-sectional area.

For this particular aspect of percutaneous interventional therapy, angioscopy may have superior utility.

INSTRUMENTS FOR COMBINED ULTRASOUND IMAGING AND PERCUTANEOUS REVASCULARIZATION

The concept of combining the elements responsible for intravascular imaging with those responsible for percutaneous revascularization has been

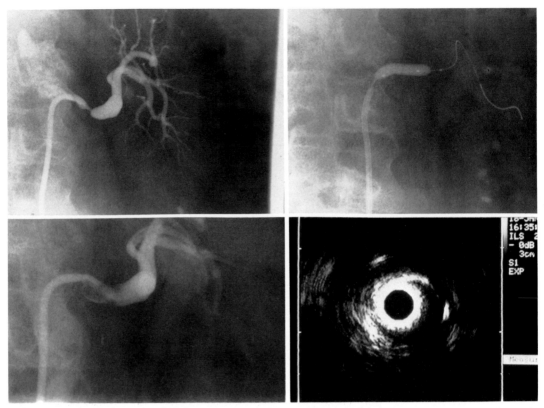

FIGURE 21–3. *Upper Left,* Angiogram recorded pre-PTRA shows high-grade stenosis in proximal left renal artery pre-PTRA. *Upper Right,* Radiograph shows guide-wire placement and balloon inflation at site of lesion. *Bottom Left,* Angiogram recorded post-PTRA shows widely patent lumen. *Bottom Right,* IVUS post-PTRA shows large crack in calcific plaque at PTRA site.

investigated previously. Intravascular ultrasound[37] and angioscopy[14–16,38] were both recognized as potential solutions to the problem of arterial perforation which complicated early clinical trials of non–wire-guided laser angioplasty. One such catheter, which was actually employed clinically, included a dedicated lumen for vascular endoscopy in addition to the lumen housing the fiberoptic elements required to transmit laser light.[39] Although this catheter retained the advantage of angioscopy for forward viewing, it also included the liability of requiring periodic evacuation of blood to record detailed images. Subsequent attempts to monitor laser ablation incorporated fluorescence spectroscopy in combination with a flash-lamp–pumped dye laser.[40] This approach eliminated the requirement for a blood-free lumen, while preserving the ability to accomplish forward imaging.

More recently, attempts have been made to combine intravascular ultrasound imaging with balloon angioplasty and/or mechanical atherectomy. Mallery et al. performed in vitro imaging with a 4.5-F balloon dilatation catheter fitted with an array of eight 20-MHz transducers mounted radially around the catheter.[41] The transducers were positioned within and midway between the two ends of a 3.0-cm polyethylene balloon; images were recorded perpendicular to the long axis of the catheter, through the balloon. Diameter measurements of pig aorta made by ultrasound reportedly correlated well with actual measurements of the aorta itself.

TABLE 21–1. CLINICAL DATA FOR 101 CONSECUTIVE PATIENTS IN WHOM IVUS WAS USED

Pt	Sex	Age	Vessel	TO	Intervention	Approach A vs R	Approach C vs I	Guiding Catheter	IVUS Catheter	IVUS Pre	IVUS Post	IVUS in lieu of Angiography
1	M	54	RCI+REI+RCF	0	PTA	R	I	0	6.6	+	+	+
2	F	74	RCI	0	PTA+Stent	R	I	+	6.6	+	+	0
3	M	63	LCI+LEI	0	PTA+Stent	R	I	+	6.6	0	+	0
4	M	84	LCI+LEI	0	PTA	R	I	0	6.6	+	+	0
5	M	58	LSF	0	PTA+Atherectomy	A	I	0	6.6	+	+	+
6	M	61	RSF	0	PTA	A	I	0	6.6	+	+	+
7	F	63	REI	0	PTA	R	I	0	6.6	+	+	+
8	M	66	REI	0	PTA	R	C	0	6.6	+	+	0
9	M	67	REI+RSF+RPOP	0	PTA+Thrombolysis	R	I	0	6.6	0	+	0
10	M	53	LCF+LSF	+	PTA	A	I	0	6.6	0	+	+
11	M	77	LSF	+	PTA	A	I	0	6.6	0	+	0
12	M	69	RCI	0	PTA	R	I	0	6.6	+	+	+
13	M	72	LSF+LPOP	0	PTA	A	I	0	6.6	+	+	0
14	M	77	LSF+LPOP+LP+LAT	+	PTA	A	I	0	6.6	+	+	+
15	M	79	LCI+LEI	0	PTA	R	I	0	6.6	+	+	0
16	F	66	LEI	0	PTA	R	I	0	6.6	+	+	+
17	F	65	RCF+RPF+LCI+LEI+LGR	0	PTA	R	C	0	6.6	0	+	0
18	M	75	RSF+RTPT+RP+RAT	+	PTA	A	I	0	6.6	0	+	0
19	M	73	RSF	+	Laser probe+PTA	A	I	0	6.6	0	+	0
20	F	71	RSF	+	PTA	A	I	0	6.6	0	+	0
21	M	62	RCI	0	PTA	R	I	0	6.6	0	+	0
22	M	75	RSF+RPOP	0	Atherectomy	A	I	0	6.6	0	+	0
23	M	75	LSF+LPT	0	PTA+Atherectomy	A	I	+	6.6	+	+	0
24	M	67	RSF+RPOP	+	PTA+Atherectomy	A	I	0	6.6	0	+	0
25	M	46	LEI	0	Atherectomy	R	I	0	6.6	0	+	+
26	M	47	REI+LCF+LSF	0	PTA	R	C	0	6.6	0	+	0
27	M	56	LSF	0	Laser probe+PTA	A	I	0	6.6	+	+	+
28	M	55	RSF+RPOP	+	PTA	A	I	0	6.6	0	+	0
29	M	67	RSF+RPOP	+	PTA	A	I	0	6.6	0	+	+
30	M	58	RSF+RPOP	0	PTA	A	I	0	6.6	0	+	0
31	M	66	LSF+LPOP	0	PTA	A	I	0	6.6	0	+	+
32	F	67	LSF	+	Laser probe+PTA	A	I	0	6.6	0	+	0
33	M	64	LEI+LCF	0	PTA	R	I	0	6.6	0	+	+
34	M	82	LSF	+	Laser probe+ Atherectomy	A	I	0	6.6	0	+	0
35	M	63	RSF+RPOP+RTPT	+	PTA+Thrombolysis	A	I	+	6.6	0	+	0
36	F	67	LR	+	PTA	R	I	0	4.8	0	+	0
37	M	64	RCI+REI+RCF	+	PTA	R	I	0	6.6	0	+	0
38	M	79	LSF+LPOP	0	PTA	R	I	0	6.6	+	+	+

(continued)

TABLE 21–1. CLINICAL DATA FOR 101 CONSECUTIVE PATIENTS IN WHOM IVUS WAS USED (Continued)

Pt	Sex	Age	Vessel	TO	Intervention	Approach A vs R	Approach C vs I	Guiding Catheter	IVUS Catheter	IVUS Pre	IVUS Post	IVUS in lieu of Angiography
39	M	70	LSF	+	PTA	A	I	0	6.6	0	+	0
40	M	77	RSF+RPOP+RP	+	Ex. Laser+PTA	A	I	0	6.6	0	+	0
41	M	74	RDF	0	PTA	R	I	0	6.6	+	+	+
42	M	72	LCI+LEI	0	PTA	R	I	0	6.6	0	+	0
43	M	68	RP	+	Ex. Laser+PTA	A	I	0	6.6	+	+	0
44	M	55	RCI+REI+RCF	0	PTA	R	I	0	6.6	+	+	+
45	M	64	RCI+REI+RCF	0	PTA	R	I	0	6.6	+	+	+
46	M	45	REI+RCF	0	PTA	R	I	0	6.6	+	+	0
47	M	69	RCI	0	PTA	R	I	0	6.6	+	+	+
48	M	72	RSF	+	Ex. Laser+PTA+Thrombolysis	A	I		6.6	0	+	0
49	M	72	RSF	0	PTA	A	I	0	6.6	0	+	+
50	M	79	RCI+RCF+LCI	0	PTA	R	C	0	6.6	+	+	0
51	M	77	REI	0	PTA	R	I	0	6.6	0	+	0
52	F	74	RDF	0	PTA	R	I	0	6.6	0	+	0
53	M	55	RSF+RPOP	0	PTA+Atherectomy	A	I	0	6.6	+	+	0
54	M	66	REI	0	PTA	R	I	0	6.6	0	+	+
55	M	68	LSF	+	PTA	A	I	0	6.6	+	+	+
56	F	74	RDF	0	PTA	R	I	0	6.6	+	+	0
57	F	45	LCI+LEI	0	PTA	R	I	0	6.6	+	+	+
58	F	69	LDF	0	PTA	R	I	0	6.6	+	+	0
59	M	55	RVG+RSF	+	Ex. Laser+PTA+Thrombolysis	R	I	0	6.6	0	+	0
60	M	52	REI	0	PTA	R	I	0	6.6	+	+	+
61	F	64	RSF+RPOP	+	PTA	A	I	0	6.6	0	+	0
62	M	72	LCI+REI	0	PTA	R	I	0	6.6	+	+	+
63	M	63	LP+LAT	+	Ex. Laser+PTA	A	I	0	6.6	0	+	0
64	F	37	LDF	0	PTA	R	I	0	6.6	+	+	+
65	F	69	LCI	0	PTA	R	I	0	6.6	+	+	+
66	M	46	RCI+REI	0	PTA	R	I	0	6.6	+	+	+
67	M	79	REI	0	PTA	R	I	0	BUIC	+	+	+
68	M	72	RCI LCI+LEI	0	PTA	R	I	0	BUIC	+	+	+
69	F	67	LEI	0	PTA+Atherectomy	R	I	0	6.6	+	+	0
70	M	59	LSF+LPOP	0	Ex. Laser+Atherectomy	A	I	0	6.6	+	+	0
71	M	66	LDF	0	PTA	R	I	0	BUIC	+	+	0
72	F	67	RSF	0	PTA+Atherectomy	A	I	0	6.6	0	+	0

Pt	Sex	Age	Vessel		Procedure							
73	M	36	LCI	+	PTA	R	C	+	6.6	+	+	0
74	M	78	RSF+RPOP	+	Ex. Laser + PTA + Atherectomy	A	I	0	6.6	0	+	0
75	F	75	RDF	0	PTA	R	I	0	6.6	+	+	0
76	M	52	RPOP	+	Ex. Laser + PTA	A	I	0	6.6	0	+	0
77	M	59	LCI	0	PTA	R	I	0	BUIC	+	+	+
78	M	69	RSF	0	PTA	A	C	0	6.6	0	+	0
79	M	76	RCI+REI+RCF+LEI	+	PTA	R	C	0	6.6	+	+	+
80	M	64	LCI	0	PTA + Atherectomy	R	I	0	BUIC	+	+	+
81	F	49	REI+RCF	0	PTA	R	I	0	4.8	+	+	+
82	F	67	LEI	0	PTA	R	I	0	6.6	+	+	+
83	F	78	REI+RCF	0	PTA	R	I	0	BUIC	+	+	+
84	F	70	LCI	0	PTA	R	I	0	BUIC	+	+	+
85	F	75	RDF	+	Atherectomy	A	I	0	6.6	0	+	0
86	F	78	RSF	0	PTA	R	I	0	6.6	+	+	+
87	M	58	REI	0	Ex. Laser + Atherectomy	A	I	0	BUIC	+	+	+
88	M	68	LSFA+LP+LPTP+LPT	+	PTA	A	I	0	6.6	0	+	0
89	M	46	RSF	+	Ex. Laser + Atherectomy	A	I	0	6.6	0	+	0
90	M	63	RSF	0	Ex. Laser + PTA	A	I	0	6.6	0	+	0
91	M	73	LSF	0	PTA	A	I	0	6.6	0	+	0
92	F	52	LCI	0	PTA	R	I	0	BUIC	+	+	0
93	M	62	LEI+LCF+LGR+LP+LAT	+	PTA + Thrombolysis	R	C	0	4.8	0	+	+
94	F	61	RSF+RPOP	0	PTA	A	I	0	6.6	+	+	0
95	M	72	RSF	+	Laser probe + PTA + Atherectomy	R	I	0	6.6	0	+	0
96	M	56	LCI	+	PTA	R	I	0	BUIC	+	+	0
97	M	71	LEI+LPF	0	PTA	R	C	+	4.8	0	+	0
98	F	30	RR	0	PTA	R	I	0	4.8	0	+	0
99	F	79	REI	+	PTA	R	C	+	4.8	+	+	0
100	F	80	LR	0	PTA	R	I	0	4.8	0	+	0
101	F	55	RSC	0	PTA	R	I	+	4.8	0	+	0
102	M	69	LR	0	PTA	R	C	0	4.8	0	+	0
103	F	71	LR	+	PTA	R	I	0	6.6	+	+	0
104	M	74	RCI+REI+RPF	0	PTA	R	I	0	4.8	0	+	0

Abbreviations: A = antegrade; B = balloon ultrasound inflation catheter; C = contralateral; Ex. = Excimer; F = female; I = ipsilateral; IVUS = intravascular ultrasound; Laser probe = hot tipped laser; LAT = left anterior tibial; LCI = left common iliac; LCF = left common femoral; LDF = left dialysis fistula; LEI = left external iliac; LGR = left graft; LP = left peroneal; LPF = left profunda; LPOP = left popliteal; LPT = left posterior tibial; LR = left renal; LSF = left superficial femoral; LTPT = left tibio-peroneal trunk; Post = following intervention; Pre = before intervention; Pt = patient; PTA = percutaneous transluminal angioplasty; R = retrograde; RAT = right anterior tibial; RCI = right common iliac; RCF = right common femoral; RDF = right dialysis fistula. REI = right external iliac; RP = right peroneal; RPOP = right popliteal; RSC = right subclavian; RSF = right superficial femoral; RTPT = right tibio-peroneal trunk; RVG = right vein graft; TO = total occlusion.

Yock et al. investigated a prototype catheter which combined a 30-MHz transducer with a modified version of the Simpson directional atherectomy catheter.[42] Preliminary experiments performed in vitro and in vivo demonstrated that this device could be used to monitor the depth to which plaque was mechanically excised.

While these two prototype devices, like the catheter employed in the present trial, were designed so that ultrasound imaging could be performed on line (i.e., during balloon inflation or mechanical atherectomy, Hodgson et al.[43] performed in vivo imaging in a series of normal canine coronary arteries with a balloon catheter on which a ring of modified phased-array transducers were positioned proximal to the balloon). The design of this device was intended to permit predilation and postdilation imaging without the requirement for multiple catheter exchanges.

Recent clinical investigation in our laboratory has confirmed that it is feasible to perform intravascular ultrasound imaging on-line during percutaneous revascularization, using a hybrid device that incorporates both diagnostic and therapeutic functions, imaging through polyethylene balloon material, the thickness of which is standard for peripheral angioplasty balloons.[44] The so-called balloon ultrasound imaging catheter (BUIC),[45] (Boston Scientific) which we have employed is illustrated in Figures 21–4 and 21–5. The catheter was used with an imaging console capable of 20-MHz imaging and 360-degree scans Diasonics) described previously in detail.[27] Briefly, the pulse repetition frequency is 10.2-kHz, the number of scans per second 10, and the number of vectors scanned in one revolution 1024. Vectors were converted, processed, and displayed through a real-time scan convertor with composite video output that allowed images to be archived on videotape or on a multiformat camera for later study.

Certain clinical data, including the site and extent of the therapeutic intervention performed in the first 10 patients in whom we investigated this device are listed in Table 21–2. In all ten patients, measurements were recorded from both the BUIC and a conventional (nonballoon) IVUS pre- and/or post-PTA and are listed individually in Table 21–3. In eight of ten patients, images recorded from the BUIC were sufficiently satisfactory to permit quantitative analysis of minimum luminal diameter (D_{min}) and luminal cross-sectional area (XSA) pre-PTA (Fig. 21–6). In the remaining two patients, artifacts resulting from subtotal evacuation of air from the angioplasty balloon and/or electrical

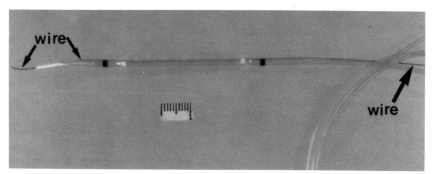

FIGURE 21–4. Design of balloon ultrasound inflation catheter (BUIC) used in the present study. Catheter is wire-guided with monorail design; wire enters distal tip of catheter, then exits side-port, reenters via dedicated port under balloon and exits port 1 cm proximal to balloon.

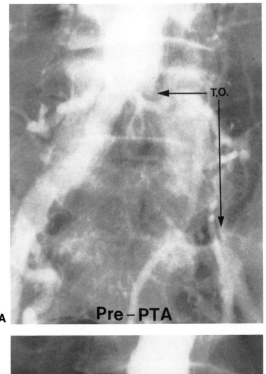

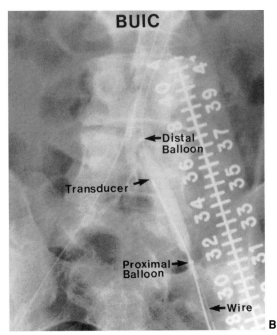

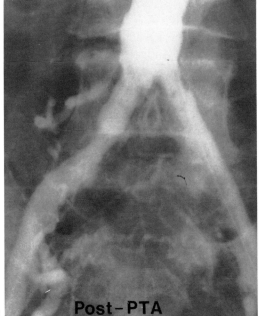

FIGURE 21–5. Angiographic cut-film depiction of BUIC used to revascularize totally occluded (T.O.) left common iliac artery (Table 21–2, patient 9). *A*, Pre-PTA. *B*, Guidewire advanced from contralateral extremity and then externalized distal to T.O. ("pull-through" technique has been used to position BUIC shown here inflated). *C*, Post-PTA.

interference compromised the diagnostic quality of the recorded image. In nine of ten patients, images recorded from the BUIC following the final balloon dilation were sufficient to permit quantitative analysis of post-PTA luminal XSA and D_{min} (Fig. 21–6). In the remaining patient, artifacts resulting from a small air bubble interfered with accurate assessment of arterial dimensions post-PTA.

As suggested from preclinical work performed in normal dogs and atherosclerotic microswine (Isner JM, Gal D, unpublished observations), the nature and mixture of material used to fill the balloon had a negligible effect on the

TABLE 21–2.   CLINICAL DATA FOR TEN PATIENTS IN WHOM BUIC WAS USED TO PERFORM PTA

Pt	Sex	Age	FCI	ABI	PTA Site	Approach	Sheath	BUIC Size (mm)	Pressure Gr (m) Pre	Post	Angio % DN Pre	Post
1	M	79	3	.44	REI	R	10 F	8 × 40	7	0	72.1	2.4
2	M	57	3	.42	LCI	R	10 F	8 × 40	27	6	100	4.3
3	M	60	3	.34	LCI	R	10.5 F	7 × 40	2	0	52.3	22.3
4	F	79	3	.39	REI	R	9 F	7 × 40	2	−2	98.9	9.8
5	F	69	3	ND	LCI	R	9 F	7 × 40	4	2	76.7	0
6	M	58	3	.51	REI	R	9 F	7 × 40	2	2	68.0	11.3
7	M	66	NA	NA	LCV	R	10 F	8 × 40	90	10	75.0	24.8
8	M	71	5	.33	RCI	R (k)	10 F	8 × 40	8	−2	52.9	0
9	M	63	3	.58	LCI	C	9 F	7 × 40	15	−2	100	31.1
10	F	53	3	.77	LCI	R	9 F	7 × 40	16	0	72.2	5.8

Abbreviations: ABI = ankle-brachial index; Angio = angiographic; BUIC = balloon ultrasound inflation catheter; C = contralateral; DN = diameter narrowing; F = female; F = French; FCI = functional classification (Rutherford[44]); Gr = gradient; k = "kissing balloon" technique; LCI = left common iliac; LCV = left cephalic vein; M = male; m = mean; NA = not applicable; ND = not done; Post = following angioplasty; Pre = before angioplasty; Pt = patient; PTA = percutaneous transluminal angioplasty; R = retrograde; RCI = right common iliac; REI = right external iliac.

quality of image obtained. The exception to this was residual air within the balloon, which when present compromised detail required for quantitative analysis. When images recorded from the BUIC were not compromised by incomplete evacuation of air from the balloon, measurements of luminal cross-sectional area and minimum diameter were nearly indistinguishable from those recorded using a nonballoon ultrasound catheter (Table 21–3); measurements recorded from the latter have been shown to correlate well with measurements derived from quantitative angiographic analysis of native normal and diseased arteries.[46–49]

All images recorded with the BUIC involved a 20-MHz transducer. While this frequency appeared satisfactory for qualitative and quantitative analysis both in the presence and absence of an inflation balloon, it remains to be determined whether frequencies investigated in other mechanical systems, specifically 30-[42] and 40-MHz[21] may yield superior results.

Assessment of recoil following balloon deflation constitutes a specific application of these quantitative findings. Recoil has long been inferred to constitute a mechanical reason for loss of gain achieved during balloon inflation.[50–53] More recently, several investigators have employed quantitative angiographic techniques to analyze the extent to which recoil complicates standard PTCA. Nobuyoshi performed coronary angiography routinely on 185 patients one day following PTCA.[54] "Restenosis" (more than 50 per cent loss of gain in absolute diameter assessed by cinevideodensitometry) was already present in 27 (14.6 per cent) of 185 patients or in 27 (11.4 per cent) of 237 lesions by 1 day and was interpreted to represent evidence of elastic recoil. Stenosis diameter among these 185 patients decreased from 1.91 ± 0.53 immediately post-PTCA to 1.72 ± 0.52 mm 1 day post-PTCA ($p < 0.001$).

Hjemdahl-Monsen et al. derived pressure-diameter curves from videodensitometric measurements made at incremental pressures (1 to 6 atm) during PTCA of 29 lesions in 27 patients.[55] Recoil (balloon diameter at 6 atm/post-PTCA luminal diameter greater than 1.0) was observed in 25 of 29 lesions and ranged from 1.02 to 2.01 (m ± SD = 1.35 ± 0.33).

Rensing et al. performed videodensitometric analysis on 151 lesions suc-

TABLE 21–3. MEASUREMENTS RECORDED FROM BUIC AND IVUS PRE-, DURING, AND POST-PTA

Pt	Pre-PTA							Balloon Inflation[a]		Post-PTA						
	Image Quality	XSA (cm²)			D_min (cm)			XSA (cm²)	D (cm)	Image Quality	XSA (cm²)			D_min (cm)		
		IVUS	BUIC	Δ	IVUS	BUIC	Δ				IVUS	BUIC	Δ	IVUS	BUIC	Δ
1	S	.11	.09	+.02	.31	.30	+.01	.38	.70	S	.28	.25	+.05	.65	.59	+.06
2	S	.05	.06	−.01	.29	.25	+.04	.50	.79	S	.47	.44	+.03	.64	.60	+.04
3	P	.09	.09	0	.29	.38	−.09	.33	.63	S	.34	.33	+.01	.61	.63	−.02
4	S	.09	.15	−.06	.38	.38	0	.33	.61	S	.17	.18	−.01	.45	.44	+.01
5	S	.10	.10	0	.35	.36	−.01	.31	.66	P	.42	.30	+.12	.57	.60	−.03
6	S	.09	.08	+.01	.33	.31	+.02	.32	.62	S	.25	.22	+.03	.55	.59	−.04
7	S	.06	.07	−.01	.26	.31	−.05	.44	.75	S	.29	.25	+.04	.53	.58	−.05
8	S	.15	.13	+.02	.33	.40	−.07	.42	.68	S	.36	.38	−.02	.66	.62	+.04
9	P	.08	.22	−.14	.35	.35	0	.42	.72	S	.23	.26	−.03	.45	.46	−.01
10	S	.10	.12	−.02	.36	.38	−.02	.34	.65	S	.31	.31	0	.56	.62	−.06

[a] Numbers listed here are maximum values among ≥1 balloon inflations listed individually in Table 21–3.

Abbreviations: Δ = mean difference; BUIC = balloon ultrasound inflation catheter; D_min = minimum luminal diameter; IVUS = intravascular ultrasound (non–balloon-catheter); P = poor; Post-PTA = post–balloon angioplasty; Pre-PTA = pre–balloon angioplasty; Pt = patient; S = satisfactory; XSA = cross-sectional area.

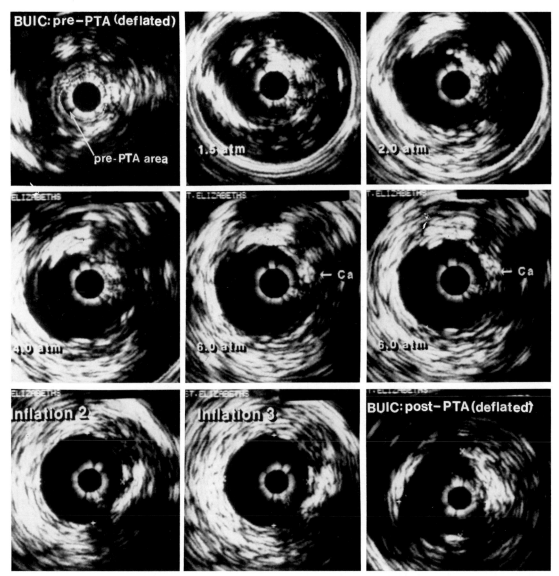

FIGURE 21–6. Serial images recorded from BUIC pre-, during, and post-PTA of common iliac arterial stenosis (patient 3, Table 21–2). *Top Left,* Image recorded from BUIC immediately prior to balloon inflation demonstrates pre-PTA cross-sectional area, indicated by inscribed circle. Subsequent images demonstrate serial expansion of balloon cross-sectional area recorded from BUIC during inflation #1 at 12.5, 2.0, 4.0, and 6.0 atm. The pair of images recorded at 6 atm demonstrates sudden yielding of arterial wall after several seconds at given inflation pressure; note movement of calcified (ca) plaque towards arrow, position of which was not changed from first to second image recorded at 6 atm. Bottom row of images illustrates cross-sectional area of BUIC at full inflations #2 and 3, and final luminal cross-sectional area recorded from BUIC immediately post–balloon-deflation.

cessfully dilated among 136 patients during balloon inflation, and directly after balloon deflation.[56] Mean cross-sectional area of the inflated balloon was 5.2 ± 1.6 mm², while mean (minimal) cross-sectional area of the dilated stenosis post balloon deflation was 2.8 ± 1.4 mm ². Thus, nearly 50 per cent of the theoretically achievable cross-sectional area was lost immediately after balloon deflation. In contrast to the findings of Nobuyoshi et al., analysis of a subset of 16 patients (18 lesions) reexamined 1 day post-PTCA disclosed no further reduction in minimum luminal cross-sectional area.

TABLE 21–4. ANALYSIS OF RECOIL FROM MEASUREMENTS RECORDED USING BUIC[a]

Pt	Inflation #1 Full Inflation D_{min}	XSA	Post-deflation D_{min}	XSA	% Recoil D_{min}	XSA	Inflation #2 Full Inflation D_{min}	XSA	Post-deflation D_{min}	XSA	% Recoil D_{min}	XSA	Inflation #3 Full Inflation D_{min}	XSA	Post-deflation D_{min}	XSA	% Recoil D_{min}	XSA
1	.70	.38	.59	.23	16	39	.69	.38	.54	.25	22	34						
2	.47	.28	.49	.25	-4	11	.60	.34	.46	.39	23	-15	.79	.50	.60	.44	24	12
3	.62	.31	.62	.37	0	-20	.63	.32	.62	.39	2	-22	.63	.33	.62	.33	2	0
4	.56	.28	.39	.15	30	46	.61	.33	.44	.18	28	45						
6	.62	.27	.55	.28	11	-4	.61	.32	.48	.31	21	3						
7	.74	.44	.34	.17	54	61	.75	.44	.56	.27	25	39	.68	.38	.58	.25	15	34
8	.68	.42	.62	.38	9	10												
9	.62	.28	.31	.14	50	50	.72	.33	.39	.15	46	55	.71	.42	.46	.26	35	38
10	.65	.34	.61	.26	6	24	.62	.34	.59	.31	5	10						

[a] Recoil could not be accurately calculated in Patient 5 in whom postdeflation images were unsatisfactory for measurements of D_{min} and XSA.
Abbreviations: BUIC = balloon ultrasound inflation catheter; D_{min} = minimum diameter; Pt = patient; XSA = cross-sectional area.

Finally, Lehmann et al. prospectively evaluated 114 lesions undergoing PTCA by quantitative angiography and found that recoil (per cent loss of diameter gained during maximum balloon inflation) averaged 34 ± 23.3 per cent, reducing calculated post-PTCA cross-sectional area from 5.65 mm^2 to 3.45 mm^2.[57]

Measurements recorded using the BUIC (Table 21–4) confirm the preceding observations made using angiographic techniques and establish that the phenomenon of recoil is common to peripheral as well as coronary angioplasty. Furthermore, because there is a nearly unavoidable delay between balloon deflation and quantitative angiographic examination post-PTCA, Rensing et al. had raised the possibility that platelet deposition and/or nonocclusive mural thrombus frequently observed at balloon angioplasty sites postmortem could not be ruled out as the basis for apparent recoil observed angiographically.[58] The present series of observations, in which ultrasound analysis of recoil was accomplished immediately upon balloon deflation, establishes conclusively that such recoil is instantaneous. Interestingly, the single patient in this series in whom clinical evidence of restenosis has thus far been observed was the patient in whom recoil was most severe.

In five instances, measurements recorded with the BUIC disclosed "negative" recoil, that is, luminal dimensions post-PTA exceeded those of the angioplasty balloon at maximum inflation. In one case, post-PTA diameter of the arterial lumen slightly exceeded that of the balloon, while post-PTA cross-sectional area was slightly less than that of the balloon. In the remaining four cases, while recoil varied from 0 to 23 per cent as a function of balloon diameter, when measured in terms of cross-sectional area, luminal area post-PTA exceeded balloon area by 4 to 22 per cent. Although not explicitly commented upon, inspection of findings reported previously by Hjemdahl-Monsen[55] and Lehmann[57] reveals several cases in which diameter measurements made by quantitative angiography were indicative of such negative recoil. Analysis of this phenomenon in the present series of cases suggests that it results from a relatively large (but non–flow-limiting) plaque fracture; this has the previously noted effect of limiting elastic recoil.

Moreover, when a radial plaque fracture is associated with a circumferential extension, the resulting cross-sectional area may in fact exceed that of the inflated balloon, despite the fact that the post-PTA minimum luminal diameter, along a selected minor axis, is slightly less than that of the inflated balloon. Because intravascular ultrasound allows direct inspection of the often complex cracked and/or dissected post-PTA lumen, diameter and cross-sectional area may both be assessed directly and independently[46–49,59,60] (Fig. 21–7). Most algorithms developed for quantitative angiography calculate cross-sectional area as a function of measured luminal diameter, and previous studies have documented that the accuracy of such algorithms may be diminished in those cases in which satisfactory orthogonal views cannot be obtained.[61] Assessment of elastic recoil postangioplasty may thus be more complicated than previously appreciated; it is in fact entirely possible that apparent recoil measured as a function of luminal diameter postangioplasty is more frequently (than previously appreciated) associated with a paradoxical increase in luminal cross-sectional area.

Finally, on-line ultrasound monitoring of balloon inflation also facilitated identification of the initiation of plaque fracture (Fig. 21–8). On-line analysis of pressure-volume curves has been investigated previously as a means of

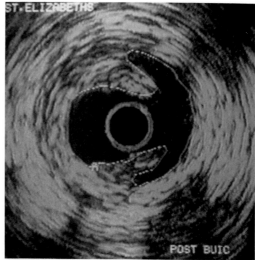

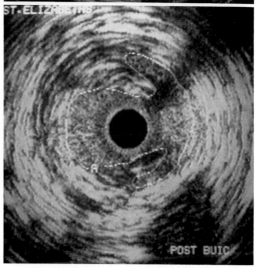

FIGURE 21–7. Irregular geometry resulting from balloon angioplasty (in this case performed using the BUIC to treat stenotic left common iliac, Table 21–2, patient 10). *Top*, Planimetered cross-sectional area post-PTA. *Bottom*, Injection of agitated saline confirms planimetry of luminal cross-sectional area.

characterizing the mechanism responsible for vascular dilation in vivo.[62] "Cracking," identified as sudden yielding of the balloon at a given inflation pressure, was less commonly observed than either patterns indicative of "stretching," or "compaction." The results of on-line ultrasound analysis of balloon inflation suggest that plaque "fracture" is proportionately more common than indicated by pressure-volume analysis, and this is further supported by post hoc ultrasound analyses,[27,49,59,60,63] and previously reported necropsy studies.[50] Moreover, in at least one patient (patient 3, Table 21–2; Fig. 21–6) we observed what graphically would appear to correspond to "sudden yielding of the balloon (and arterial wall) at a given inflation pressure" unaccompanied by evident plaque fracture during or post-PTA.

Images recorded from the BUIC disclosed that plaque fractures were initiated by dilatation at low (less than 2 atm) inflation pressures. This is consistent with previous clinical observations. Hjemdahl-Monsen et al., for example, found that most improvement in luminal size occurred at inflation pressures below 2 atm.[55] Likewise, Kahn et al. observed that full balloon

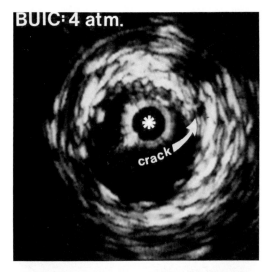

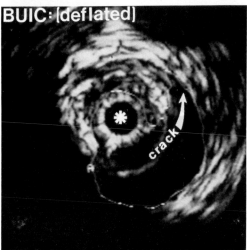

FIGURE 21–8. Example of plaque fracture (crack) observed during balloon inflation using BUIC. *Top*, Image recorded at 4 atm showing fully developed crack as seen during inflation. *Middle*, Appearance of crack immediately following balloon deflation. *Bottom*, Confirmation of crack identified with BUIC by image recorded from nonballoon intravascular ultrasound catheter (IVUS).

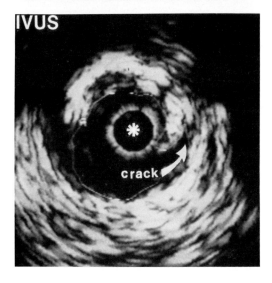

expansion as determined by fluoroscopic monitoring occurred in nearly 50 per cent of patients at inflation pressures of 4 atm or less.[64] These findings regarding the efficacy of lower inflation pressures supplement experimental data indicating a higher incidence of mural thrombus, dissection, and intimal hyperplasia as a result of higher inflation pressures. As suggested by Kleiman et al.,[65] any technique, whether it be pressure-volume or ultrasound analysis, that permits immediate, on-line recognition of plaque fracture might theoretically be employed to modify the remainder of the dilatation procedure in an attempt to prevent the development of a flow-limiting dissection.

THREE-DIMENSIONAL RECONSTRUCTION

Comparison of individual segments examined by IVUS to adjacent or more distal segments requires repeated review of serially recorded images to reconstruct, in the mind's eye, the spatial relationship of the segments of interest. For example, while one tomographic image obtained during IVUS examination may offer high-resolution definition of a plaque fracture resulting from balloon angioplasty, details regarding the longitudinal distribution of the same plaque fracture at one site relative to proximal and distal sites cannot be displayed in a single image. In contrast, conventional angiography preserves the advantage of displaying each segment in longitudinal relationship to adjacent and more distant segments; once contrast media has opacified the artery of interest, any individual segment may be compared to adjacent and distant segments, limited only by the field of view. Three-dimensional reconstruction of serially recorded tomographic images represents a possible solution to the limited spatial display features characteristic of current IVUS imaging systems.

Original attempts to perform three-dimensional reconstructions in our laboratory involved the use of software (SigmaScan, Jandel Scientific, Corte Madera, CA) that required manual morphometric tracing of each serial tomographic image followed by computer-aided reconstruction.[66] The more detail intended, the more images that were required, and consequently the more labor-intensive was the reconstruction. The principal liability of this approach, however, related to the fact that the modeling technique was based exclusively on boundary depiction and therefore allowed three-dimensional reconstruction of the lumen but not the arterial wall. Such an approach would clearly squander one of the chief assets of intravascular ultrasound; namely, the capability to image the vessel wall and thereby evaluate characteristics of the native wall, as well as pathologic alterations resulting from interventional therapies.

Automated three-dimensional reconstruction of intravascular ultrasound images was investigated in a preliminary fashion by Kitney et al.,[67] using voxel modeling. This approach considers each voxel, or volume element, as an extension to three-dimensional space of the digital image element, or pixel (picture element). Voxel modeling is a particularly attractive option for three-dimensional reconstruction of the vasculature, because it allows representation of the arterial wall rather than simply surface features that would limit the reconstruction of the arterial lumen.

More recently,[68–71] we have had the opportunity to perform three-dimensional reconstruction using a PC-based system (ImageComm Systems, Santa Clara, CA) and algorithms[72–74] designed specifically for analysis of images recorded during during IVUS examination (Omniview, Pura Labs, Brea, CA). The software employs a surface-rendering process predicated on segmented boundary formation, but includes interpolative algorithms designed to link boundary elements, and thereby preserve the capability of viewing the arterial wall as well as lumen.

Analysis of the three-dimensional reconstructions recorded in a preliminary series of 52 patients (Table 21–5) suggests that these three-dimensional images may in fact supplement analysis of conventional two-dimensional images. Use of the so-called sagittal format (Figs. 21–9 and 21–10), in particular, not only facilitates comparative analysis of adjacent tomographic images, but offers the additional advantage of displaying the ultrasound data in a longitudinal profile-type format more familiar to the angiographer. While similar in orientation to an angiogram, sagittal reconstruction substantially augments information available from conventional angiography in two important ways. First, limitless orthogonal views can be rendered by incremental rotation of the imaging plane about the reference catheter. Given the documented importance of orthogonal views in the assessment of luminal narrowing[61] on the one hand, and the logistical factors which frequently obviate the possibility of obtaining orthogonal views on the other, this feature may ultimately prove to be the principal advantage of three-dimensional reconstruction.

Second, information regarding pathologic alteration of the arterial wall is provided simultaneously with the conventional assessment of luminal diameter narrowing. Experience with several of the patients in the present series undergoing percutaneous revascularization indicates that certain features of arterial wall pathology are particularly well defined in such a longitudinal format. For example, three-dimensional reconstruction in the sagittal mode graphically demonstrated that recanalization of a lengthy total occlusion was achieved by tunneling a false lumen through calcified plaque. Such a mechanism of recanalization has been previously described in vitro[75,76] and is frequently inferred to occur in vivo,[77] but, in the present case, definition equivalent to the reconstructed ultrasound image was absent from the completion angiogram. While the individual tomographic ultrasound images indicated creation of a "double-barrel" lumen, the full extent of pathologic disruption was more immediately apparent from inspection of the sagittal reconstructions. Similarly, sagittal reconstructions of balloon-dilated nonoccluded vessels demonstrated the longitudinal distribution of barotraumatic injury (Fig. 21–10), otherwise evident as only local, isolated plaque fractures on the tomographic two-dimensional IVUS images.

Experience with the so-called cylindrical format (Fig. 21–11) suggests that this mode of three-dimensional reconstruction—particularly when the reconstructed vascular segment is hemisected—is optimally suited for those cases in which direct inspection of luminal topography is of special interest, such as analysis of implanted endovascular prostheses. Details of the "cobblestoned" neointima lining the stent cannot be appreciated angiographically or even by intravascular ultrasound, when viewed in standard video format[78]; the algorithms developed to accomplish the cylindrical reconstruction serve the dual function of both joining together the series of adjacent elements representing the neointima, and then rotating the reconstructed image 90 degrees to permit viewing of the endoluminal surface en face. The sagittal reconstruction supplements the cylindrical format by facilitating analysis of arterial contour proximal and distal to the stent; such analysis is otherwise not feasible using the unassembled tomographic images.

Alternatively, the "third dimension" of the three-dimensional software may be used as a temporal rather than spatial axis. We have utilized this option, for

example, in conjunction with the BUIC, to summate composite balloon inflation and deflation within a single image.[79]

Certain limitations of current attempts to perform three-dimensional reconstruction must be acknowledged. First, it is apparent that the quality of the three-dimensional reconstructions can only be as good as the original two-dimensional images. Details which are absent from the original recordings will likewise be absent from the reconstructed images. In those instances when calcific deposits, for example, are observed on the two-dimensional images to attenuate echoes from the subjacent plaque and/or wall, these portions of the plaque and/or wall will not be incorporated into the reconstructed image.

Second, "ring-down artifact," resulting from dead space in the acoustic transmission path and manifested on the two-dimensional image as a white halo immediately peripheral to the transducer, may obscure near-field structure in smaller, particularly stenotic vessels. In our preliminary work, such artifact was routinely masked out of the three-dimensional reconstructions; in those cases in which reconstruction is applied to two-dimensional images with little or no lumen peripheral to the transducer, such masking could overestimate three-dimensional depiction of luminal patency. Current attempts by the manufacturers of mechanical transducer systems to eliminate such artifact will hopefully resolve this issue.

Third, while major branch points, such as the aortic bifurcation, are accurately depicted in the three-dimensional reconstruction, the two-dimensional images are otherwise reassembled as a straight tube; sharp bends in the artery are not faithfully reconstructed on either the two- or three-dimensional images. While this is typically not a severe liability in evaluation of the peripheral and renal circulations, it may become more significant in the assessment of the more tortuous coronary circulation.

Fourth, three-dimensional reconstruction shares with conventional intravascular ultrasound imaging the difficulty of matching the rotational orientation of the ultrasound transducer to that of the imaged vessel. Furthermore, if the ultrasound probe is inadvertently twisted during the pullback recording, the three-dimensional reconstruction will reflect this rotational event.

Fifth, in all studies performed to date, the two-dimensional images have been acquired during a slow (approximately 0.25 cm/sec), timed catheter pullback; this strategy is intended to optimize the number of acquired images over a given segment length and provide equal representation for each portion of the artery in the reconstructed image. Such catheter pullback, however, is entirely operator-dependent and small variations in the rate of pullback may ultimately influence the three-dimensional representation. For example, if the catheter withdrawal rate is slowed during pullback through an abnormal segment of vessel, and subsequently accelerated through a more normal segment, the abnormal segment will occupy proportionally more than its true length of the resulting reconstruction. This phenomenon is particularly likely to occur when there is a tendency for the operator to slow catheter movement through abnormal segments to achieve closer inspection of morphologic disruptions. To minimize this variable in the present investigation, the sole focus of the operator performing the pullback was to observe the catheter as it was withdrawn through the sheath of guiding catheter; analysis of two-dimensional ultrasound image registration was performed before and/or after the pullback recording. This acquisition technique is currently being modified to include automated image registration that will be less operator-dependent. One such potential modification is to alter the acquisition mode such that it be based on

TABLE 21–5. CLINICAL FEATURES, ULTRASOUND EXAMINATIONS, AND THREE-DIMENSIONAL RECONSTRUCTIONS

Pt	Sex	Age	Functional Status Pre	Post	Ankle-Brachial Index Pre	Post	Vessel	Intervention	IVUS Catheter Size (Fr)	2-Dimensional IVUS Pre	Post	3-D Recon Pre (#) Sag	Cyl	Post (#) Sag	Cyl	On-line†
1	M	64	3	0	.45	.65	CIA	PTA	6.2	−	+	−	−	1	−	
2	F	69	3	1	.42	—	CIA	PTA	6.2	+	+	2	−	3	−	
3	F	53	4	0	.75	1.01	CIA	PTA	6.2	+	+	1	4	1	1	
4	M	57	3	1	.42	—	CIA	PTA	6.2	−	+	−	−	3	6	+
5	M	68	3	2	.97	—	CIA	PTA	6.2	+	+	1	1	1	2	
6	M	69	3	0	.80	1.34	CIA	PTA	6.2	+	+	3	−	5	1	+
7	F	80	4	2	.54	—	CIA	PTA	6.2	+	+	2	−	1	−	
8	M	56	3	2	.65	.87	CIA/EIA	PTA	6.2	+	+	−	−	1	1	+
9	M	72	4	2	—	—	CIA/EIA	PTA	6.2	+	+	2	−	2	−	
10	M	56	3	1	.63	.46	CIA/EIA/CFA	PTA	6.2	+	+	1	−	2	−	
11	F	63	3	1	.59	—	EIA	PTA	6.2	+	+	2	2	3	3	
12	M	67	3	3	.69	.94	EIA	PTA	6.2	+	+	1	−	1	−	
13	M	64	4	3	.58	.92	EIA	PTA	6.2	+	+	1	−	2	−	
14	F	66	5	2	.23	.94	EIA	PTA	6.2	−	+	−	−	1	−	
15	M	62	3	2	.36	.61	EIA	PTA, stent	6.2	+	+	2	−	3	−	
16	M	54	3	3	.71	.64	EIA	PTA	6.2	+	+	2	3	3	3	+
17	M	79	3	2	.44	—	EIA	PTA	6.2	+	+	1	1	2	1	
18	M	77	4	2	.48	.52	EIA	PTA	6.2	+	+	3	−	1	−	
19	F	79	4	1	.39	.40	EIA/CFA	PTA	6.2	+	+	2	1	1	−	
20	M	45	5	3	.49	.57	EIA/CFA	PTA	6.2	+	+	1	−	2	1	+
21	M	71	3	2	.39	.71	EIA/Profunda	PTA	4.8	+	+	1	−	1	−	
22	M	59	5	3	.45	.82	SFA	PTA	6.2	−	+	−	−	7	7	
23	F	75	3	0	.43	.90	SFA	Laser, PTA	6.2	−	+	−	−	4	4	

#	Sex	Age					Vessel	Treatment	Fr						†
24	M	52	3	2	.60	.88	SFA	Atherectomy	6.2	+	+	4	1	3	1
25	M	56	3	1	.49	.82	SFA	PTA	6.2	—	+	1	1	1	—
26	M	77	4	2	.30	.48	SFA/Pop A	Laser, PTA	6.2	+	+	—	—	2	—
27	M	59	3	0	.41	.92	SFA/Pop A	Laser, atherectomy	6.2	+	+	1	—	1	—
28	M	63	3	2	.40	.77	SFA/peroneal/Ant Tib	Laser, PTA	6.2	+*	—	1	1	—	—
29	M	67	3	0	.76	1.20	Pop A	Laser, PTA	6.2	+	+	2	2	3	—
30	M	55	3	0	.65	1.08	RSVG (Fem-Pop)	Lysis, laser, PTA	6.2	—	+	—	—	—	1
31	F	55	NA	NA	NA	NA	Subclavian A	PTA	4.8	—	+	—	—	1	1
32	M	75	NA	NA	NA	NA	Dialysis fistula	PTA	6.2	+	+	—	—	1	1
33	M	66	NA	NA	NA	NA	Dialysis fistula	PTA	6.2	+	+	—	—	1	1
34	F	77	NA	NA	NA	NA	Dialysis fistula	PTA	6.2	+	+	—	—	1	1
35	M	66	NA	NA	NA	NA	Dialysis fistula	PTA	6.2	+	+	—	—	1	1
36	F	75	NA	NA	NA	NA	Dialysis fistula	PTA	6.2	+	+	1	—	1	1
37	F	77	NA	NA	NA	NA	Renal artery	PTRA	4.8	—	+	—	—	2	1
38	F	80	NA	NA	NA	NA	Renal artery	PTRA	4.8	—	+	—	—	1	1
39	F	29	NA	NA	NA	NA	Renal artery	PTRA	4.8	—	+	—	—	1	1
40	M	63	NA	NA	NA	NA	Renal artery	PTRA	4.8	+	+	5	4	3	3	+
41	M	65	NA	NA	NA	NA	LAD	PTCA	4.8	—	+	—	—	1	—
42	M	65	NA	NA	NA	NA	LAD	PTCA	4.8	—	+	—	—	2	2
43	F	48	NA	NA	NA	NA	LAD	PTCA	3.5	—	+	—	—	2	2
44	M	69	NA	NA	NA	NA	LAD	PTCA	3.5	—	+	—	—	1	1
45	F	61	NA	NA	NA	NA	RCA	Laser, PTCA	4.8	—	+	—	—	5	5
46	M	64	NA	NA	NA	NA	RCA	PTCA	3.5	—	+	—	—	2	2
47	M	55	NA	NA	NA	NA	RCA	PTCA	4.8	—	+	—	—	1	1
48	M	48	NA	NA	NA	NA	RCA	PTCA	4.8	—	+	—	—	5	5
49	M	61	NA	NA	NA	NA	RCA	PTCA	4.8	—	+	—	—	2	2
50	M	59	NA	NA	NA	NA	RSVG to RCA	Laser, PTCA	4.8	+	+	—	—	5	5
51	F	59	NA	NA	NA	NA	RSVG to LAD	—	4.8	+	NA	1	1	NA	NA
52	M	52	NA	NA	NA	NA	RSVG to RCA/LAD	—	4.8	+	NA	2	2	NA	NA

Abbreviations: = Rutherford class; # = number; † = 3-dimensional reconstruction and image generation during interventional procedure; — = not done; + = done; * = ultrasound examination on superficial femoral artery only; A = artery; Ant Tib = anterior tibial artery; CFA = common femoral artery; CIA = common iliac artery; Cyl = Cylindrical; EIA = external iliac artery; F = female; Fem-pop = femoro-popliteal graft; Fr = french; IVUS = intravascular ultrasound; LAD = left anterior descending coronary artery; Lysis = thrombolysis; M = male; NA = not applicable; PTA = percutaneous transluminal angioplasty; PTCA = percutaneous transluminal coronary angioplasty; PTRA = percutaneous transluminal renal angioplasty; Pop-popliteal; Profunda = profunda femoris artery; RCA = right coronary artery; RSVG = Reverse saphenous vein graft; SFA = superficial femoral artery.

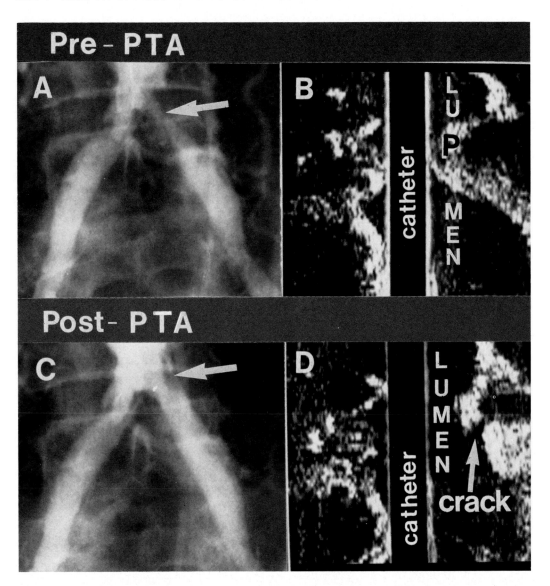

FIGURE 21–9. On-line 3D reconstruction during PTA. *A*, Pre-PTA angiogram indicates shelf-like plaque (arrow) in common iliac artery. IVUS pullbacks performed during procedure (before and after dilation) acquired 2D image sets, each of which was used to create multiple (15 to 30) sagittal views within 90 seconds of completing the pullback. One such representative reconstruction *B*, shows encroachment of lumen by plaque (P), which abuts IVUS catheter. *C*, Post-PTA angiogram demonstrates improvement in luminal diameter, with a luminal defect at the PTA site. *D*, Sagittal reconstruction generated immediately from post-PTA pullback with identical orientation to (*B*), showing obvious enhancement of luminal dimensions. A crack in the plaque at PTA site is also identified.

regular distance intervals, in contrast to the current system of time-interval–based image acquisition.

Beyond these limitations, the extent to which three-dimensional reconstruction will be employed clinically is principally dependent on two factors: the time required for reconstruction, and the prognostic implications of the resulting images. With regard to the former, image processing time has been reduced considerably through a combination of modifications in software and memory

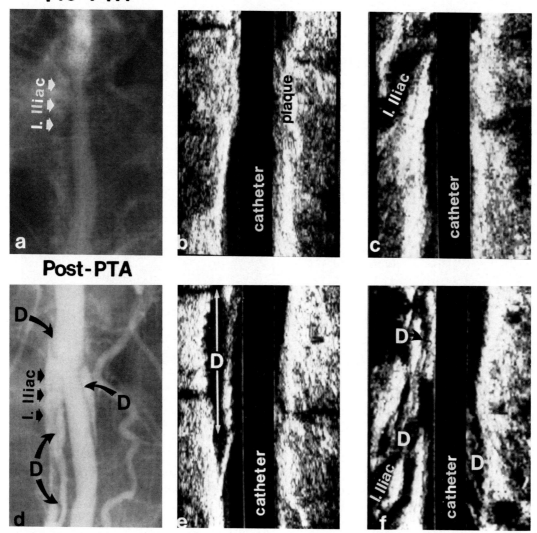

FIGURE 21–10. Sagittal 3D reconstruction of iliac artery pre- and post-PTA, demonstrating large dissection extending into internal iliac artery (I. Iliac). *a*, Pre-PTA angiogram illustrates high-grade stenosis at bifurcation of common iliac artery. I. Iliac is widely patent. *b*, Sagittal reconstruction generated from 2D IVUS pullback shows luminal narrowing at site where plaque abuts IVUS catheter. *c*, Rotation of reconstructed by image by approximately 60 degrees about longitudinal axis of IVUS catheter reveals origin and proximal portion of the I. Iliac. *d*, Post-PTA angiogram shows apparent increase in luminal diameter, with multiple fractures and dissections (D) resulting from balloon dilation. There is a suggestion that dissection extends into I. Iliac Artery. *e*, Sagittal 3D reconstruction post-PTA demonstrates enhanced luminal patency with prominent subintimal dissection (D). *f*, Rotation of reconstructed artery to same orthogonal view as *c* reveals circumferential nature of dissection, which also extends into proximal I. Iliac.

expansion. Whereas early reconstructions typically required 20 to 40 minutes to assemble, current reconstructions are routinely completed within 20 seconds of completing the pullback recording. Preliminary work[31] with yet another iteration of software has generated both sagittal and cylindrical reconstructions within 30 seconds of completing the pullback recording. It is thus realistic to expect that the time required to reconstruct and review the reconstructed images will be comparable to that currently required to review the video playback of a contrast angiogram. While reconstructions accomplished on-line

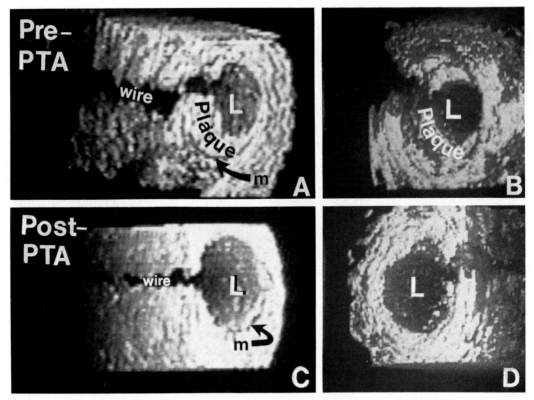

FIGURE 21–11. Cylindrical reconstruction of iliac artery pre- and post-PTA. *A,B,* Two different orientations of segment of iliac artery. Lumen (L) is narrowed by eccentric plaque. Media (m) is detected underlying the plaque; shadowing artifact from wire is also identified. *C,D,* Post-PTA, cylindrical reconstructions from same segment demonstrate increase in luminal dimensions and paucity of postdilation pathology.

in the current series were not used for the purpose of guiding therapeutic decisions, this strategy should be feasible in the future.

The extent to which three-dimensional reconstructions of two-dimensional intravascular ultrasound images will alter interventional or other therapy remains to be determined. The same, of course, remains true of the two-dimensional images as well. While the quality of the two-dimensional images has evolved to the point that they are in fact being used to make on-line decisions regarding the nature and extent of percutaneous revascularization,[59,80] prognostic implications associated with specific findings will require clinical and/or angiographic follow-up studies.[81] In the case of a dissection resulting from attempted balloon angioplasty, for example, it is conceivable that the geometric disposition of the dissection might determine whether it is likely to lead to early occlusion, later restenosis, or, in other cases, heal in a benign fashion. At present, such information cannot be adequately determined by conventional angiography, which provides too little detail regarding the plaque and/or arterial wall. Three-dimensional reconstruction of the two-dimensional examination should facilitate evaluation of the latter's prognostic utility by providing a comprehensive recapitulation of the sequentially recorded tomographic images. Ultimately, however, the utility of three-dimensional reconstruction as an adjunct to interventional procedures will need to be evaluated in prospective studies.

Finally, preliminary algorithms have already been developed to augment

the utility of three-dimensional reconstruction in two important respects. First, an automated edge-detection scheme has been incorporated which will permit automated quantitative analysis of cross-sectional area from the cylindrical reconstructions. Second, characterization of plaque composition, long an elusive goal of vascular imaging, may be facilitated by three-dimensional reconstruction. Preliminary applications of intravascular ultrasound suggest that it is more sensitive than conventional fluoroscopy for detection of vascular calcific deposits and, furthermore, is capable of distinguishing predominantly fibrotic from predominantly fatty plaque. While manual morphometric assessment of each two-dimensional frame recorded during an intravascular ultrasound examination is an impractical means by which to analyze tissue composition, preliminary applications suggest that computer-aided analyses of reconstructed three-dimensional images may make such qualitative assessment feasible.

REFERENCES

1. Vlodaver Z, Frech R, Van Tassel RA, Edwards JE: Correlations of the antemortem arteriogram and the postmortem specimen. Circulation 1973;47:162–169.
2. Grondin CM, Dyrda I, Pasternac A, Campeau L, Bourassa MG, Lesperance J: Discrepancies between cineangiographic and postmortem findings in patients with coronary artery disease and recent myocardial revascularization. Circulation 1974;49:703–708.
3. Pepine CJ, Feldman RL, Nichols WW, et al: Coronary arteriography: Potentially serious sources of error in interpretation. Cardiovasc Med 1977;2:747–752.
4. Arnett EN, Isner JM, Redwood CR, et al: Coronary artery narrowing in coronary heart disease: Comparison of cineangiographic and necropsy findings. Ann Intern Med 1979; 91:350–356.
5. Isner JM, Kishel J, Kent KM, Ronan JA Jr, Ross AM, Roberts WC: Accuracy of angiographic determination of left main coronary arterial narrowing: Angiographic-histologic correlative analysis in 28 patients. Circulation 1981;63:1056–1064.
6. Spears JR, Sandor T, Baim DS, Paulin S: The minimum error in estimating coronary luminal cross-sectional area from cineangiographic diameter measurements. Cathet Cardiovasc Diagn 1983;9:119–128.
7. White CW, Wright CB, Doty DB, et al: Does visual interpretation of the coronary arteriogram predict the physiologic importance of a coronary stenosis? N Engl J Med 1984;310:819–824.
8. Isner JM, Donaldson RF: Coronary angiographic and morphologic correlation. Cardiol Clin 1984;2:571–592.
9. Gould KL: Quantification of coronary artery stenosis in vivo. Circ Res 1985;57:341–353.
10. Zijlstra F, van Ommeren J, Reiber HC, Serruys PW: Does the quantitative assessment of coronary artery dimensions predict the physiologic significance of a coronary stenosis? Circulation 1987;75:1154–1161.
11. Marcus ML, Skorton DJ, Johnson MR, Collins SM, Harrison DG, Kerber RE: Visual estimates of percent diameter coronary stenosis: "A battered gold standard." J Am Coll Cardiol 1988; 11:882–885.
12. Clarke RH, Isner JM, Gauthier TD, et al: Spectroscopic characterization of cardiovascular tissue. Lasers Surg Med 1988;8:45–59.
13. Deckelbaum LI, Stetz ML, O'Brien KM, et al: Fluorescence spectroscopic guidance of laser ablation of atherosclerotic plaque. Lasers Surg Med 1989;9:205–214.
14. Spears JR, Marais HJ, Serur J, et al: In vivo coronary angioscopy. J Am Coll Cardiol 1983; 1:1311–1314.
15. Jakubowski A, Hickey A, Glick D, Litvack F, Grundfest W, Forrester JS: Angioscopy. In Isner JM, Clarke RH, eds: Cardiovascular Laser Therapy. New York, Raven Press, 1989;201–212.
16. White GH, White RA: Percutaneous angioscopy as adjunct to laser angioplasty in peripheral arteries (letter). Lancet 1989;2:99.
17. Sahn DJ, Barrett-Boyers, Graham K, et al: Ultrasonic imaging of the coronary arteries in open-chest humans: Evaluation of coronary atherosclerotic lesions during cardiac surgery. Circulation 1982;66:1034–1044.
18. McPherson DD, Armstrong M, Rose E, et al: High-frequency epicardial echocardiography for coronary artery evaluation: In vitro and in vivo validation of arterial lumen and wall thickness measurements. J Am Coll Cardiol 1986;8:600–606.
19. McPherson DD, Hiratzka LF, Lamberth WC, et al: Delineation of the extent of coronary

atherosclerosis by high-frequency epicardial echocardiography. N Engl J Med 1987;*316*:304–309.

20. Pandian NG, Kreis A, Brockway B, Isner JM, Sacharoff A, Boleza E: Ultrasound angioscopy: Real-time, two-dimensional, intraluminal ultrasound imaging of blood vessels. Am J Cardiol 1988;*62*:493–494.

21. Gussenhoven WJ, Essed CE, Lancee CT, et al: Arterial wall characteristics determined by intravascular ultrasound imaging: An in vitro study. J Am Coll Cardiol 1989;*14*:947–952.

22. Meyer CR, Chiang EH, Fechner KP, Fitting DW, Williams DM, Buda AJ: Feasibility of high-resolution, intravascular ultrasonic imaging catheters. Radiology 1988;*168*:113–116.

23. Yock PG, Linker DT, Thaplyal HV, et al: Real-time, two-dimensional catheter ultrasound: A new technique for high resolution intravascular imaging (abstr). J Am Coll Cardiol 1988;*2*:130A.

24. Hodgson J, Eberle M, Savakus A: Validation of a new real-time percutaneous intravascular ultrasound imaging catheter (abstr). Circulation 1988;*168*:727–731.

25. Mallery JA, Tobis JM, Gessert J, et al: Evaluation of an intravascular ultrasound imaging catheter in porcine peripheral and coronary arteries in vivo. Circulation 1988;*78*:11–21.

26. Pandian N, Kreis A, Desnoyers M, et al: In vivo ultrasound angioscopy in humans and animals: Intraluminal imaging of blood vessels using a new catheter-based high resolution ultrasound probe. Circulation 1988;*78*:II–22.

27. Isner JM, Rosenfield K, Losordo DW, et al: Percutaneous intravascular US as adjunct to catheter-based interventions: Preliminary experience in patients with peripheral vascular disease. Radiology 1990;*175*:61–70.

28. Hodgson JM, Graham SP, Savakus AD, et al: Clinical percutaneous imaging of coronary anatomy using an over-the-wire ultrasound catheter system. Int J Cardiac Imaging 1989;*4*:187–193.

29. Tobis J, Mallery J, Gessert J, et al: Intravascular ultrasound visualization before and after balloon angioplasty (abstr). Circulation 1988;*78*:II–84.

30. Graham S, Brands D, Savakus A, Hodgson J: Utility of an intravascular ultrasound imaging device for arterial wall definition and atherectomy guidance (abstr). J Am Coll Cardiol 1989;*13*:222A.

31. Rutherford RB, Flanigan DP, Guptka SK, et al: Suggested standards for reports dealing with lower extremity ischemia. J Vasc Surg 1986;*4*:80–94.

32. Isner JM, Rosenfield K, Pieczek A, et al: Clinical experience with intravascular ultrasound as adjunct to percutaneous recanalization in 101 consecutive patients. J Am Coll Cardiol 1991;*17*:125A.

33. Palmax JC, Richter G, Noeldge G, et al: Intraluminal stents in atherosclerotic iliac artery stenosis: Preliminary report of a multicenter study. Radiology 1988;*168*:727–731.

34. Chokshi SK, Meyers S, Abi-Mansour P: Percutaneous transluminal coronary angioplasty: Ten years experience. Prog Cardiovasc Dis 1987;*30*:147–210.

35. Isner JM, Donaldson RF, Fortin AH, Tischler A, Clarke RH: Attenuation of the media in coronary arteries in advanced atherosclerosis. Am J Cardiol 1986;*58*:937–939.

36. Rosenfield K, Voelker W, Losordo DW, et al: Assessment of coronary arterial stenoses post-intervention by quantitative angiography versus intracoronary ultrasound in 13 patients undergoing balloon and/or laser coronary angioplasty (abstr). J Am Coll Cardiol 1991;*17*:46A.

37. Webster WW: Catheter for removing arteriosclerotic plaque. United States patent 4,576,177 (Issued March 18, 1986).

38. Ramee SR, White CJ, Collins TJ, Mesa JE, Murgo JP: Percutaneous angioscopy during coronary angioplasty using a steerable microangioscope. J Am Coll Cardiol 1991;*17*:100–105.

39. Lee G, Ikeda RM, Stobbe D, et al: Laser irradiation of human atherosclerotic obstructive disease: Simultaneous visualization and vaporization achieved by a dual fiberoptic catheter. Am Heart J 1983;*105*:163–164.

40. Leon MB, Almagor Y, Bartorelli AL, et al: Fluorescence-guided laser-assisted balloon angioplasty in patients with femoropopliteal occlusions. Circulation 1990;*81*:143–155.

41. Mallery J, Gregory K, Morcos NC, Griffith J, Henry W: Evaluation of ultrasound balloon dilatation imaging catheter (abstr). Circulation 1987;*76*:IV–371.

42. Yock PG, Fitzgerald PJ, Jang Y-T, et al: Initial trials of a combined ultrasound imaging/mechanical atherectomy catheter. J Am Coll Cardiol 1990;*15*:105A.

43. Hodgson JMcB, Cacchione JG, Berry J, Savakus A, Eberle M: Combined intracoronary ultrasound imaging and angioplasty catheter: Initial in-vivo studies (abstr). Circulation 1990;*82*:III–676.

44. Isner JM, Rosenfield K, Losordo DW, et al: Combination balloon-ultrasound imaging catheter for percutaneous transluminal angioplasty validation of imaging, analysis of recoil, and identification of plaque fracture. Circulation 1991;*84*:739–754.

45. Crowley RJ, Couvillon LA, Abele JE: Acoustic imaging catheter and the like. United States Patent 4,951,677 (Issued August 28, 1990).

46. Hodgson J, Eberle M, Savakus A: Validation of a new real-time percutaneous intravascular ultrasound imaging catheter (abstr). Circulation 1988;*178*:II–21.

47. Nissen SE, Grines CL, Gurley JC, et al: Application of a new phased-array ultrasound imaging catheter in the assessment of vascular dimensions. In vivo comparison to cineangiography. Circulation 1990;*81*:660–666.

48. Davidson CJ, Sheikh KH, Harrison JK, et al: Intravascular ultrasonography versus digital subtraction angiography: A human in vivo comparison of vessel size and morphology. J Am Coll Cardiol 1990;*16*:633–636.

49. Gurley JC, Nissen SE, Grines CL, Booth DC, Fischer C, DeMaria AN: Comparison of intravascular ultrasound and angiography following percutaneous transluminal coronary angioplasty (abstr). Circulation 1990;*82*:III–72.

50. Waller BF: Pathology of new interventions used in the treatment of coronary heart disease. Curr Prob Cardiol 1986;*11*:666–760.

51. Liu MW, Roubin GS, King SB III: Restenosis after coronary angioplasty: Potential biologic determinants and role of intimal hyperplasia. Circulation 1989;*79*:1374–1387.

52. Sanders M: Angiographic changes thirty minutes following percutaneous transluminal coronary angioplasty. Angiology 1985;*36*:419–424.

53. Powelson S, Roubin GS, Whitworth H, Gruentzig AR: Incidence of early restenosis after successful percutaneous transluminal coronary angioplasty (PTCA) (abstr). J Am Coll Cardiol 1987;*9*:1–7.

54. Nobuyoshi M, Kimura T, Nosaka H, et al: Restenosis after successful percutaneous transluminal coronary angioplasty: Serial angiographic follow-up of 229 patients. J Am Coll Cardiol 1988;*12*:616–623.

55. Hjemdahl-Monsen CE, Ambrose JA, Borrico S, et al: Angiographic patterns of balloon inflation during percutaneous transluminal coronary angioplasty: Role of pressure-diameter curves in studying distensibility and elasticity of the stenotic lesion and the mechanism of dilation. J Am Coll Cardiol 1990;*16*:569–575.

56. Rensing BJ, Hermans WRM, Beatt KJ, et al: Quantitative angiographic assessment of elastic recoil after percutaneous transluminal coronary angioplasty. Am J Cardiol 1990;*66*:1039–1044.

57. Lehmann KG, Feuer JM, Kumamoto KS, Le Ha M: Elastic recoil following coronary angioplasty: Magnitude and contributory factors (abstr). Circulation 1990;*82*:III–313.

58. Rensing BJ, Hermans WR, Strauss BH, Serruys PW: Regional differences in elastic recoil after percutaneous transluminal coronary angioplasty. A quantitative angiographic study. J Am Coll Cardiol 1991;*17*:34B–38B.

59. Isner JM, Rosenfield K, Mosseri M, et al: How reliable are images obtained by intravascular ultrasound for making decisions during percutaneous interventions? Experience with intravascular ultrasound employed in lieu of contrast angiography to guide peripheral balloon angioplasty in 16 patients (abstr). Circulation 1990;*82*:III–440.

60. Tobis JM, Mallery JA, Gessert J, et al: Intravascular ultrasound cross-sectional arterial imaging before and after balloon angioplasty in vitro. Circulation 1989;*80*:873–882.

61. Spears JR, Sandor T, Baim DS, Paulin S: The minimum error in estimating coronary luminal cross-sectional area from cineangiographic diameter measurements. Cathet Cardiovasc Diagn 1983;*9*:119–128.

62. Jain A, Demer LL, Raizner AE, Hartley CJ, Lewis JM, Roberts R: In vivo assessment of vascular dilatation during percutaneous transluminal coronary angioplasty. Am J Cardiol 1987;*60*:988–992.

63. Losordo DW, Rosenfield K, Ramaswamy K, Harding M, Pieczek A, Isner JM: How does angioplasty work? Intravascular ultrasound assessment of 30 consecutive patients demonstrating that angiographic evidence of luminal patency is the consistent result of plaque fractures and dissections (abstr). Circulation 1990;*82*:III–338.

64. Kahn JK, Rutherford BD, McConahay DR, Hartzler GO: Inflation pressure requirements during coronary angioplasty. Cathet Cardiovasc Diag 1990;*21*:144–147.

65. Kleiman NS, Raizner AE, Roberts R: Percutaneous transluminal coronary angioplasty: Is what we see what we get? J Am Coll Cardiol 1990;*16*:576–577.

66. DeJesus ST, Rosenfield KR, Gal D, et al: Three-dimensional reconstruction of vascular lumen from images recorded during percutaneous two-dimensional intravascular ultrasound. Clin Res 1989;*37*:838A.

67. Kitney RI, Moura L, Straughan K: 3-D visualization of arterial structures using ultrasound and Voxel modelling. Int J Cardiac Imaging 1989;*4*:177–185.

68. Rosenfield K, Losordo DW, Ramaswamy K, et al: Three-dimensional reconstruction of human coronary and peripheral arteries from images recorded during two-dimensional intravascular ultrasound examination. Circulation (in press).

69. Rosenfield K, Losordo DW, Majzoubi D, Harding M, Pieczek A, Isner JM: 3-Dimensional reconstruction of coronary and peripheral vessels from 2-D IVUS images: Determination of optimal image acquisition rate during timed pullback (abstr). J Am Coll Cardiol 1991;*17*:262A.

70. Rosenfield K, Harding M, Pieczek A, et al: 3-dimensional reconstruction of balloon dilated coronary, renal, and femoropopliteal arteries from 2-D intravascular ultrasound images: Analysis of longitudinal sagittal versus cylindrical views. J Am Coll Cardiol 1991;*17*:234A.

71. Rosenfield K, Losordo DW, Palefski P, Langevin RE, Razvi S, Isner JM: On-line 3-D

reconstruction of 2-D intravascular ultrasound images during balloon angioplasty: Clinical application in patients undergoing percutaneous balloon angioplasty. J Am Coll Cardiol 1991;*17*:156A.

72. Raya SP, Udupa JK, Barrett WA: A PC-based 3D imaging system: Algorithms, software, and hardware considerations. Comput Med Imaging Graph 1990;*14*:353–370.

73. Raya SP? SOFTVU—a software package for multidimensional medical image analysis. Proc SPIE, Medical Imaging IV 1990;*1232*:152–156.

74. Raya SP: Low-level segmentation of 3D magnetic resonance brain images—a rule-based system. IEEE Trans Med Imag 1990;*9*:327–337.

75. Tobis J, Smolin M, Mallery J, et al: Laser-assisted thermal angioplasty in human peripheral artery occlusions: Mechanism of recanalization. J Am Coll Cardiol 1989;*13*:1547–1554.

76. Isner JM, Donaldson RF, Funai JT, et al: Factors contributing to perforations resulting from laser coronary angioplasty. Observations in an intact human post-mortem model of intra-operative laser coronary angioplasty. Circulation 1985;*72*:II–191–199.

77. Melchior JP, Meir B, Urban P, et al: Percutaneous transluminal coronary angioplasty for chronic total arterial occlusion. Am J Cardiol 1987;*59*:535–538.

78. Chokshi SK, Hogan J, Desai V, et al: Intravascular ultrasound assessment of implanted endovascular stents (abstr). J Am Coll Cardiol 1990;*15*:29A.

79. Isner JM, Rosenfield K, Losordo DW, Pieczek A: Intravascular ultrasound: Potential for optimizing mechanical solutions to restenosis. *In* Serruys PW, Strauss S, King S, eds: Restenosis. The Netherlands, Kluwer Academic Publishers, (in press).

80. Siegel RJ, Chae JS, Forrestr JS, Ruiz CE: Angiography, angioscopy, and ultrasound imaging before and after percutaneous balloon angioplasty. Am Heart J 1990;*120*:1086–1090.

81. Yock PG, Linker DT: Intravascular ultrasound. Looking below the surface of vascular disease. Circulation 1990;*81*:1715–1718.

22

THE USE OF ANGIOSCOPY IN THE SAPHENOUS VEIN BYPASS GRAFT

WILLIAM H. PEARCE, B. TIMOTHY BAXTER, CAROL COX ALMGREN, WILLIAM R. FLINN, WALTER J. McCARTHY, and JAMES S. T. YAO

Angioscopy is playing an increasingly important role in the operative management of patients with lower extremity ischemia. Since its introduction, angioscopy has been shown to be a useful adjunct in a variety of vascular surgical procedures including thrombectomies and femoral distal bypasses. Angioscopy affords direct visual inspection of the technical adequacy of each of these procedures. Thus, the role of angioscopy in the performance of the in situ bypass is only a natural extension of its utility.[1,2] For the first time since the original description of the in situ bypass by Hall in 1962,[3,4] angioscopy allows direct visualization of the venous valvulotomy. Hall described direct venous valve excision through multiple transverse venomities. This method of valve lysis was rapidly abandoned because of the tedious nature and length of the procedure. Since that time, a variety of instruments have been developed for transluminal retrograde valve disruption.[5] In each of these techniques, the valve leaflets are closed with retrograde pressure. Based on the belief that the valve leaf will unfold with the retrograde pressure, valve leaflets are torn blindly. Unfortunately complete valve lysis may not occur. With angioscopy, this process is closely monitored for adjacent vein-wall damage.[6,7] This chapter will review the use of angioscopy in the in situ vein bypass and discuss the advantages and disadvantages of this method of valve disruption.

EQUIPMENT

Angioscopes, cameras, monitors, and other video components are now available from a number of different manufacturers. The only equipment specific to the in situ vein bypass is a small diameter angioscope (1.5 mm) and a long flexible valvulotome. A pump-driven irrigation system is also required to provide retrograde perfusion and visualization. Unfortunately, these pumps are volume and not pressure regulated and may generate excessively high intraluminal pressures in isolated vein segment. Without side branches for decompression, pressure will rise. A minimal volume of irrigation fluid should be used to prevent overdistention of the vein. The irrigating solution is heparinized normal saline (heparin 2000 U/L). The valvulotome is 100 cm, with a detachable cutting blade (2.5 mm). This allows the instrument to be passed safely from below the blunted tip. The cutting blade is then replaced for valve incision.

OPERATIVE TECHNIQUE

Incision of the venous valves with the aid of the angioscope is performed following routine exposure of the saphenous vein, femoral vessels, and recipient popliteal/tibial vessels. The proximal venous valves are incised under direct vision. The angioscope and irrigating system are introduced either through the cut end of the saphenous vein or through large side branches. In Figure 22–1, the angioscope and irrigating system are introduced through the open end of the saphenous vein with an encircling vessel loop. Occasionally, it is difficult to maintain a water seal with the vessel loop alone and may require additional digital pressure. In Figure 22–2, the proximal anastomosis is completed, preserving several large side branches. One branch is for the introduction of the irrigation system, while the second is used for the angioscope.

Once the angioscope is inserted, the vein is gently distended. The long flexible valvulotome is inserted into the distal cut end of the vein and passed proximally into the visual field of the angioscope (Figs. 22–3a and 22–3b). With a small-diameter vein, a more proximal side branch is used to insert the cutting instrument. With gentle irrigation, blood entering from tributaries is removed and the valve leaflets and the cutting instrument can be seen. The cutting instrument is placed at the leading edge of the closed valve and the valve leaflet incised (Figs. 22–3c and 22–3d). Frequently the valve mechanism is adjacent to a side branch. With the angioscope, it is apparent how vein injury may occur

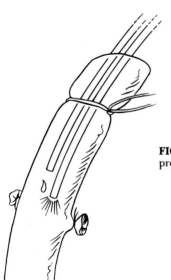

FIGURE 22–1. The angioscope and irrigation system are inserted in the proximal saphenous vein. An encircling vessel loop maintains a water seal.

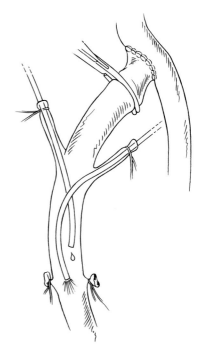

FIGURE 22–2. Angioscope and irrigating catheter are inserted via a large proximal branch of the saphenous vein.

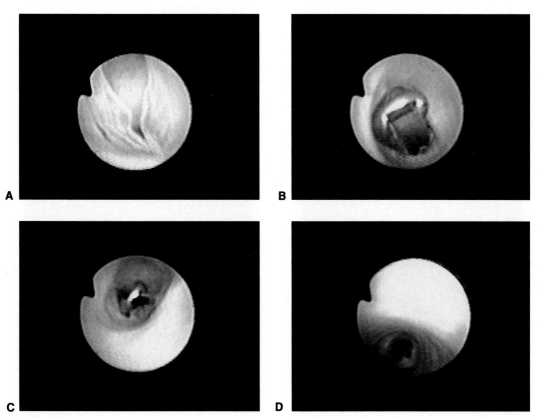

FIGURE 22–3. View through the angioscope. *A*, Partially closed valve. *B*, Valvulotome above valve. *C*, Valve incision. *D*, Completed valvulotomy.

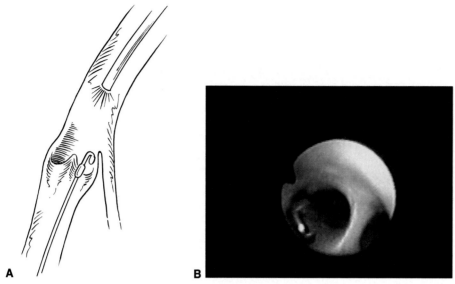

FIGURE 22–4. *A*, Frequently, a tributary of the saphenous vein enters just proximal to a venous valve. Care must be taken not to inadvertently enter this side branch. *B*, View of a tributary through the angioscope.

during the valvulotomy (Fig. 22–4). The cutting edge of the valvulotome will inadvertently lodge in the orifice of a tributary. With the angioscope it is possible to redirect the valvulotome for accurate valve incision. Once both valve leaflets have been cut, the valve mechanism is irrigated to confirm free flow.

Angioscopy also allows the identification of partially disrupted valves, sclerotic valve leaflets, and arteriovenous communications. Large venous tributaries are identified by either passing the angioscope into their lumens (no

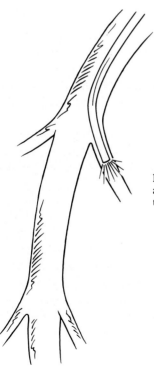

FIGURE 22–5. Large arteriovenous fistulae are identified by passing the angioscope into its lumen. The light from the angioscope may be seen through the skin and may guide dissection.

valvulotomy) or by placing the cutting instrument into their orifice. The light of the angioscope directs the dissection (Fig. 22–5). This technique is particularly useful when a long skin incision is not used to expose the vein. Instead, several small skin incisions are made to ligated arteriovenous fistulae.

The angioscope and valvulotome are passed down the vein, sequentially disrupting each valve mechanism encountered. Once all of the valvulotomies have been completed, the angioscope is withdrawn, checking each valve for function. The proximal and distal anastomoses are completed in a standard fashion.

At the completion of the procedure, angioscopy and arteriography are performed to detect any technical flaws of the distal anastomosis. Using a side branch or a catheter introducer, the angioscope and irrigating system are placed back into the vein. With proximal arterial occlusion, the vein graft is cleared of blood. Missed arteriovenous fistulae are identified and ligated. The distal anastomosis is inspected for large intimal flaps and stenoses. The angioscope is removed and a completion arteriogram is performed.

COMMENTS

The role of angioscopy in the in situ vein bypass is evolving. Presently, it is difficult to advocate the routine use of angioscopy to the experienced surgeon who has had excellent results with other techniques. However, the greatest benefit of angioscopy is the ability to visually confirm complete valve lysis. With other techniques, incomplete valvulotomy and unrecognized vein-wall trauma may occur. In a prospective study of 250 in situ bypasses, Bandyk and colleagues identified 21 early graft lesions with surveillance duplex scanning which were either retained valve leaflets, residual arteriovenous fistula, or anastomotic stenosis.[8] Furthermore, Miller et al. performed routine angioscopy following infrainguinal bypasses and found a 17 per cent incidence of retained valve leaflets and a 60 per cent incidence of residual arteriovenous fistula.[9] These partially torn valves may create turbulent blood flow and may be the site of later vein-graft stenosis.[10,11] In our own experience, angioscopy detected mid–vein-graft abnormalities in only 4 per cent of patients, all of which were unrelated to an incomplete valvulotomy. The lesions identified were sclerotic vein segments.[12] Similar results have been noted by Mehigan,[6] with one functional valve leaflet in 55 patients and 3 patent side branches.

Angioscopy offers an additional means to assess the technical adequacy of the distal anastomosis. Completion intraoperative arteriography has been the "gold standard" for evaluating the distal anastomosis and runoff vessels following lower extremity bypass. With the introduction of angioscopy, the present issue is whether this new technology offers a great enough advantage over intraoperative angiography to justify its use. In a prospective study comparing angiography with angioscopy, Baxter et al. found that completion arteriography was specific (95 per cent) but not sensitive (67 per cent) when compared with angioscopy in detecting technical problems at the distal anastomosis.[12] In 10 per cent of patients, angioscopy revealed technical problems that required an unanticipated alteration in the surgical procedure. While angioscopy appears to be useful in evaluation of the graft and the distal anastomosis, it is of no value in defining the distal anatomy. Thus completion arteriography remain essential.[12,13]

With angioscopy, this operation may be performed without a long leg incision to expose the entire vein. Several reports have demonstrated the high complication rate associated with this long incision.[14] Since it is possible to identify the major side branches with the angioscope, only small cut-downs are required for ligation. However, the below the knee incision often requires mobilization for peroneals and anterior tibial bypasses.

Despite these advantages, the angioscope may, theoretically, produce more endothelial cell damage than other methods. Therefore, it is critically important that the smallest size angioscope be used and that high distending pressures be avoided. In a small-diameter vein, this technique should probably be avoided. In addition, there is concern for fluid overload with high-flow irrigation systems. In our experience and that of others, fluid volume in excess of 1000 cc is rare for an in situ bypass. The amount of fluid usually infused is less than 500 cc, and much is lost through the open distal vein. Since this technique is relatively new, there are no long-term prospective randomized studies to clearly define the benefit or lack of benefit of this new technology. As with other new technologies, the value of the angioscope in the in situ bypass must be critically reviewed. However, preliminary reports suggest a potential benefit for its use.

ACKNOWLEDGMENT: This work was supported in part by the Alyce F. Salerno Foundation.

REFERENCES

1. Matsumoto T, Hashizume M, Yang Y, et al: Direct vision valvulotomy in in-situ venous bypass. Surg Gynecol Obstet 1987;*165*:362–364.
2. Mehigan JT, Schell WW: Angioscopic control of in-situ saphenous vein arterial bypass. *In* Moore WS, Ahn SS, eds: Endovascular Surgery. Philadelphia, WB Saunders Co, 1989;82–86.
3. Hall KV: The great saphenous vein used in-situ as an arterial shunt after extirpation of the vein. Surgery 1962;*51*:452.
4. Skagseth E, Hall KV: In-situ vein bypass. Scand J Thorac Cardiovasc Surg 1973;*7*:53.
5. Leather RP, Shah DM, Corson JP, Karmody AM: Instructional evolution of the valve incision method of in situ saphenous vein bypass. J Vasc Surg 1984;*1*:113.
6. Mehigan JT, Olcott C: Video angioscopy as an alternative to intraoperative arteriography. Am J Surg 1986;*152*:139–145.
7. Kalman PG, Sniderman KW: Salvage of in situ femoropopliteal and femorotibial saphenous vein bypass with interventional radiology. J Vasc Surg 1988;7:429–432.
8. Bandyk DF, Schmitt DD, Seabrook GR, et al: Monitoring functional patency of in situ saphenous vein bypasses: The impact of a surveillance protocol and elective revision. J Vasc Surg 1989;9:286–296.
9. Miller A, Campbell DR, Gibbons GW, et al: Routine intraoperative angioscopy in lower extremity revascularization. Arch Surg 1989;*124*:604–608.
10. Fogle MA, Whittemore AD, Couch NP, Mannick JA: A comparison of in situ and reversed saphenous vein grafts for infrainguinal reconstruction. J Vasc Surg 1987;*5*:46–52.
11. Lewine AW, Bandyk DF, Bonier PH, Towne JB: Lessons learned in adopting the in situ saphenous vein bypass. J Vasc Surg 1985;2:145–153.
12. Baxter TB, Rizzo RJ, Flinn WR, et al: A comparative study of interoperative angioscopy and completion arteriography following femorodistal bypass. Arch Surg 1990;*125*:997–1002.
13. White GH, White RA, Kopchok GE, et al: Intraoperative video angioscopy compared with arteriography during peripheral vascular operations. J Vasc Surg 1987;*6*:488–495.
14. Schwartz ME, Harrington EB, Schanzer H: Wound complications after in-situ bypass. J Vasc Surg 1988;7:802–807.

23

A COMPARATIVE STUDY OF ANGIOSCOPY AND COMPLETION ARTERIOGRAPHY AFTER INFRAINGUINAL BYPASS

WILLIAM R. FLINN, MICHAEL B. SILVA, Jr., B. TIMOTHY BAXTER, and ROBERT J. RIZZO

Infrainguinal bypass grafting is one of the most frequently performed vascular reconstructive procedures, but still remains challenging for all vascular surgeons. These procedures involve a variety of anatomic configurations including the classic femoropopliteal bypass (above and below the knee), as well as bypass to tibial and peroneal vessels, and vessels of the pedal arch. Bypass traditionally has originated at the femoral artery, but recent success has been achieved with bypass from the popliteal to distal vessels[1] or even tibial-tibial bypass.[2] While infrainguinal bypass may be performed with a prosthetic graft, the inferior patency rates of these materials below the knee[3] have led most surgeons to employ the preferential or exclusive use of autogenous vein for infrapopliteal bypass. Autogenous vein grafting also has considerable anatomic variability including the standard reversed saphenous vein (RSV), the in situ saphenous vein (ISSV), the nonreversed or "orthograde" saphenous vein, and the use of lesser saphenous, cephalic, or other upper extremity veins. Additionally, direct composite grafts and composite-sequential bypasses have been used successfully for lower limb revascularization.

This variety of reconstructive options provides a continued technical challenge that routinely includes arterial anatomoses to 1.5- to 2.0-mm vessels (some of which are significantly diseased themselves) and dissection deep within the musculature of the calf. The fate of the reconstructive procedure may also be compromised by atherosclerotic disease of the distal, or "runoff" vessels, or by a relatively hypercoagulable state in the host coagulation system. This myriad of technical and host variables seen in infrainguinal bypass grafting in many ways explains why vascular surgery has evolved as a separate specialty.

Technical defects are recognized as one of the most significant factors to threaten early graft patency following infrainguinal bypass, and graft thrombosis due to technical problems alone has been reported in 14 to 49 per cent of cases.[4–9] Typically, technical problems have included:

1. Anastomotic stenosis.
2. Distal intimal flaps in the host artery.
3. Intraluminal thrombus or platelet aggregates.
4. Kinking or errant tunnelling of the graft.
5. Inadequate valve lysis in ISSV or nonreversed vein grafts.

Vascular surgeons have rigorously pursued techniques for the detection of these technical problems during the original surgical procedure where identification and correction would presumably avoid early graft thrombosis. Intraoperative completion arteriography has been the most universally applied technique for postprocedural evaluation, becoming an almost routine part of infrainguinal bypass. Nevertheless, concerns have existed about its accuracy and risks including contrast and radiation exposure. Other techniques have included the use of electromagnetic flowmeter measurements,[10–13] B-mode ultrasonography,[14] and pulsed Doppler spectral analysis.[15,16] Uncertainty about the impact of these techniques upon operative decision-making, and their perceived technological complexities has led to a less-than-universal acceptance.

Intraoperative angioscopy has been the most dramatic recent addition to the techniques available for immediate evaluation of an infrainguinal bypass procedure. Vollmar and Junghanns[17] first reported endoscopic visualization of the arterial lumen after a bypass procedure, and the more contemporary report of Towne and Bernhardt[18] indicated the utility of this technique, but called attention to the shortcomings of available instrumentation at the time of their report in 1977. Since that time, the miniaturization of fiberoptic and video camera technology has allowed the production of angioscopes from 0.85 to 3.00 mm, small enough in diameter to use in most distal grafts. Additionally, direct coupling to a video camera has allowed viewing of the high-resolution color image without compromising the sterile field. These developments, and the expanding experience with angioscopy after infrainguinal bypass, have led some investigators to suggest that this technique may replace the use of intraoperative arteriography for most patients.[19–21]

The present section is a summary of our continued experience in the Division of Vascular Surgery at Northwestern University McGaw Medical Center with the prospective use of both completion arteriography and intraoperative angioscopy following infrainguinal bypass grafting. This review will focus particularly upon the detection of technical problems which impact surgical management and may threaten the early patency of these grafts.

EVALUATION OF FACTORS COMPROMISING EARLY GRAFT FUNCTION

While the need for some form of evaluation of the technical adequacy of each distal bypass is self-evident, the likelihood for *technical failure* differs considerably depending on the precise anatomic configuration of the reconstructive procedure and the conduit employed. Thus the impact of the method of technical assessment—arteriography or angioscopy—may vary considerably for different reconstructive procedures, and our expectations about either technique for graft evaluation are logically tempered by this realization.

Prosthetic Grafts

Infrainguinal bypass with a prosthetic graft such as polytetrafluoroethylene (PTFE) is really no more than an inert conduit between the donor vessel (usually the common femoral artery) and the recipient vessel. Thus one would not expect to discover *intrinsic* abnormalities along the course of the conduit after placement. The technical factors influencing early patency of a PTFE graft would logically be expected to be the anastomoses; particularly the distal anastomosis when grafts are performed to infragenicular vessels where the size and compliance mismatch between recipient artery and graft are the greatest. Few prosthetic grafts should ever fail due to technical problems at the proximal anastomosis, since the precise site may be chosen on the best area of the artery without regard to graft-length considerations. Thus the primary area of interest for the detection of *technical* problems after prosthetic distal bypass would be the distal anastomosis, which is addressed routinely and effectively by both completion arteriography and angioscopy.

The status of the arterial anatomy beyond the distal anastomosis may also significantly effect the early patency of a prosthetic distal bypass.[22] While this is obviously not a remediable technical problem, it may influence the use of postoperative antithrombotic therapy. In this regard, completion arteriography will give more precise anatomic detail about the runoff than will angioscopy.

There is inevitable historic bias that misadventures of tunnelling also cause early graft occlusion. Obviously, placement of a prosthetic bypass or a vein graft other than ISSV involves creation of a tunnel for the entire graft, and most favor the standard deep anatomic pathway, basically along the course of the native vessels. Nevertheless, a variety of lateral and subcutaneous routes have been employed routinely by experienced surgeons without clear demonstration that these alternative routes produce inevitable failure. While this theoretic possibility exists, it is probably unnecessary to expect that our techniques for detection of technical problems will routinely warn us of minor variations in tunnelling.

Autogenous Saphenous Vein Grafts

When a vein graft is used for infrainguinal bypass, the *entire conduit* is a potential source for technical problems. Side-branch ligation may produce strictures, especially in the smaller portions of the vein. When RSV is used, even the proximal anastomosis may produce technical problems, since this is always smallest portion of the vein. Similarly, it may be more technically challenging to create anastomosis of the larger end of the vein to a smaller distal artery, especially the infragenicular arteries.

The use of the ISSV, while increasing the utilization of autogenous vein in most surgeons' experience, also provides unique technical challenges. In these cases, the interior of the graft must be instrumented to render vein valves incompetent. This necessary instrumentation allows the potential for unsuccessful valve lysis as well as for endothelial or vein-wall damage by the instrument itself. Additionally, the vein may have been subject to previous phlebitis, with phlebosclerosis and recanalization leaving unsuitable segments within the lumen. Add to these factors the need to successfully detect and ligate residual vein-branch arteriovenous communications after arterialization.

It is clear that the technique chosen for evaluation of the technical conduct of vein bypass must be more comprehensive than that for prosthetic grafts. Completion arteriography often requires multiple exposures to obtain the necessary anatomic information, and small-diameter veins have even smaller suspicious "shadows" making interpretation challenging. Angioscopy with its direct real-time three-dimensional view of the interior of the body of the graft, where most problems occur, offers the clear advantage in these grafts; especially where decisions must be made regarding reexploration or replacement of graft segments. Additionally, it has been observed that the distal arterial runoff anatomy is less likely to compromise early patency of an autogenous graft,[23,24] so that the advantage of completion artiography in that regard is moot.

Complex Distal Revascularizations

Composite grafts using segments of vein and prosthesis or vein and vein or composite sequential bypass with proximal PTFE and a jump graft of vein are used less frequently for distal bypass. These procedures introduce at least one, and often, two or more additional anastomoses between their component parts that require technical evaluation. Frequently, these cases are also reoperative procedures to more distal infrapopliteal vessels, providing additional technical challenge. Generally, the more complex the reconstructive procedure, the more benefit to the use of precise visualization by angioscopy, although access for passage of the scope to involved segments of the graft may itself be challenging. Further, in reoperative cases *routine* use of postoperative antithrombotic therapy may be elected and may make knowledge of distal arterial anatomy, provided by the completion arteriogram, less critical to subsequent management.

NORTHWESTERN EXPERIENCE: INTRAOPERATIVE MANAGEMENT

Completion Arteriogram

Following restoration of distal arterial perfusion through the graft and achievement of hemostasis, all patients undergo routine completion arteriography after infrainguinal bypass. Single 14 × 17 inch gridded cassettes in disposable sterile covers are placed beneath the leg to allow visualization of the anatomic area of interest. A 20-gauge angiocath is introduced into the proximal portion of the graft and, with temporary inflow occlusion, single exposures are made using the distal injection of 30 to 50 cc of contrast material. The primary areas of interest for completion arteriography in most bypass procedures are the distal anastomosis, and the anatomy of the runoff vessels into the foot. When below-knee bypass is performed, this can usually be accomplished with a single exposure. When ISSV is used, more proximal exposures are routinely necessary to identify potential intrinsic abnormalities and residual vein-branch arteriovenous communications. Few patients ever require more than two films unless reexploration or other operative manipulation is performed on the basis of the findings of the original completion arteriogram. In some of these cases, another arteriogram may be performed to assess the efficacy of the manipulation.

After the performance of completion arteriography, the operating surgeon reviewed the films and made a decision concerning the need for surgical intervention based upon the standards developed at our institution.[4] Angioscopy was then performed in each case immediately after the arteriogram as described below. In the experience described in this section, and in past experience of over 1000 completion arteriograms, we have not observed an intraoperative anaphylactic reaction to contrast material or irreversible renal dysfunction in any of our patients due solely to operative arteriography.

Angioscopy

Angioscopy was performed using fiberoptic angioscopes ranging in size from 1.4 to 2.8 mm in diameter (Olympus Corp, Lake Success, NY) (Fig. 23–1). The 1.4-mm angioscope was by far the most frequently used. Its smaller size facilitates ease of insertion into the graft and allows passage through the distal portions of smaller diameter ISSV grafts; often into the native tibial vessels below the distal anastomosis and even to the ankle level without resistance. The 2.2-mm angioscope has a steerable end, which was useful in some complex grafts or in tortuous grafts with larger side branches where the nonsteerable scope might "hang up" during passage. The angioscope was coupled to a 300-watt xenon light source and a video camera, and images were continuously monitored on high-resolution television monitors and recorded on videotape.

The angioscope was introduced into the most proximal portion of the graft that was technically feasible. This was accomplished in vein grafts by passage of the scope through a side branch left intentionally long. Proximal insertion was particularly important for ISSV grafts where it was necessary to endoscopically evaluate the interior of the *entire course* of the graft. In RSV grafts where there is no concern about valves and no instrumentation of the interior of the graft, the scope was sometimes introduced preferentially into a segment of the midgraft where graft diameter and caliber of branches were larger. Prosthetic grafts were generally 6-mm PTFE, and the size of the graft relative to the size of the angioscope was obviously of less concern. Nevertheless, introduction of the larger scopes required a small dorsal incision in the graft that subsequently required suture closure. The 1.4-mm angioscope could be introduced into the PTFE grafts by first making a puncture hole with a 16-gauge angiocath; this technique also prevented excessive leakage of the irrigation fluid around the insertion site.

The key to successful angioscopy is the maintenance of a blood-free field, since even a seemingly minute amount of blood flowing into the field significantly blurs the usually excellent clarity of the image. This was accomplished in this series by the use of a dedicated angioscopy pump (Angiopump, Olympus Corp, Lake Success, NY). Warm crystalloid irrigation solution (0.9 NS with Na heparin 2000 U/L) was infused through the angiocath which had been used for the completion arteriogram. This pump was capable of delivering either high-volume or low-volume flow rates between 10 ml/min and 400 ml/min

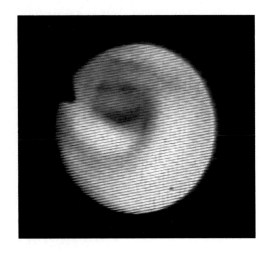

FIGURE 23–1. Angioscopic visualization of the native posterior tibial artery beyond the distal anastomosis reveals mild atheromatous disease but no significant technical abnormalities.

controlled by digital input and a bimodal foot pedal. Initial high-volume flow rates were used to "clear the field" and the low-volume rates to maintain clarity during the period of interrogation.

Following femorodistal bypass grafting, angioscopy should rarely be unsuccessful due to problems of irrigation, since surgical control of both inflow and outflow vessels has been achieved as a part of the procedure. Angioscopy was always performed with inflow occlusion of the graft proximal to the site of insertion of the scope and irrigation cannula. Variable outflow occlusion was then employed to allow maintenance of a clear field. When bypass was to a crural vessel, irrigation alone often overcame back-bleeding from the distal vessels and angioscopy could be performed without outflow manipulation. This obviously provided a much better chance of visualization of the distal vessels beyond the distal anastomosis (Fig. 23–1). When bypass was to the popliteal artery, the need for outflow occlusion was variable depending upon the luxuriance of collaterals, and was almost always necessary for above-knee femoropopliteal grafts. The need for outflow occlusion did not compromise visualization of the graft interior or the distal anastomosis, but clearly limited assessment of native arteries beyond.

Angioscopy was usually performed by passing the scope into the perianastomotic area, which was easily identifiable in the distal surgical wound by the light projecting from the tip of the scope. The field was then cleared using the irrigation fluid and the scope was passed beyond the anastomosis into the native vessel as far as possible without encountering resistance. Visual analysis and videotape recording were then performed during withdrawal of the angioscope. The perianastomotic area was visualized circumferentially with special attention to the "toe" of the graft and the transition from anastomosis to native vessel viewed end-on. These maneuvers often require rotation of the angioscope or gentle digital pressure from outside the graft to visualize the entire interior of the anastomosis. The interior of the remainder of the graft is viewed during withdrawal of the angioscope. In PTFE grafts this portion of the examination proceeded rapidly, minimizing excess irrigation. The ISSV grafts required assessment of individual valves, but identification of residual vein branches was not preferentially performed by angioscopy in our cases. Identification of persistent arteriovenous communications was performed using the completion arteriogram, and branches were ligated prior to angioscopy, again to minimize additional irrigation fluid required.

The precise volume of irrigation used in each exam was not recorded in this series. While the dedicated angioscopy pump maintains a digital readout of infusion volume, an uncertain amount of this is not delivered into the vascular space, since leakage frequently occurs around the scope or through suture holes in the graft. The majority of studies have required at least 500 ml of irrigation, and communication with the anesthesiologist managing the patient must be maintained, since this infusion occurs rapidly and is "invisible" to them. The frequently precarious cardiac status of patients with severe lower extremity arterial occlusive disease is well known, and casual intraoperative fluid administration invites postoperative cardiac decompensation.

RESULTS

This section will review our experience with the prospective comparison of completion arteriography and angioscopy in 66 cases of infrainguinal bypass grafting performed in 64 patients. This group included 30 women and 34 men whose mean age was 64 years. This group was typical for our atherosclerotic patient population; 53 per cent were hypertensive, 37 per cent had diabetes mellitus, and 72 per cent were cigarette smokers. Bypass was performed for symptoms of ischemia rest pain in 28 cases (42 per cent), for nonhealing ischemia ulceration in 12 cases (18 per cent), and for gangrene in 15 limbs (23 per cent). Ten procedures (15 per cent) were performed for debilitating claudication, and one for popliteal aneurysm.

Overall, autogenous vein was used in 35 of 66 cases (53 per cent). An ISSV graft was performed in 15 limbs, an RSV graft was used in 14 cases, a nonreversed saphenous vein graft in 2 cases, and short segments of available vein were used in 4 composite sequential bypass grafts. The remaining 31 cases had bypass with PTFE grafts. A total of 31 grafts (47 per cent) had their distal anastomosis to infragenicular vessels, including the 4 composite grafts. The remaining 35 cases had standard femoropopliteal bypass, 21 above the knee, and 14 to the popliteal artery below the knee.

Abnormal Completion Arteriograms

Intraoperative arteriograms were considered to be abnormal (and therefore an indication for reexploration of the graft) in 13 of the 66 cases (20 per cent) prior to angioscopy. These abnormal findings are listed in Table 23–1, and included seven cases with "filling defects" at or near the distal anastomosis, four vein grafts with filling defects noted in the midgraft, and distal anastomotic narrowing in two cases. Angioscopy confirmed the presence of significant morphologic abnormalities that produced the arteriographic appearance in 10 of these 13 cases. Thrombus or atheromatous debris was noted in seven cases, and perianastomotic intimal flaps in two cases (Fig. 23–2). One arteriographic filling defect was produced by platelet aggregates seen on angioscopy. Surgical correction was performed on nine of these ten defects; the platelet aggregates were small and were felt to pose no threat to early patency; the patient was treated with intravenous Dextran-40 and aspirin. Early graft thrombosis occurred in only one of these ten cases where arteriography, angioscopy, and surgical reexploration of the distal artery confirmed irremediable distal disease, and despite correction of the technical abnormality, graft failure occurred on full systemic anticoagulation.

TABLE 23–1. ANGIOSCOPIC FINDINGS IN CASES WITH ABNORMAL COMPLETION ARTERIOGRAMS

Case	Graft	Anastomosis	Findings	Angioscope
1	RSV	BK-Pop	Anast fill defect	Thrombus
2	PTFE	BK-Pop	Anast fill defect	Atherom debris
3	PTFE	AK-Pop	Anast stenosis	Confirmed
4	ISSV	Peroneal	Anast stenosis	Confirmed
5	RSV	PT	Midgraft defect	Thrombus
6	ISSV	AK-Pop	Midgraft defect	Thrombus
7	PTFE	PT	Anast fill defect	Normal
8	ISSV	AT	Midgraft defect	Normal
9	PTFE	AK-Pop	Anast fill defect	Int Flap
10	PTFE	AK-Pop	Anast fill defect	Normal
11	ISSV	Peroneal	Midgraft defect	Thrombus
12	PTFE	AK-Pop	Anast fill defect	Platelet Agg
13	PTFE	Peroneal	Anast fill defect	Atherom debris

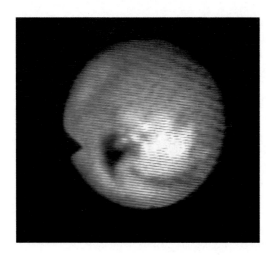

FIGURE 23–2. Angioscopy of the distal peroneal artery reveals atheromatous debris obscuring the lumen of the distal vessel. This finding clarified the appearance of a significant perianastomotic filling defect seen on completion arteriography, and surgical correction was performed.

Three grafts with abnormal completion arteriograms had no identifiable morphologic defect seen at the time of angioscopy. No reexploration was performed in these cases, and all grafts remained patent postoperatively. It should be noted that the appearance of "spasm" in the native artery (especially tibial vessels) on completion arteriography was *not* considered as a significantly abnormal arteriogram for the purpose of this study. Our early experience with angioscopy led us to disregard this finding on arteriography.

Normal Completion Arteriograms

Intraoperative arteriograms were considered by the operating surgeon to be free of significant technical problems in 53 cases (80 per cent). Subsequent angioscopy revealed major abnormalities in three grafts (5.6 per cent). All three were PTFE grafts, one above-knee femoropopliteal bypass, and two infragenicular grafts. All three cases had distal perianastomotic abnormalities on angioscopy including thrombus in one (Fig. 23–3) and intimal flaps in the two others.

Surgical reexploration confirmed these findings and correction was performed in all three cases. One infragenicular PTFE graft thrombosed postoperatively despite correction of the technical problem at the anastomosis; however, the findings in this case had been similar to the one above with irreversible distal disease and no further attempts at salvage were undertaken.

Diagnosis of Technical Defect: Impact on Early Graft Failure

Early graft thrombosis (less than 72 hours postoperatively) occurred in 5 of the 66 cases in this study (7.6 per cent), but none occluded due to identifiable technical defects. The two PTFE grafts describe in the preceding sections obviously failed due to inadequate distal runoff, although the one with an intimal flap that was only detected by angioscopy *would* have been classified as a technical failure at the time of reexploration had angioscopy not been performed. One additional graft occluded premortem in a patient with multi-system organ failure. The final two grafts (one RSV, one PTFE) that thrombosed were found to have no identifiable morphologic or anatomic cause for failure

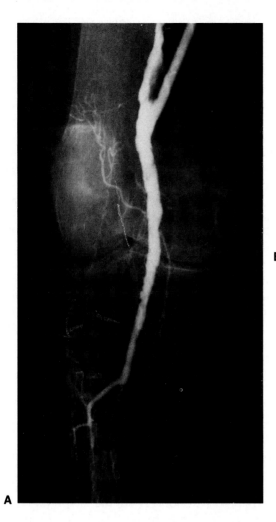

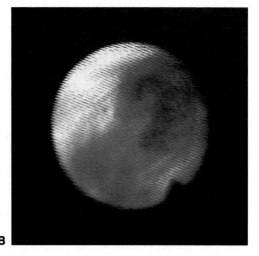

FIGURE 23–3. *A*, Completion arteriography after an above-knee femoropopliteal PTFE graft revealed significant occlusive disease in the runoff vessels, but was felt to be free of significant technical problems. *B*, Angioscopy reveals soft fresh thrombus in the popliteal artery just beyond the anastomosis which was not identified by completion arteriography. It was felt that this false-negative arteriogram might clearly have jeopardized early graft patency in this case.

at the time of reexploration. Both grafts had simple thrombectomy, and patency was maintained with systemic anticoagulant therapy.

ANALYSIS OF RESULTS

If the real-time images provided by angioscopy were used to evaluate the diagnostic accuracy of completion arteriography for the detection of technical defects following infrainguinal bypass in this study, there were three false-positive and three false-negative arteriograms. This would yield a specificity of 94 per cent and a sensitivity of 77 per cent for completion arteriography. In a logical assessment of these observations, it is useful to remember that the sensitivity of any test is basically its ability to be "positive in the presence of the disease." While a false-positive (reduced specificity) completion arteriogram may create the nuisance and frustration of an unnecessary reexploration, the *false-negative arteriogram* (reduced sensitivity) sends the patient out of the operating room with a defect which might jeopardize the patency of the graft and, potentially, the limb and life of the patient.

The angioscopic findings in this series impacted significantly upon surgical decisions in six cases (9 per cent) which is lower than the 47 per cent reported by Miller et al.,[21] the largest reported experience with angioscopy following infrainguinal bypass. The angioscopic findings in their series were predominantly uncut valve leaflets in ISSV grafts or residual vein-branch arteriovenous communications (91 of 124 findings, 73 per cent). Since intraoperative arteriograms were performed in only 13 per cent of their cases, it is uncertain what percentage of these findings would have been evident by arteriography. Additionally it should be remembered that in our experience, two patients had important surgical decisions based upon completion arteriography (i.e., decisions *not to perform reexploration*) after graft failure due solely to knowledge of the distal arterial anatomy. This component of the decision-making process would not have been available if angioscopy alone had been performed.

No graft in this series failed due to technical problems; so theoretically, the sensitivity and specificity of angioscopy was 100 per cent in this group of cases. It would, of course, be shortsighted to expect that any diagnostic test will be 100 per cent accurate, and it should be remembered that early graft occlusion did occur in 7.6 per cent of cases, a figure remarkably consistent with our previous report where only operative arteriography was used.[4] Similarly, in the report of Miller et al.,[21] early graft thrombosis occurred in 8.1 per cent of cases with routine angioscopy.

CONCLUSIONS

In 1991, the vast majority of institutions where major vascular reconstructive procedures are routinely performed have resources available for the performance of intraoperative arteriography. The equipment necessary for angioscopy is not prohibitively expensive, nor is it excessively complex to set up and operate, but it does require time and attention to detail for these procedures to be maximally effective. This is especially true concerning the day-to-day care of some of the more delicate equipment. In all but the most specialized setting, angioscopy will take more time to perform than intraoperative arteriography.

The risks of intraoperative arteriography are well known and include radiation exposure and the use of contrast material. The risks of angioscopy are less well-defined at present, but must logically include the mechanical passage of the device through a biologic conduit and into the native artery, with the potential for additional endothelial trauma. Also, this would include the volume of irrigation fluid infused. It is inconsistent to propose that the small amount of contrast used for completion arteriography would contribute to postoperative renal dysfunction and to deny that the rapid infusion of a liter of saline could be causally related to postoperative congestive heart failure or myocardial infarction. In reality, the risks of either procedure are remarkably small in comparison to the value of the information obtained, and should not discourage their routine use.

Our experience would suggest that angioscopy is most accurate for the identification and precise characterization of technical problems following infrainguinal bypass, especially intraluminal defects in autogenous grafts and in the perianastomotic area. However, only completion arteriography allows precise documentation of the distal runoff anatomy, which also may effect subsequent therapeutic decisions. It is clear that these two techniques are not mutually exclusive, but truly complementary. As the technological requirements for routine angioscopy become less demanding in routine clinical settings, this procedure will become an integral part of all infrainguinal bypass procedures.

REFERENCES

1. Veith FJ, Gupta SK, Samson RH, et al: Superficial femoral and popliteal arteries as inflow sites for distal bypass. Surgery 1981;*90*:980–990.
2. Veith FJ, Gupta SK, Ascer E, et al: Tibiotibial vein bypass grafts: A new operation for limb salvage. J Vasc Surg 1985;*2*:552–557.
3. Veith FJ, Gupta SK, Ascer E, et al: Six-year prospective multicenter randomized comparison of autologous saphenous vein and expanded polytetrafluoroethylene grafts in infrainguinal reconstructions. J Vasc Surg 1986;*3*:104–114.
4. Stept LL, Flinn WR, McCarthy WJ, et al: Technical defects as a cause of early graft failure after femorodistal bypass. Arch Surg 1987;*122*:599–604.
5. Tyson RR, Grosh JD, Reichle FA: Redo surgery for graft failure. Am J Surg 1978;*136*:165–170.
6. Whittemore AD, Clowes AW, Couch NP, et al: Secondary femoropopliteal reconstruction. Ann Surg 1981;*193*:35–42.
7. Craver JM, Ottinger LW, Darling RC, et al: Hemorrhage and thrombosis as early complications of femoropopliteal bypass grafts: Causes, treatment, and prognostic implications. Surgery 1973;*74*:839–845.
8. Mulherin JL, Allen TR, Edwards WH, et al: Management of early postoperative complications of arterial repairs. Arch Surg 1977;*112*:1371–1374.
9. Brewster DC, LaSalle AJ, Robinson JG, et al: Femoropopliteal graft failures: Clinical consequences and successes of secondary reconstructions. Arch Surg 1983;*118*:1043–1047.
10. Terry HJ, Allan JS, Taylor GW: The relationship between blood-flow and failure of femoropopliteal reconstructive arterial surgery. Br J Surg 1972;*59*:549–551.
11. Mannick JA, Jackson BT: Hemodynamics of arterial surgery in atherosclerotic limbs: I. Direct measurement of blood flow before and after vein grafts. Surgery 1966;*59*:713–720.
12. Cappelan C, Hall VK: Intraoperative blood flow measurements with electromagnetic flowmeter. Prog Surg 1969;*8*:102–123.
13. Stirnemann P, Triller J: The fate of femoropopliteal and femorodistal bypass grafts in relation to intraoperative flow measurement: An analysis of 100 consecutive reconstructions for limb salvage. Surgery 1982;*100*:38–44.
14. Sigel B, Coelho JC, Flanigan DP, et al: Detection of vascular defects during operation by imaging ultrasound. Ann Surg 1982;*196*:473–480.
15. Bandyk DF, Zierler RE, Thiele BL: Detection of technical error during arterial surgery by pulsed Doppler spectral analysis. Arch Surg 1984;*119*:421–428.
16. Bandyk DF, Cato RF, Towne JB: A low flow velocity predicts failure of femoropopliteal and femorotibial bypass grafts. Surgery 1985;*98*:799–809.
17. Vollmar JF, Junghanns K: Die Arterioskopie, eine neue Moglichkeit der intraoperativen Erfolgsbeurteilung bei rekonstruktiven Gefaßeingriffen (Farbfilm). Langenbecks Arch Klin Chir 1969;*325*:1201–1212.
18. Towne JB, Bernhard VM: Vascular endoscopy: Useful tool or interesting toy. Surgery 1977;*82*:415–419.
19. Mehigan JT, Olcott C: Video angioscopy as an alternative to intraoperative arteriography. Am J Surg 1986;*152*:139–145.
20. Miller A, Campbell DR, Gibbons GW, et al: Routine intraoperative angioscopy in lower extremity revascularization. Arch Surg 1989;*124*:604–608.
21. Miller A, Stonebridge PA, Jepson SJ, et al: Continued experience with intraoperative angioscopy for monitoring infrainguinal bypass grafting. Surgery 1991;*109*:286–293.
22. O'Mara CS, Flinn WR, Neiman HL, et al: Correlation of foot arterial anatomy with early tibial bypass patency. Surgery 1981;*89*:743–751.
23. Buchbinder D, Pasch AR, Rollins DL, et al: Results of arterial reconstruction to the foot. Arch Surg 1986;*121*:673–677,
24. Corson JD, Karmody AM, Shah DM, et al: In situ vein bypasses to distal tibial and limited outflow tracts for limb salvage. Surgery 1984;*96*:756–763.

24

ANGIOSCOPY-ASSISTED THROMBOEMBOLECTOMY

THOMAS J. FOGARTY and GEORGE D. HERMANN

BACKGROUND

Thromboembolectomy

The advent of the embolectomy balloon catheter in 1963 simplified the treatment of acute arterial occlusion by providing an expedient means to remove large amounts of soft thrombus from the arterial system.[1] At that time, the majority of clot that was removed was embolic in origin, due primarily to cardiac disorders such as mitral valve stenosis, and myocardial infarction. This clot was usually soft in consistency and was relatively easy to remove with minimal need for arterial visualization. Today, however, there is an increased incidence of clot formation of thrombotic origin. Peripheral atherosclerotic disease can create sites for adherent thrombus formation which can grow slowly for a considerable period of time before precipitating an occlusive event. Also, arterial grafts (bypass grafts as well as hemodialysis grafts) are subject to thrombosis, and can be difficult to remove completely with the simple blind technique using a standard balloon embolectomy catheter.

As a result, there are many instances today where optimal clot removal is facilitated by direct intraluminal visualization. Angioscopy is an excellent tool to assist in the thrombectomy technique, particularly in cases of adherent clot of thrombotic origin, typically found in synthetic grafts and atherosclerotic vessels.

Angioscopy

There are a variety of barriers that have prevented the widespread adoption of angioscopy by vascular surgeons. First of all, the sources of angioscopy equipment change relatively frequently. For example, Baxter Edwards, a leading manufacturer and innovator in angioscopes for the surgeons, recently decided to focus only on the coronary applications. Also, it is not uncommon for manufacturers of catheter-based systems to use the peripheral circulation as a training/proving ground for instruments for coronary applications. Once the products are approved for coronary applications, manufacturers focus on the coronary market and reduce attention to the vascular surgeon. Other players such as Boston Scientific and Vascucare have muted their enthusiasm for angioscopy for a variety of business reasons. The most prominent remaining player in angioscopy for the surgeon is Olympus, a company which manages a wide range of reusable scopes for several specialities including gastroenterology,

TABLE 24–1. TROUBLESHOOTING IMAGE ARTIFACT DURING ANGIOSCOPY

Symptom	Possible Cause	Solution
White image	Catheter tip is against vessel wall. Excessive light is reflecting back to camera.	Reorient the tip. In addition to manipulating the catheter, external palpation on the skin can reorient the tip sufficiently.
Red image	Image is obscured by blood in the visual field.	Control infusion of blood by external clamping, or occlusion balloon.
		Provide a route for the blood to escape as the infused saline irrigant displaces the blood.
		Increase the irrigation flow rate or irrigation pressure.
	Clot is adhering to the tip of the angioscope.	Remove angioscope and clean tip.
Dark image	Insufficient light for size of vessel.	Turn up light intensity at the light source.
		Decrease diameter of vessel by temporary external compression on the artery.
Blurry image	Camera is out of focus.	Adjust camera focus to sharpen the perimeter edge of the image.
		Remove angioscope and refocus on a known image (e.g., a printed word or surgical forceps)
	Moisture condensation at optical connections.	Disconnect optical connections, wipe them with a sterile cotton swab.
Black dots in image	Broken optical fibers.	Cannot be corrected. Handle the angioscope gently to prevent further deterioration.

urology, and general surgery. Newer companies such as Intramed are emerging to focus on the vascular market and there will probably be additional angioscopy manufacturers in the near future.

In addition to instability from the supply end, there are also barriers from the user end. First of all, vascular surgeons are a careful and somewhat skeptical group when it comes to new technology. Recent disappointments with laser angioplasty, for example, have left many surgeons with a particularly healthy skepticism toward new endovascular technologies. The other barrier is that an angioscope is not a therapeutic tool per se; it is an enabling tool. Therefore its utility is less obvious to the user. At first glance angioscopy doesn't appear to allow the surgeon to treat the previously untreatable patient. It merely allows the surgeon to see something that could not be seen before. But before angioscopy has clinical utility, the surgeon must decide on what exactly is being seen, and also how seeing it will translate to better patient care. Also, cost is a barrier. Reusable scopes cost in the $10,000 range, and even the less expensive, disposable angioscopes still require the same capital investment for the ancillary equipment (light source, camera, video monitor, irrigation system, portable cart) which easily runs an additional $20,000. In many states, current reimbursement policies don't have a place for angioscopy, making it even more difficult for an institution to justify the purchase price of the system. And finally, there is a learning curve associated with the use of the system. There are a variety of types of artifacts that a user will typically encounter, which if not properly identified and corrected, render the angioscope ineffective (Table 24–1).

ADVANTAGES OF ANGIOSCOPY FOR THROMBOEMBOLECTOMY

In spite of the barriers listed above, angioscopy has utility for a variety of peripheral vascular procedures,[2,3] and can be particularly useful during thromboembolectomy. For this application, angioscopy is used primarily to assess the completeness of removal of intraluminal material and has several important advantages over arteriography. First of all, angioscopy allows the surgeon to see intraarterial pathology directly. Arteriography allows the surgeon to make only an educated guess based upon the flow of contrast material as viewed from one or two side-viewing planes. This fundamental difference eliminates the uncertainty of how completely the surgeon has performed the thrombectomy and clarifies the nature of residual intraluminal material. Hazy or questionable areas on the arteriogram can be assessed definitively (e.g., as plaque, flaps, or thrombus). Also, areas that appear adequately patent from an angiographic perspective may contain latent thrombus or flaps which, if undetected, may require reoperation later.

With experience, it is possible that angioscopy can be used as an alternative to arteriography in many instances, particularly for acute arterial occlusion. Because of their emergency nature, thrombectomy procedures are performed at all hours of the day or night, at times when a radiologic technician may not be available. Angioscopy does not require the presence of a technician, as long as the operating room personnel have been familiarized with setting up the equipment.

DESCRIPTION OF ANGIOSCOPY EQUIPMENT

The primary components of an angioscopy system are described in Figure 24–1.

Angioscope

The viewing end of a typical angioscope is shown in Figure 24–2. It consists of a flexible catheter that contains a saline irrigation lumen, a fiberoptic light bundle, and a fiberoptic image bundle. At the proximal end are attachment ports that allow connection to a video monitor, light source, and a saline irrigation system. The angioscope can be either disposable (Baxter Edwards, Santa Ana, CA; Intramed, San Diego, CA) or reusable (Olympus, Lake Success,

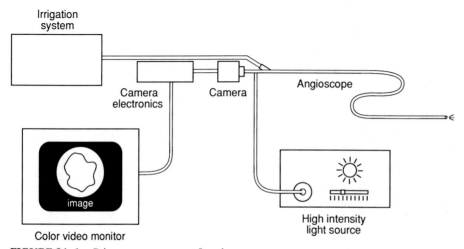

FIGURE 24–1. Primary components of angioscopy system.

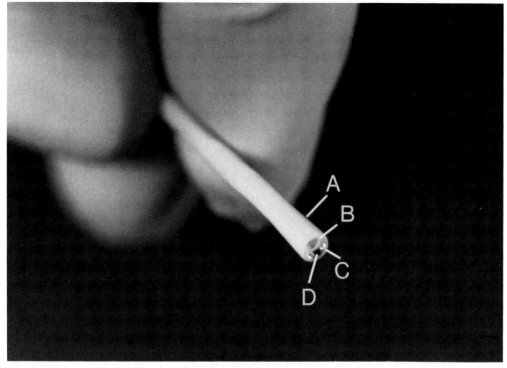

FIGURE 24–2. Viewing end of a typical angioscope. *A*, 7F catheter body. *B*, Saline irrigation port. *C*, One of two fiberoptic light bundles. *D*, Fiberoptic imaging bundle.

NY). Both styles have their advantages. Disposable angioscopes not only require less capital investment, but they also have no image degradation due to broken fibers. With multiple use, reusable angioscopes develop broken optical fibers, which manifest as black dots that obscure the image. Also, with disposable units, angioscopy can be performed on two or more successive patients because there is no "down time" during sterilization of the angioscope. On the other hand, if angioscopy is performed routinely at an institution, it may be more cost-effective to employ a reusable angioscope.

Angioscopes are also available in several sizes, from less than 1 mm to over 3 mm in diameter. As a general rule, the larger scopes have a higher resolution image. The smaller scopes are easier to maneuver in tortuous vessels and distal locations, and often contain no irrigation channel.

Camera System

The purpose of the camera system is to take the image from the proximal end of the scope and convert it to a video image for viewing on the video monitor. It receives the image from the fiberoptics and converts it to a digitized electrical signal that is delivered via a cable to the video monitor. Most angioscope manufacturers provide the camera system as part of their angioscopy system. Some manufacturers provide adaptors so that other cameras (e.g., from an arthroscopy system borrowed from the orthopedic unit) can be used with their angioscopes. This can be an appeal cost-saving maneuver for the vascular surgeon who is interested in getting started in angioscopy.

Light Source

As with the camera systems, most angioscope manufacturers provide a light source as part of their angioscopy system. It consists of a small box containing a high-intensity light bulb and a cooling fan. A flexible fiberoptic cable connects the light source to a port at the proximal end of the angioscope. It is important that the light source be sufficiently bright, especially when using the smaller scopes. A light source for one type of scope (e.g., an arthroscopy light source) may not provide sufficient light intensity for an angioscope. Flexible scopes with fiberoptics require more light than the rigid-rod lens scopes used frequently in urology and arthroscopy. Also, the larger the vessel the angioscope is placed in, the more light that is needed. For example, a scope placed in an 8-mm iliac vessel requires significantly more light than would be required in a 4-mm popliteal vessel.

Video Monitor

A color video monitor is another essential component of an angioscopy system. Early angioscope designs had eyepieces for direct viewing into the scope instead of video monitors, like the urologist's cystoscope. This viewing method usually proves cumbersome for the mobile vascular surgeon in a sterile operating room environment. Today, it is customary to view the angioscopic image on a video monitor. As with the other components mentioned above, angioscope manufacturers provide a monitor as part of their system, but other monitors can be substituted fairly easily.

Irrigation Systems

Irrigation systems are perhaps the most overlooked component of a successful angioscopy system. Whereas much of the angioscope technology was based on developments in other surgical areas (e.g., gastrointestinal endoscopy, arthroscopy, urology), the vascular system is distinctly different from these other fields because the region to be visualized is usually filled with blood, a completely opaque fluid. Irrigation systems tend to lag behind the other components in technical sophistication. This is due in part to the inability to share experience from the use of scopes in other anatomical systems (e.g., urology, gastroenterology). For an angioscopy system to be effective, the angioscopist must have a properly functioning irrigation system and understand the strengths and limitations of the various systems available. There are three types of irrigation systems that are currently being used today (Fig. 24–3).

The first type is a saline bag with a line attached to the irrigation port on the angioscope. The bag may be suspended from a pole to provide a constant pressure source. As an alternative, the bag can be squeezed by an assistant or by a pressurized blood pressure cuff. With this setup, irrigation pressures are low and can be insufficient to clear the visual field of blood. Also, an additional hand is required to initiate and terminate the flow of saline.

An alternative irrigation system that is becoming increasingly popular is a roller pump. More sophisticated than a saline bag, the roller pump is activated by a foot switch, which eliminates the need for coordinating the irrigation flow via an assistant. The volume flow rate can also be set to the desired level. In addition, the volume of fluid infused into the patient can be monitored automatically. When the foot pedal is depressed, the pump starts pumping at

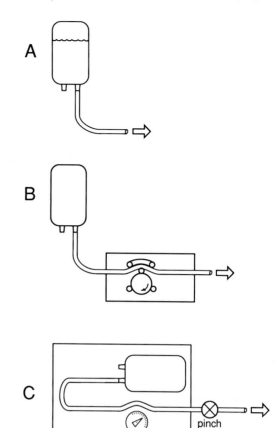

FIGURE 24–3. Styles of irrigation systems. A, Simple saline bag. B, Roller pump. C, Pressurized saline with pinch valve.

a flow rate determined by the user. Total volume infused can be tallied on a digital readout. Other features include a high- and low-flow setting. Miller et al. provide an excellent description of the advantages and features of a roller pump irrigation system for angioscopy.[4]

Roller pumps are not without drawbacks, however. First of all, when the foot pedal is initially activated, there is noticeable infusion of saline at low pressure before the roller pump gets up to speed and delivers saline at sufficient pressure. This low-pressure saline is of insufficient pressure to displace the blood column in the visual field, yet it is still infused into the patient. This "ramp-up" phenomenon accounts for a cumbersome delay before the blood is cleared. It also means that extra fluid is pumped into the patient. The second and more worrisome shortcoming of roller pumps is that they are not pressure-dependent. Instead, they are volume-dependent. When the foot pedal is activated, the pump will administer saline at the prescribed flow rate regardless of the pressure encountered. In instances where there is a closed system in the blood vessel (e.g., proximal clamping with distal obstruction and no side branches), there is no place for the displaced blood to go when saline is infused. This results in a dramatic increase in intraarterial pressure when saline is infused that can lead to damage of the vessel. There is no effective means to compensate for this with the current roller pumps, since they are not a pressure-dependent irrigation system.

The third type of irrigation system used today is a saline bag within a pressure vessel, with an electronic foot-activated on/off switch that operates a pinch valve. A conventional saline bag is placed within a tank that is filled with pressurized air from the operating room air line or separate air compressor. A regulator can be adjusted to vary the tank pressure. Typically, 25 to 30 psi is sufficient pressure to provide clear visualization in the ileofemoral system and below. To irrigate, the foot pedal is pressed on demand, as with the roller pump. The flow rate can be adjusted, but unlike the roller pump, the flow rate is adjusted by varying the pressure. This irrigation system is pressure-dependent and hence is automatically protected against generating dangerously high pressures inside the blood vessel. Also, there is more instantaneous delivery of saline on demand, with virtually no ramp-up time during saline delivery.

Ancillary Equipment

In addition to the essential items listed above, there are several ancillary pieces of equipment that can be quite worthwhile to the angioscopist. The first is a cart on which all the components of the angioscopy system may be consolidated. The cart allows for rapid setup as well as portability among operating rooms. Another useful piece of equipment is a tape recorder. It provides basic documentation and also allows the angioscopist to review images both during and after the procedure.

NEW TOOLS FOR MORE COMPLETE THROMBOEMBOLECTOMY

The ability of the angioscope to detect residual material on the inside of a graft or native vessel after thrombectomy has helped prompt the need for more thorough thrombectomy tools. Two such tools have been recently developed.[5] One is a corkscrew-shaped adherent clot catheter, and the other is an open helical wire graft thrombectomy catheter (Baxter Healthcare Corporation, McGaw Park, IL).

Adherent Clot Catheter

The working end of the adherent clot catheter is described in Figure 24–4. It is a flexible catheter with a variable-pitch spiral cable, covered with a latex membrane. A handle at the proximal end allows the surgeon to adjust the pitch of the corkscrew membrane from the fully collapsed 3-mm diameter position, to a tight spiral configuration with a diameter of up to 10-mm. Although used in much the same manner as a conventional balloon embolectomy catheter, it engages clot by a slightly different mechanism. Whereas a balloon catheter is inflated distal to the clot and is withdrawn to push the clot toward the arteriotomy for removal, the adherent clot catheter is expanded within the region of clot. The clot material is engaged within the interstices of the corkscrew and withdrawn toward the arteriotomy for removal.

In use, the adherent clot catheter is passed in a low-profile position through the clot and advanced distally. The spiral membrane is then retracted to a larger diameter and the catheter is withdrawn. Just as with the regular balloon embolectomy catheter, the spiral membrane can be continuously adjusted in diameter in response to the resistance encountered by the surgeon as the catheter is being withdrawn.

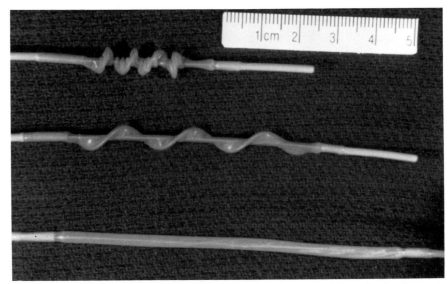

FIGURE 24–4. Working end of adherent clot catheter, collapsed for introduction (bottom), partially retracted (middle), and fully retracted (top).

Graft Thrombectomy Catheter

The working element of the graft thrombectomy catheter is shown in Figure 24–5. Its construction is similar to the construction of the adherent clot catheter: Adjustable-pitch spiral wire loops are expanded and retracted via a handle at the proximal end. Unlike the adherent clot catheter, however, the graft thrombectomy catheter has no latex covering over the spiral wires. Also, the wires are more stiff, they expand to a larger diameter (up to 20-mm), and they are shorter in length. As a result, this catheter is more aggressive at removing material than other embolectomy/thrombectomy catheters, and is to be used specifically on synthetic grafts. The device is also used in the same basic manner as the adherent clot catheter. The catheter is passed into the vessel in the collapsed low-profile position and advanced to the site of adherent material. The wires are then expanded by retracting the knob on the handle of the catheter until resistance to further expansion of the wires is encountered.

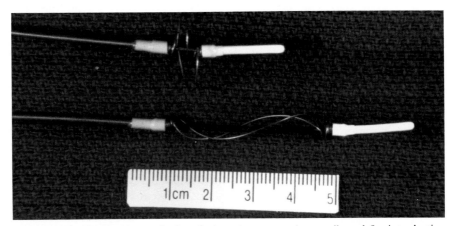

FIGURE 24–5. Working end of graft thrombectomy catheter collapsed for introduction (bottom) and fully retracted (top).

The catheter is then withdrawn with the wires in the expanded position, adjusting the diameter as necessary during retraction of the catheter. Both catheters can remove soft fresh clot, but are specifically designed to remove adherent, rubbery mature clot as well as more stringy material such as intimal hyperplasia or the disrupted neointima that can be encountered in synthetic grafts.

SURGICAL TECHNIQUE

Graft Thrombectomy

The following is description of an angioscopy-assisted thrombectomy of an occluded aortobifemoral Dacron bypass graft.

The angioscopy cart is wheeled adjacent to the sterile area. The sterile angioscope is hooked up to the saline irrigation line and camera coupler. The saline line is purged of air by running the saline supply until a steady stream emerges from the angioscope tip. The angioscope is focused and white balanced and is placed on a sterile area, ready for use.

A standard cutdown is performed at the groin level and the distal anastomosis is dissected free. A transverse incision is made into the graft and a standard #5 or #6 embolectomy balloon catheter is passed proximally as far as possible and is withdrawn inflated, in an attempt to remove any soft fresh thrombus. If material is removed, the conventional embolectomy balloon is passed repeatedly until no more material can be removed.

It is not uncommon for flow to remain weak or nonexistent after conventional balloon thrombectomy in these types of grafts. A more aggressive thrombectomy tool is often required to facilitate adequate removal. In preparation for angioscopy, a deflated #8-22 occlusion balloon catheter is threaded through the spiral wire of the graft thrombectomy catheter and then passed up into the aortic section of the graft. The occlusion balloon is then inflated and retracted until the surgeon feels the balloon seat against the bifurcation. This maneuver provides hemostatic control as additional material is removed. The occlusion balloon also prevents dislodged thrombotic material from migrating down the other branch of the iliac bifurcation. The graft thrombectomy catheter is then passed into the graftotomy and is guided along the body of the occlusion balloon to a site immediately distal to the inflated occlusion balloon. The coil regions of the catheter are expanded and the catheter is withdrawn through the graftotomy. Material adhering to the wire coils of the catheter is removed before the catheter is passed again, and the process is repeated. The proximal section of the graft is thrombectomized first before attempting thrombectomy of the distal section of the graft. If significant material is removed, the occlusion balloon is deflated momentarily to determine if flow through the proximal region of the obstruction has improved. If so, the graft thrombectomy catheter is removed and the angioscope is passed to the proximal region and the walls of the graft are inspected for completeness of removal (Fig. 24–6). The inflated 8-22 occlusion balloon preserves the effectiveness of the saline irrigation by preventing torrential infusion of arterial blood into the region to be visualized. If additional material is detected by the angioscope, the location is noted by observing the linear distance of the tip of the angioscope from the graftotomy. The angioscope is removed and the graft thrombectomy catheter is inserted and thrombectomy is attempted at that location. The surgeon alternates between using the thrombectomy catheter and the angioscope

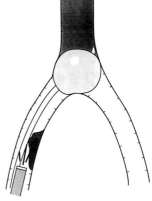

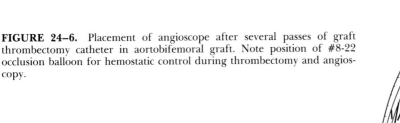

FIGURE 24–6. Placement of angioscope after several passes of graft thrombectomy catheter in aortobifemoral graft. Note position of #8-22 occlusion balloon for hemostatic control during thrombectomy and angioscopy.

until the proximal region is sufficiently cleared of intraluminal material. Attention is then turned to the distal portion of the graft where several additional iterations between the thrombectomy catheter and angioscope are performed until the graft is completely free of thrombus. The distal anastomotic site is then inspected with the angioscope and any corrective measures are implemented before initiating closure of the graftotomy. Prior to the closing stitches of the graftotomy, the occlusion balloon is deflated and removed. The graftotomy closure is completed and the groin incision is closed in standard fashion.

Adherent Thrombus in Native Vessel

The following is a description of an angioscopy-assisted thrombectomy of the SFA and popliteal artery containing fresh thrombus with underlying mature adherent clot.

After the angioscopy system is prepared for use, a groin incision is made over the femoral triangle. Clamps are applied to the deep femoral and the proximal SFA. An arteriotomy is made in the common femoral artery immediately proximal to the origin of the deep femoral artery. The major vessels of the femoropopliteal system are thrombectomized with standard #3 or #4 embolectomy balloon catheters. It is helpful to reconstruct the anatomic location of the soft clot removed by placing the clot segments on a towel outside the body. Reconstructing the clot gives insight as to where residual material may remain. At this point in the procedure, the angioscope is placed into the arteriotomy and is passed to the distal popliteal. The walls of the vessel are inspected for any residual material that remains (e.g., adherent clot, intimal flap). It is important that during irrigation, the flow of saline irrigant should be pulsatile, so that flaps can be more easily detected. Under a steady flow of saline, flaps can appear motionless and may therefore be much more difficult to detect. It is quite common to encounter a flap worth removing or additional adherent material that was missed on earlier passes. The angioscope allows the surgeon to direct efforts at a specific area. Often, a flap can be removed once its specific location is identified by noting the depth of insertion of the angioscope. Should additional adherent clot be identified angioscopically, removal is facilitated with the use of the adherent clot catheter (Fig. 24–7).

One of the most striking features of angioscopy is that it shows considerably more surface detail than an arteriographic image. A sizeable segment of adherent clot may barely be detected on fluoroscopy but can be quite prominent

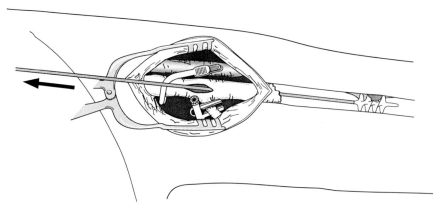

FIGURE 24–7. Removal of residual clot segment with adherent clot catheter after conventional balloon thrombectomy and angioscopic inspection.

with the angioscope. The surgeon must be prudent in the degree to which he/she tries to irradicate every intraluminal surface defect.

When satisfied with the degree of removal of material, closure of the arteriotomy can be initiated. Restoration of patency in the SFA and popliteal segments are confirmed angioscopically. Visualization of runoff vessels can be confirmed via arteriography. The groin incision is closed in standard fashion.

SUMMARY

In spite of some of the current barriers to using angioscopy in vascular surgery, this method of visualization has real utility in thromboembolectomy procedures. Angioscopy allows the surgeon to be more thorough with conventional embolectomy procedures. In addition, with the help of some recently designed thrombectomy tools, angioscopy can allow the surgeon to thrombectomize regions that were previously not amenable to a catheter-based approach. With the growing trend toward less-invasive procedures, angioscopy provides opportunities for new less-invasive procedures in the surgical environment.

REFERENCES

1. Fogarty TJ, Cranley JJ, Krause RJ: A method for extraction of arterial emboli and thrombi. Surg Gynecol Obstet 1963; *116*:241–244.
2. White RA, White GH: A color atlas of endovascular surgery: Interventional techniques in vascular disease. Philadelphia; JB Lippincott, 1990; 113–127.
3. Crew J: Angioscopy for in-situ bypass grafting. *In* White GH, White RA, eds: Angioscopy: Vascular and Coronary Applications. Chicago, Year Book Medical Publishers, 1989; 65–71.
4. Miller A, Lipson WE, Isaacsohn JL, et al: Intraoperative angioscopy: Principles of irrigation and description of a new dedicated irrigation pump. Am Heart J 1989; *118*:391–399.
5. Fogarty TJ, Monofort SY, Hermann GD, et al: New techniques and instrumentation for the management of adherent clot in native and synthetic vessels. Curr Surg 1991; *48*:123–126.

25

THE USE OF ANGIOSCOPY IN LASER ANGIOPLASTY

JAMES M. SEEGER

Laser energy transmitted through fiberoptics can be used to ablate atherosclerotic plaque. However, to date, this new technique for treating peripheral vascular disease has been relatively ineffective. In part, the limited success of laser angioplasty is due to inadequate arterial imaging and poor guidance of laser energy during the recanalization procedure. Real-time assessment of the arterial wall during laser recanalization is necessary to limit arterial wall injury and perforation. Determination of the composition of the occluding lesion prior to laser angioplasty is required for selection of the proper type and amount of laser energy for precise atheroablation. Careful inspection of the newly created channel after recanalization must be done to assure that an adequate lumen has been re-established and to detect luminal abnormalities that may cause acute recanalization failure. Without arterial imaging techniques that can provide this information, laser angioplasty is likely to fail.

Techniques currently used to investigate arterial pathology and to direct laser energy during laser angioplasty include fluoroscopy, contrast angiography, and angioscopy. Systems which use laser-induced fluoroscopy to guide laser angioplasty have also been investigated.[1,2] Unfortunately, reliable discrimination of normal arterial wall and atherosclerotic plaque has been difficult, and the incidence of arterial wall injury during recanalization has not been reduced significantly using "smart" laser systems. Intraluminal ultrasound, which provides real-time assessment of arterial wall pathology,[3] currently cannot be used simultaneously with laser angioplasty. However, the potential of this technique for imaging the arterial wall during endovascular procedures such as laser angioplasty appears great.[4]

Laser angioplasty of occluded arteries guided by fluoroscopy and contrast angiography is essentially a blind procedure. Fluoroscopy can be used to visualize a laser probe/fiber within an artery if the fiber is capped with a radiopaque material. However, the wall of the artery being treated and the relationship of the laser probe to that artery cannot be seen, particularly in an area of occlusion. Even if the artery to be treated is patent, contrast arteriography only outlines the arterial lumen and the arterial wall is visualized as a negative image. The type of plaque present, the thickness of the plaque to be removed, and its relationship to the remaining normal arterial wall cannot be defined.

In addition, detection of significant luminal abnormalities, which can occur after balloon or laser angioplasty, is suboptimal using contrast angiography.[5]

Conversely, angioscopy provides excellent assessment of luminal detail after arterial recanalization and allows identification of occlusion type (thrombotic or atherosclerotic), based on surface characteristics and color. Visual aiming of the laser energy is also possible, although this is limited by difficulty in directing the end of angioscopes which do not have deflecting tips. However, angioscopy cannot be used to determine plaque thickness or to define the boundary between the plaque being ablated and the normal arterial wall. Regardless, angioscopy has been found to be an important adjunct to laser angioplasty, and this chapter will review what has been learned about the use of angioscopy with laser angioplasty and discuss its current and future role as an imaging and guidance system for this new therapy of peripheral vascular disease.

BACKGROUND AND CLINICAL RESULTS

Advances in fiberoptic catheter construction, development of video cameras specifically adapted for angioscopy, and better systems for clearing blood from the field of view have allowed widespread application of angioscopy to patients with peripheral vascular disease. Angioscopes range in diameter from 0.85- to 2.9-mm so that almost all vessels in the coronary or peripheral vascular system can be examined. Most angioscopes have channels that allows irrigation at the working end of the angioscope to improve clearing of blood from the visual field, and some newer angioscopes have systems for angulation of the angioscope tip, which increases the field of view. Minimal focal lengths range from 2.0- to 6.5-mm, and spacial resolution at a focal length of 5-mm is greater than 20 μm.[6]

Clearing the intraluminal visual field of blood is essential for successful angioscopy. Dedicated pumps for the irrigation of heparinized saline are now available. Unlike the pressurized blood bags used in the initial studies of angioscopy, use of a dedicated pump allows: (1) clearing of blood from the field of view more quickly, (2) maintenance of this clear field longer, and (3) limits the amount of infused fluid to an average of less than 500 cc per procedure.[7,8] More importantly, such pumps have allowed successful use of angioscopy in percutaneous procedures such as percutaneous laser angioplasty where it is difficult or impossible to occlude flow of blood into the area being visualized. A potential further advance in obtaining a clear field for angioscopy was reported by Silverman et al.[9] who used carbon dioxide (CO_2) gas to displace blood from the arterial lumen during angioscopy. Use of CO_2 gas during simulated percutaneous angioscopy in animals provided a shorter time interval from onset of infusion to total blood clearance from the field of view, a longer duration of a clear field once blood was displaced, and a greater percentage of viewing fields totally cleared of blood compared to heparinized saline infused from a pressure bag. However, the use of CO_2 gas infusion to displace blood during angioscopy is still experimental and has not undergone human trials.

As initially envisioned, laser angioplasty would be done using laser energy delivered through laser fibers passed through small, flexible fiberoptic angioscopes. Occluding atherosclerotic plaque would be identified and laser energy visually directed to ablate that plaque. The newly created lumen would then be visually inspected to determine the adequacy of laser recanalization and to detect remaining abnormalities requiring further treatment.

The use of this technique was first investigated in the initial Food and Drug Administration- (FDA)-approved feasibility study of laser angioplasty reported by Abela and Seeger et al. in 1986.[10] Angioscopically guided laser angioplasty of 13 occluded superficial femoral arteries was attempted in 11 patients undergoing femoral popliteal bypass. Optical wave guides or metal-capped laser probes were backloaded into a 2.8-mm angioscope. The angioscope was then advanced to the point of obstruction in the superficial femoral artery and the occlusion visualized. The laser fiber or probe was positioned as close to the center of the cross-section of the obstruction as possible, and lasing was initiated using argon ion laser energy. Passage of the laser probe through the obstruction was observed if possible. Once the artery had been recanalized, the 2.8-mm angioscope containing the laser fiber was removed and a smaller 1.7-mm angioscope introduced to inspect the newly created channel. At the completion of this procedure, the arterial segment that had been treated was removed and processed for microscopic examination.

Results of this preliminary study documented advantages and disadvantages of the use of angioscopy for arterial imaging and laser guidance during laser angioplasty. Good images of the point of obstruction were obtained in 5 of the 11 patients. In four of the remaining six patients, intermittent images were obtained owing to difficulty in maintaining the visual field clear of blood. This study was done prior to the introduction of dedicated pumps for flushing blood from the visual field, and use of such a pump would likely have significantly improved these results. In the remaining two patients, camera malfunction prevented viewing. In those patients in whom images could be obtained, the site of obstruction was identified and the type of occlusion determined. Atherosclerotic plaque was seen to occlude 9 of 12 arteries (Fig. 25–1A) and fresh thrombus was identified in one (Fig. 25–1B). Significant atherosclerosis and small intimal flaps not seen on preoperative angiography were also identified proximal to the site of occlusion (Fig. 25–1C).

Eleven of thirteen totally occluded arteries were recanalized in the eleven patients. Using the angioscope, it was possible to align the laser probe coaxial to the arterial walls prior to attempted recanalization (Fig. 25–2A). However, once lasing was begun, it was not possible to follow the laser probe into the obstruction, as the channel created by the laser probe was not large enough to accommodate the 2.8-mm angioscope. Perforation occurred in six patients owing to deflection of the laser probe into the subintima and through the arterial wall. All perforations occurred distal to the point of entry of the laser probe into the occlusion, outside the field of view on the angioscope.

After recanalization, the new lumen was inspected using the 1.7-mm angioscope in all patients. Charring along the arterial wall could be seen in all cases and occasional flecks of calcium could be identified within the new channel (Fig. 25–2B). In addition, in one case, recanalization of the entire length of the arterial obstruction was confirmed by passage of the angioscope through the new lumen into the patent distal artery (Fig. 25–2C). Vessels occluded with fresh thrombus were seen to have inadequate lumens after laser recanalization, as passage of the laser fiber into the thrombus produced only slight shrinking of the thrombus. None of the arterial perforations were identified by postangioplasty angioscopy.

Subsequent to this initial feasibility study, a therapeutic clinical trial of laser

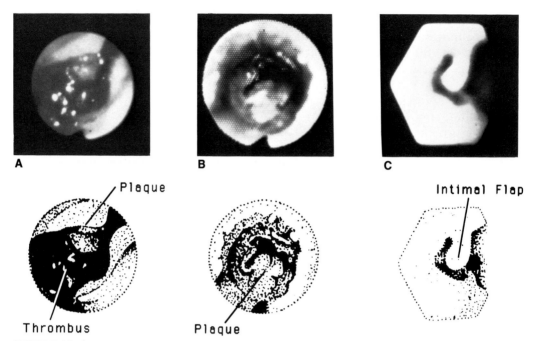

FIGURE 25–1. *A,* Angioscopic view of an atherosclerotic occlusion of a popliteal artery. The atherosclerotic occlusion is irregular, lobulated, and yellowish. *B,* Angioscopic view of thrombus totally occluding a superficial femoral artery. The thrombus is characteristically smooth, glistening, and reddish-brown. It is easily differentiated from an atherosclerotic occlusion. *C,* Angioscopic view of intimal flap; these are common in areas of atherosclerosis, particularly proximal to an area of occlusion. (From Seeger JM, Abela GS: Angioscopy as an adjunct to arterial reconstructive surgery: A preliminary report. J Vasc Surg 1986; *4*:315–320, with permission.)

angioplasty has been done in 84 carefully selected patients. The majority of these patients underwent percutaneous laser angioplasty, which limited the use of angioscopy as an adjunct to these procedures. However, angioscopy was successfully used in 17 patients. Angioscopy prior to attempted laser angioplasty was useful in detecting thrombus that could not be treated using laser angioplasty and in detecting false channels that had been created by attempts at passage of a guide wire through all obstructions prior to laser angioplasty. Once such a channel was present, attempted laser angioplasty was abandoned because the laser probe passed preferentially into the false channel. Inspection of the recanalized lumen after laser angioplasty identified intraluminal flaps in the new channel that required removal, and in a few cases, documented the recanalized lumen to have been created in the subintimal plane. However, as previously demonstrated, angioscopy could not be used to guide the laser probe through the area of occlusion, and fluoroscopy and contrast angiography were required during this part of the procedure.

Findings similar to these have been reported by White et al.[11] They investigated 30 patients undergoing 23 intraoperative and 7 percutaneous laser angioplasty procedures. Angioscopy was used in all cases. Patients were divided into two groups, 24 with diffuse superficial femoral and popliteal artery disease and occlusions 4 to 30 cm in length, and 6 with localized disease and lesions less than 3 cm in length. In 16 of the 24 patients with diffuse disease, it was not possible to pass the angioscope to the point of obstruction. This was due to disease in the superficial femoral artery proximal to the area of arterial occlusion, which usually had not been detected by angiography. In the remaining

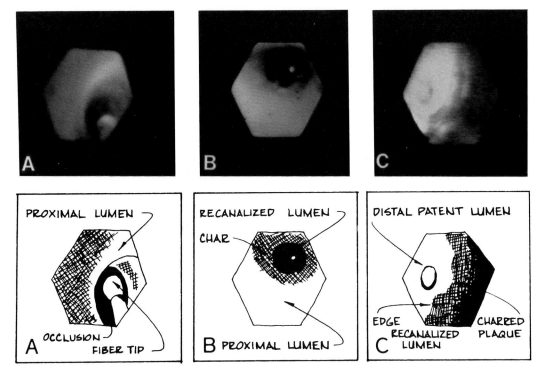

FIGURE 25–2. *A*, Angioscopic view of a 2-mm laser probe is seen in the center of the artery just proximal to an area of total occlusion. The angioscope has been rotated and angled showing the laser probe at the 5 o'clock position. *B*, Angioscopic view of the new lumen created by laser angioplasty. The new channel is seen as a dark tunnel in the right upper quadrant. The bright spot in the center of the new lumen is due to light reflection from saline perfusate. Charring can be seen around the edges of the lumen from the lasing process. *C*, Angioscopic view of the communication between the charred, recanalized vascular segment and the patent distal artery seen at the 9 o'clock position. Charring within the newly created vascular lumen is seen. (From Abela GS, Seeger JM, Barbieri E, et al: Laser angioplasty with angioscopic guidance in humans. J Am Coll Cardiol 1986; *8*:184–192, with permission.)

eight patients, passage of the angioscope to the point of arterial occlusion was possible, but at times, it was difficult to differentiate severe stenosis from occlusion. Despite these problems, in patients in whom angioscopy could be done, its use was valuable in preventing placement of the laser probe into collateral vessels, false channels, or arterial wall dissections. However, as previously reported by us, the laser probe could not be visualized once it entered the area of obstruction, and perforation could not be prevented using angioscopy for guidance of the laser probe.

In contrast, visualization of the entire laser recanalization procedure was possible in all six patients with localized disease. In addition, investigation of the new channel after laser angioplasty was possible in 88 per cent of these patients. Charring, retained thrombus, and intimal flaps could be seen, and the size of the new lumen estimated. Intimal flaps were seen in 81 per cent and charring in 87 per cent of the new channels. None of these abnormalities were detected by angiography. Angioscopy was also used to direct endovascular removal of large intimal flaps in three patients and retrieval of detached laser probe tips from two patients. Identification of large amounts of retained thrombus, large intimal flaps which could not be removed, and narrow recanalized lumens were associated with early arterial reocclusion.

Other investigators have also demonstrated the value of the use of angioscopy with laser angioplasty. Grundfest et al.[6] reported that angioscopy could be used to aim the laser delivery system and to inspect the new channel after lasing in five patients. Koga[12] reported visualization of the point of obstruction in occluded arterial venous dialysis shunts in 23 of 28 patients undergoing laser angioplasty for treatment of this problem. Prior to attempted laser angioplasty, it was possible to determine whether thrombotic occlusions were old or new, and after the procedure, the completeness of recanalization could be assessed. Finally, Lee reported successful use of angioscopy to direct coronary laser angioplasty in one patient[13] and peripheral laser angioplasty plus atherectomy in one patient.[14]

Based on these findings, angioscopy appears to be of value during laser angioplasty. It is most useful in patients with localized arterial occlusions, which is also the type of disease in which laser angioplasty is also most successful. In patients with this type of disease, lesion type can be identified, probe advancement into false channels or collateral vessels can be prevented, and newly created channels can be examined for size and for intimal defects that could lead to rethrombosis. Furthermore, angioscopy can be used to direct removal of retained thrombus or large intimal flaps that predispose the recanalized artery to acute re-occlusion. However, angioscopy cannot be used to guide laser probes through arterial occlusions or to reduce the incidence of arterial wall injury and perforation during laser angioplasty.

USE OF ANGIOSCOPY TO QUANTIFY ARTERIAL LUMEN SIZE

Determination of lumen size during and after laser angioplasty is important to the success of the procedure. Contrast angiography, which is the technique currently used to assess lumen size, can be very misleading. Angiography produces a two-dimensional arterial image in two planes, at most. Eccentric and irregularly shaped arterial lumens are difficult to assess in this manner and lumen size can be overestimated. Angioscopy can overcome these problems by providing a cross-sectional image of the lumen of an artery. However, magnification is inherent in the angioscopic image, dependent on the distance between the angioscope and the site being studied, and techniques which correct for magnification must be developed.

This problem has been investigated by Lee et al.[15] and Friedl and Abela et al.[16] Lee examined 11 diseased coronary artery sites in patients undergoing coronary artery bypass grafting. The angioscope was positioned coaxial to the artery, approximately 1 mm from the stenotic area to be measured. Cross-sectional areas were obtained using caliper measurements from the angioscopic image. The measured area was corrected for magnification using a factor previously determined by directly measuring the degree of magnification at 1 mm of an object of known size. These measurements were then compared to similar measurements taken from coronary angiograms. Correlation between the two sets of measurements was good, with a correlation coefficient of 0.90.

Friedl and Abela et al.[16] used a more sophisticated system to quantify angioscopic images and obtained even better results. They coupled a computer image processing system to an angioscope and compared measurements of cross-sectional areas of stenotic arteries obtained in vitro using this system to

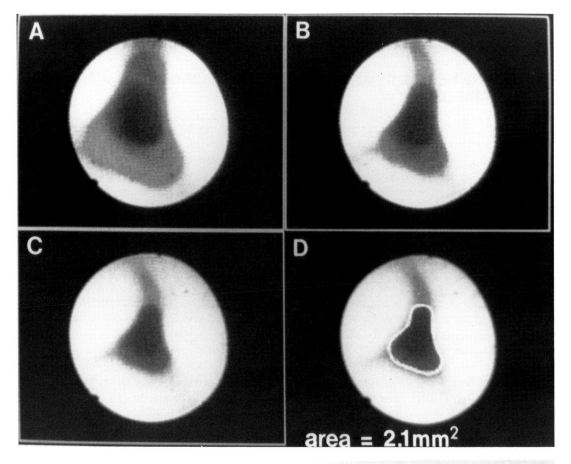

area = 2.1mm²

FIGURE 25–3. *A*, Photograph of the computer screen taken during quantitative angioscopy. The top left quandrant contains the closest view of the stenosis being measured, the top right image was taken 1 mm back, and the bottom left image was taken 2 mm back from the initial image. The bottom right image is that of the third view with the lumen boundaries traced by the operator. The computer reported a cross-sectional area of 2.1 mm². *B*, Photograph of the cross-section of the vessel at the level of the stenosis which was measured using quantitative angioscopy. During processing, the constrictive area has changed shape slightly and the "folds" in the computer view appear more prominent. The area measured by a planimetry is 1.9 mm. (From Friedl SE, Abela GS, Tomaru T, et al: Quantitative endovascular angioscopy. SPIE Optical Fibers and Med IV 1989; 1067:197–202, with permission.)

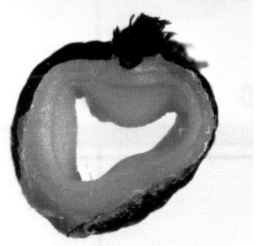

area = 1.9mm²

planimetry measurements from histologic specimens (Fig. 25–3). The distance between the end of the angioscope and the site to be measured was determined by assessing differences in lumen size produced by moving the angioscope a known distance. The correlation coefficient of the two measurements was 0.94 and the average error was 15 per cent. Thus, with proper image-analysis equipment and techniques, angioscopy can be used to quantify arterial lumen size very accurately.

THE FUTURE OF ANGIOSCOPICALLY GUIDED LASER ANGIOPLASTY

A unique catheter system for laser angioplasty has recently been developed by Medilase, Inc., Minneapolis MN[17] (Fig. 25–4). This system incorporates both angioscopy and laser delivery in the same catheter. Catheters range in size from 4.5- to 6-F, and each catheter contains separate imaging fibers, laser delivery fibers, and an irrigation channel. Aiming of the laser energy is done visually, and pulsed-dye laser energy is used for plaque ablation. Initial versions of the catheter do not have a system for angulating the catheter tip, and laser energy can only be directed straight ahead.

Riley et al.[18] has reported the initial evaluation of the safety and effectiveness of the use of this catheter system for laser angioplasty in nine patients undergoing femoropopliteal bypass. Partial or complete recanalization of occluded superficial femoral arteries was possible in five of nine arteries. Improper catheter alignment to the laser precluded angioscopic visualization and laser firing in two patients. In the other two, dense, fibrotic plaque which could not be penetrated by the pulsed-dye laser was encountered. Perforations occurred in two of the five arteries that were recanalized. One perforation was thought to be mechanically induced, while the other occurred during lasing.

Complete recanalization of these arteries was not attempted in this phase I safety trial. Regardless, the lack of adequate arterial wall imaging using angioscopy alone, and the inability to direct laser energy toward the arterial wall made this impossible. Planned modifications of this unique delivery catheter will incorporate intraluminal ultrasound and either a deflectable catheter tip or an angled laser fiber that can be rotated so that laser energy can be applied circumferentially to the artery. These modifications should improve the possibility that this catheter could be used for total arterial recanalization without adjunctive balloon angioplasty. In addition, in the future, a thulium: yttrium aluminum garnet (YAG) laser, which can penetrate fibrotic plaque, will be used with this delivery catheter.

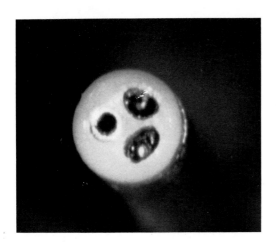

FIGURE 25–4. Medilase catheter tip. This new catheter contains three channels including the laser fiber seen at the top right, the illumination and imaging bundle seen at the bottom right, and irrigation port seen to the left. (From Reilly MK, Perry MO, Nanney LB: True ablation of atheromatous plaques with laser energy—a phase I safety study. Ann Surg 1991; 213:440–445, with permission.)

SUMMARY

In summary, an imaging/guidance system which allows precise aiming of laser energy, real-time visualization of the arterial wall during lasing, and detailed assessment of the arterial lumen before and after treatment will be necessary if laser angioplasty is to be successfully used for treatment of peripheral vascular disease. Angioscopy has been shown to provide excellent luminal detail of occluded arteries and to allow aiming of laser light at occluding atherosclerotic plaque. In addition, the type of occluding lesion can be identified and laser probe advancement into collaterals or false channels can be prevented using this technique. Angioscopy after successful laser angioplasty also detects defects not identified by angiography which can lead to vessel reocclusion. However, angioscopy cannot be used to assess the thickness of occluding atherosclerotic plaque or to determine the boundary between atherosclerotic plaque and the underlying, more normal, arterial wall. Thus its use does not prevent arterial wall injury or perforation during laser angioplasty.

Recent introduction of a new catheter system that combines angioscopy and laser delivery in a single catheter that can be made deflectable and into which intraluminal ultrasound may be incorporated may overcome these problems. Such a system could provide accurate, real-time arterial wall imaging before, during, and after laser angioplasty, and could allow treatment of occluded arteries using laser energy alone. This should be a significant step in endovascular therapy of peripheral vascular disease, because in animals, laser angioplasty without balloon dilatation appears to limit arterial wall injury and intimal thickening,[19] which leads to restenosis and recanalization failure.

REFERENCES

1. Geschwind HJ, Dubois-Rande J, Shafton E, et al: Percutaneous pulsed laser-assisted balloon angioplasty guided by spectroscopy. Am Heart J 1989; *117*:1147–1152.
2. Leon MB, Almagor Y, Bartorelli AL, et al: Fluorescence-guided laser-assisted balloon angioplasty in patients with femoral popliteal occlusions. Circulation 1990; *81*:143–155.
3. Tabara M, Kopchok G, White RA: In vitro and in vivo evaluation of intraluminal ultrasound in normal and atherosclerotic arteries. Am J Surg 1990; *160*:556–560.
4. Graham S, Brands D, Sarahus A, Hodgson J: Utility of an intravascular imaging device for arterial wall definition and atherectomy guidance (abstr). J Am Coll Cardiol 1989; *13*:222a.
5. Stept LL, Flinn WR, McCarthy WJ, et al: Technical defects as cause of early graft failure after femoral distal bypass. Arch Surg 1987; *122*:599–604.
6. Grundfest WS, Litvack F, Sherman T, et al: Delineation of peripheral and coronary detail by intraoperative angioscopy. Ann Surg 1985; *202*:394–400.
7. Miller A, Campbell BR, Gibbons GW, et al: Routine intraoperative angioscopy and lower extremity revascularization. Arch Surg 1989; *124*:604–608.
8. Baxter BT, Rizzo RJ, Flinn WR, et al: A comparative study of intraoperative angioscopy and completion arteriography following femoral distal bypass. Arch Surg 1990; *125*:997–1002.
9. Silverman SH, Mladinich CJ, Hawkins IF, et al: The use of carbon dioxide gas to displace flowing blood during angioscopy. J Vasc Surg 1989; *10*:313–317.
10. Abela GS, Seeger JM, Barbieri E, et al: Laser angioplasty with angioscopic guidance in humans. J Am Coll Cardiol 1986; *8*:184–192.
11. White GH, White RA, Colman PD, Kopchok GE: Experimental and clinical applications of angioscopic guidance for laser angioplasty. Am J Surg 1989; *158*:495–501.
12. Koga N, Sato T, Baba T, et al: Angioscopy in transluminal balloon and laser angioplasty in the management of chronic hemodialysis fistulae. Trans Am Soc Art Int Organs. 1989; *35*:193–196.
13. Lee G, Reis RL, Chan MC, et al: Clinical laser recanalization of coronary obstruction. Angioscopic and angiographic documentation. Chest 1986; *90*:770–772.
14. Lee G, Morelli R, Long JB, et al: Combined laser-thermal and atherectomy treatment of peripheral arterial occlusion: Documentation by angioscopy and angiography. Am Heart J 1989; *118*:1324–1327.

15. Lee G, Garcia JM, Corso PJ, et al: Correlation of coronary angioscopic to angiographic findings in coronary artery disease. Am J Cardiol 1986; *58*:238–241.

16. Friedl SE, Abela GS, Tomaru T, et al: Quantitative endovascular angioscopy. SPIE Optical Fibers and Med IV 1989; *1067*:197–202.

17. Goldman ML, Wan CS, Shaw DW, et al: The Yucatan microswine model of atherosclerosis for evaluation of a tunable dye laser system. Lasers Surg Med 1989; *1*(suppl):13.

18. Reilly MK, Perry MO, Nanney LB: True ablation of atherosclerotic plaques with laser energy—a phase I safety study. Ann Surg 1991; *213*:440–445.

19. Abela GS, Crea F, Seeger JM, et al: The healing process in normal canine arteries and in atherosclerotic monkey arteries after transluminal laser irradiation. Am J Cardiol 1985; *56*:983–988.

V
INTERVENTIONAL TECHNOLOGY

26

PERCUTANEOUS BALLOON ANGIOPLASTY FOR ARTERIOSCLEROSIS OBLITERANS: Long-Term Results

ROBERT B. RUTHERFORD and JANETTE DURHAM

Although transluminal dilation for lower extremity arteriosclerotic occlusive arterial disease was introduced as early as 1964 by Dotter,[1] and the balloon catheter in 1974 by Grüntzig and Hopf,[2] extended experiences with long-term follow-up did not begin to accumulate until the mid 1980s. Now, in the early 1990s we are in a position to assess the benefit of percutaneous transluminal balloon angioplasty (PTA), not just in terms of overall results, but with specific regard to type of lesion, anatomic site, length and degree of occlusion, condition of the adjacent segment and the downstream vessels ("runoff"), associated risk factors, indications for intervention, and the initial hemodynamic result. This will be the focus of this chapter.

The value of an analysis of the long-term results of PTA goes beyond its intrinsic merit in predicting outcome and allowing these results to modify future application. These results can also serve as the "gold standard" for newer percutaneous endovascular procedures (e.g., laser "angioplasty," atherectomy, and other forms of mechanical recanalization). Initially at least, many of these procedures were justified, primarily on the basis of claimed dissatisfaction with PTA results, especially for longer lesions. Also because many of these procedures still employ balloon dilation as the final maneuver, their scientific "control" should be PTA alone. Finally, there is the need to compare PTA results with those of conservative therapy (exercise, rheologic drugs), on the one hand, and open surgical revascularization on the other, in selecting the most appropriate therapeutic option for a given patient. The actual comparison of these three basic options is beyond the scope of this chapter; however, it should be pointed out that this weighing of alternatives should *not* be done by simple comparison of *overall* results for patients with peripheral arterial occlusive disease. These three basic modes of therapy are likely to be applied to significantly different patients in regard to clinical status, lesion characteristics, and other factors that affect outcome. Furthermore, articles on these three forms of therapy, by vascular internists, interventional radiologists, and vascular surgeons, may employ quite different reporting standards.[3] The common ploy of using historical controls, carefully selected to compare unfavorably with the newly introduced technique, can no longer be tolerated, while focused studies of contemporary experiences, contrasting results with specific and comparable lesions are acceptable. Of course, randomized prospective trials, comparing different modes of therapy on similar patients/lesions are the most desirable, and more studies such as the recent Oxford, England[4] and New Zealand[5] trials of PTA versus conservative (exercise) therapy in claudicators with discreet femoropopliteal occlusive disease, and the Veterans Administration cooperative study of PTA versus surgical treatment,[6] are needed.

THE EFFECT OF DIFFERING REPORTING STANDARDS ON LATE SUCCESS RATES

A number of reporting practices profoundly affect the long-term success rates appearing in the literature. One is the practice of eliminating initial failures in determining long-term patency. This has a greater impact in femoropopliteal PTA where a 15 to 26 per cent early failure rate has been reported to occur.[7] For example, eliminating a 20 per cent initial failure rate and reporting a 60 per cent cumulative success rate obscures the fact that less than half (48 per cent) of patients in which treatment was employed received long-term benefit. These hypothetical figures are not unusual, particularly for some of the newer endovascular procedures. On the other hand, a point can be made that failure to even pass a lesion with a guidewire, unassociated with any significant complication, should not be counted against PTA. While this qualifies under "intent to treat," it is unlikely that vascular surgeons count limb salvage cases where the planned bypass could not be carried out because exploration of the distal artery showed it not to be feasible. More debatable is the situation in which the lesion was passed and dilated with apparent (angiographic) success, but because of the severity of additional downstream disease, there was no clinical improvement or detectable hemodynamic benefit. One may dismiss this as being due to the patient's disease, or count it as an error in judgment, but it will affect long-term success rates if initial hemodynamic failures are excluded, along with technical failures, in calculating these rates. Since almost all of these cases ultimately fail, they will either show up as initial (hemodynamic) failures, or decrease the cumulative patency rate if included among initial successes because of angiographic evidence of successful dilation.

The criteria of success, of listing a patient as "improved" or of counting the dilated segment as "patent," do have a major impact on late-outcome reports. The difference between "soft" (subjective) and "hard" (objective, hemodynamic) criteria is best appreciated by considering outcome after iliac PTA. "Palpable femoral pulses and symptomatic improvement" may seem like reasonable criteria, but most iliac PTAs are performed for stenosis, so pulses are usually palpable *prior to dilation* and, if several years intervene and the patient has become more sedentary, or simply walks more slowly because of arthritis, deteriorating cardiopulmonary status, or other health reasons, the subjective perception may be that claudication is still improved. On the other hand, some demand both a categorical improvement in clinical status *plus* a persistent improvement in the ABI of at least 0.10. A superficial femoral occlusion could intervene, downstream from a still patent dilated iliac segment, resulting in demonstrable clinical and hemodynamic deterioration [decreased ankle-brachial index (ABI)]. This occurred, during a 3-year follow-up, in 16 per cent of cases in the initial experience with iliac PTA at the University of Colorado. Only by using the thigh-brachial index, derived by using a regular sized upper thigh cuff, was this potential misinterpretation of PTA failure avoided. By using varying criteria then appearing in the literature, we could vary the 3-year success rate for our iliac dilations from 52 to 86 per cent and for femoropopliteal PTA from 27 to 63 per cent.[8]

Clearly, uniform objective reporting standards need to be adopted and complied with. Suggested standards have been recommended by the Joint Committee of the SVS/ISCVS[9]. Recently the Journal of Vascular and Interventional Radiology has also adopted these standards with little modification.[10] Widespread compliance is a future goal, but does not impact on most of the papers quoted in this article. We will therefore either not cite misleading data, or point out significant weaknesses in certain reports.

PTA FOR AORTOILIAC OCCLUSIVE DISEASE

Overall Results for Aortoiliac Occlusive Disease

Six articles contribute long-term patency data for aortoiliac occlusive disease treated by balloon angioplasty which used objective hemodynamic data, in addition to clinical improvement, to determine patency status (Table 26–1).[6,11–15] As already pointed out, using the ABI to judge the patency of proximal revascularization will underestimate patency in patients who develop hemodynamically significant disease downstream from the site of angioplasty. On the other hand, the lack of objective patency criteria has contributed to overly optimistic estimates of PTA success. The truth lies somewhere between. Two of these reports, by Johnston et al.[13] and Wilson et al.,[6] included primary technical failures in their patency analysis. Patency rates, corrected for technical failures, for the other authors are presented in brackets in order to allow full comparison.

The initial technical success of aortoiliac angioplasty in these six studies ranges from 94 to 96 per cent. The easy access to the lesion from a retrograde femoral approach, the large vessel diameter, the rapid blood flow through the iliac artery, and the low thrombosis rate following dilatation, all contribute to this high success rate. Initial clinical success, based on improvement in leg hemodynamics, after a technically successful angioplasty ranges from 89 to 97 per cent, resulting in a mean overall success rate (30 days) for all six studies of 92 per cent. One-, three-, and five-year cumulative patencies, *including initial failures,* range from 74 to 96 per cent (mean 84 per cent), 61 to 89 per cent (mean 76 per cent), and 59 to 83 per cent (mean 74 per cent), respectively. Differences in primary patency, reporting methods, and patient selection explain these wide ranges in long-term data. To generalize, one can expect a 4 per cent technical failure rate compounded by an additional hemodynamic failure of 4 per cent, for an overall initial success rate of 92 per cent. During the first year there is a further 10 per cent failure rate, with approximately 3 per cent per year failure in subsequent years. This is shown in Figure 26–1, along with the data points from Table 26–1.

TABLE 26–1. PATENCY FOLLOWING ILIAC ANGIOPLASTY

Study Number	Author (Year)	Number of Patients	Initial Success (Technical/Clinical)	Cumulative Patency Reported (Corrected) in Years			
				1	2	3	5
1.	Kumpe[11] (1982)[a]	71 A	.96/.93	.88(.82)	.82(.76)	.82(.76)	
		B	.96/.85	.73(.62)	.55(.47)		
2.	Van Andel[12] (1985)	154	.96/NR	.98(.94)	.93(.89)	.91(.87)	.86(.83)
3.	Johnston[13] (1987)[b]	684	NR/.91 A	.80	.80	.70	
			CI	.79	.69	.65	.59
			EI	.74	.62	.51	.48
4.	Wilson[6] (1989)	81	.89	.74	.71	.61	
5.	In der Maur[14] (1990)	157	NR/.97	.99(.96)	.96(.93)	.92(.89)	.84(.81)
6.	Stokes[15] (1990)	70	.94/.89	.85(.79)	.74(.69)	.67(.63)	.34(.32)

[a] Reported same patients by thigh-brachial index (A) and ankle-brachial index (B) criteria.
[b] Reported separately aortic (A), common iliac (CI), and external iliac (EI) lesions.
NR, Not reported.

Although the initial failures of PTA are greater than for surgical therapy, the durability of an iliac angioplasty, once the artery is successfully dilated, is similar to reconstructive surgery. The Veterans Administration Cooperative Study, the only prospective randomized trial comparing surgical and angioplasty treatments of iliac disease, demonstrated this similarity of results in the early follow-up period.[6] The lesions treated in this study tended to be less severe than is typically reported in surgical series because of the requirement for all patients entered in the study to have lesions amenable to both therapies. Therefore, while the bottom line results of angioplasty can appear similar, arterial disease treated by surgical reconstruction is typically more severe.

Factors Influencing Outcome of Proximal (Aortoiliac) PTA

There are two main reasons that make accurate analysis of factors effecting the patency of iliac PTA difficult: preselection bias and the tendency to exclude

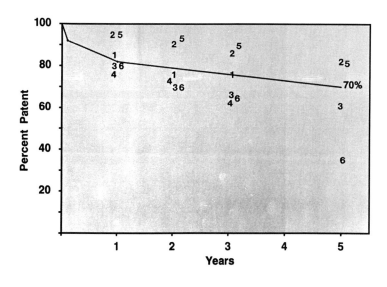

FIGURE 26–1. Composite patency curve for iliac PTA, based on the literature, and particularly on the data from reports featured in Table 26–1, indicated by study number. Note closeness of curve to data from report number 1.

initial failures from cumulative patency evaluation. The latter is much less of a factor in series in which the former plays a dominant role, since the more favorable the lesion selected, the lower the initial failure rate. Eliminating early failures can not only make a series with liberal selection criteria look reasonably successful, but it can obfuscate analysis of the factors that affect patency, since the unfavorable lesions will generally fail early. Jorgenson et al. demonstrated this in a large series of patients treated for limb salvage.[16] Lesion length, degree of stenosis, and runoff were all statistically significant variables affecting iliac patency when technical failures were included in the patency analysis. Since these same factors tended to affect early patency, their significance could not be demonstrated when the technical failures were removed from consideration. This lack of unselected treatment groups and patency analysis after the exclusion of technical failures, both of which pervade the literature, prevents convincing (i.e., statistically significant) conclusions to be drawn about those variables which affect patency. Nevertheless, these factors are well recognized and will be summarized below.

Effect of Clinical Status

Because focal iliac occlusive disease tends to produce symptoms of claudication, the majority of patients who undergo iliac PTA are treated for disabling claudication. A role for aortoiliac angioplasty in limb salvage has been established for high–operative-risk patients, but these are in the decided minority. These same patients should also have lesions that are technically more difficult to treat percutaneously. Hasson supports this perception with a review of the morbidity and mortality of PTA.[17] Clinical indication significantly predicted poor outcome, claudication having clearly the best outcome. Johnson's data, which reflects a population of patients who were primarily treated for claudication, predicts a 12 to 14 per cent difference in 3-year patency for a common iliac stenosis treated for limb salvage compared to the same type of lesion in patients with claudication.[13]

Two other reports document this difference because of the large number of limb salvage patients included in their experiences. Jorgenson et al. reported a series of 34 patients with iliac lesions who all were in a limb salvage situation.[16] Although the technical and 1-year success rates were only slightly worse than in claudicators treated by the same group, 82 per cent versus 89 per cent and 80 per cent versus 85 per cent, respectively, the 2-year patencies diverged by 10 per cent, widening further to 20 per cent at 3 years (60 per cent versus 79 per cent).[16,18] Stokes et al. reported the results of 70 iliac angioplasties, all in diabetics. Patients in the limb salvage category had a 5-year patency of 29 per cent compared with 70 per cent for claudicators.[15]

Effect of Anatomic Site

The anatomic site of the lesion has been shown convincingly to effect angioplasty results, so much so that most authors separate lesions into suprainguinal and infrainguinal arteries when reporting results, as we have. Differences may also exist within the aortoiliac segment itself. Odurny et al. reported 1- and 5-year patency data of 80 per cent and 70 per cent for 25 aortic lesions treated with angioplasty.[19] Yakes et al. reported a series of 32 aortic lesions with only 3 failures after a mean follow-up time of 2 years.[20] Johnston et al. separately analyzed aortic, common iliac, and external iliac lesions. Aortic and common iliac lesions responded significantly better than external iliac lesions, which surprisingly did not perform differently than femoropopliteal lesions.[13] In an analysis of 66 early iliac PTAs, the senior author noted an almost 20 per cent (89.5 per cent versus 70 per cent) patency difference in common versus external iliac dilations at 3 years, but most of this difference could be explained by a difference in early failure (13.5 per cent).[8]

Effect of Degree of Occlusion, Lesion Length, and Extent of Disease

When evaluating the six studies outlined in Table 26–1, it is important to consider the type of lesion treated, including indication for treatment, anatomical site of the lesion, degree of occlusion, and lesion length. The similarity of treated lesions among all these studies is striking, with the vast majority of lesions being short (less than 10 cm), iliac stenoses in patients with disabling claudication (Table 26–2). This homogeneity reveals the selection bias for focal lesions that still dominates the indications for iliac angioplasty. The poor technical results of early experiences with dilation of stenoses longer than 10 cm and complete iliac occlusions has dissuaded most investigators from continuing to treat these lesions with angioplasty alone, and because of a lack of sufficient data, the long-term patency for such lesions, even if successfully dilated, is difficult to estimate. When these latter lesions are included in a report of iliac angioplasty, one can suspect that the clinical indication is limb salvage and the patients overall condition is poor.

Johnston et al. presented the only convincing argument that outcome differences exist between short stenosis and occlusions.[13] He also demonstrated multifocal disease to have a poorer outcome than discrete disease. Other authors have been unable to show any difference between stenosis and occlusions, short versus long lesions, or single versus multiple lesions.[15,21] Colapinto et al. reported the treatment of 64 iliac occlusions, 37 greater than 5 cm in length, with a 78 per cent technical success rate and a 78 per cent cumulative patency at 4 years, similar to PTA of iliac stenosis.[22] Thus degree of occlusion, lesion length, and disease extent all clearly affect initial patency. How much these factors affect patency once a lesion is successfully dilated is less clear.

TABLE 26–2. FRACTIONS OF PATIENTS WITH FACTORS THOUGHT TO AFFECT PATENCY, FOR SIX STUDIES PRESENTED IN TABLE 26–1

Study Number	Indication		Site		Degree of Occlusion		Lesion Length
	C	LS	CI	EI	S	O	
1.	.80	.13	.53	.42	.94	.06	
2.	.90	.10			1.00	.00	.91 <2 cm
3.	.88	.12	.55	.43	.88	.12	
4.	.72	.28					1.00 <10 cm
5.	.80	.20			1.00	.00	1.00 < 3 cm
6.	.37	.63			1.00	.00	1.00 < 8 cm

C, claudication; CI, common iliac; S, stenosis; LS, limb salvage; EI, external iliac; O, occlusion.

Effect of Poor Runoff

The effect of downstream arterial occlusive disease is difficult to evaluate when, as they often do, investigators chose a hemodynamic criteria for patency that is affected by downstream disease, namely the ankle-brachial index. Preexisting femoropopliteal disease may mask a successful iliac dilation, and the subsequent development of distal disease may incorrectly suggest iliac PTA failure. Kumpe and Jones clearly demonstrated this when they reported both thigh and ankle measurements following iliac PTA and showed differences in patency estimates using these two endpoints of nearly 20 per cent at 1 year and 30 per cent at 2 years (Table 26–1).[11] To demonstrate the importance of runoff, serial evaluation of both thigh and ankle pressures is necessary, although duplex scanning may also help with this dilemma in the future.

Two studies reveal the impact of poor runoff on the ABI following iliac PTA. Runoff status was found to be a significant outcome predictor in both Johnston's univariate and multivariate analysis of patency, causing a 15 per cent difference in patency at 5 years.[13] Stokes demonstrated only 76 per cent patency at 1 year in diabetic patients with poor runoff compared to 95 per cent patency in patients with good runoff.[15] The difference at 5 years was 20 per cent compared with 77 per cent!

Effect of Diabetes

Because it is the characteristic of diabetic arteriosclerosis to involve the infrapopliteal vessels more than the proximal vessels, a higher proportion of diabetics would be expected to present for iliac PTA with multilevel disease, poor runoff, and limb-threatening ischemia. Stokes et al., in a 5-year evaluation of diabetic patients, including 127 who underwent iliac PTA, found 85 per cent patency at 1 year and 34 per cent at 5 years, the latter well below that reported by other authors for nondiabetic patients.[15] Seventy-one per cent of their patients presented in a limb salvage condition. When only those patients with good runoff and claudication were considered, patency was near 70 per cent at 5 years, similar to nondiabetic populations. Thus any effect of diabetes on PTA results is due to the additional distal disease, not diabetes itself.

Predicting Results for Iliac PTA

Taking into account the overestimation of iliac angioplasty success by using soft patency criteria and eliminating initial failures, and underestimation by using hemodynamic criteria that fail to distinguish progression of downstream disease, it is possible to predict overall 5-year patency following iliac angioplasty. Initial technical and hemodynamic success for percutaneous dilatation should be around 92 per cent (technical and hemodynamic failures each accounting for 4 per cent). A further 10 per cent of patients will fail early in the first year, (82 per cent 1-year patency), and another 12 per cent will fail over the next 4 years, for a 5-year patency of 70 per cent. As seen in Figure 26–1, the results of Kumpe and Jones,[11] using the thigh-brachial index (TBI) as an index of patency, came closest to the composite patency curve.

The clinical indication for the procedure, the anatomic site, and the condition of the runoff will significantly affect these results, and one can extrapolate in either direction from the composite results curve. For example, procedures performed for claudication will have improved results from the average 5-year patency of 70 per cent by approximately 10 per cent; if performed for limb salvage the results can be expected to decline by 10 per cent (i.e., 80 and 60 per cent, respectively). Patency for aortic and external iliac lesions will vary above and below common iliac results by 10 per cent. Runoff, specifically occlusion of the superficial femoral artery, may lower results by about 20 per cent at 5 years. Occlusions, stenosis greater than 10 cm, and multifocal disease will all also have lower initial and early patency results, but the patency at 5 years for these lesions is still unknown. Thus, we can expect the best results following dilatation of focal, common iliac stenoses in claudicating patients with patent superficial femoral arteries (80 to 85 per cent patency at 5 years). Changing any of these variables will result in worse results, and the effect of multiple variables will be additive. In the worst scenario, patency would probably drop to 40 to 50 per cent by 5 years.

PTA FOR INFRAINGUINAL OCCLUSIVE DISEASE

The results of PTA get progressively worse as one proceeds distally in the lower extremity in terms of technical success, degree of hemodynamic improvement, and long-term durability. Although the same can be said for arterial bypass, it is to a much lesser degree. In fact, the overall results of femoropopliteal PTA are such that it has difficulty competing with conservative therapy for the claudicator (i.e., exercise programs[4,5]). Therefore, one must carefully consider those factors which favorably influence PTA outcome in order to take advantage of its lesser mortality and morbidity versus bypass on the one hand, and justify its greater cost and morbidity over an exercise program for the claudicator on the other. Finally, analysis of the results of PTA for femoropopliteal occlusive disease, particularly for the longer lesions, should serve as the basis for evaluating other endovascular procedures (e.g., laser angioplasty, atherectomy).

Comparison with iliac disease holds some interesting numerical implications. As Martin[23] has pointed out, symptomatic femoropopliteal occlusive disease outnumbers aortoiliac disease by between 2:1 and 5:1, being closer to the latter in series made up only of candidates for intervention. In addition, if one accepts his premise that the main value of PTA is on short (less than 5 cm) occlusive lesions, his data indicate that 94 per cent of iliac stenoses and 30 per cent of iliac occlusions fall within these limits, but only 79 per cent of femoropopliteal stenoses and 9 per cent of occlusions would qualify. This and the fact that the less favorable occlusions outrank stenoses in the femoropopliteal segment by *at least* 2:1, explain why the use of PTA (in comparison to arterial bypass) even in "liberal" institutions has plateaued at around 35 per cent and, barring more effective new technology, is not likely to go higher. Finally, in spite of a predominance of up to 5:1 of femoropopliteal lesions in candidates for intervention, the worse initial and late results, the greater length of lesions, and the high proportion of occlusions all combine to make selection of bypass over PTA more likely at the femoropopliteal level. This is reflected in a lower proportion of femoropopliteal compared to iliac dilations in most series. For example, in the large University of Toronto experience, femoropopliteal dilations made up only 25.7 per cent of the total.[24]

Overall Results for Femoropopliteal Lesions

There are more than 40 articles in the literature which present the results of femoropopliteal (FP) PTA, and although some contribute worthwhile information on specific aspects, less than a third of them yield meaningful data on long-term patency. Some of these results, primarily those with serial data over time, are summarized in Table 26–3. In studying PTA results, two North American series are particularly noteworthy because of their large number of patients and their careful, in-depth analysis using objective criteria: the University of Toronto series[13] reported by Johnston, and the University of Pennsylvania experience summarized by Berkowitz.[25,26] In addition, Adar[27] has recently made a meaningful contribution to our understanding of FP-PTA results by subjecting what he considered the most complete and informative reports to confidence profile analysis, producing a composite estimate of the durability of FP-PTA success with time, including a separate breakdown for those treated for claudication and for limb salvage (see Table 26–4). Estimates from these combined data projected an early (30-day) overall success rate of 86 ± 3 per cent with continuing "patency" at 6 months of 73 ± 4 per cent, at 1 year of 66 ± 5 per cent, at 2 years of 61 ± 4 per cent, at 3 years at 58 ± 6 per cent, and at 5 years of 60 ± 5 per cent. In general, reports from European centers present a more favorable impression of PTA durability than those from North America, and this is reflected in Adar's projections. The suggested explanations—greater skill or selectivity versus more demanding criteria of success or treating more difficult lesions—cannot be easily reconciled. What is apparent from Adar's figures, however, is that there is still a much greater technical failure rate compared to that for dilating iliac stenoses, and that after a high restenosis rate over the first year, averaging 13 per cent at 6 months and 20 per cent by 12 months, the patency curve flattens out in the range of 60 per cent by 2 years with minimal additional fall thereafter. For most North

TABLE 26–3. LONG-TERM PATENCY OF FEMOROPOPLITEAL PTA[a]

Study Number	Author	Years				
		1	2	3	4	5
Initial failures excluded						
	Krepel[31]		.77			
	Gallino[48]		.71	.70		
	Schneider[49]	(.74)[b]	.70			.70
	Waltman[50]	.86	.84		.70	(.67)[b]
	Greenfield[44]	.89	.84	.73	.69	.68
Initial failures included						
1.	[c]Gallino[48]	.63	.62			
2.	Berkowitz[25]		.67	.61		
3.	[c]Waltman[50]	.73	.70	.63		
4.	[c]Greenfield[44]	.72	.68	.62		.58
5.	[d]Adar[27]	.66	.61	.58		.59
6.	[e]Johnston[13]	.63	.53	.50	.44	.40

[a] From Stokes KR, et al: Five-year results of iliac and femoropopliteal angioplasty in diabetic patients. Radiology 1990; *174*:977–982.
[b] From other article by same author(s).
[c] Adjusted for initial failure rate by Adar et al.[27]
[d] Estimated from the literature (including most of the above studies) using confidence profile analysis.
[e] Also required improvement in clinical grade.

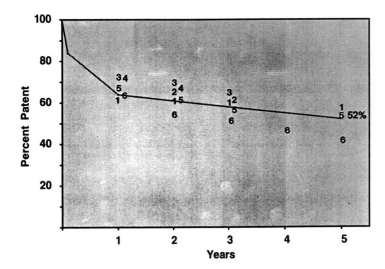

FIGURE 26–2. Composite patency curve for femoropopliteal PTA, based on the literature, and particularly on the data including initial failures from reports featured in Table 26–3, indicated by study number. Note closeness of curve to data from report number 5.

American experiences, this late plateau is closer to 40 per cent. Figure 26–2 shows a composite patency curve for femoropopliteal PTAs using data and taking the latter into consideration. The 52 per cent, 5-year patency rate represents a compromise between data from European and North American literature and reflects the gradually improving results from more discriminating patient selection and improving technique.

Effect of Clinical Status: Claudication versus Limb Salvage as an Indication

Table 26–4 shows Adar's data on this important consideration, with a close to 20 per cent difference seen between the results of these two groups by 3 years and with clearly widening confidence limits. Much of this difference relates to lower technical and early (clinical) success rates in the limb salvage (LS) group versus the intermittent claudication (IC) group, but it results in 5-year success rates of 60 and 40 per cent for FP-PTA performed for IC and LS, respectively. The early data (e.g., a 70 per cent 1-year patency) are interesting when viewed against the early patency rates for other endovascular procedures now being reported, for they have been promoted as better alternatives to PTA and, although meaningful comparisons must take the degree of occlusion and length of lesion into consideration, it would appear that for the most part, they have not lived up to expectations.

TABLE 26–4. COMPARISON OF SUCCESS/PATENCY RATES FOR FEMOROPOPLITEAL PTA: CLAUDICATION VERSUS LIMB THREAT[a]

Length of Follow-up	Claudication (%)	Limb Threat (%)
30 days	89.1 ± 2.5	76.8 ± 4.0
6 months	81.1 ± 2.7	60.7 ± 4.4
1 year	69.8 ± 4.2	50.3 ± 6.4
2 years	63.7 ± 8.1	46.6 ± 6.5
3 years	62.4 ± 9.1	43.1 ± 7.2

[a] Adapted with permission from Adar R, et al: A confidence profile analysis of the results of femoropopliteal percutaneous transluminal angioplasty in the treatment of lower-extremity ischemia. J Vasc Surg 1989; *10*:57–67.

Effect of Degree of Occlusion

In general, the PTA results for total occlusion are 10 to 20 per cent worse than for stenoses in the femoropopliteal segment. In fact, Jorgensen et al.[23] have reported only half of the long-term success for occlusions as stenoses (26 per cent versus 52 per cent) with an early rethrombosis rate of 41 per cent for the former. Graziani,[29] on the other hand, showed an almost threefold difference in the technical success and late patency rates in favor of PTA for femoropopliteal versus iliac total occlusions (73 per cent versus 28 per cent technical success and 66 per cent versus 22 per cent "late" patency). They claim that, as relatively poor as are the results of dilating femoropopliteal occlusions, the results for complete iliac occlusions are even worse. However, the preliminary use of thrombolytic therapy may change this impression.[30] Berkowitz[26] showed an 18 to 20 per cent difference between the late results for stenosis and occlusion for lower extremity PTA (48 per cent versus 28 per cent at 5 years), with two thirds of this difference being apparent from the outset in initial success rates of 88 per cent versus 74 per cent, respectively. The Toronto group[13] has presented similar data for femoropopliteal PTA, with a 17 per cent difference in 5-year patency for those done for stenosis and for occlusion with good runoff, whether the indication was IC (53 per cent versus 36 per cent) or LS (38 per cent versus 21 per cent). Fourteen to eighteen per cent differences were seen in the poor-runoff group at 5 years (40 per cent versus 22 per cent for IC and 24 per cent versus 10 per cent for LS).

Effect of Length of Lesion

Not unexpectedly, the shorter the lesion dilated, the better the results. Krepel's 5-year results (excluding initial failures) show this for both stenoses and occlusions, with a greater difference seen for the latter.[31] Using 3 cm as the dividing point, their 5-year patency was 89 per cent for short versus 26 per cent for long occlusions. Using 2 cm to separate short from long stenoses, the 5-year patencies were 77 per cent and 54 per cent, respectively. Jeans[32] reported a more detailed breakdown, with a steadily decreasing 5-year success rate for longer occlusions (37 per cent for 0 to 4 cm, 43 per cent for 4 to 9 cm, 29 per cent for 9 to 14 cm, and 17 per cent for greater than 14 cm). These latter results *include* early failures.

Effect of Poor Runoff

Poor runoff adversely effects the outcome of PTA just as it does for bypass. Krepel's 5-year patencies for FP-PTA were 77 per cent for good runoff and 59 per cent for poor runoff.[31] Johnston's 5-year results,[13] which include initial failures and stricter criteria for success, are in the range of 50 per cent for good runoff and 25 per cent for poor runoff. In this series, there was a 13 to 14 per cent difference related to runoff, whether performed for claudication versus limb salvage, or stenosis versus occlusion. The Cleveland Clinic experience, reported by Graor,[33] shows a steady dropoff in intermediate patency of femoropopliteal dilations as the number of patent infrapopliteal vessels decreased from 3 (75 per cent) to 2 (63 per cent) to 1 (43 per cent). In the University of Colorado early experience, the late success rate (at 3 years) was 65 per cent for good and 44 per cent for poor runoff, after excluding initial failures.[8]

Extent of Diseases in the Treated Arterial Segment

This focuses on the evidence of disease *adjacent* to the dilated lesion in the same arterial segment. However, length of (dilated) lesion and extent of adjacent disease commonly go together and, therefore, there is considerable cross-correlation. In the previously mentioned series from Holland by Krepe,[31] an 83 per cent 5-year success rate was reported for initially successful femoropopliteal dilations in which the lesion was discrete, as opposed to 62 per cent for diffusely involved segments. In the same series, stenoses with an eccentric lumen had a 77 per cent 5-year success rate versus 69 per cent for concentric stenoses. In the University of Colorado experience, when a single FP lesion was dilated, the 5-year patency was 55 per cent versus 18 per cent when multiple lesions were dilated in that same segment.[8]

The Effect of Calcification

Calcification in and around the occlusive lesion does not, in itself, appear to adversely affect long-term patency. In fact, in the University of Colorado experience,[8] calcified lesions fared somewhat better (59 per cent versus 42 per cent patency at 3 years).

The Effect of Diabetes

Diabetes appears to correlate with worse results following transluminal angioplasty if one looks at overall results where iliac and femoropopliteal disease are lumped together. However, this is because of the characteristically different distribution of lesions in diabetics; that is, they have proportionately fewer of the more favorable proximal iliac lesions and more disease in the infrapopliteal (runoff) vessels. In our series and others where the results are separated by anatomic site, there is no difference at either level for diabetics versus nondiabetics, but in one large series, while no difference was found for iliac dilations, diabetics had only a 53 per cent success rate with femoropopliteal dilations versus 85 per cent for nondiabetics.[34] Again, if there is an effect of diabetes, it probably relates to the frequent presence of infrapopliteal occlusive lesions which produced "poor runoff."

Effect of Initial Hemodynamic Response on Ultimate Success

It seems almost axiomatic that the degree of hemodynamic improvement should correlate positively with late success (durability). Ordinarily, a poor hemodynamic response to the dilation of an isolated lesion means incomplete restoration of luminal patency, so that very little restenosis will be required to result in failure detectable by objective criteria. In contrast, a poor hemodynamic response to successfully dilating a lesion proximal to significant residual distal occlusive disease may be due to either inadequate dilation or the distal disease, although usually the latter. Even if the dilation site can be shown to be functionally patent by discriminating noninvasive testing, its late success rate can be expected to be worse because of the poor runoff (see above). Thus, a poor initial hemodynamic response correlates with poor patency for several reasons. We and others[11,35–39] have reported that the rate of late deterioration or failure is considerably higher in those with lesser degrees of initial hemodynamic improvement. In our experience, iliac PTAs with marked hemodynamic improvement enjoyed an 85 per cent 3-year functional patency rate compared to 65 per cent for those only minimally or moderately improved.[8] For FP-PTAs, it was observed that none of the minimally improved cases were still patent at 6 months. Furthermore, gradations of initial hemodynamic improvement were identified within the FP group with a satisfactory initial result which, in retrospect, correlated with durability. Those who sustained their initial good response (average late ABI 1.0 or above) had an initial ABI increase of from 0.68 to 1.04. Those who later deteriorated (to an average ABI of 0.75) had a mean initial ABI response of from 0.51 to 0.96, while those that ultimately failed (all by 9 months) had an initial ABI increase from 0.38 to 0.85. These data indicate that, while either poor runoff or incomplete dilatation contributed to failure in the latter group, deterioration was primarily a restenosis phenomenon.

Effect of Combinations of Factors which Adversely Affect Outcome

Many of the above-mentioned factors are present in varying combinations in a given patient, and estimating their combined impact is a much more difficult task. Cambria et al.[40] reported that claudication (versus LS), focal lesion (versus long stenosis or occlusion), immediate restoration of pulses, good runoff, and no diabetes were all favorable predictors of long-term success after lower extremity PTA, but clearly the last three and probably the first of these characteristics are, to a large degree, interdependent. Jeans et al.,[32] in an analysis of PTA results with a commendable 97 per cent follow-up, showed that when femoropopliteal stenosis was combined with good runoff, the 3-year patency rate was 78 per cent, whereas at the other extreme, when femoropopliteal occlusion was associated with poor runoff, only 25 per cent were still patent at 3 years. Berkowitz[25] performed an analysis of factors significantly affecting PTA outcome, citing four: length of lesion, clinical status, degree of occlusion, and presence of diabetes, each of which resulted in a 15 to 25 per cent difference in 5-year patency, but his data combined iliac and femoropopliteal lesions. Johnston et al. made a similar analysis, but used the Cox linear regression method to predict outcome after PTA and also identified four factors—clinical status, location of lesion dilated, degree of occlusion, and "runoff"—as dominating the analysis, with 5-year patencies for femoropopliteal dilations ranging between 53 per cent and 10 per cent from the best to the worst scenario.[13] The degree of occlusion appeared to make a greater difference in patency (20 to 22 per cent at 3 and 5 years) than runoff (15 to 17 per cent at 3 and 5 years).

Predicting Outcome of Femoropopliteal PTA

While Adar's confidence profile analysis of FP-PTA, giving approximately 60 per cent and 40 per cent for 5-year success rates for IC and LS, respectively, is encouraging, it contains a preponderance of European data. Multifactorial analysis, featured in several key North American experiences cited above, which characteristically include initial failures and stricter criteria of success, suggests to the authors that a 60 per cent 5-year patency after FP-PTA represents the best scenario (i.e., a claudicator with a discreet stenosis and good runoff) and that one should probably subtract 12 to 15 per cent from the 5-year patency for each of these three major negative factors. Thus, a limb salvage patient with a total occlusion and poor runoff could only expect a 15 per cent ± 5 per cent 5-year success rate. The reason composite data from many series yield a close to 50 per cent 5-year patency for femoropopliteal PTA (see Fig. 26–2) is that most patients selected for PTA are claudicators with discrete lesions and good runoff. It also must be realized that limb salvage rates will run consistently higher than actual patency rates, just as they do for bypass. For example, Milford et al.[7] reported a 43 per cent 2-year overall limb salvage rate for femoropopliteal PTAs, which increased to 64 per cent in those whose PTA was technically successful and demonstrated initial hemodynamic improvement. Thus, limb salvage rates, in those who have FP-PTA for limb-threatening ischemia, characteristically run 20 per cent to 30 per cent higher than true patency rates by 5 years.

PTA FOR INFRAPOPLITEAL ARTERY OCCLUSIVE DISEASE

Now that the soft, low-profile catheters developed for coronary dilation have been modified for tibial use, PTA of infrapopliteal arteries is becoming increasingly common, but to date there are only about a half dozen series reported, and even those have only 1 to 3 years follow-up. Horvath, from Linz, Austria,[41] reports 103 tibial lesions dilated, with a 96 per cent technical success and a cumulative patency of 80 per cent at 1 year, 75 per cent at 2 years, and 65 per cent at 3 years. Schwarten[42] reports a 97 per cent technical success rate and an 83 per cent 2-year limb salvage rate in a group of patients who were essentially all smokers with threatened limbs, two thirds of whom were diabetics. Brown[43] and Greenfield[44] report 75 per cent and 81 per cent 1-year LS rates, respectively, but Sprayregen[45] and Tamura[46] et al., report only 40 and 33 per cent success rates at 1.5 and 2 years, respectively. The reason for these marked differences is not clear, but it is suspected that the latter reports focused on evidence of patency (i.e., continued improvement) and not mere avoidance of amputation. Unfortunately, many of these PTAs were done as one or more of several dilations performed for multilevel disease.[47] This, and the difficulty of assessing the individual patency of one of three peroneal/tibial vessels, precludes accurate appraisal of the patency of tibial PTA from the current literature.

SUMMARY

The long-term results of PTA for lower extremity arteriosclerotic occlusive disease gathered from current literature reflect a wide range of success rates, partly due to differing reporting standards and differing patient/lesion mixes. It is not only necessary to separate PTA results for anatomic site (since femoropopliteal PTAs have twice the immediate and early failure rates of iliac PTA's) (Fig. 26–3), but within each category, degree of occlusion, length of lesion, and runoff status all clearly influence outcome, and initial hemodynamic response also has predictive value. Fortunately, the relative impact of most of these factors on success rate is now well documented, which allows one to extrapolate on either side of the composite average and predict outcome with reasonable accuracy for specific lesions and clinical settings. These estimates, when initial technical and hemodynamic failure rates are also taken into consideration, should help guide choice of therapy, as well as provide standards

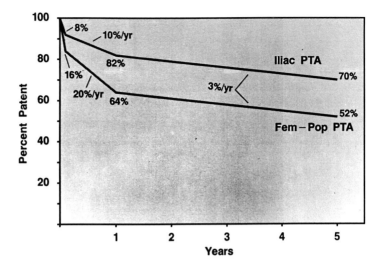

FIGURE 26–3. Composite patency curve for iliac and femoropopliteal PTA. Note that the initial and early failure rates for the femoropopliteal group are twice that of the iliac group; however after the first year the failure rates for both groups are similar.

against which the results of other new percutaneous endovascular revascularization techniques may be compared.

REFERENCES

1. Dotter CT, Judkins MP: Transluminal treatment of arteriosclerotic obstruction. Description of a new technique and a preliminary report of its application. Circulation 1964;*30*:654.
2. Grüntzig A, Hopff H: Perkutane Rekanalisation chronischer arterieller Verschlusse mit einem neuen Dilatations-Katheter. Dtsch Med Wochenschr 1974;*99*:2502.
3. Rutherford RB: Standards for evaluating the results of interventional therapy for peripheral vascular disease. Circulation 1991;*83*:(suppl 2):6–11.
4. Creasy TS, McMillan PJ, Fletcher EWL, et al: Is percutaneous transluminal angioplasty better than exercise for claudication?—Preliminary results from a prospective randomized trial. Eur J Vasc Surg 1990;*4*:135.
5. Van Rij AM, et al: Information presented at the XIXth World Congress of the International Society for Cardiovascular Surgery, Toronto, Canada, September 8, 1989.
6. Wilson SE, Wolf GL, Cross AP: Percutaneous transluminal angioplasty versus operation for peripheral arteriosclerosis. Report of a prospective randomized trial in a selected group of patients. J Vasc Surg 1989;*9*(1):1–9.
7. Milford MA, Weaver FA, Lundell CJ, et al: Femoropopliteal percutaneous transluminal angioplasty for limb salvage. J Vasc Surg 1988;*8*(3):292–299.
8. Rutherford RB, Patt A, Kumpe DA: The current role of percutaneous transluminal angioplasty. *In* Greenhalgh KM, Jamieson CW, Nicolaides AN, eds: Vascular Surgery: Issues in Current Practice. London, Grune & Stratton, 1986;229–244.
9. Rutherford RB, Flanigan DP, Gupta SK, et al: Suggested standards for reports dealing with lower extremity ischemia. J Vasc Surg 1986;*4*:80–94.
10. Rutherford RB, Becker GJ: Standards for evaluating and reporting the results of surgical and percutaneous therapy for peripheral arterial disease. JVIR 1991;*2*:169–174.
11. Kumpe DA, Jones DN: Percutaneous transluminal angioplasty. Appl Radiol 1982;*11*:29–40.
12. van Andel GJ, van Erp WF, Krepel VM, Breslau PJ: Percutaneous transluminal dilatation of the iliac artery: Long-term results. Radiology 1985;*156*:321–323.
13. Johnston KW, Rae M, Hogg JS, et al: 5-year results of a prospective study of percutaneous transluminal angioplasty. Ann Surg 1987;*206*(4):403–413.
14. In der Maur GTD, Boeve J, Kerdel MC, et al: Angioplasty of the iliac and femoral arteries. Initial and long-term results in short stenotic lesions. Eur J Radiol 1990;*11*(3):163–167.
15. Stokes KR, Strunk HM, Campbell DR, et al: Five-year results of iliac and femoropopliteal angioplasty in diabetic patients. Radiology 1990;*174*:977–982.
16. Jorgensen B, Henriksen LO, Karle A, et al: Percutaneous transluminal angioplasty of iliac and femoral arteries in severe lower limb ischaemia. Acta Chir Scand 1988;*154*(11–12):647–652.
17. Hasson JE, Archer CW, Wojtowycz M, et al: Lower extremity percutaneous transluminal angioplasty: Multifactorial analysis of morbidity and mortality. Surgery 1990;*108*:748–754.

18. Henriksen LO, Jorgensen B, Holstein PE, et al: Percutaneous transluminal angioplasty of infrarenal arteries in intermittent claudication. Acta Chir Scand 1988;*154*(10):573–576.

19. Odurny A, Colapinto RF, Sniderman KW, et al: Percutaneous transluminal angioplasty of abdominal aortic stenoses. Cardiovasc Intervent Radiol 1989;*12*:1–6.

20. Yakes WF, Kumpe DA, Brown SB, et al: Percutaneous transluminal aortic angioplasty: Techniques and results. Radiology 1989;*172*:965–970.

21. Walden R, Siegel Y, Rubinstein, et al: Percutaneous transluminal angioplasty. A suggested method for analysis of clinical, arteriographic and hemodynamic factors affecting the results of treatment. J Vasc Surg 1986;*3*(4):583–590.

22. Colapinto RF, Stronell RD, Johnston WK: Transluminal angioplasty of complete iliac occlusions. AJR 1986;*146*:859–862.

23. Martin EC: Introduction. Circulation 1991;*83*(2)(suppl I):1–5.

24. Morin JF, Johnston KW, Wasserman L, et al: Factors that determine the long-term results of percutaneous transluminal dilatation for peripheral arterial occlusive disease. J Vasc Surg 1986;*4*(1):68–72.

25. Berkowitz HD, Spence RK, Frieman DB, et al: Long-term results of transluminal angioplasty of the femoral arteries. *In* Dotter CT, Grüntzig A, Schoop W, Zietler E, eds: Percutaneous Transluminal Angioplasty. Berlin, Springer-Verlag, 1983;207–214.

26. Berkowitz HD: Percutaneous arterial dilation for atherosclerotic lower extremity occlusive disease. *In* Ernst CB, Stanley JC, eds: Current Therapy in Vascular Surgery. 2nd ed. Philadelphia, BC Decker, 1991;473–475.

27. Adar R, Critchfield GC, Eddy DM: A confidence profile analysis of the results of femoropopliteal percutaneous transluminal angioplasty in the treatment of lower-extremity ischemia. J Vasc Surg 1989;*10*:57–67.

28. Jorgensen B, Meisner S, Holstein P, et al: Early rethrombosis in femoropopliteal occlusions treated with percutaneous transluminal angioplasty. Eur J Vasc Surg 1990;*4*(2):149–152.

29. Graziani L: Percutaneous recanalization of total iliac and femoropopliteal artery occlusions. Eur J Radiol 1987;*7*(2):91–93.

30. Motarjeme A: Thrombolytic therapy in arterial occlusions and graft thrombosis. Semin Vasc Surg 1989;*2*(3):155–178.

31. Krepel VM, van Andel GJ, van Erp WRM, et al: Percutaneous transluminal angioplasty of the femoropopliteal artery: Initial and long term results. Radiology 1985;*156*:325–328.

32. Jeans WD, Armstrong S, Cole SE, et al: Fate of patients undergoing transluminal angioplasty for lower limb ischemia. Radiology 1990;*177*(2):559–564.

33. Graor RA, Young JR, McCandless M, et al: Percutaneous transluminal angioplasty: Review of iliac and femoral dilatations at the Cleveland Clinic. Cleve Clin Q 1984;*51*(1):149–154.

34. Lally ME, Johnston KW, Andrews D: Percutaneous transluminal dilation of peripheral arteries: An analysis of factors predicting early success. J Vasc Surg 1984;*1*:704–709.

35. Kalman PG, Johnston KW: Outcome of a failed percutaneous transluminal dilation. Surg Gynecol Obstet 1985;*161*:43–46.

36. Lu CT, Zarins CK, Yang CF, et al: Percutaneous transluminal angioplasty for limb salvage. Radiology 1982;*142*:337–341.

37. Johnston KW, Colapinto RF, Baird RJ: Transluminal dilation: An alternative? Arch Surg 1982;*117*:1604–1609.

38. Glover JL, Bendick PJ, Dilley RS, et al: Efficacy of balloon catheter dilatation for lower extremity atherosclerosis. Surgery 1982;*91*:560–565.

39. Katzen BJ: Percutaneous transluminal angioplasty for arterial disease of the lower extremities. AJR 1984;*142*:23–25.

40. Cambria RP, Faust G, Gusberg R, et al: Percutaneous angioplasty for peripheral arterial occlusive disease. Correlates of clinical success. Arch Surg 1987;*122*(3):283–287.

41. Horvath W, Oertl M, Haidinger D: Percutaneous transluminal angioplasty of crural arteries. Radiology 1990;*177*(2):565–569.

42. Schwarten DE: Clinical and anatomical considerations for nonoperative therapy in tibial disease and the results of angioplasty. Circulation 1991;*83*(suppl I):86–90.

43. Brown KT, Schoenbert NY, Moore ED, et al: Percutaneous transluminal angioplasty of infrapopliteal vessels: Preliminary results and technical considerations. Radiology 1988;*169*:75–78.

44. Greenfield AJ: Femoral, popliteal, and tibial arteries: Percutaneous transluminal angioplasty. AJR 1980;*135*:927–935.

45. Sprayregen S, Sniderman KW, Sos TA, et al: Popliteal artery branches: Percutaneous transluminal angioplasty. AJR 1980;*135*:945–977.

46. Tamura S, Sniderman KW, Beinart C, et al: Percutaneous transluminal angioplasty of the popliteal artery and its branches. Radiology 1982;*143*:645–648.

47. Dake MD, Katzen BT: The current state of percutaneous transluminal angioplasty in peripheral vascular disease. *In* Veith FJ, ed: Current Critical Problems in Vascular Surgery, Vol 2. St. Louis, MO, Quality Medical Publishing, Inc., 1990;145–154.

48. Gallino A, Mahler F, Probst P, Nachbur B: Percutaneous transluminal angioplasty of the arteries of the lower limbs: A 5 year follow-up. Circulation 1984;*70*:619–623.

49. Schneider E, Grüntzig A, Bollinger A: Long-term patency rates after percutaneous transluminal angioplasty for iliac and femoropopliteal obstructions. *In* Dotter CT, Gruntzig A, Schoop W, Zeitler E, eds: Percutaneous Transluminal Angioplasty. Berlin, Springer-Verlag, 1983;175–180.
50. Waltman AC, Greenfield AJ, Novelline RA, et al. Transluminal angioplasty of the iliac and femoropopliteal arteries. Arch Surg 1982;*117:*1218–1221.

27

EXCIMER LASER TREATMENT OF FEMORAL ARTERY ATHEROSCLEROSIS

WALTER J. McCARTHY, ROBERT L. VOGELZANG,
WILLIAM H. PEARCE, WILLIAM R. FLINN, and JAMES S.T. YAO

Physicians have been intrigued by the possibility of removing occluding atherosclerotic plaque since the pathophysiology of ischemia was understood. Surgical arterial endarterectomy was devised to this end and has addressed specific occluding lesions with some success. In the modern era of vascular surgery, bypass of occluding lesions with autologous tissue or even prosthetic material has become the standard to which all other techniques must be compared. Recently, the advent of a group of procedures loosely termed "endovascular surgery" has ushered in the possibility of relieving arterial occlusions without direct surgical exposure or anesthetic-related morbidity. These procedures, usually performed percutaneously from a distant site, either disrupt atheroma mechanically or dislodge it by thermal or other means.

The era of endovascular treatment allowing reshaping of atherosclerosis without direct surgical exposure might be dated from November 1964 when Charles Dotter and Melvin Judkins published their work on arterial dilatation.[1] Their technique involved passing graduated Teflon dilating catheters over a guide wire and effectively opening some arterial stenoses. The concept of working within an artery to relieve stenosis was further advanced by Andreas Gruentzig, who performed the first percutaneous transluminal coronary balloon angioplasty in September 1977.[2] Gruentzig had treated 169 patients in Zurich by October 1980, and a decade later the worldwide acceptance of this technique is well known.[3] Balloon catheter angioplasty has subsequently been used to treat atherosclerotic stenoses of virtually every artery and is now familiar to all vascular surgeons.

There are at least three well-established limitations of balloon angioplasty. These include difficulty in passing a guide wire through totally occluded arterial lesions and thus the inability to position the balloon catheter. Immediate elastic restenosis following the balloon angioplasty or failure to achieve any dilatation due to calcification are problems sometimes encountered. Finally, if the balloon angioplasty is initially successful, biological regrowth restenosis quite reliably occurs in 25 to 30 per cent of patients in the early follow-up period.

To address these three basic problems, a number of mechanical and thermal devices have been developed for atheroma manipulation.[4] These include high-speed rotary atherectomy catheters, side-biting atherectomy catheters, and devices conceived to ablate atheroma by ultrasonic vibration. In addition, it is feasible to ablate atheroma with energy transmitted in the form of laser light, and virtually all available laser wavelengths have been tried in this capacity. Early on in the experimenting with lasers and arteries, argon and carbon dioxide (CO_2) lasers and those derived from neodynium: yttrium-aluminum-garnet (Nd-YAG) sources predominated.[5,6] These were chosen largely because they were available for medical purposes and also because at least the argon and Nd-YAG wavelengths could be transmitted through available flexible fiberoptic cables. Carbon dioxide laser can be used to ablate atheroma, but to date, a flexible wave guide has not superseded the rigid wave guides usually employed. Lasers have been used in large clinical series not only as direct contact devices whereby the laser energy is in contact with atheroma, but also as heating devices. A number of ingenious heated caps allow the actual energy in the laser light to be thermally converted, and then may be pushed through occluding atheroma. There are even caps that split the light, allowing some laser energy to impact on tissue and some to heat the cap itself. The purpose of this chapter is not to review the complex, divergent, and ever-changing field of laser-assisted atherectomy, but rather to focus on the use of a specific group of lasers referred to as excimer lasers and their use in arteries.

Excimer lasers are relatively new in the medical arena and have tremendous theoretical appeal. They are able to vaporize tissue without generating significant heat,[7-9] calcified material is relatively susceptible, and passage through fiberoptic systems is possible with appropriately long pulse widths.[10] Excimer is a contraction of the two words "excited dimer." Inert gases from the same column in the periodic table, argon, xenon, or krypton, are combined with the halogens chloride or fluorine. Electrical energy is used to ionize these atoms, and an excited state of the inert gas plus the halogen is then formed. This returns to a lower energy state, and the alternating process generates the characteristic wavelength of the laser. Excimer lasers are thus available using ArF at 193 nm, KrCl at 222 nm, XeCl at 308 nm, and XeF at 351 nm.[11] These wavelengths are all in the ultraviolet range, which explains their excellent absorption by tissue and also at least a theoretic concern regarding cellular mutagenicity. Excimer lasers are all delivered in a pulsed mode, not in the continuous-wave form. Background laboratory work supports the clinical findings of excellent tissue penetration with minimal thermal effect.[12-17]

EXCIMER LASER TECHNIQUE

The experience at Northwestern University with the excimer laser and the femoral location is based on a xenon chloride pulsed 308-nm instrument purchased from Advanced Interventional Systems of Irvine, California.[18] This is the first commercially available excimer laser for angioplasty in the United States. The unit is magnetically switched, using 200-nsec pulses at between 10 and 40 Hz. The long pulse width is critical and is one of the engineering contributions of this unit. Previously, shorter pulse widths with the same energy had rapidly destroyed existing fiberoptic catheters. With the longer pulse width, the burst of energy is essentially spread out and does not destructively stress the conducting fiber.

Three separate catheters have been utilized for treatment in the Northwestern experience. Specifically, for complete arterial occlusion and the inability to pass a guide wire, a 7-F balloon catheter with a 2-cm × 4- to 7-mm balloon is available. This is used to centrally position a 600-μm single fiber 3.3-F (1.1-mm) fiberoptic tip. The concept is that the balloon is first inflated within the proximal patent artery and thus stabilizes and centrally locates the laser fiber. The activated laser fiber can then be passed manually down through the occluded vessel. For patients with a complete arterial occlusion, the balloon catheter is first positioned proximal to the lesion in question. The laser fiber is guided with fluoroscopic control and is advanced at a rate of less than 1 mm/sec into the arterial occlusion. Obviously, the risk of perforation is higher with this relatively blind end-on approach, and in an attempt to limit this problem, the laser catheter is never advanced more than 2 cm beyond the end of the balloon tip. Once the 2-cm progress is made, the balloon-centering device can be deflated and then advanced over the laser catheter. The process can be repeated until the occluded arterial segment has been completely penetrated. After a central channel is achieved, a standard guide wire can be positioned to allow conventional balloon angioplasty (Fig. 27–1).

Two over-the-wire fibers are available, and are used if a guide wire can be

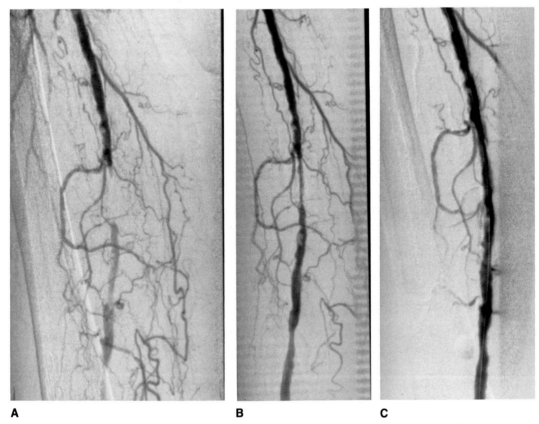

A   B   C

FIGURE 27–1. *A*, This superficial femoral artery occlusion caused the patient to present with toe gangrene. *B*, The excimer laser was easily passed through the occlusion, but the resulting channel was obviously of inadequate caliber for good hemodynamic result. *C*, After conventional balloon angioplasty, the superficial femoral artery occlusion attained good anatomic patency.

initially placed (Fig. 27–2). A 6.6-F (2.2-mm) device composed of multiple separate fibers is used over a 0.018-inch guide wire. A smaller 4.7-F catheter can also be used over a 0.018-inch wire if a smaller diameter is appropriate. This device uses 12 200-μm fibers. With the catheters available, the maximum lumen generated with laser alone is 2.2 mm. Thus, for all femoral or popliteal applications, the lumen must be expanded using conventional balloon angioplasty. When an over-the-wire catheter is used, the 0.018-inch wire is first

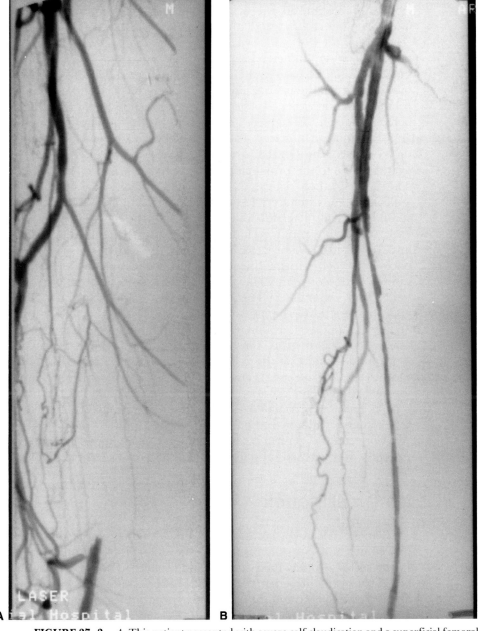

A   B

FIGURE 27–2. *A,* This patient presented with severe calf claudication and a superficial femoral artery occlusion from its origin at the common femoral to the adductor hiatus. *B,* It was possible to traverse this entire area with the excimer laser and then complete balloon angioplasty for reasonable anatomic success. This patient, however, went on to thrombose the recently treated artery and required femoropopliteal bypass.

positioned through the stenotic lesion. Then the laser catheter can be advanced to the area just proximal to the stenotic region. The laser is then activated and the catheter advanced to ablate the lesion.

The individual laser fiberoptic catheters are purchased from Advanced Interventional Systems and are not reusable. After the laser has had time to equilibrate, the actual energy output at the fiberoptic tip is calibrated using a meter built into the laser unit. The output at the completion of the procedure (or if changes are made in power output) is also measured by the meter. Calibration is set to emit 35 to 50 mJ/mm^2.

At our institution, the general approach to all arterial occlusions is to first attempt guide-wire passage and use every possible trick and technique to be successful with the guide wire. Thus, the lesions addressed with the end-on balloon-centered catheter are truly those inaccessible to a guide wire. If the guide wire can be passed, then an over-the-wire catheter is always used. These over-the-wire catheters are much less prone to perforation than the balloon-centered end-on variety. In the usual setting, a complete aortogram is performed before the laser procedure, and then using the ipsilateral femoral approach, an 8-F introducer is placed. Patients are heparinized with 5000 units of heparin on a routine basis. Once a wire has been passed, the laser catheter is advanced over the wire to the proximal portion of the arterial stenosis or occluded area. The laser is then activated and passed forward by hand at the rate of approximately 1 mm/sec. Experience has shown that treatment for 10 to 20 seconds is ideal. The slow rate of advancement was selected so that the laser itself would cut through occluding tissue rather than dilatation being performed in a Dotter-like dilator capacity. Usually the catheter is passed several times once a channel is formed, to completely sculpt the stenotic surface. In every case to date, conventional balloon angioplasty has been used following the initial laser channeling. This technique is well known and uses catheters of appropriate size for the measured arterial diameter.

One supposed advantage of excimer laser is its ability to pass 'hrough calcified arterial disease. The experience from our initial review is that this is well founded and that the catheter could always be passed once a guide wire was placed. The excimer seemed to cut through tissue with little difficulty, and the rate of catheter advance was usually limited only by the agreed upon 1 mm/sec rate. The calculated actual laser on-time ranged from 18 to 306 seconds for the initial patients studied and reported.

Conventional aspirin treatment using 325 mg/day is recommended for all patients. This is based on policies established for balloon angioplasty.

PATIENT SELECTION

Patient selection has much to do with the outcome of interventional procedures and can sway results in either a favorable or unfavorable direction. In the series of individuals studied and treated at Northwestern, there are two broad categories of patients. The first group includes those who presented with intermittent claudication but are reluctant to undergo femoropopliteal bypass. These patients often agree to a laser-assisted angioplasty. Patients from this group are generally younger and have much less severe occlusive disease than those with limb-threatening ischemia. The second group of patients studied are those presenting with limb-threatening ischemia, including rest pain, foot gangrene or ulceration, and multiple severe medical disabilities (Fig. 27–3).

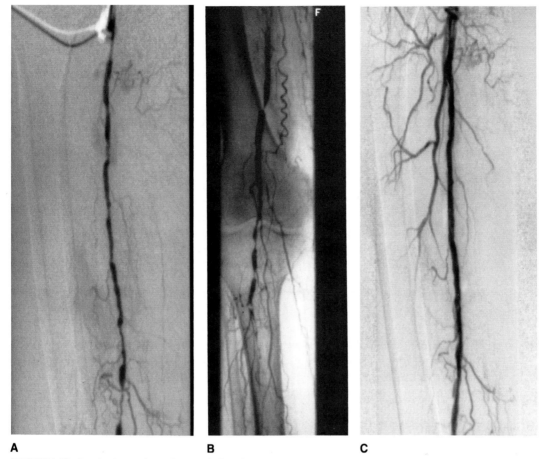

A   **B**   **C**

FIGURE 27–3. *A,* A number of very challenging cases were attempted in the initial series. Included is this elderly renal dialysis patient with severe foot ischemia. She was deemed too unstable for an operative procedure. *B,* Besides superficial femoral artery stenosis, the tibial runoff below the popliteal level was extremely limited. *C,* With a combination of laser angioplasty and conventional balloon angioplasty, good anatomic patency was accomplished with some increase in distal limb perfusion.

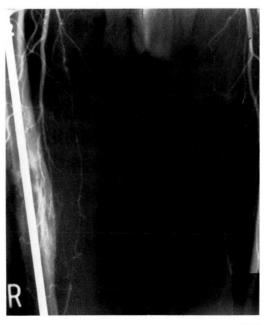

FIGURE 27–4. This patient with severe limiting claudication seemed ideal for treatment, as guide-wire and over-the-wire laser therapy were easily achieved. Despite early anatomic and hemodynamic success, this long superficial artery stenosis went on to restenose and then occlude. The rapid restenosis of long superficial femoral artery stenotic lesions was common in the Northwestern experience.

These individuals are those felt to be at extremely high risk for an anesthetic and operative intervention. Therefore, in an attempt to reduce their overall morbidity, we advised a percutaneous procedure. Thus, the second group represents the most debilitated of all vascular patients with femoral occlusive disease, and the first group represents those with the least severe disease.

Other than degree of systemic atherosclerotic disease, the case selection also depends on actual atherosclerotic lesion dimensions. At the beginning of the present series, *all* femoral popliteal stenoses and occlusions were considered candidates for treatment. It was perceived that perhaps the laser would show some dramatic advantage over conventional balloon angioplasty and allow the treatment of these previously untreatable lesions. After a number of attempts to open very long stenoses or occlusions, it became apparent that the immediate patency rate was not acceptable (Fig. 27–4). Therefore, later in the trial, lesions of more moderate length were used as a definition for treatment.

RESULTS OF TREATMENT

We have decided to present follow-up data as a percentage of initially technically successful treatments which remained patent. This is somewhat deceiving in that it reduces the denominator by subtracting lesions unsuccessful at first technical attempt. However, because this experience represented learning not only with the technique but also with patient selection, such an analysis seemed rational. That is, as earlier described, initially treated long occlusions, which are now known to be hopelessly difficult for this technique, can be subtracted and do not confuse the follow-up data.

Twenty-six superficial femoral artery lesions in twenty-three patients were treated over an 11-month period. Fifteen of these (58 per cent) were initially technically successful, as demonstrated by angiographic information and change in ankle-brachial index. Short lesions (less than 5 cm) were more successfully dealt with (83 per cent) than the longer lesions (greater than 10 cm). Long lesions were successfully treated in only 22 per cent.

We noticed that lesions in which a guide wire could be passed were most commonly successful (68 per cent). Overall, 11 of 21 total arterial occlusions were successfully treated and 4 of 5 stenotic lesions were treated. One of the persistent problems encountered with this series was a high perforation rate (Fig. 27–5). This was seen in six individuals, and of those, half developed arteriovenous fistula demonstrated by the fluoroscopic control. The fascinating thing about these perforations and fistulas was that they all were completely benign. The fistulas closed spontaneously within a short time, and none of the perforations required surgical exploration. This was surprising to us, but is explained by the small (1.1-mm) perforations involved.

Follow-up was available for all patients and was documented by frequent office visits and blood flow studies. The number of initial technical successes was 15, of which eight thrombosed during the follow-up period out to 14 months. That is to say that 47 per cent remained patent with a mean follow-up of 9.5 months, ranging from 1.5 to 14 months. In reviewing the eventual outcome for patients with failed procedures, it is interesting that five of them went on to femoropopliteal bypass to relieve their claudication. One of the five had the operation on the same day because of increasing leg ischemia related to embolic occlusion of the below-knee popliteal. Five patients decided that they would rather continue to claudicate than have a bypass procedure done.

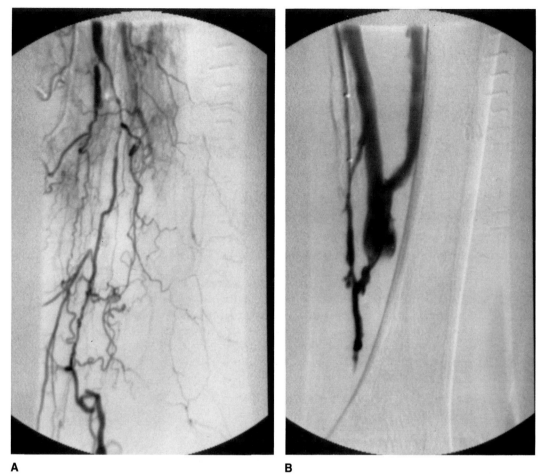

A   **B**

FIGURE 27–5. *A,* This patient presented with limb ischemia and a long superficial artery occlusion. *B,* Successful advance through most of the occlusion was accomplished using the balloon-centered end-on excimer laser. Unfortunately, the laser perforated in Hunter's canal, an area typical from our experience. The rapid filling of the common femoral vein can be easily delineated. In our series, all instances of arteriovenous fistula caused by laser perforation closed spontaneously without any specific therapy.

One of the initial failures was too medically ill for a tibial bypass procedure and had an elective above-knee amputation performed.

COMPLICATIONS FROM LASER ANGIOPLASTY

Laser-assisted angioplasty is a complicated technical exercise and requires reliable surgical backup. Macroembolization to the popliteal artery was seen in three of the patients treated. One of these had the femoropopliteal bypass described above, one was successfully treated with urokinase infusion, and the other was not a candidate for surgical bypass and underwent leg amputation as previously arranged. Overall, 3 limbs were lost of the 26 treated, but none were unanticipated or as a result of the laser intervention. They were simply patients with severe medical disease where the percutaneous angioplasty was attempted as a last resort. Six femoral hematomas were demonstrated in this group, two of which required an operative intervention for suture repair. One complete superficial femoral artery occlusion occurred after laser treatment, and this was successfully treated with urokinase. Perforations were frequent (6 of 26) as were arteriovenous fistulas (3 of 6), but these were all benign and required no surgical therapy.

FOLLOW-UP AND RESTENOSIS FROM OTHER SERIES

Excimer laser angioplasty is a recent addition to medical technology, and detailed, reliable follow-up is limited. Besides the recently reported experience from Northwestern University, information from the Cedars-Sinai Medical Center reported by Litvack et al. is useful.[19] The Cedars-Sinai group, responsible for the early clinical use of the AIS laser, has contributed much to the development of this technology. Besides using the laser in femoropopliteal occlusions and stenoses, this group has also evaluated excimer laser use for coronary lesions. Their work, reported in *Radiology,* is of interest. Thirty patients with femoropopliteal occlusions (22) or stenoses (9) were treated. Of that group, 77 per cent were initially successful. This compares to a 58 per cent initial success rate among the patients treated at Northwestern. The difference, most likely, is due to a more ambitious selection of patients in our series. Litvack reported a similar better result treating shorter lesions and was successful in only one of three lesions longer than 15 cm. Reliable follow-up was obtained for patients who had favorable outcomes, and the authors report that 7 of 24 (29 per cent) returned with a restenosis after a mean follow-up of 9 months. In the Northwestern series, 53 per cent of those patients initially treated successfully were seen back with restenosis with a similar 9-month follow-up. These differences again may be explained by different lesion description in the two series.

There is great interest in this technology related to coronary artery angioplasty. Again, review of the subject is hindered by lack of detailed angiographic follow-up. Coronary angioplasty is more difficult than peripheral to follow by nonangiographic means. Reporting from the medical center at the University of Tuebingen, Haase and associates detail angiographic follow-up of 107 patients treated with an excimer laser for coronary artery disease.[20] They have attempted to differentiate between those patients who required only the bare-fiber excimer laser for correction of their lesion and those who had additional balloon angioplasty. With 6-month follow-up, they determined that 32 per cent of patients treated with only laser restenosed compared to 56 per cent of patients who also required balloon angioplasty. The conclusion that the balloon angioplasty detracts from the bare-fiber treatment is tempting, but actually two different patient populations are represented. Those treated with additional balloon angioplasty had failed an attempt with the laser alone, and therefore their lesions were somehow different.

Margolis has described the follow-up of 958 patients initially treated for coronary disease with the same laser used in the Northwestern series.[21] His multicenter group treated 1151 lesions and had follow-up on 446 patients at 6 months. Of the initial group, 129 had required an additional intervention, either with coronary artery bypass or angioplasty. An additional 189 coronary angiograms were obtained, of which 32 per cent defined a restenosis. A combination of those patients with restenosis and those patients requiring reintervention suggests a significant percentage of early failure. One conclusion of the Margolis study is that higher tip energies of 50 to 59 mJ/mm^2 may be advantageous over lower energy levels. Detailed follow-up of patients described in the numerous acute studies published recently in the English and German literature will certainly define this therapeutic modality more clearly in the next year. It appears to cardiac angiographers that the excimer laser may provide a distinct advantage for coronary lesions unfavorable for conventional balloon angioplasty.[22] These include lesions longer than 10 mm, restenoses, complete occlusions, and possibly lesions with an ostial location.[23]

CONCLUSIONS

Experience from this series and that reported by others suggest that the 308-nm excimer wavelength is ideal for transecting atherosclerotic disease. We found only minor resistance in tissue, rapid catheter passage, and little difficulty with apparently calcified lesions. Troubles with arterial perforation predominated the experience. This is not surprising, as the guidance by a central balloon is extremely crude. Future instrument generations with this wavelength will need to address guidance and may utilize new developments such as intra-arterial ultrasound.

Patency, once initial technical success was achieved, was not outstanding. Our experience compares to that reported by others in the coronary vasculature. With the present catheter producing a maximum 2.2-mm plaque penetration, the accompanying balloon angioplasty predominates the surface effect. Once this balloon angioplasty takes place, the lumen presented to flow has little to do with the initial excimer laser contact. In the future, a large laser catheter capable of producing channels big enough to "stand alone" without balloon angioplasty will allow more critical analysis of this technique. It may be that ultimately biologic alteration of the newly formed luminal surface will be necessary to prevent rapid restenosis.

ACKNOWLEDGMENTS: This work was supported in part by the Veterans Administration Research Service and the Division of Research Resources, National Institutes of Health (Grant No. RR00048), and the Alyce F. Salerno Foundation

REFERENCES

1. Dotter CT, Judkins MP: Transluminal treatment of arteriosclerotic obstruction: Description of a new technic and a preliminary report of its application. Circulation 1964;30:654–670.
2. Gruentzig A: Transluminal dilatation of coronary-artery stenosis. Lancet 1978;1:263.
3. Gruentzig AR, King SB, Schlumpf M, Siegenthaler W: Long-term follow-up after percutaneous transluminal coronary angioplasty: The early Zurich experience. N Engl J Med 1987;316:1127–1132.
4. Wholey MH, Jarmolowski CR: New reperfusion devices: The Kensey catheter, the atherolytic reperfusion wire device, and the transluminal extraction catheter. Radiology 1989;172:947–952.
5. White RA, White GH: Laser thermal probe recanalization of occluded arteries. J Vasc Surg 1980;9:598–608.
6. Choy DSJ: History of lasers in medicine. Thorac Cardiovasc Surg 1988;36:114–117.
7. Clarke RH, Isner JM, Donaldson RF, Jones G: Gas chromatographic-light microscopic correlative analysis of excimer laser photoablation of cardiovascular tissues: Evidence for a thermal mechanism. Circ Res 1987;60:429–437.
8. Isner JM, DeJesus SR, Clarke RH, et al: Mechanism of laser ablation in an absorbing fluid field. Lasers Surg Med 1988;8:543–554.
9. Isner JM, Gal D, Steg PG, et al: Percutaneous, in vivo excimer laser angioplasty: Results in two experimental animal models. Lasers Surg Med 1988;8:223–232.

10. Litvack F, Grundfest WS, Goldenberg T, et al: Pulsed laser angioplasty: Wavelength power and energy dependencies relevant to clinical application. Lasers Surg Med 1988;*8:*60–65.
11. White RA, Grundfest WS: Lasers in Cardiovascular Disease. Chicago, Year Book Medical Publishers, 1987.
12. Sartori M, Henry PD, Sauerbrey R, et al: Tissue interactions and measurement of ablation rates with ultraviolet and visible lasers in canine and human arteries. Lasers Surg Med 1987;*7:*300–306.
13. Isner JM, Rosenfield K, Losordo DW: Excimer laser atherectomy: The greening of Sisyphus. Circulation 1990;*81:*2018–2021.
14. Cross FW, Bowker TJ: The physical properties of tissue ablation with excimer lasers. Med Instrum 1987;*21:*226–230.
15. Haina D, Landthaler M: Fundamentals of laser light interaction with human tissue, especially in the cardiovascular system. Thorac Cardiovasc Surg 1988;*36:*118–125.
16. Steg PG, Rongione AJ, Gal D, et al: Pulsed ultraviolet laser irradiation produces endothelium-independent relaxation of vascular smooth muscle. Circulation 1989;*80:*189–197.
17. Isner JM, Donaldson RF, Deckelbaum LI, et al: The excimer laser: Gross, light microscopic and ultrastructural analysis of potential advantages for use in laser therapy of cardiovascular disease. J Am Coll Cardiol 1985;*6:*1102–1109.
18. McCarthy WJ, Vogelzang RL, Nemcek AA Jr, et al: Excimer laser-assisted femoral angioplasty: Early results. J Vasc Surg 1991;*13:*607–614.
19. Litvack F, Grundfest WS, Adler L, et al: Percutaneous excimer-laser and excimer-laser-assisted angioplasty of the lower extremities: Results of initial clinical trial. Radiology 1989;*172:*231–335.
20. Haase KL, Mauser M, Baumbach A, et al: Restenoses after excimer laser coronary atherectomy. Circulation 1990;*82*(suppl III):672.
21. Margolis JR, Krauthamer D, Litvack F, et al: Six-month follow-up of excimer laser coronary angioplasty registry patients. J Am Coll Cardiol 1991;*17:*218A.
22. Cook SL, Eigler NL, Shefer, et al: Excimer laser coronary angioplasty of lesions not favorable for balloon angioplasty. J Am Coll Cardiol 1991;*17:*218A.
23. Reeder GS, Bresnahan JF, Bresnahan DR, Litvack F: Excimer laser coronary angioplasty in patients with restenosis after prior balloon angioplasty. Circulation 1990;*82*(suppl III):672.

28

HOT-TIP LASER ANGIOPLASTY: A Three-Year Follow-up Study

DAVID ROSENTHAL

Laser angioplasty is an evolving technology which has progressed from a theoretical concept to a potential clinical adjunct in the treatment of patients with atherosclerotic occlusive disease. Because current thermal laser delivery systems create only a small channel in the artery, balloon angioplasty appears necessary to dilate any residual stenosis, thereby allowing sufficient blood flow for symptom relief.[1,2] To evaluate the efficacy, safety, and midterm benefits of superficial femoral artery thermal laser-assisted balloon angioplasty (LABA) a multicenter study was performed.

MATERIALS AND METHODS

Between September 1986 and January 1989, 584 patients underwent 602 superficial femoral artery (SFA) thermal laser-assisted balloon angioplasties. Three hundred eighty-two patients were men, and the mean age of all patients was 68 years (range, 37 to 82 years). Three hundred ninety-seven patients (66 per cent) were cigarette smokers, 319 (53 per cent) had coronary artery disease, 307 (51 per cent) had hypertension, and 138 (23 per cent) patients had diabetes mellitus. The indications for LABA were intermittent claudication in 439 (73 per cent), rest pain in 115 (19 per cent), and gangrene in 48 (8 per cent) of the 602 limbs treated. Two hundred ninety-two (49 per cent) procedures were performed for multifocal stenotic disease of the SFA (greater than 80 per cent arteriographic diameter reduction), 258 for occlusion of the SFA, and 52 for both SFA stenoses and occlusion. Stenotic lesions were classified as less than 3 cm, 4 to 7 cm, or greater than 7 cm in length (Table 28–1).

Two hundred eleven LABA were performed by femoral artery cutdown, and 391 were performed via percutaneous arterial puncture. An 8.5-F introducer sheath was placed into the superficial femoral or common femoral artery. Under fluoroscopic control, intraoperative arteriography demonstrated the location and extent of the arterial lesion, and a .035-inch metallic guide wire was passed to, or through, the occlusion, whenever possible. If the guide wire

Portions of this paper are reprinted from Rosenthal D, Pesa FA, Gottsegen WL, et al.: Thermal laser balloon angioplasty of the superficial femoral artery: A multicenter review of 602 cases. J Vasc Surg 1989; 14:152–159.

TABLE 28–1. STUDY GROUP

Indication (n = 602)	Lesion Length (cm)		
	<3	4–7	>7
SFA stenoses (292)	64	75	153
SFA occlusions (258)	53	106	99
SFA stenosis and occlusion (52)	3	18	31

initially traversed the lesion, laser angioplasty was commenced with a 2.5-mm Laserprobe (Trimedyne, Inc, Tustin, CA). If, however, the lesion could not be crossed with a guide wire, a 2-mm or 2.5-mm Laserprobe was used to create a channel through which the .035-inch guide wire could then be passed. Five- or ten-second pulses of 8 to 12 watts of laser energy from a continuous-wave laser energy source were then delivered, and the Laserprobe was advanced through the lesion with a continuous motion. Repeat arteriography was performed to determine the luminal diameter produced by the Laserprobe and to evaluate distal vessels for possible embolism. The arterial segment was then dilated by conventional balloon angioplasty followed by angioscopy or arteriography to document arterial patency.

Laser-assisted balloon angioplasty was deemed successful if the ankle-brachial index (ABI) increased by 0.25. During follow-up (range, 1 to 30 months; mean, 11.3 months), SFA patency was assessed by segmental Doppler studies. Laser-assisted balloon angioplasty was considered failed when hemodynamic information indicated closure (ABI less than .15 of the highest postoperative index). After LABA, the patients were discharged on a regimen of 325 mg dipyridamole daily. All patients were followed-up by office visits every 3 months during the first year and semiannually thereafter. Statistical analysis was performed by the actuarial life-table method to determine patency rates over time.[3]

RESULTS

Laser-assisted balloon angioplasty successfully recanalized 84 per cent (218 of 258) of occluded superficial femoral arteries (Table 28–2). This technique also enlarged the luminal diameter of 95 per cent (278 of 292) of stenotic vessels, so that less than 20 per cent residual stenosis remained (Table 28–3). With the use of LABA, 80 per cent (42 of 52) of both stenotic and occluded arteries were successfully treated (Table 28–4). This yielded an overall initial angiographic success rate of 89 per cent (538 of 602) and there was no

TABLE 28–2. LIFE-TABLE ANALYSIS OF SFA OCCLUSIONS HAVING LABA

Interval (Mo.)	No. of SFAs at Risk at Start	Lost to Follow-up	No. of Failed LABA	Interval Patency Rate (%)	Cumulative Patency (%)	Standard Error (%)
0–0	258	0	40	100	100	0.0
0–6	218	19	21	89.9	90.3	1.6
6–12	178	26	16	90.3	87.5	2.3
12–18	136	11	8	93.8	79.0	3.1
18–24	117	18	29	73.1	74.2	3.4
24–30	62	3	30	50.4	54.2	4.6

TABLE 28–3. LIFE-TABLE ANALYSIS OF SFA STENOSES HAVING LABA

Interval (Mo.)	No. of SFAs at Risk at Start	Lost to Follow-up	No. of Failed LABA	Interval Patency Rate (%)	Cumulative Patency (%)	Standard Error (%)
0–0	292	0	14	100	100	0.0
0–6	284	17	20	92.7	92.7	1.4
6–12	247	28	5	97.6	85.9	2.0
12–18	214	12	10	94.8	83.9	2.2
18–24	192	20	15	90.4	79.6	2.5
24–30	157	24	23	79.1	71.9	3.0

significant difference in results between centers. Laser-assisted balloon angioplasty was unsuccessful in 64 (11 per cent) superficial femoral arteries (SFA).

Complications related to LABA occurred in 10 per cent (62) of patients, and were most frequently noted in heavily calcified, long segment occluded arteries (Table 28–5). Perforation, the most common complication, occurred in 5 per cent (31) of patients, but only six perforations resulted in bleeding that required surgical repair. Thromboses occurred in 18 SFAs, dissection in 7, and embolization in 6. Because of a thromboembolic complication, operation was necessary in 4 per cent (24) of patients and consisted of above-knee femoropopliteal bypass (14), arterial repair (6), or thromboembolectomy (4). In the entire series, only one limb amputation was necessary as a result of a complication related to LABA. This was due to an SFA-popliteal dissection, which resulted in an embolic "shower" to poor quality tibial runoff vessels in a diabetic patient.

In follow-up extending to 30 months (mean, 11.3 months; range, 1 to 30 months), 60 per cent of arteries have remained patent and the patients asymptomatic with improved Doppler indices (0.25 ± 20) (Table 28–6; Fig. 28–1). Sixty-four arteries could not be recanalized and were considered initial failures. Two hundred other LABA sites thrombosed during late follow-up, and 137 of these patients underwent above-knee femoropopliteal bypass. After late failure in patients in whom the initial indication for LABA was limb salvage, 42 in situ femoropopliteal/tibial bypasses were performed for recurrence of limb salvage symptoms. Nine patients had below-knee amputations after late LABA failure; however, these patients were not deemed surgical candidates because of absent tibial "runoff" when LABA was initially performed for limb salvave.

Midterm (more than 30 days) patency was also evaluated in relation to the type of lesion; that is, occlusion (Table 28–2; Fig. 28–2) versus stenosis (Table 28–3; Fig. 28–2) or both stenosis and occlusion (Table 28–4; Fig. 28–2). In

TABLE 28–4. LIFE-TABLE ANALYSIS BOTH OF SFA STENOSES AND OCCLUSIONS HAVING LABA

Interval (Mo.)	No. of SFAs at Risk at Start	Lost to Follow-up	No. of Failed LABA	Interval Patency Rate (%)	Cumulative Patency (%)	Standard Error (%)
0–0	52	0	10	1.000	100	0.0
0–6	42	3	10	.75	75	5.7
6–12	29	6	2	.92	57	5.7
12–18	21	4	11	.41	52	7.8

TABLE 28–5. COMPLICATIONS RELATED TO LABA

	Number	%
Perforation	31	5
Thrombosis	18	3
Dissection	7	1
Embolization	6	1
Total	62	

TABLE 28–6. LIFE-TABLE ANALYSIS OF SFAS HAVING LABA

Interval (Mo.)	No. of SFAs at Risk at Start	Lost to Follow-up	No. of Failed LABA	Interval Patency Rate (%)	Cumulative Patency (%)	Standard Error (%)
0–0	602	0	64	100	100	0.0
0–6	538	39	51	90.2	90.2	1.2
6–12	448	60	23	94.5	81.3	1.6
12–18	365	27	29	91.7	76.8	1.9
18–24	309	38	44	84.8	70.5	2.1
24–30	227	27	53	75.1	59.8	2.5

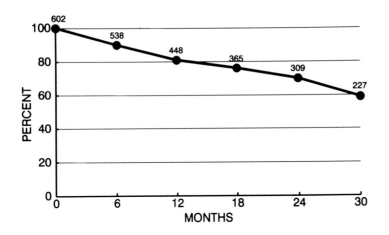

FIGURE 28–1. Cumulative patency of superficial femoral artery laser-assisted balloon angioplasties. Numbers at intervals indicate arteries at risk.

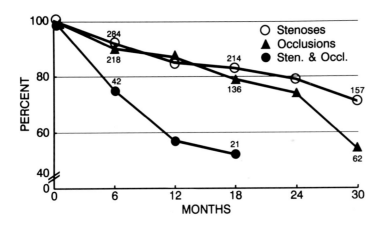

FIGURE 28–2. Cumulative patency of superficial femoral artery laser-assisted balloon angioplasties performed for stenoses, occlusions, or stenoses and occlusion. Numbers at intervals indicate arteries at risk.

TABLE 28–7. LIFE-TABLE ANALYSIS OF SFA STENOSES HAVING LABA

Interval (Mo.)	No. of SFAs at Risk at Start	Lost to Follow-up	No. of Failed LABA	Interval Patency Rate (%)	Cumulative Patency (%)	Standard Error (%)
			≤3 cm			
0–0	64	0	1	100	100	0.0
0–6	63	5	2	96.6	98.4	1.5
6–12	56	11	0	100	95.1	2.7
12–18	45	6	2	95.2	95.1	3.1
18–24	37	7	3	91.0	90.6	4.5
24–30	27	7	5	78.7	82.5	6.6
			4–7 cm			
0–0	75	0	3	96.0	100	0.0
0–6	72	6	6	91.3	96.0	2.2
6–12	60	12	1	98.1	87.6	3.9
12–18	47	3	3	93.4	86.0	4.6
18–24	41	7	2	94.6	80.3	5.5
24–30	32	8	5	82.1	76.0	6.5
			≥7 cm			
0–0	153	0	10	93.0	100	0.0
0–6	143	6	12	91.4	93.4	1.9
6–12	125	5	4	96.7	85.4	2.9
12–18	116	3	5	95.6	81.7	3.2
18–24	108	6	10	90.4	78.1	3.5
24–30	92	9	13	98.8	70.6	3.9

TABLE 28–8. LIFE-TABLE ANALYSIS OF SFA OCCLUSIONS HAVING LABA

Interval (Mo.)	No. of SFAs at Risk at Start	Lost to Follow-up	No. of Failed LABA	Interval Patency Rate (%)	Cumulative Patency (%)	Standard Error (%)
			≤3 cm			
0–0	53	0	3	94.0	100	
0–6	50	6	3	93.6	94.0	3.2
6–12	41	8	3	91.9	88.0	4.7
12–18	30	5	2	92.7	80.8	6.4
18–24	23	6	5	75.0	74.9	7.8
24–30	12	1	5	56.5	56.2	10.7
			4–7 cm			
0–0	106	0	15	86.0	100	0.0
0–6	91	7	6	93.1	85.8	3.3
6–12	78	10	4	94.5	79.9	4.0
12–18	64	3	2	96.8	75.5	4.6
18–24	59	6	8	85.7	73.1	4.9
24–30	45	2	15	65.9	62.7	5.7
			≥7 cm			
0–0	99	0	22	78.0	100	0.0
0–6	77	6	12	83.7	77.7	4.1
6–12	59	8	9	83.6	65.1	5.0
12–18	42	3	4	90.1	54.5	5.6
18–24	35	6	16	50.0	49.1	6.0
24–30	13	0	10	23.0	24.5	6.1

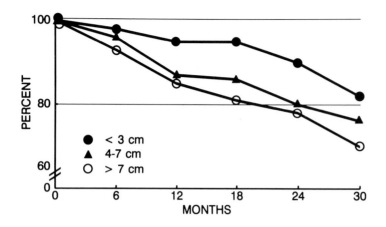

FIGURE 28–3. Cumulative patency of superficial femoral artery laser-assisted balloon angioplasties performed for stenoses by lesion length.

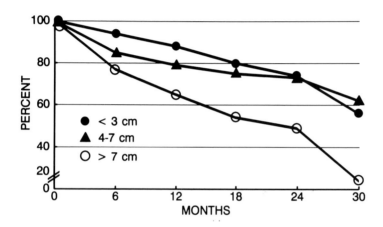

FIGURE 28–4. Cumulative patency of superficial femoral artery laser-assisted balloon angioplasties performed for occlusions by lesion length.

general, stenosed vessels (Table 28–7; Fig. 28–3) remained patent better than occluded vessels (Table 28–8; Fig. 28–4), and short lesions (less than 3 cm) both for SFA stenoses and occlusions remained patent better than longer lesions (greater than 7 cm) (Figs. 28–3 and 28–4).

DISCUSSION

The role and benefits of thermal laser-assisted balloon angioplasty using "hot-tip" laser probe remains controversial. The objective of this multicenter study was to evaluate the safety, efficacy, and midterm results of superficial femoral artery thermal laser-assisted balloon angioplasty.

Initial clinical results with thermal LABA suggest that it is a safe technique.[1,2,4,5] In this review, the complication rate associated with LABA was 10 per cent (62 patients), which is similar to other reported rates for femoral LABA.[6–9] Indeed, only one limb amputation occurred as the result of a LABA complication. This was in a diabetic patient who suffered an SFA-popliteal dissection and subsequent "trashing" of poor quality tibial runoff vessels.

Late occlusion of the LABA site did not result in limb loss nor compromise alternative reconstructive operations, as only a short segment of artery around the angioplasty site thromboses and the abundant collateral network appears to protect the remaining artery. During follow-up, 200 LABAs occluded and

137 patients underwent above-knee femoropopliteal bypass. Of the 137 patients, 116 (85 per cent) had recurrence of the same claudication symptoms that were present when LABA was performed. Twenty-one patients (15 per cent) who required femoropopliteal bypass, however, had worsening of symptoms when the LABA site reoccluded. At repeat arteriography, 10 of these 15 patients had longer segment occlusions than were present when the initial LABA was performed, and five patients had worsening of distal occlusive disease. Another 42 patients had in situ femoropopliteal/tibial bypasses performed for recurrence of limb-salvage symptoms when the LABA site occluded. The initial indication for LABA in these 42 patients was limb salvage. In general, thrombosis of the LABA site caused the recurrence of symptoms, not limb loss. As with all endovascular (and surgical) techniques, complication rates are directly proportional to the operator's experience. In experienced hands, superficial femoral artery LABA appears to be a safe procedure.

The overall 30-month cumulative patency rate of 60 per cent in this series is equal to or greater than that reported for conventional SFA balloon angioplasty when evaluated on the basis of type and length of lesion, as well as method of data analysis. For example, the 12-month patency rates with short (less than 3 cm) stenoses and short occlusions in this series were 95.1 per cent and 88.0 per cent, respectively (Tables 28–7 and 28–8). These rates are considerably higher than those obtained in balloon angioplasty series, in which the 12-month patency rates range between 72 and 81 per cent for stenoses[10,11] and 67 and 93 per cent for short occlusions.[10,12] The 12-month patency rate for medium length (4 to 7 cm) occlusions treated with LABA (Table 28–8) was 79.9 per cent, and the rate for occlusions longer than 7 cm, was 65.1 per cent, both of which are better than the patency rate for occlusions longer than 3 cm treated by balloon angioplasty[12] (Table 28–9). Although the patency rates for occlusions longer than 3 cm appear to be better in two of the balloon angioplasty series, their results are not comparable to ours because they did not consider a SFA "redilitation" for a restenosed or occluded vessel as a failure.[10,11] Only a randomized prospective trial comparing LABA and balloon angioplasty alone can resolve this controversy.

Finally, these and virtually all published results for balloon angioplasty are based only upon *initially successful* angioplasties; inability to cross a lesion or to reduce the angiographic percentage of stenosis is considered a failure and these procedures are *excluded* from calculations of long-term patency. The results of LABA in this study are superior to those of SFA balloon angioplasty because *all* patients, regardless of initial success or failure, were included in the life-table analysis. One possible explanation for the higher patency rates after laser thermal angioplasty is that the laser partially removes the atheromatous lesion

TABLE 28–9.   TWELVE-MONTH PATENCY RATES FOR SFA LABA VERSUS BALLOON ANGIOPLASTY

	Stenosis (%)			Occlusions (%)		
	<3 cm	4–7 cm	>7 cm	<3 cm	4–7 cm	>7 cm
LABA (n = 292)	95.1	87.6	85.4	(n = 258) 88	79.9	65.1
Balloon Angioplasty						
Hewes[10] (n = 50)	85	100	38	(n = 41) 67	100	68
Murray[11] (n = 116)	82.4	(<7 cm)	23.1	(n = 77)	85.9	(all occlusions)
Krepel[12] (n = 127)	83	62 (>3 cm)		(n = 37)	50 (>3 cm)	

and leaves behind a smoother arterial surface. Undue thrombogenesis resulting from thermal injury after laser angioplasty does not seem to be a clinically significant cause of failure.[1]

Our study demonstrates that thermal LABA was best suited for the treatment of localized SFA lesions, which inherently limits the number of patients who will benefit from this procedure. The 24.5 per cent patency rate for occlusions longer than 7 cm at 30-month follow-up was poor (Table 28–8). Although the study design did not delineate the length of the 99 occlusions longer than 7 cm, data were available indicating that 65 long-term failures had occlusions between 10 and 18 cm. For the best long-term results, it seems a long-segment SFA occlusion should be treated by femoropopliteal bypass when symptoms warrant.

This study demonstrates that superficial femoral artery LABA is safe and efficacious. The promising midterm benefits for short-segment occlusive lesions warrant further investigation. The most appropriate method to report long-term patency results of endovascular interventional techniques remains controversial. It seems logical, however, to evaluate the durability of LABA once a successful procedure has been accomplished, rather than evaluating the operator's ability to recanalize an artery.

Laser angioplasty is not the panacea many people thought it would be, and it will not revolutionize the treatment of lower extremity arterial occlusive disease. As experience grows and technology improves we will learn which concepts to embrace and which to disregard, but in this study, thermal LABA was most successful in claudicant patients with short-segment (less than 7 cm), noncalcific lesions. This will inherently limit the number of patients who will currently benefit from this procedure, but to more thoroughly understand and evaluate the role of LABA in the treatment of SFA occlusive disease, a randomized prospective trial comparing no treatment, balloon angioplasty, and LABA, must be done. Until then, LABA offers the benefits of a minimally invasive treatment technique, but careful patient selection is necessary to ensure good results with minimal risks.

ACKNOWLEDGMENTS: Felix A. Pesa, M.D., Ohio Heart Institute, Youngstown, Ohio; Warrem L. Gottsegen, M.D., Doctors Hospital of Jefferson, Metairie, Louisiana; John R. Crew, M.D., San Francisco Heart Institute, Seton Medical Center, Daly City, California; Charles A. Moss, M.D. and Robert Walsky, M.D., Vascular Institute of New Jersey, Emerson, New Jersey contributed patients to this study.

REFERENCES

1. Seeger JA, Abela GS, Silverman SH: Initial results of laser recanalization in lower extremity arterial reconstruction. J Vasc Surg 1989;9:10–16.
2. Sanborn TA, Greenfield AJ, Guben JK, et al: Human percutaneous and intraoperative laser thermal angioplasty: Initial clinical results as an adjunct to balloon angioplasty. J Vasc Surg 1988;5:83–90.
3. Dickson WJ, Brown MB, Engleman L, et al: DMDP Statistical Software. Regents University of California, 1985.
4. Cumberland DC, Sanborn TA, Taylor DI, et al: Percutaneous laser thermal angioplasty: Initial clinical results with a laserprobe in total peripheral artery occlusions. Lancet 1986;1:1457–1459.
5. Kateen BT, Kaplan JD, Schwarten DM, et al: Complications of "Hot Tip" laser assisted angioplasty (abstr). Circulation 1988;78(suppl II):II–417.
6. Thomas HM, Siragusa V, Bowers JA, et al: Percutaneous laser assisted balloon angioplasty of lower extremity arterial disease in a free standing laboratory. Diagn Ther 1989;16:216–223.

7. Criado FJ, Queral LA, Patten P, et al: Laser angioplasty in the lower extremities: An early surgical experience. J Vasc Surg 1990:*11*:532–535.
8. White RA, White GH: Laser thermal probe recanalization of occluded arteries. J Vasc Surg 1989;*9*:598–608.
9. Leachman DR: Hot tip laser angioplasty. A review of the Texas Heart Institute experience. Tex Heart Inst J 1989;*16*:207–215.
10. Hewes RC, White RI, Murray RR, et al: Long-term results of superficial femoral artery angioplasty. Am J Radiol 1986;*146*:1025–1029.
11. Murray RR Jr, Hewes RC, White RI Jr, et al: Long-segment femoropopliteal stenoses: Is angioplasty a boon or a bust? Radiology 1987;*162*:473–476.
12. Krepel VM, van Andel GJ, van Erp WFM, et al: Percutaneous transluminal angioplasty of the femoropopliteal artery: Initial and long-term results. Radiology 1985;*156*:325–328.

29

LONG-TERM RESULTS OF SIMPSON ATHERECTOMY

LUIS A. QUERAL, FRANK J. CRIADO, PEGGY PATTEN, and
CHERYL D. MEYERS

The Simpson[1,2] Atherocath (Devices for Vascular Interventions, Redwood City, CA) is an interesting device designed for the transluminal extraction of discrete atherosclerotic lesions. As an alternative to balloon angioplasty, its potential advantages include the avoidance of significant intimal cracking and dissection, and the mechanical ablation of atheromatous material. Although these features are attractive, the promise of a decreased restenosis rate remains unproven.

This clinical study began in December 1988, when we decided to utilize the Simpson peripheral atherectomy device in our endovascular unit for the transluminal treatment of symptomatic discrete lesions of the superficial femoral (SFA) and popliteal arteries.

Immediate and two-year follow-up results are herein reported.

MATERIALS AND METHODS

Between December 1988 and December 1990, 68 patients were treated with Simpson atherectomy for lower extremity arterial insufficiency at the Maryland Vascular Institute, Union Memorial Hospital, Baltimore, Maryland. The average age of patients was 66 years (range, 52 to 86). There were 41 males and 27 females. Risk factors for this series included cigarette smoking (n = 49), coronary artery disease (n = 24), hypertension (n = 26), and diabetes mellitus (n = 18).

A total of 77 atherectomies (77 limbs) of the SFA and popliteal arteries were atherectomized. Indications for the procedure were claudication in 62 cases (81 per cent), and critical ischemia in 15 patients (19 per cent). The latter was clinically defined by the presence of nonhealing ulceration, rest pain, or frank gangrene. Patients were evaluated by continuous wave (CW) Doppler tracings of the major lower extremity arteries and by segmental pressures measured at the ankle level. Ankle-brachial indices (ABIs) were determined prior to subjecting the patients to angiography. Color flow Duplex scanning was performed in routine fashion at the initial evaluation of patients during the last 6 months of the study period.

Preoperative angiography revealed a complete obstruction in 31 cases, multiple stenotic lesions in 30 cases, and single stenotic lesions in 16. Patients were pretreated with acetylsalicylic acid (ASA) 325 mg/day beginning 48 hours before atherectomy. A percutaneous approach was utilized in 68 patients, and open surgical exposure in the other 9. The procedures were done in a dedicated surgical vascular suite equipped with sophisticated high-quality x-ray imaging (International Surgical Systems, Phoenix, AZ). Anesthesia consisted of local groin infiltration with 1 per cent lidocaine (Xylocaine) supplemented with intravenous sedation. The latter was administered by members of the department of anesthesia and consisted of midozolam HCI (Versed) and fentanyl citrate (Sublimaze). The employed dosages of these drugs varied depending on patient response and anesthesiologist preference.

PROCEDURAL TECHNIQUE

A guide wire was inserted into the common femoral artery (CFA) or proximal SFA via antegrade percutaneous puncture or open surgical exposure. An introducer sheath of appropriate caliber (8- or 9-F) was tracked over the wire and advanced antegrade into the upper SFA. Once the sheath was in place, anticoagulation with 5000 units of heparin was effected. A size 7-, 8-, or 9-F device was then passed through the sheath and advanced downstream to the target lesion. Proper placement of the metallic housing-cutter unit was aided by "road mapping." At least two passes with the cutter were effected in each quadrant of the cross-sectional arterial circumference. When the specimen chamber became full, the device was withdrawn, emptied, and reintroduced (Fig. 29–1). Completion angiography was obtained in all cases. In patients with

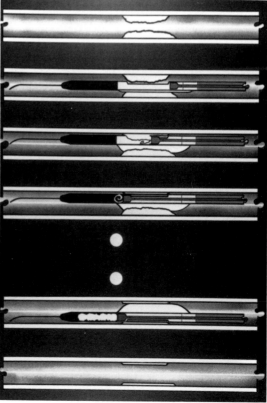

FIGURE 29–1. An atheromatous vessel is depicted at the top of this illustration. The Simpson Atherocath is positioned and atherectomy carried out after inflation of the balloon. The plaque is collected in a contiguous chamber. Lastly, the Atherocath is withdrawn and the vessel is noted to be devoid of atheroma.

total obstructions, a pilot channel was first created by either laser probe or wire crossing. Following the procedure, the patient was transferred to the recovery room with the sheath still in place. Sheath removal was done within 1 hour of completion of the atherectomy. The heparin was not reversed.

FOLLOW-UP

Patients were tested in our noninvasive laboratory within 2 weeks after the procedure. Ankle brachial indices were calculated at that time and CW Doppler recordings made. Duplex color flow imaging of the atherectomized arterial segments was also obtained. This protocol was repeated at 3-, 6-, 12-, 18-, and 24-month intervals. Determination of success was based on an increase in ABI of 1.5 or more and the visualization of the treated arterial segment by duplex scanning.

RESULTS

This study focuses on the outcome of the atherectomy in each of the limbs treated. It is for this reason that 77 procedures are described in 68 patients; obviously, 9 patients had atherectomies performed in both lower extremities. Immediate anatomical success was angiographically defined as a postatherectomy residual stenosis of 20 per cent or less of the artery's normal diameter. Initial success rate was 94 per cent (72 of 77). The five immediate failures were due to inability to cross an occluded lesion (n = 3), and incapacity to cut a densely calcified atherosclerotic plaque (n = 2).

Postatherectomy evaluation involved both clinical and hemodynamic data. Clinical success was defined as improvement or resolution of preprocedural symptomatology. A hemodynamic success depended on a rise in ABI of greater than 0.15. There was no discrepancy between clinical and hemodynamic criteria. The success rate progressively diminished to 76 per cent at 3 months, 70 per cent at 6 months, 66 per cent at 12 months, 55 per cent at 18 months, and 44 per cent at 24 months. These figures were calculated from the raw data and interpreted using life-table analysis. A total of 36 patients have been followed-up for 24 months (Fig. 29–2). There was one postoperative death secondary to myocardial infarction that occurred approximately 2 weeks after the patient

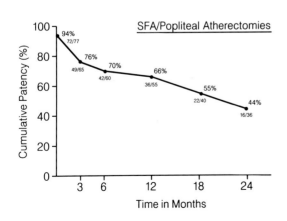

FIGURE 29–2. This graph denoted by life-table method the SFA/popliteal patency of Simpson atherectomy. An initial group of 77 patients were followed, and at 2 years, 36 patients were available for evaluation.

underwent the procedure. One patient required a below-knee amputation, and six others required bypasses to correct severe ischemia during the study period. Only seven patients were lost to follow-up. There were four groin hematomas noted, but none required surgical evacuation. Clinically significant distal embolization did not occur during the study period.

DISCUSSION

Results of atherectomy with the Simpson atherectomy device have been previously published.[3,4] This chapter, however, represents the first account of this treatment modality by a surgical team.

The Simpson atherotome was designed to remove obstructive atheroma transluminally without the need for a major surgical procedure. It works best when applied to focal or discrete lesions. For this reason, its use is appropriate for a relatively small number of patients.[5] Accordingly, our experience is limited to patients with favorable superficial femoral and popliteal arterial disease. Patients with iliac lesions were not subjected to atherectomy, since they respond very well to balloon angioplasty.

Patient selection for major surgical arterial reconstructive procedures has traditionally been based on the presence of limb-threatening ischemia. Patients with claudication have been considered surgical candidates only when their disability severely effected their socioeconomic status. Such patient selection excluded from effective treatment the majority of claudicators who have alternatively been placed on risk-factor control regimes and an exercise program. Such a conservative approach to atherosclerotic occlusive disease of the lower extremities is beginning to change on the one hand because today's geriatric population has become less tolerant of restrictions in their lifestyles; and on the other hand because the newly developed catheter-based procedures can effectively alleviate leg ischemia with a very low morbidity and mortality. The majority of patients entered in this study (62 of 77) had claudication as the only indication for therapy. It is thus quite apparent that the primary goal of treatment was symptom relief so as to allow full walking capacity. Critical leg ischemia, on the other hand, requires revascularization by surgical bypass in the vast majority of instances.

Directional atherectomy emerged as a technique offering distinct potential advantages over balloon angioplasty in the treatment of discrete atherosclerotic lesions of the SFA/popliteal arteries. This is an important consideration, since the immediate success rate and long-term durability of balloon angioplasty has been questioned for these arterial segments. Advantages of atherectomy include the avoidance of major intimal cracking and dissection, and true atheroablation, which would appear to be an important theoretical goal. One can certainly obtain some of the best angiographic "cosmetic" results after atherectomy. Routine postatherectomy angioscopy has shown, however, that intimal defects, polypoid residual lesions, and minor dissections are not uncommon. These may be the result of the concomitant "angioplasty effect" caused by inflating the device balloon even though inflation pressures were kept at 3 atm or less. It is our contention, and that of others,[6,7] that balloon dilatation may account for as much as 50 per cent of the luminal enlargement effected by directional atherectomy.

The atherectomies in this series were performed by two surgeons (Criado/Queral) in a dedicated operating room suite with excellent x-ray imaging capabilities. This setting permits arterial access by either a percutaneous or an open surgical route. Our preference is for percutaneously cannulating the femoral artery, and this was effectively done in 68 cases. However, nine cases were performed by surgical cutdown. This so-called "open" approach is particularly desirable in obese patients (n = 4), because the rigid housing on the Simpson Atherocath device makes its insertion into the femoral artery very difficult by the percutaneous technique. Other indications in our "open" group included the need for iliac balloon angioplasty (n = 3), and SFA origin disease which required patch angioplasty (n = 2).

A very high immediate success rate was obtained (94 per cent). This should probably be attributed to careful patient selection and newly available wires that allow easy crossing of total occlusions and complex stenoses. A laser "hot-tip" catheter (Trimedyne, Inc, Tustin, CA) was also employed (n = 8) when mechanical attempts at crossing the target area failed. There were only five immediate failures in this series (5.4 per cent). This subset of patients included were in the total obstruction category (n = 2) and the multiple stenotic group (n = 3) (Fig. 29–2).

Subsequent hemodynamic failures occurred primarily in patients whose SFA/popliteal arteries exhibited multiple stenoses (Table 29–1). The success rate for this group was 30 per cent at the end of the follow-up period. Reasons for this very significant failure rate are at present speculative and include incomplete atherectomy, deep cuts with luminal exposure of the arterial wall media,[8,9] and the presence of extensive calcification. Based on these results, we no longer employ Simpson atherectomy for those patients with multiple SFA/popliteal stenoses.

Total obstructions of less than 5.0 cm in length fared better after initial success (29 of 31). The two instances of early failures involved the inability to cross the lesion in one, and a heavily calcified lesion in the other. The patency in this group at 2 years was 52 per cent (16 of 31). The causes of failure noted were often a restenosis at the treated site and at other locations in the SFA/popliteal vessels. A clear-cut pattern has not been observed at this time. A key question is the possibility of the procedure accelerating occlusive disease at sites not previously affected. Longer follow-up may shed some light on this area.

Patients treated for single stenosis did remarkably well, with patency in 14 of 16 cases, or 88 per cent. All of these cases were claudicants, who have been very happy with their ability to ambulate without discomfort. Their lifestyles have undoubtedly been enhanced. The two failures in this subgroup have gone back to their preprocedural state and are being closely monitored. All failures once detected have to be clinically addressed. Of the five patients with immediate failures noted, two chose to undergo femoropopliteal bypasses as a corrective measure. This procedure was performed during the same hospitalization, and

TABLE 29–1. CUMULATIVE PATENCY OF ATHERECTOMY[a]

Angiography	Success (%)
Single stenosis	88
Multiple stenoses	30
Obstructions <5.0 cm	52
Totals	44

[a] Vessel patency is computed based on angiographic presentation.

both patients did well. The other patients in our series who failed to maintain patency were managed on an individual basis. One patient underwent a distal bypass which failed after a short period with a resultant below-knee amputation. Another four patients had successful bypasses and are doing well. Other patients who were catalogued as failures continue to be closely monitored. We had a total of seven patients lost to follow-up.

Upon close examination of the accumulated data, our overall low 2-year patency of 44 per cent (36 cases followed for that period) is largely attributed to failures on patients with multiple stenoses. The avoidance of such lesions is an important "lesson" and we no longer recommend interventional therapy in this subgroup. Conversely, single stenotic lesions are very aptly treated by Simpson atherectomy. Relief of presenting symptoms is both rapid and dramatic. Patient and surgeon satisfaction is high, although long-term results (2 years or more) are not yet available.

The results noted on the group of patients with short obstructions (5.0 cm or less) is puzzling, and we have not reached a clear-cut opinion regarding these. It does appear that extensive calcification is a contraindication to atherectomy because the lesion cannot be effectively cut by the Simpson device. It is also important to fully ablate the causative lesion, and angioscopy has been noted to identify cases that required more atherectomizing although the angiographic appearance was benign. Routine angioscopy is recommended for this reason. However, a significant number of failures in this subgroup are enigmatic and without mechanical explanation appears possible. Perhaps the procedure stimulates either rethrombosis, pseudointimal hyperplasia or both.

It is important to note that failures did not result in deterioration of the patients' preprocedural status. Lower extremity arterial perfusion was not harmed by unsuccessful atherectomy. All 31 failures resulted in a return of the ABI to baseline level.

Complications in the series consisted primarily of four groin hematomas that were clearly noticeable but which did not require surgical evacuation. These four patients had percutaneous procedures, and two were obese. The other two had extensive calcifications at the puncture site in the common femoral artery. These patients are best approached by open technique. One patient did have a myocardial infarction and died during the postprocedure period. All of the atherectomies were done under local anesthesia supplemented by intravenous sedation administered by an anesthesiologist. The drugs commonly utilized provide both pain relief (Fentanyl) and memory loss (Versed). This unique combination makes the experience a benign one for the patient. We have rarely heard complaints. This contrasts sharply with what the same patients report after standard angiography done without adequate sedation.

No attempt has been made to calculate the monetary cost involved in the management of this group of patients. However, it is worth mentioning that hospital stay was generally less than 48 hours. Patients are routinely admitted the same day of the procedure and discharged the following day after morning rounds by the attending physician. The return to normal activity was encouraged after a period of home convalescence of 3 to 5 days. The patient's acceptance of the procedure appears to the authors to be most enthusiastic.

In conclusion, the Simpson Atherocath has been an effective tool in augmenting the arterial perfusion of ischemic limbs in selected patients with discrete atherosclerotic lesions of the superficial femoral and popliteal arteries. However, this procedure is ineffective when applied to patients harboring multiple stenoses. Lastly, a longer follow-up time is needed to determine the appropriateness of Simpson atherectomy in treating short obstructions. Long-term results are pending.

REFERENCES

1. Simpson JB, Johnson DE, Thapliyal HV, Marks DM, Braden LJ: Transluminal atherectomy: A new approach to the treatment of atherosclerotic vascular disease (abstr). Circulation 1985;72(suppl III):111–146.
2. Simpson JB, Johnson DE, Braden LJ, Gifford HS, Thapliyal HV, Selmon Mr: Transluminal coronary atherectomy (TCA): Results in 21 human cadaver vascular segments (abstr). Circulation 1986;74(suppl II):II–202.
3. Simpson JB, Robertson GC, Selmon MR: Percutaneous coronary atherectomy (abstr). Circulation 1988;78(suppl II):II–326.
4. Johnson DE, Selmon Mr, Simpson JB: Primary stenoses and restenoses excised byperipheral atherectomy (abstr). J Am Coll Cardiol 1988;11:173A.
5. Simpson JB, Zimmerman JJ, Selmon MR, et al: Transluminal atherectomy: Initial clinical results in 27 patients (abstr). Circulation 1986;74(suppl II):II–203.
6. Schwarten DE, Katzen BT, Simpson JB, Cutliff WB: Simpson catheter for percutaneous transluminal removal of atheroma. AJR 1988;150:799–801.
7. Simpson JB, Selmon MR, Robertson GC, et al: Transluminal atherectomy for occlusive peripheral vascular disease. Am J Cardiol 1988;61:96G–101G.
8. Selmon MR, Robertson GC, Simpson JB: Restenosis in peripheral transluminal atherectomy (abstr). Circulation 1988;78(suppl II):II–1073.
9. Johnson DE, Robertson GC, Simpson JB: Coronary atherectomy: Light microscopic and immunohistochemical study of excised tissues (abstr). Circulation 1988;78(suppl II):II–327.

30

ILIAC ARTERY ANGIOPLASTY AND STENTS: A Current Experience

MICHAEL C. DALSING, KAREN O. EHRMAN, DOLORES F. CIKRIT, STEPHEN G. LALKA, and ALAN P. SAWCHUK

One accepted method of treating iliac artery occlusive disease is by percutaneous transluminal angioplasty (PTA). Technological advancements in balloon construction and delivery techniques have continually improved the overall results of this procedure.[1] Some lesions, however, cannot be approached successfully, even with these improvements. An early suggestion by Dotter that an intraluminal stent might improve the results of PTA was largely ignored until the limitations of PTA became obvious.[2] Our experience at Indiana University has demonstrated to our satisfaction that early technical failures and post-PTA restenosis are a problem in a significant number of patients.[3,4] In the mid-1980s, Julio Palmaz reported a very favorable canine experiment using a balloon expandable stent.[5] We became involved in the clinical trial of this device in May 1987 for the treatment of symptomatic patients with iliac artery stenosis.

MATERIALS AND METHODS

Device

The Palmaz stent is a slotted, uninconstructed, stainless-steel hollow tube measuring 3 mm in diameter and 3 cm in length in the nondilated state. (Fig. 30–1). The wall thickness is 0.12 mm. It can be expanded to a diameter of 8 to 12 mm with only a modest postdilatation reduction in length such that the device is 26 mm long at a diameter of 12 mm. The dilation essentially expands the parallel slots into a rectangular shape to obtain the desired stent configuration when expanded (Fig. 30–1).

Inclusion and Exclusion Criteria

Certainly not all PTA procedures require the addition of an intravascular endoskeleton for acceptable results.[3,4,6–14] However, there are two circumstances

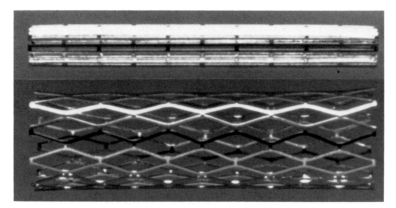

FIGURE 30–1. Photograph of the stent in an unexpanded (*top*) and then expanded state (*bottom*). Note the parallel slotted stent design at rest which becomes a rectangular shape on expansion.

which might be improved by stent placement, and which were accepted as indications for stent placement in this study. An ineffective angioplasty result was demonstrated by a greater than 30 per cent residual diameter stenosis or a residual pressure gradient of 10 mm Hg or more at rest or a 15 per cent or greater change in the femoral-brachial systolic pressure index with vasodilation, and was considered an appropriate indication for stent placement. Such unacceptable results can be seen in vessels with elastic recoil, PTA-induced dissection, spasm, acute thrombosis, or a combination of any of these.[1,3,6,7,14,15] Recurrent stenosis following an initially successful PTA may define a high-risk group of patients prone to recurrent luminal narrowing after a second attempt at angioplasty. These patients were also considered candidates for stent placement.

Absolute contraindications to stent deployment were extravasation at the target site (perforation), severe vessel tortuosity which precluded safe balloon and stent placement, aneurysmal disease at the proposed site of stent placement, as well as severe vascular calcification which precluded PTA. Relative contraindications were mild vessel tortuosity, impaired pain sensation owing to an increased difficulty in determining potential problems during stent deployment, a diseased common femoral artery of less than 5 mm in diameter (which may suggest the need for open operative placement), poor runoff status, severe hypertension, and/or a hypercoagulable state. Severe hypertension could lead to difficulty in controlling bleeding from the puncture site, and a hypercoagulable state could lead to early thrombosis of the stented area. Prolonged anticoagulation may improve the results in the latter case as well as in the case of patients with poor runoff. Of course, surgical correction of distal arterial occlusive disease would also improve runoff status, and might be considered if deemed appropriate by the patient's clinical presentation.

Technique

The equipment required for iliac artery Palmaz stent placement is shown in Figure 30–2. Figure 30–3 is an artists depiction of the entire stenting procedure. A standard Seldinger approach allowed access through the common femoral artery to the iliac artery. A routine balloon angioplasty was preformed at the target site to demonstrate that the vessel could be dilated, to avoid

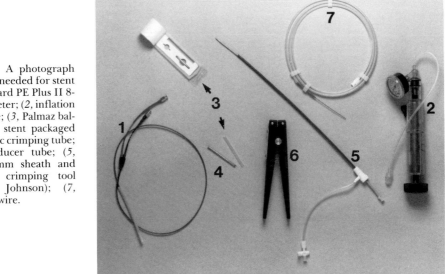

FIGURE 30–2. A photograph of all equipment needed for stent placement: (*1*, Bard PE Plus II 8-mm balloon catheter; (*2*, inflation device—any type; (*3*, Palmaz balloon-expandable stent packaged with a clear plastic crimping tube; (*4*, metal introducer tube; (*5*, Cook 10-F 30-mm sheath and introducer; (*6*, crimping tool (Johnson and Johnson); (*7*, 0.035-cm guide wire.

stenting a lesion having a good result with PTA (exclusive of restenosis patients), and to widen a channel for sheath placement thereby avoiding plaque trauma when a stent is required. A guide wire was constantly maintained across the area of vessel narrowing until the decision to proceed or to forego further intervention was made. If a stent was required, the second stage of the procedure was begun.

The stent was manually mounted on a Bard PE Plus II (USCI, Billerica, MA) 8-mm balloon catheter and will be designated the stent-balloon assembly. The clear plastic crimping tube was placed over the stent and the stent was secured to the balloon by a special crimping tool. The security of the stent placement onto the angioplasty balloon was confirmed by a lack of movement on manual testing. A 10-F 30-cm-long Cook sheath (Bloomington, IN) with introducer was inserted over the guide wire and into the vessel. It was advanced to a point just proximal to the iliac target lesion. A metal introducer tube was placed over the stent-balloon assembly to protect the stent from being dislodged as it was placed through the sheath's hemostatic valve. Once the stent-balloon assembly was safely in the sheath, the metal tube was pulled from the hemostatic valve and pushed to the distal end of the balloon angioplasty catheter. The stent-balloon assembly was now advanced in the sheath to lie adjacent to the target lesion. The stent's stainless-steel construction made it easily visible on routine fluoroscopy or radiograph (Fig. 30–4). The sheath was pulled back to expose the entire stent-balloon assembly to the vessel lumen. The balloon was inflated at 8 to 12 atm to dilate the stent and adjacent vessel to an 8-mm diameter. If the desired lumen diameter was larger, as determined by angiographic measurement of the normal iliac artery, a balloon catheter change was required. The current balloon was deflated, gently rotated clockwise to detach it fully from the stent, and removed from the sheath. A larger diameter balloon angioplasty catheter was then placed through the sheath to the stented area and dilated to acquire the desired diameter. This was done as often as required for an optimal result.

All patients were administered 325 mg of aspirin the day prior to intervention. Preintervention pelvic angiography confirmed the presence of iliac

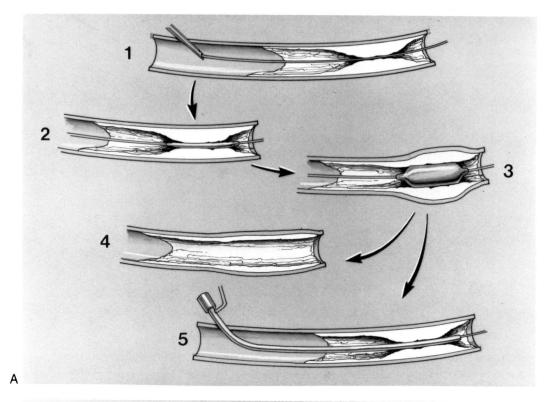

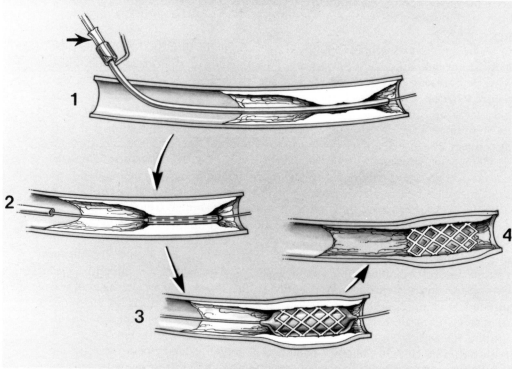

FIGURE 30–3. *A,* Seldinger access (*1*) to the vessel with guide wire passed across the lesion; (*2*) angioplasty balloon placed for predilatation; (*3*) balloon angioplasty performed and if successful the procedure may be terminated (*4*), or the decision may be made to place a stent (*5*), in which case, a Cook 10-F 30-cm-long sheath is advanced past the target lesion. *B,* The stent-balloon assembly (*1*) is placed into the sheath with the use of the metal introducer tube (*arrow*); (*2*), the stent-balloon assembly is advanced to oppose the target lesion and the sheath is pulled back to expose the stent-balloon assembly to the vessel lumen; (*3*), dilatation is performed and, (*4*) the balloon is removed leaving the stent in its proper location.

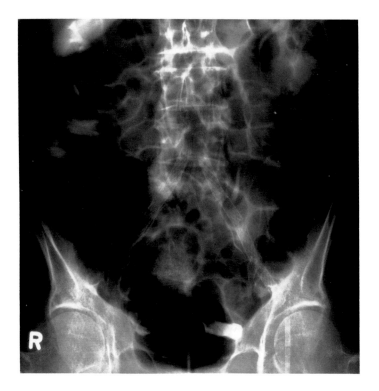

FIGURE 30–4. Plain radiograph of multiple overlapping stents in the left common and external iliac artery and in the right common iliac artery. Note the radiodensity of the stent, which aids in proper placement.

disease, and intravascular pressure measurements of the gradient across the lesion confirmed its hemodynamic significance. The patient received a 5000- to 8000-unit heparin bolus prior to any PTA intervention. The result of the initial PTA was often analyzed by the residual pressure gradient to determine if a stent was needed. If more one than one stent was required, the first was usually placed most cephalad, but this was not mandatory. Following stent placement, the residual pressure gradient was measured by a standard angiographic catheter, which replaced the balloon catheter. After an acceptable result was obtained, the catheter, guide wire, and sheath were removed and the puncture site controlled with direct manual compression. Each patient was maintained on 325 mg aspirin for at least 3 months.

The experimental protocol for this study was FDA-approved and the institutional review board approved both its implementation and the consent form which was used. Informed consent was obtained from each patient, with specific explanation of the experimental nature of the device and possible risk and benefits. Patient characteristics and noninvasive hemodynamic measurements were obtained on each patient prior to angiography. Clinical follow-up involved obtaining a history, lower extremity vascular physical examination, and a hemodynamic noninvasive study involving at least an ankle-brachial index (ABI). This evaluation was performed at 2 weeks, and at 1, 3, 6, 9, and 12 months, and then twice yearly thereafter. A pelvic radiograph and angiography was scheduled for 3 and 6 months post–stent placement, respectively.

Patients

From May 1987 through March 1991, 32 patients have participated in the iliac artery stent protocol at the Indiana University Medical Center. There were 24 male and eight female patients, with an average age of 61.8 ± 8.4 years (range, 44 to 76). Associated conditions included 20 patients with cardiovascular disease (seven had a previous coronary artery intervention), seven with cerebral vascular disease, eight with chronic pulmonary disease, and six were afflicted with significant renal compromise (serum creatinine above 1.5). All patients were (ten) or are (22) currently cigarette smokers. Obesity was recorded in seven patients, hypertension in 19, and diabetes in six, of whom two required insulin. Previous vascular interventions were common. Eleven patients had had a prior iliac PTA, of which five were bilateral. Three patients required a previous femorofemoral bypass graft and five a femoropopliteal or femorotibial graft. One patient had both a femorofemoral and femoropopliteal bypass graft. Except for one patient whose femoropopliteal graft had occluded prior to consulting us, each of the other grafts were at risk of failure secondary to inflow disease. One patient had had a previous aortoiliac endarterectomy and a superficial femoral artery atherectomy.

Thirty-seven limbs required a stent procedure. Symptoms per limb were lifestyle-limiting and worsening claudication in 23, rest pain in nine, and ulceration or gangrene in five. The preintervention ABI was 0.63 ± 0.28, reflecting the preponderance of patients with claudication. The specific indication for stent placement was an immediate technical failure in 25 cases: elastic recoil (four), dissection (ten), or an unacceptable PTA result based upon a residual stenosis or a residual pressure gradient (11). The procedure was planned as an adjuvant to angioplasty for restenosis in 12 cases. More than one stent (Fig. 30–4) was required for the desired effect in 24 cases, for a total of 95 stent deployments. The average number of stents per limb was 2.6 ± 1.6 (range, 1 to 7).

Specific radiographic and angiographic findings defined the lesions treated in a more precise manner. Fourteen iliac vessels demonstrated significant calcification which, however, did not preclude a balloon angioplasty. The target iliac artery lesion was located on the left side in 16, and on the right in 21. In five patients, the occlusive lesion was obviously bilateral. The location in the iliac artery requiring stent placement was the common iliac artery only in ten limbs, the external iliac artery only in 11, and traversed both segments in 16 limbs. The per cent diameter stenosis measured at the most stenotic area on biplanar angiography was 84.1 ± 13.7 per cent (range, 50 to 100 per cent) The minimal average luminal diameter of the occlusive disease was 2.0 ± 1.6 mm and the mean pressure gradient across the narrowing was 32.1 ± 17.7 mm Hg. The length of the vessel involved with the occlusive process averaged 4.1 ± 4.2 cm. Runoff status was classified as per the Adhoc Committee on Reporting Standards[16] and was generally very good, with a resistance value of less than 4 for 26 limbs, and 4 or higher for 11 limbs.

Results

Two patients (6.25 per cent), accounting for three limbs, expired during the first month of follow-up. One patient expired from an allergic reaction to the radiologic contrast material resulting in multisystem failure and death within 6 days. This patient required thrombectomy of one stented limb secondary to hypotension and thrombosis of that limb. The other mortality was a patient who expired from a myocardial infarct 3 weeks after the stent procedure had been completed. Electrocardiogram (ECG) and creatinine phosphokinase (CPK) isoenzyme measurements confirmed that no immediate myocardial infarction had occurred, and were obtained because of chest pain experienced during the procedure.

One other patient was classified as an immediate procedural failure. He experienced a perforation during the initial PTA of the iliac artery, and a detachable occlusive balloon was placed in the artery to prevent hemorrhage. Within a few days, a femorofemoral bypass graft was constructed to relieve the patient's symptoms, which had not been made worse by the PTA.

One patient required operative placement of a sixth stent to resolve a problem with dissection. This patient experienced a complication of the procedure, since the operative placement of the stent under local anesthesia had not been planned, but the event was not classified as a treatment failure. There were four other procedural complications including three groin hematomas, one of which required a 2-unit blood transfusion, and one arteriovenous fistula. The fistula did not require urgent operative repair, but was repaired at a later date.

There were two planned operative exposures of the common femoral artery for stent placement. In one case, a femorofemoral bypass graft was constructed at the time of stent placement. A dissection plane extending past the stent was unrecognized, and the postoperative ABI was not improved as much as would have been expected. Postoperative angiography confirmed that dissection was the cause of the luminal compromise. However, after 1 month of follow-up and with the patient on sodium warfarin (Coumadin), the luminal obstruction resolved as demonstrated by an improvement in the ABI and clinical symptoms. There were no problems with the second planned operative exposure.

The stent procedure resulted in a decrease of the mean pressure gradient across the lesion to 1.0 ± 2.1 mm Hg (n = 19). The postintervention ABI measured within a few days of the procedure increased to 0.82 ± 0.28 (Fig. 30–5). The clinical status of the patients was evaluated as per the criteria suggested by the Adhoc Committee on Reporting Standards[16] (Table 30–1). One of the patients, designated as a degree-of-clinical-improvement 0, experienced an unsuccessful stent procedure secondary to perforation as described previously. The patient classified as a degree -1 did not return until 5 months after stent placement, at which time by both angiographic and clinical criteria it was confirmed that the stented iliac artery was occluded.

Within 1 month of stenting, four limbs in four patients underwent

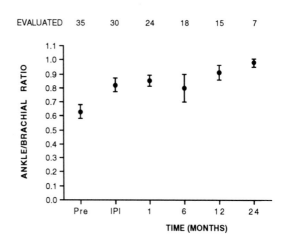

FIGURE 30–5. Average ankle-brachial index with standard error of the mean for preintervention (Pre), immediately postintervention (IPI), and at 1, 6, 12, and 24 months after stent placement. "Evaluated" indicates those patients available for study at that particular time. For the 12- and 24-month intervals, the raw data was obtained $\pm$ 3 months of the time indicated.

TABLE 30–1. THE CHANGE IN OVERALL CLINICAL STATUS PER LIMB FOLLOWING STENT PLACEMENT[a]

Clinical Status		Number of Limbs			
Degree	Description	0–1 Month	6 Months	12 Months	24 Months
+3	Asymptomatic and ABI > 0.90	16	15	10	6
+2	1+ Category and ABI > 0.10 ↑	6	3	3	—
+1	1+ Category or ABI > 0.10 ↑	5	1	1	1
0	No Δ category and ABI < 0.01 Δ	5	—	1	—
−1	1− Category or ABI > 0.10 ↓	1	—	—	—
−2	1− Category or unexpected minor amputation	0	1	—	—
−3	>1− Category or unexpected major amputation	0	—	—	—
Procedural mortality		3 (2 Patients)			

[a] The clinical and hemodynamic data for the 12- and 24-month periods of study represent a time interval of ± 3 months.

reconstruction for disease distal to the stented iliac artery. This consisted of one profundoplasty, one femorofemoral bypass graft, and two cases of femorodistal in situ grafting. These interventions were accounted for when reporting the resistance values for runoff, since this is the outflow affecting the stented iliac artery shortly after deployment. There would be four more patients with a resistance of 4 or greater if we had ignored these subsequent early interventions. The 1-month ABI for the 24 patients available for evaluation was 0.85 ± 0.21. The pelvic radiographs obtained at 3-month follow-up demonstrated no instance of stent migration. One patient died of complications of a necrotizing pneumonia 3 months following the stenting procedure. One patient required a below-knee amputation 4 months after iliac artery stent intervention because of distal disease. This patient had refused further distal intervention.

Six months after stent placement, clinical and hemodynamic improvement was evident in the majority of patients (Table 30–1; Fig. 30–5). The 6-month angiogram was usually obtained within a month or two of the planned date. There were six abnormal angiographic findings (28.6 per cent) in the 21 patients available for this part of the study. One patient demonstrated an angiographic stenosis of 63.2 per cent in the stented area of the iliac artery at 3-month follow-up. Redilatation with a balloon catheter successfully corrected the stenosis to approximate the normal luminal diameter. One stent failure was observed as complete occlusion of the iliac artery on the stented side with a diminished ABI (0.13) and worsening clinical symptomatology. These changes were found at approximately 6 months of follow-up and the procedure was considered a failure prior to its entrance into Table 30–1 and Figure 30–5 for the 6-month tabulation. Two patients experienced an iliac artery stenosis of less than 50 per cent on angiographic study, one above and one below the stented area. No intervention was performed in these two patients. One other patient demonstrated an angiographic stenosis of 66.7 per cent distal to the stented area; PTA increased the luminal area to 6 mm and resolved the intraluminal pressure gradient. This patient was the one patient categorized as a degree-of-clinical-improvement −2 by clinical evaluation at 6 months (Table 30–1). The final patient experienced recurrent, severe claudication at 3 months after stent deployment. Angiography demonstrated a more than 75 per cent

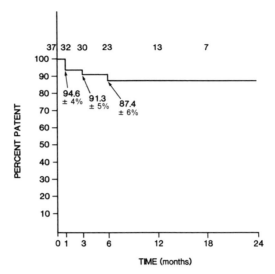

FIGURE 30–6. Life-table analysis of stent patency for the 37 limbs treated with a Palmaz balloon-expandable stent procedure.

luminal diameter reduction immediately below the stented artery. The patent refused percutaneous treatment and underwent a successful aortobifemoral bypass graft 6 months after the original stent placement.

One patient expired at 8 months following stenting of the iliac artery from a massive cerebral vascular accident. At 1 year, the hemodynamic and clinical results (Table 30–1; Fig. 30–5) were similar to those observed at 6 months. Between the first and second year, one patient required an additional iliac stent placed distal to the previous one, and also required a superficial femoral artery atherectomy to relieve his vascular symptoms entirely. At 2-year follow-up, seven limbs were available for analysis. The results, both hemodynamic and clinical, are shown in Table 30–1 and Figure 30–5.

Overall, there were four stent failures (10.3 per cent). Figure 30–6 is the patency statistics for the stent procedures as analyzed by the life-table method. There were two procedure-related deaths (three limbs), for a procedural

TABLE 30–2. CHARACTERISTICS OF PATIENTS EXPERIENCING A STENT FAILURE

Characteristics	Patient			
	14	19	24	26
Male		x	x	x
Diabetics			x	
HBP			x	
Renal				
Indication	CL	CL	CL	CL
Location	C&E	E	C&E	C&E
Length (cm)	6	6	4	3
% Stenosis	90%	100%	85%	95%
Side	L	R	R	L
Runoff[a]	0	6	0	6
Why stent	GR	GR	RS	Dis
Number of stents	2	1	4	3
Complication	Allergic RX hypotension-thrombosis	Perforation	RS at stent	Occluded
Time	3 Days	Immediate	3 Months	6 Months

[a] See test.

CL, claudication; E, external iliac artery; C, common iliac artery; GR, gradient/residual stenosis; RS, restenosis; Dis, dissection.

mortality of 6.25 per cent. Table 30–2 highlights the specifics for each case of stent failure to aid in clarifying the risk factors involved with failure. The seven early procedural complications (18.9 per cent) required four surgical (10.8 per cent) interventions, either early or delayed. Even with a patent stent, three aortoiliac interventions were required to maintain the desired clinical result.

Successful results of stenting for elastic recoil were obtained in 100 per cent (4 of 4) of cases, with a follow-up ranging from 8 to 24 months. Only one of the ten cases performed for dissection was unsuccessful, with follow-up ranging from 0.13 to 35 months. Two of eleven (18.2 per cent) iliac artery stents performed for an unacceptable PTA result and 1 of 12 (8.3 per cent) performed for restenosis were failures. The period of study ranged from 3 to 28 months and 2 to 18 months, respectively, for these last two indications of stent placement.

DISCUSSION

Before becoming involved in a new experimental protocol, two questions must be considered. Is the new device or drug needed? Is the device or drug you are considering the best available for a clinical trial?

Percutaneous transluminal angioplasty in the iliac arterial system is an accepted method of treating localized occlusive disease, with success rates at 1 year ranging from 50 to 93 per cent.[4,6,8,9,11,12,14] Two problem areas do exist: early technical failure and restenosis. Initially unsuccessful attempts at PTA have been reported to range from 6 to 15 per cent of all cases.[4,6,9,10,11] Our own early experience demonstrated a 13.7 per cent technical failure rate when PTA was performed in the iliac/common femoral artery.[3] Our involvement in the Veterans Administration Cooperative Study confirmed this finding when more modern balloon angioplasty catheter designs were used (15.5 per cent).[4] Approximately 25 per cent of these technical failures were in vessels where angioplasty was possible, but did not result in an acceptable lumen postinter-vention.[3,6] These cases may have been salvaged by an endoskeletal support (stent). The underlying cause of these early technical failures may involve spasm, acute thrombosis, dissection, elastic recoil, or any combination of these problems.[1,3,6,7,14,15]

Recurrent symptoms resulting from a PTA restenosis also occur.[3,4,6,8–10,14,15,17] Our own early experience with PTA demonstrated a 50 per cent restenosis at an average follow-up of 9.4 ± 4.5 months.[3] The overall experience of PTA failures suggests a rapid initial decline in the first 6 to 12 months of follow-up, with a more gradual decline thereafter.[3,4,6,8,9,10] Recurrent disease at the precise site of a previous PTA has been clearly documented by several investigators.[3,6,8,14,17] The reason for the restenosis appears to be fibromuscular hyperplasia or, at a later time, atherosclerosis.[18] Such a rapid progression of the disease process suggests that stents may also be useful in this setting. This is a somewhat controversial area, since second-attempt angioplasty results are not statistically different than primary PTA results.[14,17] However, there is a trend to a less-desirable outcome with reangioplasty,[14,17] and therefore stents have the potential to be useful in this setting.

At the time of original protocol evaluation, a number of stent designs were available for study. Nitinol wire-constructed stents (a thermal expansion device) were formed at high temperature as coils, and then straightened at room temperature for easy delivery to the target lesion. Neointimal thickening tended to narrow the stented lumen over an 8-week period in the canine model.[19]

Self-expanding stents were likewise being investigated. Maass et al. evaluated several steel alloy spiral spring designs in calf and canine models.[20] No stent migration or acute thrombosis was noted, but the delivery system was large and cumbersome. In the early 1960s, Wright et al. were involved with investigations of a stent constructed as a zig-zag arrangement of surgical stainless-steel wire.[21] Migration of the stent and acute thrombosis were not significant problems in a 30-stent canine experiment; however, incomplete contact with the vascular wall did result in an incomplete and delayed endothelial coverage of the stent.

The early Palmaz experiments were not without problems. In 1985, a canine experiment using his initial balloon-expandable stent reported one complete and two partially clotted stents, with eight stents doing well for up to 8.5 weeks.[22] In a longer follow-up of 18 canine stents, two demonstrated acute thrombosis and two occluded within 4 weeks. Furthermore, six stents were involved with a 30 per cent or more luminal narrowing over a 34-week period of observation.[23] This original stent was a continuous, woven stainless-steel design with cross-points soldered to resist radial collapse. These soldered points increased the local wall thickness to 405 μm from a 150 to 200 μm thickness in the remainder of the wall. An experimental study of a more streamlined model resembling the present stent design was reported in 1986.[5] It was constructed as a continuous stainless-steel wire arranged in eight rows of staggered, offset slots. The result without adjuvant anticoagulant or antiplatelet therapy was impressive. Twenty rabbits with artificially generated atherosclerotic plaque had the resultant stenosis corrected by stenting. All stents were patent up to 6 months following deployment, and no angiographic or histologic narrowing was observed in the area of stent deployment. Near-complete neointimal coverage was observed at 1 week following placement of the stents. There was continuous growth of this neointima over a 24-week period of study, but the majority of neointimal growth was noted in the first 8 weeks.

The Palmaz stent design seemed best from our perspective in a practical sense as well. It was delivered and deployed by standard PTA techniques requiring no difficult technical training. It was visible angiographically, which facilitated proper placement (Fig. 30–4). It was also versatile such that one size could be made to accommodate several luminal diameters. Biocompatibility and reasonable expansion characteristics were addressed experimentally, and were found acceptable.[5]

Based on these initial considerations, an experimental study of stents using the Palmaz design seemed reasonable and warranted. Furthermore, limiting the indications for stent placement to only those angioplasty sites experiencing a technical problem or being performed for restenosis would define a group of patients who would conceivably require more than the standard treatment for acceptable results. We could feel comfortable with this protocol, since the alternative was interventional failure in many cases.

Four PTA procedures required a stent placement because of elastic recoil which had resulted in minimal improvement in the vascular obstruction. The inherent arterial wall elasticity tends to promote this recoil to a deforming force such as balloon angioplasty.[24] Eccentric lesions, especially where one wall is relatively devoid of plaque, may be prone to this problem because no stiff plaque is present in the wall to eliminate recoil following balloon deflation.[15] All of these cases treated by stent placement, in our experience, have been successful for a period of observation ranging from 8 to 24 months. Stents may prove valuable in the treatment of this cause of immediate PTA failures.

Angioplasty-induced dissection as a technical problem can lead to stenosis or total occlusion of the lumen. Ten cases of PTA-induced dissection required stent placement in this series. These patients experienced a decreased blood flow through the vessel and would probably have required operative intervention if stents were not available. It is also interesting that when dissection played a part in stent requirement, generally two or more stents were needed to solve the problem. One case (10 per cent) had an initially poor clinical and hemodynamic result, was not further treated, and was proven to have progressed to total occlusion at approximately 6 months following stent placement. All other cases were found to have continued patency with a follow-up ranging from 4 days to 35 months. Certainly not all PTA-induced dissections will result in failure,[25,26] but early hemodynamic compromise would be most logically treated promptly if a low-risk device to do so was available. Stents may be especially useful in accomplishing this goal.[27] Possibly 2 per cent of all iliac PTA procedures demonstrate a significant dissection plane and may eventually define a population of patients where a stent would be needed.[9,25] On the basis of a recent experience, angioplasty-induced iliac artery dissection may be even more frequent and may approach a 5 per cent rate of occurrence.[27]

Technical failures seen as the inability of a PTA to affect an adequate hemodynamic and angiographic result also fail to demonstrate improvement in the clinical symptoms. These cases defy an easy classification, such as being designated examples of elastic recoil but the two categories may overlap somewhat in a practical sense. Such unacceptable PTA results do not seem to be a rare occurrence, since approximately 25 per cent of patients treated by PTA alone have a postprocedural gradient of 10 mm Hg or greater at rest.[11,12] Furthermore, the ability to correct this pressure gradient should be clinically beneficial.[11,28,29] Based on these facts, this group of patients may become a major contingent of those requiring a stenting procedure for optimal results. Eleven of our present cases are examples of this situation. Since all would be considered failures based upon the PTA results, an 81.8 per cent success rate over the period of this study seems acceptable. The failures include one case of occlusion following a severe hypotensive episode (patient died), and one case of PTA perforation prior to stent placement which required control for hemorrhage. In view of the actual reasons for failure, these results may seem even more respectable.

The success of the stenting procedure to maintain a widely patent iliac artery when performed for early technical failure is 22 of 25 cases, or 88 per cent. Considering the fact that these cases would have otherwise been considered immediate failures, such a technical result is excellent. However, our ultimate enthusiasm must be tempered by the risks of the procedure, which will be discussed later.

The last reason for stent deployment is a PTA failure secondary to restenosis. Iliac artery restenosis following a PTA is reported in 3.3 to 17 per cent of cases.[5,9,14] The majority of the restenosis problems occur in the first 6 months to 1 year after the original intervention.[4,6,8–10,14,15,17] Twelve cases in the present series were performed for this indication, and one has failed (8.3 per cent). This may not seem to be an improvement over the results of primary iliac PTA, but one should keep in mind that the patients stented are a highly select group. These patients have already demonstrated a propensity to restenosis, and although redilatation results are not statistically different from primary PTA results, there does appear to be a trend to lower patency in the secondary procedures.[14,17] It is hypothesized that the stent may decrease the restenotic process by forming a relatively smooth flow surface which prevents the proliferative injury response.[29] However, the accumulation of hyperplastic neointimal tissue noted in early experimental studies would suggest the possibility of such a buildup in the human artery, and was observed in one stent failure.[5] It is interesting that the only documented case of stented iliac artery restenosis would occur in a patient already shown to have the propensity for a hyperplastic response to injury of the vascular lumen.

The overall success of stenting iliac artery occlusive disease is 87.4 per cent as analyzed by the life-table method. The number of limbs available for analysis diminishes rapidly, however, and the results must be considered preliminary.

No obvious patient or specific characteristic of the iliac artery stenosis could be used to determine the likelihood of stent success or failure (Table 30–2). Clearly, more patients must be evaluated before such an analysis of predictive factors can be made. In a larger series of the Palmaz stent experience, it was also commented that the analysis of predictive factors for stent failure must await sufficient data acquisition.[30]

Seven stent procedures (18.9 per cent) were burdened with a complication, and five of these (13.5 per cent) required more than simple careful observation for a successful resolution. If all complications are included, 10 to 31 per cent of iliac PTA procedures will have a complication associated with the procedure, and 1.8 to 6 per cent will require aggressive intervention to correct the problem.[4,11,25] Certainly, our complication rate is not excessive in view of this information, but the requirement for aggressive treatment may be greater. The larger sheath and multiple balloon exchanges may result in complications requiring more frequent operative interventions or blood transfusions. One patient experienced two of the seven complications, requiring a 2-unit transfusion for a groin hematoma and surgical repair of an acquired arteriovenous fistula. This particular patient is a small woman whose small vessels reflect her small size. Certainly, the relative contraindication to a percutaneous approach when faced with a small common femoral artery (less than 5 mm) may apply to this woman and may highlight the need to take these precautions to heart. In addition, operative correction of aortoiliac occlusive disease is not without reported complications, and range from a 4 to 30 per cent incidence.[31-34] Major problems were encountered in only 9 to 13 per cent of these cases.[32,33] Again, the complication rate of the stent procedure is not prohibitive based on a comparison to surgical intervention, but may suggest a higher rate of complications requiring aggressive treatment. With a larger experience, better patient selection and technical expertise may eliminate some of these problems. In fact, in a larger reported series of stent procedures, the overall complication rate has decreased to 11.7 per cent.[30]

No vascular intervention is without the risk of a procedural mortality. The two deaths occurring within 30 days of the stent procedure reflect the systemic nature of atherosclerotic vascular disease, a myocardial infarction, and the risk of a radiologic contrast injection, an allergic reaction. The patient suffering the cardiac death had had no recent cardiac symptoms prior to the procedure. The patient with a contrast reaction had had no previous allergic history. Although the stent procedure itself was not the cause of death, the classification as a procedural mortality is warranted, since we did decide to treat these patients with the use of a stent. Whether this procedural risk will remain at 6 per cent cannot be determined at this early stage of study. The ultimate procedural mortality will have to reflect the less than 3 per cent risk of operative intervention and the less than 1 per cent PTA mortality risk for the treatment of aortoiliac occlusive disease.[6,4,8,11,31-34]

CONCLUSION

This initial experience with the Palmaz stent suggests that it can be a valuable adjuvant to PTA when used to salvage cases otherwise deemed immediate technical failures: PTA-induced dissections, elastic recoil, and technically unsuccessful PTA attempts. In these cases, 88 per cent of these cases have maintained a patent status during this period of the study. Percutaneous transluminal angioplasty restenosis may also be favorably influenced, demonstrating a 91.7 per cent patency rate. In all cases, longer follow-up will be required to verify the overall benefit, but life-table analysis would suggest an 87.4 per cent patency rate for the duration of this study. There is significant morbidity and mortality associated with this early experience with stent use in the iliac arterial system. Improvements in the procedural risk are likely to occur with experience and technical refinements, but for the present, these facts must be considered when evaluating risk versus benefit of the procedure for any given patient. It is clear that a larger and more extensive experience is the only way to determine the ultimate role of the Palmaz stent in the treatment of iliac artery occlusive disease.

REFERENCES

1. Becker GJ, Katzen BT, Dake MD: Noncoronary angioplasty. Radiology 1989;*170*:921–940.
2. Dotter CT: Transluminally-placed coilspring endarterial tube grafts. Invest Radiol 1969;*4*:329–332.
3. Glover JL, Bendick PJ, Dilley RS, et al: Efficacy of balloon catheter dilatation for lower extremity atherosclerosis. Surgery 1982;*91*:560–565.
4. Wilson SE, Wolf GL, Cross AP: Percutaneous transluminal angioplasty versus operation for peripheral arteriosclerosis. J Vasc Surg 1989;*9*:1–9.
5. Palmaz JC, Windeler SA, Garcia F, et al: Atherosclerotic rabbit aortas: Expandable intraluminal grafting. Radiology 1986;*160*:723–726.
6. Spence RK, Freiman DB, Gatenby R, et al: Long-term results of transluminal angioplasty of the iliac and femoral arteries. Arch Surg 1981;*116*:1377–1386.
7. Lu C, Zarins CK, Yang C, et al: Percutaneous transluminal angioplasty for limb salvage. Radiology 1982;*142*:337–341.
8. Johnston KW, Rae M, Hogg-Johnston SA, et al: 5-year results of a prospective study of percutaneous transluminal angioplasty. Ann Surg 1987;*4*:403–413.
9. Stokes KR, Strunk HM, Campbell DR, et al: Five-year results of iliac and femoropopliteal angioplasty in diabetic patients. Radiology 1990;*174*:977–982.
10. Cambria RP, Faust G, Gusberg R, et al: Percutaneous angioplasty for peripheral arterial occlusive disease. Arch Surg 1987;*122*:238–287.
11. Kadir S, White RI, Kaufman SL, et al: Long-term results of aortoiliac angioplasty. Surgery 1983;*94*:10–14.
12. Walden R, Siegel Y, Rubinstein ZJ, et al: Percutaneous transluminal angioplasty. J Vasc Surg 1986;*3*:583–590.
13. Colapinto RF, Stronell RD, Johnston WK: Transluminal angioplasty of complete iliac obstructions. AJR 1986;*146*:859–862.
14. Gallino A, Mahler F, Probst P, et al: Percutaneous transluminal angioplasty of the arteries of the lower limbs: A 5 year follow-up. Circulation 1984;*4*:619–623.
15. Krepel VM, van Andel GJ, van Erp WFM, et al: Percutaneous transluminal angioplasty of the femoropopliteal artery: Initial and long-term results. Radiology 1985;*156*:325–328.
16. Rutherford RB, Flanigan DP, Gupta SK, et al: Suggested standards for reports dealing with lower extremity ischemia. J Vasc Surg 1986;*4*:80–94.
17. Kalman PG, Johnston KW: Outcome of a failed percutaneous transluminal dilation. Surg Gynecol Obstet 1985;*161*:43–46.
18. Simpson JB, Selmon MR, Robertson GC, et al: Transluminal atherectomy for occlusive peripheral vascular disease. Am J Cardiol 1988;*61*:96G–101G.
19. Cragg AH, Lund G, Rysavy JA, et al: Percutaneous arterial grafting. Radiology 1984;*150*:45–49.
20. Maass D, Zollikofer CL, Largiader F, et al: Radiological follow-up of transluminally inserted vascular endoprostheses: An experimental study using expanding spirals. Radiology 1984;*152*:659–663.

21. Wright KC, Wallace S, Charnasangavej C, et al: Percutaneous endovascular stents: An experimental evaluation. Radiology 1985;*156;*69–72.
22. Palmaz JC, Sibbitt RR, Reuter SR, et al: Expandable intraluminal graft: A preliminary study. Radiology 1985;*156:*73–77.
23. Palmaz JC, Sibbitt RR, Tio FO, et al: Expandable intraluminal vascular graft: A feasibility study. Surgery 1986;*99:*199–205.
24. LeVeen RF, Wolf GL, Turco MA: Morphometric changes in normal arteries and those undergoing transluminal angioplasty. Invest Radiol 1983;*18:*63–67.
25. Gardiner GA, Meyerovitz MF, Stokes KR, et al: Complications of transluminal angioplasty. Radiology 1986;*159:*201–208.
26. Gardiner GA Jr, Meyerovitz MF, Harrington DP: Dissection complicating angioplasty. AJR 1985;*145:*627–631.
27. Becker GJ, Palmaz JC, Rees CR, et al: Angioplasty-induced dissections in human iliac arteries: Management with Palmaz balloon-expandable intraluminal stents. Radiology 1990;*176:*31–38.
28. Flanigan DP, Ryan TJ, Williams LR, et al: Aortofemoral or femoropopliteal revascularization? A prospective evaluation of the papaverine test. J Vasc Surg 1984;*1:*215–223.
29. Palmaz JC, Richter GM, Noeldge G, et al: Intraluminal stents in atherosclerotic iliac artery stenosis: Preliminary report of a multicenter study. Radiology 1988;*168:*727–731.
30. Palmaz JC, Garcia OJ, Schatz RA, et al: Placement of balloon-expandable intraluminal stents in iliac arteries: First 171 procedures. Radiology 1990;*174:*969–975.
31. Piotrowski JJ, Pearce WH, Johes DN, et al: Aortobifemoral bypass: The operation of choice for unilateral iliac occlusion? J Vasc Surg 1988;*8:*211–218.
32. Szilagyi DE, Elliott JP, Smith RF, et al: A thirty-year survey of the reconstructive surgical treatment of aortoiliac occlusive disease. J Vasc Surg 1986;*3:*421–436.
33. Bunt TJ: Aortic reconstruction vs extra-anatomic bypass and angioplasty. Arch Surg 1986;*121:*1166–1171.
34. Couch NP, Clowes AW, Whittemore AD, et al: The iliac-origin arterial graft: A useful alternative for iliac occlusive disease. Surgery 1985;*97:*83–87.

31

PRELIMINARY CLINICAL RESULTS OF ROTARY ATHERECTOMY

SAMUEL S. AHN, DARWIN ETON, and JOHN T. MEHIGAN

The Auth Rotablator (Biophysics International, Bellevue, WA) is a flexible catheter-deliverable atherectomy device with a variable sized, football-shaped metal burr on the distal tip (Fig. 31–1). The burr is studded with multiple diamond chips (22 to 45 μm size) that function as microblades. The burr comes in various sizes, ranging from 1.25 to 6.0 mm in diameter. During the recanalization process, progressively bigger burrs are used, depending on the artery size. The burr rotates at 100,000 to 200,000 rpm, is powered by a pressurized nitrogen gas tank, and tracks along a central guide wire. The guide wire must first traverse the lesion before rotational atherectomy can proceed. The high-speed rotation allows the diamond microchips to preferentially attack hard calcified atheroma while leaving the underlying normal elastic tissue intact (diminishing the risk of perforation). The pulverized particles are generally smaller than red blood cells and pass harmlessly through the circulation[1,2] and are depicted in Figures 31–2 through 31–4. The device leaves a smooth intraluminal surface with smooth distal endpoints and intact collateral orifices (Figs. 31–5 and 31–6). However, under scanning electron microscopy, denuded endothelium and etched grooves in the media can be seen, and imply that increased local thrombogenicity and the risk of restenosis from intimal hyperplasia are not obviated.

In the early experimental studies using the Auth Rotablator on harvested and intact human cadaver arteries, the Auth Rotablator was effective in recanalizing 16 of 22 cadaveric vessels. Five of the failures were in occluded segments, and one was in a stenotic segment. Causes for failure included inability to pass the guide wire (three), inability to pass the burr (one), guide-wire perforation (two), and burr perforation (one).[1,2]

After we completed these animal and cadaver experiments, prospective phase-II clinical trials were initiated at several centers. We will report the short- and long-term results of peripheral rotary atherectomy from the two institutions, UCLA and Stanford, that have the largest experience.

UCLA SERIES

Demographics

Between August 1987 and October 1989, 20 patients underwent 25 atherectomies of their femoral, popliteal and/or tibial arteries. The average age

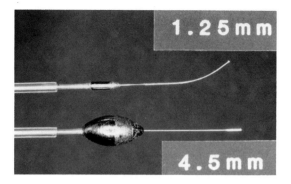

FIGURE 31–1. Atherectomy burr and guide wire. Burrs of 1.25 and 4.5 mm diameter, respectively, are shown. Note diamond microchips embedded in distal half of burr. Also note the coaxial spring-tip (top) and semirigid (bottom) guide wires. (Reproduced with permission from Ahn SS, Auth D, Marcus DR, Moore WS. Removal of focal atheromatous lesions by angioscopically guided high-speed rotary atherectomy: Preliminary experimental observations. J Vasc Surg 1988; 7(2):292–300.)

was 69 years, ranging from 49 to 89. There were 15 males and 5 female patients. Their risk factors for atherosclerosis were hypertension in 17 patients (85 per cent), coronary artery disease in 11 (55 per cent), diabetes mellitus in 10 (50 per cent), cigarette smoking history in eight (40 per cent), and hyperlipidemia in three (15 per cent). Indications for intervention were claudication in 11 cases (44 per cent), ulcer or gangrene in eight cases (33 per cent), rest pain in five cases (20 per cent), and asymptomatic failing graft in one case (4 per cent). Furthermore, in 17 of the 25 cases (68 per cent), the patient had at least one previous vascular reconstructive procedure.

Lesion Characteristics

The ankle-brachial index ranged from 0 to 0.73, mean 0.41. The per cent stenosis of the lesions to be treated ranged from 50 to 95 per cent (mean 90 per cent) in 20 of the cases. Occlusions were treated in the other five cases. The length of the lesions to be treated ranged from 1 to 40 cm, mean 14 cm. The lesion length was less than 7 cm in 12 cases, and greater than 10 cm in 13 cases, giving a median length of 10 cm for the 25 cases.

Technique

All atherectomy procedures were performed in the operating room by a multidisciplinary team—a vascular surgeon and an interventional cardiologist and/or an interventional radiologist working together.

After exposing the artery proximal to the atherectomy lesion, an introducer sheath ranging in size from 9 to 14 F (depending upon the artery size and the

FIGURE 31–2. Coulter counter analysis of atherectomized particles. Vertical axis is the distribution of particles. Horizontal axis is the relative threshold in size of particles. *PPT Small* = precipitate of particles generated by 2.5 mm burr; *PPT Large* = precipitate of particles generated by 4.5 mm burr; *SNT Small* = supernatant of centrifuged colloidal suspension generated by 2.5 mm burr; *SNT Large* = supernatant of centrifuged colloidal suspension generated by 4.5 mm burr. Note that particles are generally smaller than 10 µm. (Reproduced with permission from Ahn SS, Auth D, Marcus DR, Moore WS. Removal of focal atheromatous lesions by angioscopically guided high-speed rotary atherectomy: Preliminary experimental observations. J Vasc Surg 1988; 7(2):292–300.)

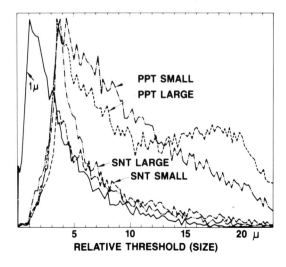

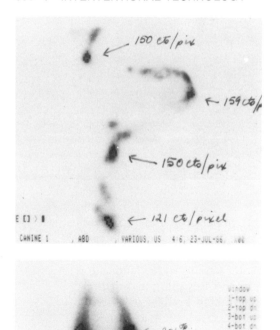

FIGURE 31–3. Radionuclide scan of dog injected with technetium 99m–labeled atherectomized particles. Note that most particles pass through the leg and accumulate in the lung, liver, and spleen, the reticuloendothelial system. (Reproduced with permission from Ahn SS, Auth D, Marcus DR, Moore WS. Removal of focal atheromatous lesions by angioscopically guided high-speed rotary atherectomy: Preliminary experimental observations. J Vasc Surg 1988; 7(2):292–300.)

burr size used) was inserted into the artery through an open arteriotomy. This sheath prevented repeated arterial trauma generated by multiple passages of the atherectomy device, angioscopes, catheters, and guide wires. The sheath's hemostatic valve also prevented back-bleeding, thus minimizing blood loss.

Prior to atherectomy, the lesion characteristics were documented angiographically in each of the 25 cases, and were inspected angioscopically in the operating room in 16 cases. A 0.014-inch atraumatic high-torque floppy guide wire was passed through the stenosis under fluoroscopic, and occasionally, angioscopic, control. A 4-F guide catheter was then inserted over the guide wire. The atraumatic guide wire was exchanged for the stiffer 0.009-inch

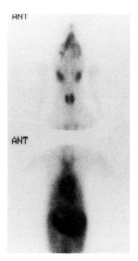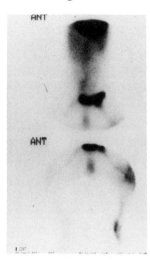

FIGURE 31–4. Radionuclide scan of control dog injected with technetium 99m in saline solution. Note accumulation of technetium radioactivity in the parotid gland, thyroid, heart, stomach, bladder, and joints. (Reproduced with permission from Ahn SS, Auth D, Marcus DR, Moore WS. Removal of focal atheromatous lesions by angioscopically guided high-speed rotary atherectomy: Preliminary experimental observations. J Vasc Surg 1988; 7(2):292–300.)

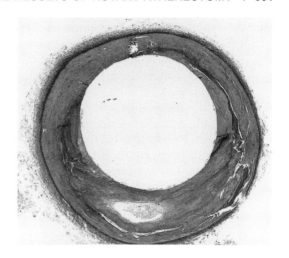

FIGURE 31–5. Photomicrographs of successfully atherectomized artery seen on cross section. Note smooth, highly polished, intraluminal surface denuded of intima and endothelial cells (hematoxylin-eosin stain; original magnification × 40). (Reproduced with permission from Ahn SS, Auth D, Marcus DR, Moore WS. Removal of focal atheromatous lesions by angioscopically guided high-speed rotary atherectomy: Preliminary experimental observations. J Vasc Surg 1988; 7(2):292–300.)

diameter atherectomy guide wire that comes with the Auth Rotablator system. The guide catheter was then exchanged for the atherectomy burr and drive shaft. Under fluoroscopic control, the burr was positioned just proximal to the obstructive lesion. The atherectomy turbine was connected to a pressurized nitrogen tank. The pressure was adjusted between 40 and 50 psi, thereby maintaining the burr rotational speed between 100,000 and 175,000 rpm. A 1-L solution of 0.9 per cent normal saline mixed with 100 cc of low molecular weight dextran-40 and 300 mg of papaverine was infused through the atherectomy irrigation port. Atherectomy commenced and the burr was advanced with a rapid to-and-fro, staccato-like motion through the obstructing lesion. A burr size approximately half the diameter of the native artery was used initially. After the first burr passed through the lesion, it was exchanged over the guide wire with one 0.5 or 1 mm diameter larger. This procedure was repeated until the residual luminal stenosis was less than 25 per cent.

Results were documented with completion angiography in each of the 25 cases. Completion angioscopy was performed in 16 cases. The procedure time, defined as the time from arteriotomy to arteriotomy closure was 15 to 240 minutes, mean 87 minutes. The actual atherectomy rotary time was 0.5 to 30 minutes, mean 8.9 minutes. The burr sizes used were 1.7, 2.0, 2.5, 3.0, 3.5,

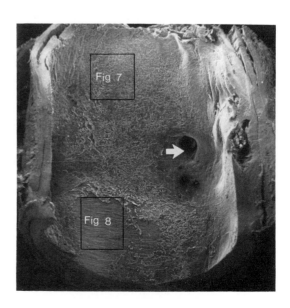

FIGURE 31–6. Scanning electron microscopy of sagittal section of a successfully rotary atherectomized popliteal artery (magnification × 40). Note smooth contoured luminal surface and intact patent geniculate branch orifice (arrow). Areas pictured in Figures 31–7 and 31–8 are boxed. (Reproduced with permission from Ahn SS, Arca MJ, Marcus DR, Moore WS. Histologic and morphologic effects of rotary atherectomy on human cadaver arteries. Ann Vasc Surg 1990; 4:563–569.)

4.0, and 4.5 mm. Simultaneous vascular reconstructive procedures were performed in 14 cases. These procedures included aortobifemoral bypass (three), common femoral or external iliac endarterectomy (five), profundaplasty (one), and femoropopliteal bypass (five). Atherectomy alone was performed in 11 cases.

Intravenous dextran (25 cc/hr) mixed with papaverin (15 mg/hr) was administered perioperatively for 24 to 48 hours in the first 12 cases. However, after observing early thrombosis in five patients, the next 13 patients received full heparinization for 24 to 48 hours. All patients received preoperative and long-term postoperative aspirin.

Data Analysis

Definition of success was divided into three categories: (1) initial intra-operative technical success, (2) in-hospital clinical success, and (3) late success or failure. The definition of initial intraoperative technical success was reduction of residual stenosis to less than 25 per cent with no significant flaps, dissections, or perforations visualized by completion intraoperative angiography of the atherectomized artery. The definition of in-hospital clinical success was: (a) intraoperative technical success; (b) postoperative improvement in the ankle-brachial ratio by 0.15 or more; (c) the presence of a palpable pulse immediately distal to the atherectomized segment; and (d) clinical improvement of tissue perfusion as manisfested by improved capillary refill, skin color, and warmth. All four of the above criteria had to be met. Late success was defined as persistence of the above criteria. Late failure was defined as recurrent or persistant preoperative symptoms, loss of previously palpable distal pulses, a decrease of ankle-brachial ratio by more than 0.15, and/or angiographic evidence of arterial stenosis 50 per cent or more.

Nineteen of the twenty-five patients had a follow-up angiogram, usually for clinical evidence of atherectomy failure. Of the six patients without follow-up angiogram, two patients had clinical evidence of failure and underwent amputation at 1 and 3 months, respectively, because of persistent nonhealing ulcers. Two patients underwent surgical exploration because of clinical evidence of failure but without angiographic documentation; these two patients had surgical documentation of their failures. One patient considered to have a technical and clinical success had no symptoms, normal ankle-brachial indices, and readily palpable pedal pulses. One patient had rapid healing of multiple previously nonhealing ulcers and subsequently remained asymptomatic with maintenance of a ankle-brachial index of 0.9.

The patients who underwent simultaneous vascular reconstructive procedure were considered to have atherectomy failure regardless of whether their atherectomized segment failed or the bypass reconstruction failed, since the two vascular beds were adjacent to each other and often depended upon each other for clinical success. In fact most of these patients did fail, and all of these failures were associated with a significant clinical deterioration. All failures in this group were documented by angiography and/or surgical reexploration.

All patients had physical examination and ankle-brachial indices in the recovery room, at 24 hours, and prior to discharge. Following discharge, all patients were followed at regular intervals during a period of 15 to 41 months, mean 26 months. Any deterioration in the patient's clinical status including decrease in postoperative Doppler pressure, loss of a palpable pulse, return of symptoms, or clinical evidence of decreased perfusion led to an angiogram or surgery to establish the etiology of failure.

Intraoperative Results

Technical success was achieved in 23 of 25 cases (92 per cent), and in 39 of 42 (93 per cent) arterial segments. The atherectomy device was equally effective in the superficial femoral, popliteal, and tibial arteries. We were successful in recanalizing 13 of 14 superficial femoral arteries, 14 of 15 popliteal arteries, and 12 of 13 tibial arteries. Two of the superficial femoral artery (SFA) lesions met the criteria for technical success but underwent balloon dilatation of a short residual segmental lesion to achieve the final desired result.

The two intraoperative failures were due to technical problems. In the first patient, the guide wire traversed a popliteal artery occlusion in a subintimal plane. This intimal dissection was unrecognized because of inadequate fluoroscopy equipment (which was replaced for subsequent cases). This problem was identified intraoperatively and the patient was treated immediately with a femoropopliteal artery bypass. In the second patient, a 3.0-mm burr was selected to treat a lengthy 95 per cent superficial femoral artery stenosis. This burr was probably too large for the initial recanalization and was advanced too rapidly. The burr became entangled within the artery and could not be removed transluminally. The burr became disconnected from the drive shaft when we attempted to pull the burr out of the artery. This patient required a cut-down of the above-knee popliteal artery to remove the burr, and femoropopliteal artery bypass was performed.

We failed to recanalize a peroneal artery because of the inability to pass the guide wire across a preocclusive peroneal artery orifice. However, the popliteal and anterior tibial artery stenoses were successfully atherectomized, and thus this patient was counted as a technical success.

Postoperative In-Hospital Results

There were five early thromboses. One patient developed thrombosis of an inadequate proximal vein interposition graft, but the atherectomized peroneal artery was patent on reexploration. The other four cases were each found to have a hypercoagulable state (two heparin-induced thrombocytopenia, one lupus anticoagulant, and one mixed). These were unsuspected preoperatively and were diagnosed as part of the evaluation of the thrombotic event. Heparin-induced thrombocytopenia was documented by identifying antiplatelet antibody with the heparin aggregation platelet test. A positive lupus anticoagulant was identified on serologic assay. One patient had multiple hypercoagulable abnormalities identified, including the presence of the lupus anticoagulant, heparin-induced thrombocytopenia, and disseminated intravascular coagulopathy (DIC). Disseminated intravascular coagulopathy was diagnosed on the basis of a positive protamine sulfate test, increased fibrin degradation product, and decreased fibrinogren level. This patient required a below-knee amputation. Histologic sections of the amputated limb showed microthromboemboli, consisting of aggregated red and white blood cells, platelet, and atheroma in the small arterioles.

Each of these five patients who developed early thrombosis in the hospital had an initial improvement of ankle-brachial index of greater than 0.15 during the first 24 hours following the procedure. However, within a week these patients developed clinical evidence of thrombosis manifested by decreased perfusion, loss of palpable pulse, and/or decrease of ankle-brachial pressure of at least 0.15. All five of these patients were documented to have thrombosis by either angiogram or surgical exploration.

Complications

The in-hospital complications include the intimal dissection and burr entanglement mentioned in the operative results section. There was one other equipment breakage; namely, a disconnection of the guide-wire spring tip. This guide-wire fragment was retrieved transluminally using an angioscopically guided flexible grabber. There were no perforations.

There were four cases of hemoglobinemia and microscopic hemoglobinuria documented by serum and urine chemistry tests. These patients presented with tea-colored urine, which resolved within 8 hours. There were no electrolyte abnormalities or renal insufficiency in any of these patients. The creatinine and blood urea nitrogen (BUN) remained unchanged from preoperative values, and the urine output remained brisk. There was one groin-wound hematoma and one groin-wound infection.

There were three cases of clinically insignificant microthromboemboli that were diagnosed by the clinical findings of multiple small maculopapular cutaneous lesions randomly distributed over the foot and/or the thigh. These lesions resolved spontaneously within 1 to 3 weeks without any clinical sequelae. Two patients, however, developed clinically significant thromboemboli. One patient had undergone atherectomy of a long superficial femoral artery stenosis, and developed extensive patches of diffuse petechiae and skin necrosis on his thigh consistent with thromboembolism. The other had a mixed hypercoagulable state (described above) and required an amputation following thrombosis of the atherectomized segment.

With the two early technical failures and five early thromboses, the in-hospital clinical success rate was 18 of 25 (72 per cent).

Long-Term Results

Late failure was observed in 14 additional cases. Intimal hyperplasia was clearly documented angioscopically in two SFA-treated cases during secondary vascular reconstructions at 3 and 5 months, respectively. Two popliteal artery occlusions occurred in cases where the SFA alone was atherectomized. During secondary reconstructions at 5 and 9 months, respectively, the popliteal artery segment was explored through a posterior approach and repaired with an interposition vein graft in one case, and a popliteal thrombectomy with tibial patch angioplasty in the other. In both instances, intimal hyperplasia of the popliteal artery was identified and presumed to be secondary to the guide-wire trauma during atherectomy and/or the subsequent hemodynamic changes postatherectomy. The other late failure occurred 2 to 18 months postoperatively, and the angiograms suggested intimal hyperplasia in all cases.

The 2-year primary patency rate of the 25 cases was 12 per cent, and the secondary patency rate was 29 per cent. The primary patency rate of the 18 cases with in-hospital success (modified primary patency) was 66 per cent at 6 months, but the 2-year patency dropped to 17 per cent.

Further analysis revealed that the cases in which claudication was the indication for atherectomy was only slightly better than the primary patency of the cases in which limb threat was the indication for treatment. The difference between these two groups was not statistically significant.

The shorter lesions (less than 7 cm) had a slightly higher patency rate after 12 months than the longer lesions (greater than 10 cm). However, this difference was not statistically significant.

Cases involving atherectomy alone had a better intermediate patency rate at 1 and 6 months compared to the cases in which the patient underwent a simultaneous vascular reconstruction. The difference between these two groups was statistically significant ($p < 0.02$).

The first 12 cases in this series were treated with perioperative dextran and papaverin and had generally worse results than the last 13 cases that were treated with perioperative heparin; but this difference was not statistically significant ($p > 0.1$).

Only two patients clearly benefited from the rotary atherectomy procedure. One of these was an 89-year-old woman with multiple nonhealing ulcers and diffusely stenotic superficial femoral, popliteal, and tibial artery disease. She was not a suitable candidate for percutaneous balloon angioplasty because of the diffuse nature of the disease, nor was she a candidate for vascular reconstruction because of her cardiovascular status. However, she underwent successful atherectomy of the entire superficial femoral, popliteal, and proximal tibial arteries with subsequent complete healing of her ulcers. She died 6 months later from complications of a hip fracture that occurred during one of her daily walks.

The other patient that clearly benefited in this study had multiple thromboembolic events to the distal limb and had diffusely ulcerated but patent superficial femoral, popliteal, and proximal tibial arteries with no other cardiac or vascular abnormalities noted on echocardiogram, Holter monitor testing, and angiography. Percutaneous balloon angioplasty was contraindicated in this patient with thromboembolic symptoms; open endarterectomy would have been difficult and associated with significant morbidity; and bypass with exclusion of diseased segments could have caused significant vascular compromise to the gastrocnemius muscles and other popliteal fossa structures with possible interval gangrene. Rotary atherectomy resulted in complete resolution of his lesions and the patient remained asymptomatic with palpable pulses and normal ankle Doppler pressures at 2 years' follow-up.

STANFORD SERIES

Demographics

Thirty-eight patients underwent 42 atherectomy sessions of iliac (one common and one external iliac), superficial femoral (24), profunda femoral (one), popliteal (11), anterior tibial (four), tibioperoneal (one), posterior tibial (one), and peroneal (ten) arteries. Four sessions were combined with surgical reconstruction of an ipsilateral segment and were excluded from data analysis. The average age was 65. There were 28 male and 14 female patients. Their risk factors for atherosclerosis were hypertension in 35 patients (83 per cent), coronary artery disease in 29 (69 per cent), diabetes mellitus in 19 (45 per cent), and history of cigarette smoking in 28 (67 per cent). Indications included stable claudication (45 per cent), severe disabling (less than 100 ft) claudication (10 per cent), or ischemic limb threat (45 per cent). Preprocedure evaluation revealed 29 (69 per cent) of patients to be favorable, eight (19 per cent) unfavorable, and five (12 per cent) prohibitive candidates for conventional surgical reconstruction with respect to vascular anatomy, conduit availability, and medical condition.

Technique

All atherectomy procedures were performed by the senior cardiologist. Half were treated percutaneously and half were treated in the operating room.

The same procedure was followed as was described in the UCLA series. The one difference was that balloon angioplasty was frequently performed on the arterial segment immediately after creation of a satisfactory lumen in the Stanford series. Systemic heparin was used for 12 to 24 hours after the procedure.

Prior to atherectomy, the lesion characteristics were documented angiographically. Arterial pulses were recorded. The majority of patients underwent Doppler measurement of the ankle-brachial index (ABI). Arteriograms were performed following atherectomy, along with serial ABI. A blinded review of preatherectomy and postatherectomy angiograms was performed by three to five interventional radiologists and resulted in a consensus opinion as to arteriographic success of the procedure. Hemodynamic success was defined by the development of a new palpable pulse or an improvement in ABI of more than 0.15. Clinical success at 6 months was defined by a greater than 100 per cent increase in claudication distance, relief from rest pain, or healing of an ischemic ulcer.

Immediate Results

Of the 38 Rotablator procedures followed, immediate angiographic and hemodynamic success were obtained in 18 cases (46 per cent). Immediate angiographic success associated with hemodynamic failure were seen in nine cases (24 per cent). Both immediate angiographic and hemodynamic failure were seen in two cases (5 per cent). Intraprocedure failure of atherectomy was seen in the remaining nine cases (24 per cent).

Of the nine intraprocedure failure of atherectomy cases, six (67 per cent) had been considered "favorable" surgical candidates, one an "unfavorable" candidate, and two were deemed "prohibitive" candidates. Six of these patients had ischemic limb threat, and three had stable claudication. The complications that resulted in procedure failure in these patients were: aortic dissection following iliac atherectomy (emergent aortobifemoral bypass required for retroperitoneal hemorrhage); peroneal perforation (leading to below-knee amputation); three cases of foot ischemia and sepsis (leading to below-knee amputation in two and femoropopliteal bypass in the third); and four cases of dissection of the superficial femoral artery, one of which was also complicated further by perforation of the posterior tibial artery (all treated surgically by femorodistal bypass grafting). Overall, two of the limb losses were attributable to the device (the third below-knee amputation was attributed to nature of disease despite atherectomy failure because the patient was a prohibitive surgical candidate). Two life-threatening complications, the aortic dissection and one of the ischemic foot/sepsis cases, were also attributed to the device.

Complications

Minor complications occured in eight patients (25 per cent). Four experienced transient hemoglobinuria resolving without sequelae in 12 to 24 hours. Nonhemodynamically significant SFA dissection was noted angiographically in two patients who were simply observed without sequellae. Superficial femoral artery perforation and creation of intimal flaps occured in one patient, who was also observed without sequellae. A femoral pseudoaneurysm occurred at the femoral puncture site in one patient, which resolved spontaneously.

There was no significant difference in the incidence of complications or efficacy of atherectomy between percutaneous and open atherectomy.

Results at 6 Months

Of the 18 cases having immediate angiographic and hemodynamic success, only 11 (61 per cent) remained clinically and hemodynamically improved at 6 months. Seven (39 per cent) deteriorated both angiographically and hemodynamically. Four (22 per cent) experienced recurrent symptoms and required an adjunctive intervention.

Of the nine cases having immediate angiographic success associated with hemodynamic failure, six (67 per cent) required an adjunctive intervention, one failed hemodynamically but improved clinically (increase in claudication distance), one patient died, and the last was lost to follow-up.

Of the two cases having both immediate angiographic and hemodynamic failure, both were poor surgical candidates and no further intervention was undertaken. Both died within 6 months of unrelated causes, and with unchanged symptoms

Of the 19 patients treated with the Rotablator alone for claudication, 18 (95 per cent) had an immediate increase of 100 per cent or greater in claudication distance, and 11 of 18 (61 per cent) maintained this at 6 months. Of the five patients treated with the Rotablator alone for ischemic ulceration, only one healed his ulcer by 6 months. Of the seven patients treated with ischemic rest pain, only one was pain free at 6 months without requiring another intervention. Eleven patients had another angiogram during the 6-month interval. Nine had occluded the atherectomized segment.

The combined success rate at 6 months for all patients was 29 per cent. The complication rate was 21 per cent. Three perforations (7 per cent) occurred, two requiring emergent bypass and one resulting in below-knee amputation.

DISCUSSION

Endovascular surgery has recently emerged as a possible adjunct or alternative to conventional peripheral arterial reconstruction.[3] There are now four endovascular techniques available to recanalize atherosclerotic arteries: balloon dilatation, laser recanalization, thromboendarterectomy, and atherectomy. Percutaneous transluminal balloon angioplasty (PTA) has become an established effective method for treating short stenoses in the iliac and superficial femoral arteries; however, it has proved less effective in the treatment of occlusions or of long complex stenoses.[4–8] Laser-assisted balloon angioplasty (LABA) is still under development. So far, the long-term results of LABA have been suboptimal due to a high restenosis rate.[9–12] Semiclosed mechanical endarterectomy using the Hall oscillating endarterectomy instrument has a 55 to 75 per cent 2-year cumulative patency rate for iliac and femoral arterial segments, but its efficacy in the smaller popliteal and tibial arteries drops to less than 33 per cent.[13] Furthermore, this technique still requires dissection of the proximal and distal endpoints, tacking of the distal intima, and patch angioplasty of the distal arteriotomy. Mechanical atherectomy, the selective removal of atheroma from atherosclerotic diseased arteries combines the relative simplicity of balloon angioplasty and the atheroma removal capability of endarterectomy.

There are at least 12 different atherectomy devices currently under development. Four have undergone previous preliminary clinical trials and have received FDA approval for general clinical use. These four include the Simpson Peripheral Atherocath (Devices for Vascular Intervention Inc, Redwood, CA), the Kensey catheter (now known as the Trac-Wright catheter: Dow

Corning Wright, Arlington, TN), the transluminal extraction catheter (TEC: InterVentional Technologies Inc, San Diego, CA), and most recently, the Auth Rotablator (Heart Technology Inc, Bellevue, WA).

The Auth Rotablator effectively recanalized 80 to 90 per cent of the arteries attempted. Unlike previous studies of other atherectomy devices, over half of the cases in the UCLA study involved limb-threatening ischemia and lesion length longer than 10 cm. The Simpson Atherocath has been reported to have an initial success rate of 87 per cent in patients presenting predominantly with claudication and whose lesions were generally shorter than 7 cm.[14] Snyder et al. reported that the Kensey atherectomy device was initially successful in only 14 of 23 cases (61 per cent) in patients with lesions comparable in severity to those described in the UCLA Rotablator series.[15,16] Wholey et al. reported using the transluminal extraction catheter to achieve an initial success rate of 92 per cent in 126 lesions in 95 patients who were 90 per cent claudicants and had lesions generally less than 3 cm.[17] Thus, the Auth Rotablator appears equally, if not more, capable than these other devices in achieving initial technical success.

The UCLA intermediate in-hospital success rate of 72 per cent is also similar to that reported for other atherectomy devices, but is significantly worse than bypass grafting. In addition to the two early technical failures reported in the UCLA series, five patients developed early in-hospital thrombosis of the atherectomized limb. These thrombotic events occurred despite dextran and papaverine. It is interesting that four of these patients with early thrombosis had one or more hypercoagulable states, which was unsuspected preoperatively and diagnosed only postoperatively during evaluation of the thrombotic event. Thus, it is unclear how much the hypercoagulable state contributed to the early thrombosis and how much the atherectomy procedure itself caused the thrombotic complication. It is tempting to speculate that the Auth Rotablator possibly initiated the hypercoagulable state, but Whittimore et al. reported that as many as 15 to 20 per cent of patients undergoing routine vascular reconstructive procedures have an underlying hypercoagulable state.[18] Furthermore, it is important to note that the subsequent 13 patients treated with perioperative heparin did not develop early thrombosis, suggesting that heparin effectively prevents these early thrombotic complications. The Stanford series reported results in a population that received perioperative heparin. Thrombosis was not as high as in the first 12 UCLA patients treated without heparin.

The two UCLA patients who developed clinically significant embolic complications (i.e., thigh skin loss and below-knee amputation, respectively) deserve further discussion. In our previous cadaver experiments, the particles generated from rotary atherectomy were generally smaller than red blood cells, passed harmlessly through the canine capillary circulation, and were taken up mostly by the lung, liver, and spleen.[1] However, there were some larger singular or aggregated particles in the 20- to 40-μm range which would not pass through the capillary circulation. These larger particles were generated by the larger 4.5-mm burr, but not the smaller 2.5-mm burr; the larger burr, having larger diamond chips, generated larger particles. Not surprisingly, in the current clinical study, all three of the minor emboli and both of the major emboli cases involved atherectomy of long superficial femoral artery segments treated with burr sizes 4.0 and/or 4.5 mm in diameter.

Furthermore, the atherectomy procedure was performed using an open technique in which the inflow was clamped, thus reducing blood flow and promoting stasis, which in turn could have encouraged aggregation of small particles into larger particles. On the other hand, we may be observing simply a mass effect of a large atheroma particle burden; both of the patients who suffered embolic tissue loss underwent atherectomy of long superficial femoral artery lesions resulting in a large atheroma particle burden that may have overwhelmed the ability of the distal capillary circulation to clear the embolic debris. It is also interesting that one of these patients developed disseminated intravascular coagulopathy. One could speculate that this coagulopathy was precipitated by fat emboli from the atheromatous debris.

One unexpected complication in this clinical series was the development of hemoglobinuria and hemoglobinemia in both the UCLA and the Stanford series. All four patients in the UCLA series had long superficial femoral artery lesions, a rotary atherectomy time of greater than 8 minutes, and the use of burr sizes 4.0 mm or 4.5 mm. This hemoglobinuria is most likely caused by the vortex action created by the high-speed rotating burr, which disrupts the red blood cells. Since a larger burr has a greater circumference, it rotates at a faster circumferential speed than the smaller burrs at any given rpm, creating a greater sheer stress. This has been documented in vitro (Auth D, personal communication). Thus selection of smaller sized burrs and limiting the rotary atherectomy time (preferably less than 5 minutes) may decrease or eliminate this complication. Fortunately, the hemoglobinuria was transient, and caused no clinical sequelae. However, the potential for renal insufficiency must be considered.

Since all four cases of hemoglobinemia and hemoglobinuria, and all five cases of thromboembolic complications in the UCLA series occurred in the cases involving long superficial femoral artery lesions requiring long rotary atherectomy times and use of the larger 4.0- by 4.5-mm burrs, one should avoid rotary atherectomy of long SFA lesions that require long atherectomy time and burrs 4.0 mm or larger.

The low incidence of perforation and late aneurysmal changes was predicted by our previous experimental studies, which suggested that the elastin fibers of the arterial wall remained intact.[12,13] In fact, differential cutting prevented perforation in one patient despite the fact that the guide wire (and thus the burr rotating over the guide wire) were in a subintimal plane. We also found that selection of an oversized burr or a too-rapid progression of burr sizes prevented efficient and safe atherectomy, as demonstrated in the patient whose burr became lodged in the SFA and broke off. Thus proper guide-wire placement, proper selection of burr sizes, and gradual increase in burr diameter are crucial.

Despite the satisfactory early technical results, the long-term primary and secondary patency rates of atherectomized arteries were dismal. Even the later group of 13 cases in the UCLA series that had perioperative heparin, no early thrombosis, and no technical failure had a poor 8 per cent patency rate at 2 years. Furthermore, all late failures occurred between 2 and 18 months postatherectomy, highly suggestive of intimal hyperplasia rather than thrombosis (which occurs within 1 to 7 days) or progression of underlying atherosclerosis (which occurs after 2 years). In four cases, intimal hyperplasia was clearly documented postatherectomy by vascular endoscopy (two cases), and by direct surgical inspection (two cases). In the latter two cases, the occluded popliteal arteries with the intimal hyperplasia were distal to the atherectomy sites, suggesting the possibility of guide-wire injury distal to the atherectomy burr. Of note is that the guide wire was seen periodically to undulate under fluoroscopy during burr rotation. Also, the other late failures had angiographic findings highly suggestive of intimal hyperplasia (i.e., smooth, tapered narrowing of the atherectomized artery).

Thus, intimal hyperplasia may be the biggest unsolved problem facing rotary atherectomy. Previous histologic studies of atherectomized arteries showed endothelial peeling and abrasion of medial smooth muscles of atherectomized arteries.[13] Despite the smooth polished luminal surface of the atherectomized artery seen on inspection, intimal and medial injury invariably occurred and incited intimal hyperplasia. Even claudication patients with short lesions were not spared.

The adverse influence of simultaneous vascular reconstruction on the atherectomy results was statistically apparent. This difference may reflect the fact that the patients undergoing simultaneous vascular reconstruction have multilevel disease with more advanced complex lesions. Another possibility is that the prolonged low flow state in the distal atherectomized artery present during the proximal bypass procedure allowed subclinical thrombosis formation on the freshly denuded luminal surface. The patency curves of the group that underwent simultaneous vascular reconstruction versus atherectomy alone showed the most disparity at the 1-month interval, suggesting thrombosis rather than intimal hyperplasia as the cause of the numerous early failures in the vascular reconstruction group.

The Stanford series only has 6-month follow-up data to this point. However, several important observations were able to be drawn. Patients with claudication received the greatest benefit acutely, with a 95 per cent clinical success rate; dropping, however, to 61 per cent by 6 months. This was in marked contrast to the 9 per cent clinical success rate for patients with limb-threatening ischemia. The combined success rate for the Stanford series was a dismal 29 per cent. Immediate and 6-month hemodynamic success rates in patients considered good surgical candidates were 52 and 33 per cent, respectively. These are inferior to the 5-year patency rate of 75 per cent reported by Taylor et al. for reversed vein infrainguinal bypass grafting.[19] Lastly, two thirds of the major complications reported in the Stanford series were observed in "favorable" surgical candidates.

The Auth Rotablator has early results comparable to other atherectomy devices. The 6-month patency rate of cases treated with atherectomy alone was 73 per cent in the UCLA series; and the 6-month patency rate of all the patients with in-hospital success was 66 per cent. Simpson et al. reported that patients with initial success treated with the Simpson Atherocath had at least a 36 per cent restenosis rate at 6 months; and only 69 per cent of these successfully treated patients, or 50 per cent of the total patient population, continued to have improved exercise tolerance at the 6-month follow-up interval.[14] Snyder et al. reported for the Kensey catheter a cumulative 1-year patency rate of 37.5 per cent and a 6-month patency rate of 63.9 per cent for the patients with initial success. The long-term results of the TEC catheter have not been reported. Finally, one should note that the TEC device and Simpson catheter treated favorable lesions 7 cm or less in patients predominantly with claudication. In the UCLA Rotablator series, the lesions averaged 10 cm in length, and the majority of patients had limb threat.

It is also quite possible that the late patency results of other atherectomy devices would appear similarly poor when proper long-term follow-up is reported. One should note that reporting our results at a 12-month follow-up interval would have erroneously overestimated the overall benefit of this procedure. Thus, atherectomy data previously reported, and having only 6- or

12-month follow-up, must be viewed skeptically. Indeed, premature reporting of endovascular device results is misleading and should be avoided.

The role of the rotary atherectomy in the treatment of peripheral arterial occlusive disease is limited by its early thromboembolic complications and dismal late patency rates. Perhaps rotary atherectomy could be useful in very selected and unusual cases where a patient has a short life expectancy or has lesions that are not suited for standard balloon angioplasty or vascular reconstruction. Such lesions would include hard calcified atheroma that cannot be dilated by balloon angioplasty, or ulcerated atheroma with embolic manifestations in which balloon angioplasty is contraindicated as demonstrated by the two patients in the UCLA study that benefited from rotary atherectomy. Another hypothetical benefit would be the "buying of time" to clear infection in an ischemic limb without suitable autogenous conduit with which to bypass, in anticipation of future prosthetic bypassing.

In conclusion, rotary atherectomy is still experimental and is not recommended for general use. The problem of late restenosis secondary to intimal hyperplasia must be solved first. However, the field of endovascular surgery is still in its infancy, and one should not be discouraged by these poor results. Instead, further rigorous investigation should be vigorously pursued to solve the intimal hyperplasia problem and to refine endovascular technology.

REFERENCES

1. Ahn SS, Auth D, Marcus D, Moore WS: Removal of focal atheromatous lesions by angioscopically guided high-speed rotary atherectomy: Preliminary experimental observations. J Vasc Surg 1988;7:292–300.
2. Ahn SS, Arca M, Marcus D, Moore WS: Histologic and morphologic effects of rotary atherectomy on human cadaver arteries. Ann Vasc Surg 1990;4:563–569.
3. Moore WS, Ahn SS, (eds): Endovascular Surgery. Philadelphia, WB Saunders Co., 1989.
4. Zeitler E, Richter EI, Roth EJ, et al: Results of percutaneous transluminal angioplasty. Radiology 1983;146:57–60.
5. Cumberland DC: Percutaneous transluminal angioplasty. Clin Radiol 1983;34:25–38.
6. Lally ME, Johnston KW, Andrews D: Percutaneous transluminal dilation of peripheral arteries: An analysis of factors predicting early success. J Vasc Surg 1984;1:704–709.
7. Doubilet P, Abrams HL: The cost of underutilization: Percutaneous transluminal angioplasty for peripheral vascular disease. N Engl J Med 1984;310:95–102.
8. Stanton AW: A perspective of percutaneous transluminal angioplasty. Cardiovasc Clin 1983;13:245–259.
9. White RA, White GH: Laser thermal probe recanalization of occluded arteries. J Vasc Surg 1989;9:598–608.
10. Wright JG, Belkin, Greenfield AJ, et al: Laser angioplasty for limb salvage: Observations on early results. J Vasc Surg 1989;10:29–38.
11. Perler BA, Osterman FA, White RI, Williams GM: Percutaneous laser probe femoropopliteal angioplasty: A preliminary experience. J Vasc Surg 1989;10:352–357.
12. Seeger JM, Abela GS, Silverman SH, Jablonski SK: Initial results of laser recanalization in lower extremity arterial reconstructions. J Vasc Surg 1989;9:10–17.
13. Lerwick ER: Oscillating loop endarterectomy for peripheral vascular reconstruction. Surgery 1985;97:574–584.
14. Simpson JB, Selmon MR, Robertson GC, et al: Transluminal atherectomy for occlusive peripheral vascular disease. Am J Cardiol 1988;61:96–101.
15. Snyder SO, Wheeler JR, Gregory RT, et al: Kensey catheter: Early results with a transluminal endarterectomy tool. J Vasc Surg 1988;8:541–543.
16. Desbrosses D, Petit H, Torres E, et al: Percutaneous atherectomy with the Kensey catheter: Early and midterm results in femoropopliteal occlusions with the Kensey dynamic angioplasty catheter. Radiology 1989;172:95–98.
17. Wholey MH, Smith JAM, Godlewski BS, Nagurka M: Recanalization of total arterial occlusions with the Kensey dynamic angioplasty catheter. Radiology 1989;172:95–98.
18. Donaldson MC, Weinberg DS, Belkin M, et al: Screening for hypercoagulable states in vascular surgical practice: A preliminary study. J Vasc Surg 1990;11:825–831.
19. Taylor LM, Edwards JM, Porter JM: Present status of reversed vein bypass grafting: Five-year results of a modern series. J Vasc Surg 1990;11:193–206.

32

THE IMPACT OF NONOPERATIVE THERAPY ON THE CLINICAL MANAGEMENT OF PERIPHERAL ARTERIAL DISEASE

FRANK J. VEITH

Nonoperative therapy of arterial disease may be defined as including all conservative noninterventional treatments and those which are interventional but which do not require traditional open surgical operation. The latter nonsurgical endovascular interventions include percutaneous transluminal balloon angioplasty (PTA) and techniques to ablate atherosclerotic plaque using a variety of laser energy systems or atherectomy devices. Although these endovascular interventions may be performed percutaneously, they can also be carried out via direct surgical access to an artery at a point remote from the site of proposed treatment. In general, most of the laser systems and some of the atherectomy devices have been used in combination with balloon angioplasty to enhance luminal restoration of the occluded or narrowed arterial segment being treated.

One purpose of this chapter is to consider the impact of percutaneous transluminal balloon angioplasty (PTA) and other, newer endovascular techniques with laser or atherectomy devices on the treatment of lower limb ischemia produced by aortoiliac and infrainguinal arteriosclerosis. A second purpose is to examine the role of conservative, noninterventional treatment, which in many instances amounts to nontreatment, in the management of this common disease entity.

To achieve these goals it is necessary to review briefly the natural history of the various clinical stages of lower limb ischemia resulting from arteriosclerosis as well as the current ability to deal with this process by open surgical operations which include, primarily, bypass procedures. With these facts in mind, we can evaluate the role and potential impact of conservative noninterventional treatment and the nonoperative endovascular interventions in managing atherosclerotic lower limb ischemia. To this end, the following questions must be addressed. How can these endovascular interventions better *or worsen* the natural history of the disease process? Should they justify a change in the indications for intervention? Can they replace or facilitate standard operative treatment? To answer these questions we need to know the relative safety and efficacy, both short- and long-term, of standard operations, the newer endovascular treatments, and conservative treatment for various stages of the disease process. In most instances, precise data to answer these complex questions with certainty is not available. The following discussion will therefore largely be an expression of opinion based on reasonable extrapolations of what is currently known about an extraordinarily common and usually benign disease process and its response to standard operative treatment and PTA. It will also highlight gaps in knowledge that need to be filled to provide precise answers to the questions posed. Finally, it will address the issue of who, by virtue of their experience in dealing with this disease process, is best qualified to treat it and provide definitive answers to these questions.

NATURAL HISTORY, STAGING, AND TREATMENT OF LOWER EXTREMITY ISCHEMIA: ROLE OF CONSERVATIVE TREATMENT AND NONTREATMENT

Arteriosclerosis may involve the infrarenal aorta, the iliac arteries, the common femoral artery and its branches, the above-knee and below-knee popliteal artery, any of the infrapopliteal arteries including their terminal branches, or any combination of these arteries. This involvement generally begins early in adult life and progresses slowly to the point where a flow-reducing stenosis or occlusion occurs in one or more of the arteries below the renal segment of the aorta. As the average age of our population increases, the number of individuals with this hemodynamically significant infrarenal arteriosclerosis also increases.

Obviously, this disease is associated in varying degrees with arteriosclerotic involvement elsewhere in the body, and this fact must constantly be considered when making therapeutic decisions in afflicted patients. It is this consideration that should guide the physician correctly to seek palliation rather than cure and to attempt a lesser intervention or operation that maintains function rather than one that will restore a normal circulation. The generalized and slowly progressive nature of the disease process and the imperfect results of all interventional treatments should also deter any who might be unwisely tempted to treat asymptomatic or minimally disabling arteriosclerotic occlusive lesions. In the management of the increasingly common entity of lower extremity arteriosclerosis, diagnostic and therapeutic restraint and the desire to minimize risks and avoid doing harm must be paramount principles if the disease is not producing major functional impairment or tissue necrosis. On the other hand, despite the advanced age and poor generalized condition of the afflicted population, aggressive intervention for both diagnosis and treatment is justified if limb loss is truly possible as a result of the disease process.

The reserve of the human arterial system is enormous. Hemodynamically significant stenosis or major artery occlusions can exist in the infrarenal arterial tree with no symptoms or with only minimal symptoms. This is particularly true if collateral pathways are normal or the patient's activity level is limited by coronary arteriosclerosis or other disease processes. Accordingly, the most common manifestation of a short segmental occlusion of the superficial femoral artery, the most common site of major arteriosclerotic involvement below the inguinal ligament, will be mild intermittent claudication. Similarly, this lesion will often be totally asymptomatic, and this is usually the case if only one or two tibial arteries are occluded without other significant lesions. Thus the usual patient who presents severe disabling intermittent claudication or tissue necrosis has multiple sequential occlusions or so-called "combined-segment" disease with hemodynamically significant lesions at the aortoiliac level and the superficial femoropopliteal level, or either or both of these combined with severe infrapopliteal disease as well.

Staging

Patients with hemodynamically significant infrarenal arteriosclerosis may be classified into one of five stages depending on their clinical presentation as indicated in Table 32–1. Patients in stage III and stage IV are those with so-called "critical ischemia" and whose limbs may be considered imminently threatened, although some patients with mild ischemic rest pain may remain stable for many years, and an occasional patient with a small patch of gangrene or an ischemic ulcer will heal their lesion with conservative in-hospital treatment.[1] With the exception of these few patients, invasive diagnostic procedures such as angiography are usually justified for those with stage III and IV disease, which is usually associated with disease and significant lesions at several levels.

Rest pain as an isolated symptom in patients with infrainguinal arteriosclerosis can be difficult to evaluate unless it is accompanied by other findings. Many patients with significant arterial lesions have pain at rest from causes other than their arteriosclerosis, such as arthritis or neuritis. Such pain will not be relieved by even a successful revascularization. Significant ischemic rest pain must be associated not only with decreased pulses but also with other objective manifestations of ischemia such as atrophy, decreased skin temperature when compared to the other extremity, and rubor and relief of pain with dependency. In some patients with a complex etiology to their rest pain, it may be necessary to perform a noninvasive laboratory and angiographic evaluation before the predominant cause of the symptom can be determined and appropriate treatment instituted. Every patient with pain at rest and decreased pulses is not a candidate for angiography and an arterial intervention. Some of these patients will be relieved by appropriate treatment for gout or osteoarthritis. Others can be well managed with simple analgesics and reassurance that their limb is not in jeopardy. Such reassurance generally suffices for patients with stage I disease and those with stage II disease who are elderly (older than 80 years) or at high

TABLE 32–1. STAGING OF INFRARENAL ARTERIOSCLEROSIS WITH HEMODYNAMICALLY SIGNIFICANT STENOSIS OR OCCLUSIONS

Stage	Presentation	Invasive Diagnostic and Therapeutic Intervention at Present
0	No signs or symptoms	Never justified
I	Intermittent claudication (>1 block) No physical changes	Usually unjustified
II	Severe claudication (<1/2 block) Dependent rubor Decreased temperature	Sometimes justified Not always necessary May remain stable
III	Rest pain, atrophy, cyanosis, dependent rubor	Usually indicated but may do well for long periods without revascularization
IV	Nonhealing ischemic ulcer or gangrene	Usually indicated but not always

risk because of intercurrent disease or atherosclerotic involvement of other organs such as the heart, the kidneys, or the brain.

This conservative approach to patients with stage I involvement from lower extremity arteriosclerosis is widespread among surgeons, albeit not universally so.[2] Conservatism appears to be clearly justified by the numerous reports of the benignancy and slow progression of stage I disease to more advanced stages.[3–5] Without treatment, 10 to 15 per cent of patients in stage I will improve over 5 years, and 60 to 70 per cent will not progress over the same period. The 10 to 15 per cent who do worsen, are in our opinion, best treated with a primary nonoperative intervention or operation after their disease progresses. This conservative approach to stage I disease is justified by the greater surgical difficulty encountered when a procedure for claudication fails in the early or remote postoperative period and the patient then has a threatened limb, a situation that we have observed all too frequently.

The fact that some patients in stage II and a few in stage III or stage IV may remain stable and easily managed without operation for protracted periods of 1 or more years justifies a cautiously conservative noninterventional approach to selected patients in these stages.[1] This often requires hospitalization so that the patient and the progress of his ischemia can be assessed. Moreover, this conservative approach is particularly indicated if the patient is elderly and a poor surgical risk from a systemic and a local point of view. An example of this would be an octogenarian with intractable congestive failure in whom a difficult distal small vessel bypass would be required to alleviate stage III signs and symptoms. Close observation can and often should be the preferred management for such a patient for several months or even years; however, we would not hesitate to revascularize such a patient when his rest pain became intolerable or he developed a small progressive patch of gangrene.[6]

PRESENT STATUS OF SURGICAL TREATMENT FOR LOWER EXTREMITY ISCHEMIA

Details of this are presented elsewhere in this volume and are beyond the scope of this chapter. However, several generalities concerning arterial surgery for lower limb ischemia are relevant to the theme of this chapter and the questions already posed.

One such generality is that most patients who currently require treatment for severe limb-threatening lower extremity ischemia have a pattern of arterial disease that is amenable to some form of bypass operation. In the past, many patients were thought to have arteries that were "unsuitable for reconstruction" because of extensive, multilevel occlusive disease in the leg arteries. However, we and others have shown that, with appropriate commitment, high-quality arteriography, and use of technical innovations, very few patients with lower limb ischemia cannot be revascularized successfully. In one study published in 1981, we found that only 6 per cent of patients with threatened limbs had arteries unsuitable for a bypass operation.[6] With more recent technical improvements, particularly use of distal origin, short vein grafts, and the ability to perform bypasses to arterial segments in the ankle region or foot, less than 1 per cent of previously unoperated cases and less than 2 per cent of all patients with limb-threatening ischemia are unsuitable for some operative attempt at limb salvage, with more than an 80 per cent chance of initial success.[7,8] On the other hand, many of these very distal small artery limb salvage operations are difficult, time consuming, and technically demanding. If the ischemia is associated with extensive necrosis or infection in the foot, multiple debridements and protracted hospitalizations may be required. Nevertheless, these are usually successful and result in limb salvage and normal ambulation, a state often not achieved after major amputation.[6] For this reason, most vascular surgeons currently believe that aggressive efforts at limb salvage are worthwhile. This is true even if the patient with a threatened limb has multiple risk factors that might appear to increase operative mortality and limit life expectancy. With improved anesthetic management and perioperative intensive care, it has been possible to perform long, complex operations on patients with severe coronary artery disease, recent congestive heart failure, diabetes, and advanced age, with an acceptably low 30-day operative mortality of 2 to 5 per cent.[6,9,10]

A second generality is that all interventions that manipulate arteries, including operations, carry risks. In addition to the obvious risks of provoking a myocardial infarction or thrombosis or bleeding from instrumented arteries, surgical operations may be complicated by wound infection. When this involves an arterial suture line or graft it may be difficult to treat, result in further arterial occlusions, and require complex revascularizations and protracted hospitalization. Moreover, any reconstructive arterial procedure, even if initially successful, can be complicated by subsequent failure with thrombosis.[11] When this occurs immediately after operation, it may be due to an imperfect repair or the choice of the wrong procedure. Late failure, usually within 2 to 20 months of operation, may be produced by the healing process in the traumatized artery or the arterial graft. Such fibrointimal hyperplasia can occur after any manipulation of a blood vessel. Its etiology is poorly understood, but fortunately its occurrence is not universal. Late failure, after 2 years, is usually due to progression of arteriosclerosis.[11] All these processes produce a substantial late failure rate for arterial reconstructions, particularly those to the popliteal or infrapopliteal arteries. Because of this, most vascular surgeons generally have a conservative attitude regarding arterial interventions for anything less than critical stage III or stage IV ischemia, and this is certainly true when an arterial reconstruction extending below the popliteal artery is required. This conservatism is further supported by the fact that failure of a primary arterial intervention is sometimes associated with ischemia greater than that originally present, necessitating secondary interventions, which are often rendered difficult by scarring, obliteration of previously patent arterial segments, and sometimes, infection. Nevertheless, when such difficult reoperative procedures are required, appropriate strategies and operative techniques have been developed so that they can be carried out effectively with resulting benefit to most patients.[11,12]

A third generality, which is related to some of the foregoing points, is that patients whose arteries are easy to operate upon, in terms of having relatively normal arteries proximal and distal to a single severe stenosis or occlusion, probably do not require any operation, since they will have relatively nondisabling claudication. In contrast, patients who have stage III or IV ischemia that requires revascularization usually have arteries that are difficult to operate on by virtue of having diffuse disease, often with calcification and thick diseased walls in even their patent arterial segments.

A fourth therapeutic generality is that the arterial intervention, when performed in these very ill, end-stage disease patients with complex multilevel peripheral arteriosclerosis, should be the simplest procedure possible to salvage the patient's extremity or relieve the patient's most troublesome symptom. If the patient has stage II or III ischemia or trivial necrosis in the foot, correction of the most proximal hemodynamically significant lesion will generally suffice, even if multiple distal occlusions remain. Only if extensive necrosis or infection are present in the distal limb is it usually necessary to restore straight-line arterial flow to the foot to achieve healing.[6,13]

IMPACT OF NONOPERATIVE INTERVENTIONS ON PATIENTS PRESENTLY UNDERGOING OPERATION

To Replace Operation

In light of all the foregoing considerations, it is clear that we believe that patients who presently have valid indications for operative therapy, if they have one (or more) hemodynamically significant lesion suitable for treatment by PTA at this time, should have that technique used to treat that lesion. This applies to stenoses and short (less than 5 cm) occlusions of the common and external iliac arteries, the superficial femoral and popliteal arteries, and the tibial arteries.[6,14] Although the success rates of PTA for such lesions in mostly stage III and IV ischemia varies depending on the nature and location of the lesion, the criteria of success, and the presence of associated lesions, it is high enough to warrant such treatment. The morbidity of the procedure is less than 8 per cent, and the mortality is less than 1 per cent.[15] More than 50 per cent of the patients will derive benefit for at least 2 years, and when complications or early or late failure occur, they can be managed by operative intervention generally no more complex and risky than if the PTA had not been performed.[15] However, these good results in this group of patients with diffusely diseased arteries requires close collaboration and cooperation between the radiologist and the vascular surgeon.[15,16] The proportion of operative candidates who can be treated by PTA varies depending on the aggressiveness of the radiologist and how far from the ideal short, stenotic lesion he is willing to extend his or her attempts at PTA. Success rates vary inversely with the radiologist's boldness, and complication rates vary directly. We as surgeons remain enthusiastic about these extended indications for PTA in these patients because they usually apply to those who would be difficult, high-risk operative candidates as well. Presently, approximately one third of our limb-salvage operative candidates undergo PTA of one or more lesions. Some of these patients never require operation.

To Facilitate Operation

Approximately two thirds of our patients undergoing PTA, or one quarter of all our limb salvage operative candidates, require an operation after the PTA. Most of these operations are bypass procedures to overcome a lesion other than the one treated by PTA, and some may be required because a PTA fails or has a complication. Percutaneous transluminal balloon angioplasty of significant iliac lesions are often performed proximal to a distal operative procedure originating from the common femoral artery. Complex aortofemorodistal operations are thereby avoided, and treatment simplified and rendered less risky in this group of patients with multiple systemic risk factors and complex multilevel disease. The enthusiasm that we and others had for this approach many years ago has now been verified by recent late observations showing durable long-term results.[6,17,18] More recently, we have also used PTA to treat popliteal and tibial lesions distal to a bypass when the distal lesions were impairing healing of the foot.[14]

Another way that PTA can facilitate or improve operative treatment is to correct a hemodynamically significant lesion that develops in, proximal to, or distal to a bypass graft without yet causing graft thrombosis. This condition, which we have termed a "failing graft," must be treated or the graft will thrombose (fail). This treatment may be by operation or PTA.[19] We currently favor PTA for short inflow and outflow lesions and stenoses smaller than 1.5 cm in vein grafts. Although others have had poor results with PTA of vein-graft stenoses, some of our patients have had arteriographically good results for 3 to 6 years.

Other New Nonoperative Interventions

To date, most laser systems have facilitated balloon angioplasty by enabling passage of a guide wire through otherwise impassable occlusions, and ather-ectomy devices have restored luminal patency by excising plaque, thereby removing lesions that might otherwise be treated by balloon angioplasty. Larger diameter laser systems, which can ablate sufficient plaque to restore an adequate arterial lumen, are just beginning clinical trials. All these methods are interesting and attractive because of their promise of effective treatment with a lower morbidity. All therefore deserve to be tried clinically. However, it is well known that all arterial trauma induces a healing response and that this may lead to fibrointimal hyperplasia. This in turn may not only overcome the benefit of the therapeutic intervention, it may also produce more extensive luminal obliteration than was present before the treatment and thereby worsen the patient. Poor 1-year patency results after hot-tip laser-assisted balloon angioplasty[20–22] and mixed anecdotal reports after various atherectomy device treatments underscore this potential risk. It is mandatory, therefore, that all clinical trials with newer endovascular interventions include late arteriographic follow-up extending for at least 2 years after the procedure. Until such observations are available to allow comparison of the newer method with operative treatment and standard PTA to treat various lesions in various stages of the disease, the exact role of these newer technologies in the management of lower limb ischemia cannot be defined.

IMPACT OF NONOPERATIVE INTERVENTIONAL TREATMENTS ON THE THRESHOLD FOR THERAPY

Because PTA of ideal iliac and superficial femoral artery lesions is simple, reasonably safe, and reasonably durable, it seems logical to extend the indications somewhat beyond those for operation. This is particularly true for short stenoses in otherwise undiseased arteries. Patients with such lesions and stage I or stage II disease certainly may be subjected to PTA. However, complications and failures can occur, and patients should be informed of the risks and that the treatment is not intended to prevent disease progression, since it does not, but only to relieve the symptom. On this basis we have performed PTAs on a few patients who we would not have subjected to operation. However, the number of such individuals is small, constituting less than 1 per cent of our treated patients. The philosophy underlying this therapeutic restraint is reinforced by recent data showing that conservative therapy for claudication may offer benefits equal to PTA after several years.[23] This underscores our belief that arteriosclerotic medical regimens to delay progression of arteriosclerosis may be more important than PTA for patients with stage I disease. However, this remains unproven.

The relative simplicity of other new endovascular treatments using laser and atherectomy devices with or without PTA has prompted many physicians and surgeons to recommend the extension of indications and the lowering of therapeutic thresholds for lower limb arteriosclerosis. Some surgeons, radiologists, and particularly, cardiologists new to the peripheral vascular field and armed with these new techniques and devices, have used them routinely to treat stage I and even stage 0 disease detected incidentally during physical examination or coronary arteriography. Their rationale is that such treatment may prevent disease progression, an assumption for which there is not one shred of evidence. This practice is to be condemned at this time. The mid- and long-term safety and efficacy of these newer treatments remain totally unknown. Even if they are successful immediately, they can initiate a healing process in the artery that causes late failure, or worse, an acceleration of the occlusive process and ultimately net harm to the patient. Therapeutic thresholds should not be lowered until clinical trials demonstrating mid- and long-term safety and efficacy are available. Moreover, these trials must include arteriographic follow-up at least 2 years after the intervention.

QUALIFICATIONS AND CREDENTIALING OF INDIVIDUALS WHO SHOULD TREAT PERIPHERAL VASCULAR DISEASE PATIENTS

The introduction of many new devices that can potentially treat peripheral atherosclerotic lesions has provoked much interest in the field of lower extremity ischemia. However, the mere presence of a flow-reducing lesion in the infrarenal arterial tree does not mean that it should be treated. Those who care for this disease entity should be familiar with the natural history of all stages of the disease. They should be aware of other manifestations of arteriosclerosis and other disease processes that are rampant in this patient population. Most importantly, they should be aware of the relative benignancy of the disease in most patients and how effective conservative treatment and nontreatment can be. Finally, they should be aware of how difficult it can be to treat effectively some patients with true limb-threatening ischemia.

To determine qualifications and credentialing requirements for specialists who should treat lower limb ischemia goes beyond the scope of this chapter. However, a few relevant points can be made. For years, vascular surgeons have managed the vast majority of lower extremity circulatory problems. They have administered both operative and nonoperative treatment for these patients, and they are aware of the value of conservative treatment. Clearly, vascular surgeons should be among those who continue to care for these patients in the future, and an article on guidelines for hospital privileges in this specialty has recently appeared.[24] One year of special training in this field is the fundamental requirement for credentialing and hospital privileges in vascular surgery.

With the introduction of PTA, interventional radiologists have become involved in the management of patients with lower limb ischemia. Generally, these radiologists work in close collaboration with vascular surgeons. They provide the surgeon with high-quality arteriograms, they collaborate in joint therapeutic decisions, and individuals from the two complimentary specialties help to take care of each other's complications. Interventional radiologists, too, have 1 year of specialized training devoted in large part to the diagnosis and management of lower limb ischemia. Clearly, they too should continue their role in the management of these patients.

More recently, cardiologists have professed an interest in these patients, and they have begun to treat them interventionally.[25] Clearly, cardiologists can contribute to improved care. They know about coronary artery disease and its management, and they may be able to bring special expertise in the use of the newer endovascular devices, some of which were specifically designed for use in the coronary arteries. However, if cardiologists wish to become involved in the care of peripheral vascular disease, they too should fulfill two requirements. First, they should have 1 year of training during which they have broad exposure to peripheral vascular disease patients of all stages, including those that require all kinds of treatment—nontreatment, conservative, nonoperative interventional, operative, and a combination of these modalities. Second, they should work together as part of a team which includes interventional radiologists, vascular surgeons, and cardiologists. Only in that way will patients with lower extremity ischemia get the safest, least meddlesome, and most effective management.

SUMMARY

Nonoperative therapy includes conservative noninterventional and endovascular interventional modalities. The latter includes PTA and a variety of laser systems and atherectomy devices. This chapter considers the role and impact of all nonoperative treatments in the perspectives of the natural history of lower extremity arteriosclerosis and its current surgical (operative) treatment. Nonoperative treatments may replace or facilitate surgical treatment in operative candidates. Nonoperative methods may also justify treatment in patients who cannot or should not be subjected to operation. Facts and opinions relating to these uses of nonoperative treatments are presented. The issue of qualifications and credentialing of individuals who should be treating patients with lower extremity ischemia from peripheral arteriosclerosis is discussed.

REFERENCES

1. Rivers SP, Veith FJ, Ascer E, Gupta SK: Successful conservative therapy of severe limb threatening ischemia: The value of non-sympathectomy. Surgery 1986;99:759–762.
2. Donaldson MC, Mannick JA: Femoropopliteal bypass grafting for intermittent claudication. Is pessimism warranted? Arch Surg 1980;115:724–727.
3. Boyd AM: The natural course of arteriosclerosis of the lower extremities. Proc R Soc Med 1962;55:591–593.
4. Coran AG, Warren R: Arteriographic changes in femoropopliteal arteriosclerosis obliterans: A five year follow-up study. N Engl J Med 1966;274:643–645.
5. Imparato AM, Kim GE, Davidson T, Crowley JG: Intermittent claudication: Its natural course. Surgery 1975;78:795–797.
6. Veith FJ, Gupta SK, Samson RH, et al: Progress in limb salvage by reconstructive arterial surgery combined with new or improved adjunctive procedures. Ann Surg 1981;194:386–401.
7. Veith FJ, Ascer E, Gupta SK, et al: Tibiotibial vein bypass grafts: A new operation for limb salvage. J Vasc Surg 1985;2:552–557.
8. Ascer E, Veith FJ, Gupta SK: Bypasses to plantar arteries and other tibial branches: An extended approach to limb salvage. J Vasc Surg 1988;8:434–441.

9. Rivers SP, Scher LA, Gupta SK, Veith FJ: Safety of peripheral vascular surgery after recent myocardial infarction. J Vasc Surg 1990;*11:*70–76.

10. Taylor LM, Edwards JM, Porter JM: Present status of reversed vein bypass: Five year results of a modern series. J Vasc Surg 1990;*11:*207–215.

11. Veith FJ, Gupta SK, Ascer E, Rivers SP, Wengerter K: Improved strategies for secondary operations on infrainguinal arteries. Ann Vasc Surg 1990;*3:*85–90.

12. Bartlett ST, Olinde AJ, Flinn WR, et al: The reoperative potential of infrainguinal bypass: Long-term limb and patient survival. J Vasc Surg 1987;*5:*170–179.

13. Veith FJ, Gupta SK, Daly V: Femoropopliteal bypass to the isolated popliteal segment: Is polytetrafluoroethylene graft acceptable? Surgery 1981;*89:*296–303.

14. Bakal CW, Sprayregen S, Scheinbaum K, Cynamon J, Veith FJ: Percutaneous transluminal angioplasty of the infrapopliteal arteries: Results in 53 patients. Am J Roentgen 1990;*154:*171–174.

15. Samson RH, Sprayregen S, Veith FJ, et al: Management of angioplasty complication, unsuccessful procedures and early and late failures. Ann Surg 1984;*199:*234–240.

16. Franco CD, Goldsmith J, Veith FJ, et al: Management of arterial injuries produced by percutaneous femoral procedures. J Cardiovasc Surg 1989;*30:*7.

17. Alpert JR, Ring EJ, Freiman DB, et al: Balloon dilatation of iliac stenosis with distal arterial surgery. Arch Surg 1980;*115:*715–717.

18. Brewster DC, Cambria RP, Darling RC, et al: Long-term results of combined iliac balloon angioplasty and distal surgical revascularization. Ann Surg 1989;*210:*324–330.

19. Veith FJ, Weiser RK, Gupta SK, et al: Diagnosis and management of failing lower extremity arterial reconstructions. J Cardiovasc Surg 1984;*25:*381–384.

20. Wright JG, Belkin M, Greenfield AJ, et al: Laser angioplasty for limb salvage: Observations on early results. J Vasc Surg 1989;*10:*29–38.

21. Perler BA, Osterman FA, White RI, Williams GM: Percutaneous laser probe femoropopliteal angioplasty: A preliminary experience. J Vasc Surg 1989;*10:*351–357.

22. Harrington ME, Schwartz ME, Sandborn T, et al: Expanded indications for laser assisted balloon angioplasty in peripheral artery disease. J Vasc Surg 1990;*11:*146–155.

23. Van Rij AM, Packer SGK, Morrison ND: Angioplasty for claudicants with femoropopliteal disease. J Cardiovasc Surg 1989;*30:*88.

24. Moore WS, Treiman RL, Hertzer NR, Veith FJ, et al: Guidelines for hospital privileges in vascular surgery. J Vasc Surg 1989;*10:*678–682.

25. DeMaria AN: Peripheral vascular disease and the cardiovascular specialist. J Am Coll Cardiol 1988;*12:*869–870.

33

INTERVENTIONAL TECHNOLOGY: Intraoperative Strategies and Techniques

GEORGE ANDROS

Of all surgical devices created for diagnosis and treatment, no group is undergoing more rapid evolution than endovascular tools. With this development has come an equally rapid and costly obsolescence or extinction of once-promising instruments. Still after more than two decades of vigorous efforts to design better transluminal methods for arterial disobliteration, only balloon angioplasty has survived as an effective and proven therapeutic modality.

During this period of trial-and-error testing of new modalities, balloon catheters have been refined and new indications for their applications have emerged. One such application is intraoperative or open transluminal balloon angioplasty (OpTA), usually performed concomitantly with an inflow or outflow bypass procedure. As the result of strategic planning, diagnostic angiography and percutaneous transluminal balloon angioplasty (PTA) can frequently be combined into a single procedure. By analogy, we contend that OpTA will become increasingly appropriate therapy, because it promises to spare patients a second or even third intervention. There are, however, conceptual and technical impediments to the coupling of surgical and endovascular procedures. This chapter will deal with the methods and limitations as well as the strategies and tactics of concomitant open revascularization and transluminal procedures for the treatment of chronic severe arteriosclerosis of the lower extremities.

RATIONALE FOR OPERATIVE TRANSLUMINAL BALLOON ANGIOPLASTY AND OTHER ENDOVASCULAR TECHNIQUES

Vascular surgeons are accustomed to operating on patients with disabling claudication, rest pain, and gangrene. Generally speaking, these patients require open revascularization, usually in the form of a bypass. Very severe ischemia is often associated with tandem lesions, and it may be possible that one of the lesions in a series of obstructions may be amenable to balloon angioplasty. This approach confers the benefit of either decreasing the scope of the operative procedure or performing one operation where two might otherwise be necessary

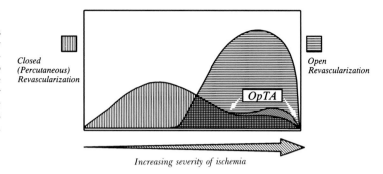

FIGURE 33–1. Percutaneous transluminal balloon angioplasty and open revascularization patients divide themselves into two categories: PTA for less-severe and open revascularization for more-severe ischemia. It is in the more-severe category for patients with tandem lesions that OpTA is indicated.

Closed (Percutaneous) Revascularization

OpTA

Open Revascularization

Increasing severity of ischemia

(Fig. 33–1). Patients with mild to moderate claudication usually have symptoms because of a short stenosis or a short, poorly collateralized occlusion. Such lesions are ideally suited to balloon angioplasty. This rough dichotomy of patients into those with mild lesions and symptoms receiving balloon angioplasty and those with more severe problems undergoing open revascularization has been observed by other investigators.[1] Open transluminal balloon angioplasty is indicated for the treatment of tandem arteriosclerotic lesions of the aortoiliac and femoropopliteocrural arterial segments; it should be reserved for severe chronic ischemia. The combination of angioplasty with open revascularization such as bypass for acute and subacute arterial occlusions is a useful strategy. However, it usually requires the use of intraoperative thrombolytic therapy and is, therefore, beyond the scope of this chapter. Other disobliteration methods such as atherectomy,[2–4] laser angioplasty,[5,6] and intraluminal stents[7,8] will only be touched upon. Each of these devices comes in many varieties, and some have had considerable clinical application. Moreover, insertion and use of the instruments is sometimes facilitated by the surgical exposure of the femoral artery. Simpson atherectomy has been shown to be effective in the management of iliac and superficial femoral artery lesions, primarily short eccentric stenosis.[2] However, since no studies to date have demonstrated the superiority of atherectomy over balloon angioplasty, it has been excluded from consideration. With the departure of hot-tip laser-assisted angioplasty from the endovascular scene, the use of laser devices is now centered around a growing collection of instruments delivering various laser energies.[9] As these are presently investigational, their application in a strategic sense is conjectural. At least two types of stents have been investigated and both are seeking FDA approval. As of this writing, neither has been released for unrestricted clinical application.

TYPES OF OpTA

There are three strategic contexts in which OpTA is performed. Open transluminal balloon angioplasty is *obligatory* if access to the femoral artery is precluded by obesity or scarring. Cutdown on the common femoral artery is sometimes essential because the guide wire and catheter cannot traverse a lesion in the proximal superficial femoral artery. Such orificial lesions may be continuations of femoral bifurcation occlusive disease. Surgical exposure (and usually femoral endarterectomy) allows otherwise uncrossable lesions to be traversed by the guide wire and balloon catheter. The Fogarty-Chin[10] extrusion balloon catheter cannot be inserted percutaneously; it is, therefore, an *obligatory* OpTA device at this time. An over-the-guide wire catheter is currently in

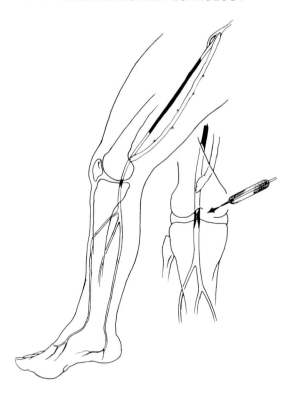

FIGURE 33–2. Common femoral to suprageniculate bypass with intraoperative balloon angioplasty of midpopliteal stenosis.

development. *Elective* OpTA is performed when, for example, an iliac balloon angioplasty is coupled to a femorodistal bypass graft rather than performing PTA concomitantly with angiography. Infrequently, retrograde iliac balloon angioplasty and antegrade superficial femoral or popliteal balloon angioplasty can be simplified and performed in one procedure using femoral artery cutdown. Open transluminal balloon angioplasty is most often indicated as an *adjunctive* procedure concomitant with a bypass. This category resembles the aforementioned elective OpTA. Occasionally, a superficial femoral artery balloon angioplasty is performed at the time of aortofemoral bypass. Efficiency and ready acceptance by patients are two desirable aspects of combined procedures. Potential complications at the puncture site are avoided. We have employed outflow OpTA of a midpopliteal stenosis in cases where the saphenous vein is too short to extend from the common femoral to the infrageniculate popliteal artery (Fig. 33–2); likewise, balloon angioplasty of midpopliteal stenoses permits the surgeon to use a synthetic bypass graft and terminate at the suprageniculate popliteal artery.

DETERMINANTS OF EFFECTIVE OpTA

To date, no studies have objectively compared OpTA to percutaneous transluminal balloon angioplasty (PTA) in terms of durability; however, our experience and that of others suggests that they are equivalent. From these cases we have developed some clinical guidelines to ensure successful OpTA.

Preoperative Assessment

Preoperative assessment (angiographic and hemodynamic) should determine the contribution that each of the tandem lesions makes to the overall hemodynamnic deficit. Just as the success of balloon angioplasty is assessed by post-treatment angiography, likewise, the selection of appropriate lesions is dependent on high-quality pre–balloon angioplasty arteriography. Cut film is preferred and oblique views should be obtained wherever necessary. Duplex scanning is useful to determine the hemodynamic significance of stenoses based upon velocity measurements.[11] Changes in velocity profiles and Doppler waveforms are useful in postoperative assessment, but this technology generally is not applicable intraoperatively. When iliac and superficial femoral lesions are each reducing peripheral perfusion, duplex-derived velocities may be the only noninvasive way to determine the significance of each lesion. Finally, whenever possible, pressure gradients across stenoses should be measured before and after OpTA.

Sequence of Procedures

Because adequate inflow is indispensable, retrograde (inflow) OpTA must precede outflow revascularization (bypass). Whether the intended bypass graft is a femorofemoral or femorodistal graft, adequate aortoiliac inflow must be obtained (Figs. 33–3 and 33–4). This is obviously effected via a retrograde femoral approach. Balloon angioplasty of the common and superficial femoral arteries may be indicated if the saphenous vein is inadequate in length, as

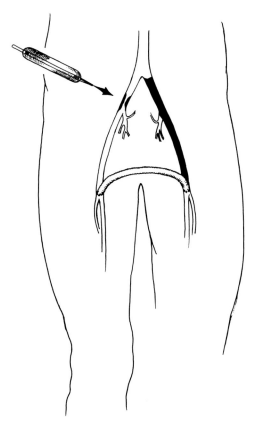

FIGURE 33–3. Open transluminal balloon angioplasty of iliac artery stenosis via the proximal (common femoral) anastomotic site prior to femorofemoral bypass.

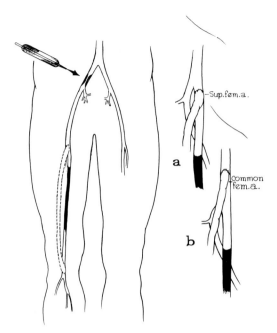

FIGURE 33–4. Iliac OpTA to provide inflow to a femoropopliteal bypass. *A*, With the graft originating from the superficial femoral artery, flow is allowed to continue into the deep femoral artery as the proximal anastomosis is performed. *B*, Graft originating from the common femoral artery.

previously mentioned. However, other options such as the creation of a composite autogenous graft using arm or short saphenous vein or the use of the deep femoral artery as a more distal inflow site should be considered. In cases where a distal popliteal to paramalleolar bypass graft is proposed, retrograde angioplasty of the popliteal or superficial femoral artery is possible (Fig. 33–5). A staged angioplasty and subsequent distal bypass is preferred, but if only focal stenoses are dilated, effective and durable inflow with OpTA can be anticipated.

Outflow OpTA is problematic. It is performed after the inflow bypass procedure has been completed and should be reserved for cases where the operative indication is ischemic rest pain or gangrene. Customarily, we limit

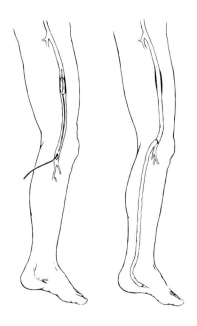

FIGURE 33–5. Inflow OpTA of superficial femoral artery stenosis prior to popliteoplantar bypass. *A*, Inflow OpTA via popliteal anastomotic site. *B*, Completed popliteoplantar bypass.

outflow OpTA to the superficial femoral artery in cases of aortofemoral bypass graft and to the mid and distal popliteal artery in cases of femoropopliteal bypass. Infrapopliteal OpTA, although feasible, should be replaced with either postoperative PTA or popliteal to distal bypass using an autogenous conduit. Of course, if the saphenous vein is satisfactory, in situ saphenous vein bypass graft beginning at the femoral artery and terminating as far as the ankle and foot is preferable to a combined inflow bypass and outflow OpTA.

In the past we have staged the OpTA procedure and the femorodistal bypass graft with vein harvesting, dissection of the proximal and distal anastomotic sites, and creation of the tunnel, all to be completed before inflow iliac balloon angioplasty was performed. At present it is our policy to cut down first on the artery to be used as the inflow site, usually the common femoral artery. After the administration of 3000 to 4000 units of heparin, inflow OpTA is performed, the quality of the pulse is assessed, and pressure gradients are measured. The OpTA procedure alone may be enough to relieve mild claudication, but treatment of more severe disease dictates the addition of a concomitant distal bypass graft. The bypass procedure is then performed in its entirety. We were previously reluctant to do the complete vascular dissection in a heparinized patient, but have found that the attendant bleeding is increased only slightly.

Luminal Access and the "Hemodynamic Stent"

Arterial access should be obtained with a needle or sheath so that the hemodynamic stenting affect of flow and pressure are maintained. It is preferable to maintain blood flow and arterial distension before, during, and after OpTA and during the subsequent distal bypass graft (the hemodynamic stent). There are three techniques for obtaining access to the arterial lumen via the surgically exposed artery at the intended proximal anastomotic site.[12] First, a #18 thin-walled entry needle may be used to puncture only the anterior wall of the artery or graft. With pulsatile flow established, the guide wire is passed and the needle is exchanged for an appropriate sized dilator, which is in turn exchanged for the balloon angioplasty catheter. Whenever possible, the pressure gradient should be measured. Second, if more than a simple balloon angioplasty is intended with multiple exchanges of guide wires and catheters, it is advisable to use a sheath introducer. This device also controls annoying bleeding around the puncture site that occurs when only a needle and a guide wire are employed. Third, Fogarty has developed a sheath introducer with an occlusive pinch-valve (Fig. 33–6). The device is inserted over a guide wire, and once in a place, expands to occlude inflow; consequently, the hemodynamic stenting effect of flowing blood is lost. This disadvantage is compensated for by the presence of a valve which permits easy exchange of multiple endovascular devices such as guide wires, catheters, angioscopes, atherectomy devices, and so forth. Its use is desirable if multiple techniques are contemplated, but is seldom necessary if only balloon angioplasty is done. With the occlusion of arterial inflow, angioscopic assessment is facilitated. These expandable sheaths may be used antegrade or retrograde.

Guide Wires and Balloon Catheters

Endovascular devices such as guide wires and balloon catheters can traumatize as well as treat. Because OpTA is reserved almost exclusively for stenoses,

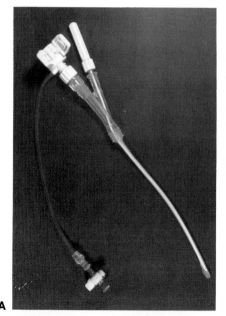

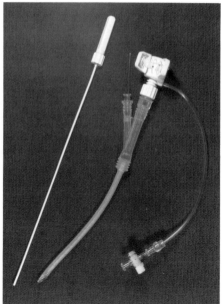

A

B

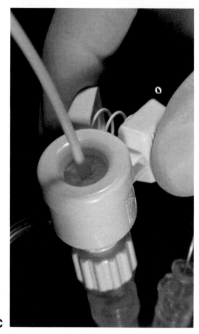

C

FIGURE 33–6. Fogarty expandable sheath. *A,* Sheath with opdurator in place prior to insertion. *B,* Expanded sheath with opdurator removed. *C,* Hemostatic pinch-valve with endovascular device in position.

these lesions are easily crossed with most guide wires. Simple floppy guide wires usually suffice to cross lesions; occasionally Wholey wires or Terumo glide wires are mandatory. In general, we use an 0.035-inch diameter guide wire with a #18 thin-walled entry needle and standard 5-F balloon angioplasty catheters. The guide wire should be passed only a few inches beyond the lesion undergoing dilatation; guide-wire movement within the vessel should be minimized. Balloons 4 cm in length are normally employed. With lesions 1 to 2 cm in length, the balloon is placed astride the lesion and is inflated to the manufacturers prescribed pressure limit for 60 seconds (after the disappearance of the waste), deflated for 30 seconds, and reinflated for 60 seconds. If the lesion is longer than 4 cm, the dilated areas are overlapped to encompass the entire stenotic segment. Normally, mild distension of 1 to 2 cm of adjacent artery is tolerated. If the lesion is 6 to 7 cm in length, a 10-cm-long balloon catheter is selected. Lesions longer than this are generally treated with a form of therapy other than OpTA. Balloons are distended with a half-and-half mixture of contrast and saline delivered with standard inflating devices. The balloon must be scrupulously deflated and evacuated of contrast before it is moved or withdrawn from the artery, to avoid mural trauma.

Restenosis is the most frequent late complication of balloon angioplasty. We have been surprised to observe that after 6 months, the stenosis occurs frequently in an area remote from the originally dilated segment. This has suggested to us that the guide wires and balloon catheters may in some way destabilize plaques that were not stenosed and caused them to become progressive, hemodynamically significant lesions. As a result of this experience, we prefer to perform OpTA using Terumo glide wires and low-profile balloon catheters, believing that they will be less traumatic to unaffected segments of the artery.

Imaging for OpTA

The most critical determinant of successful peroperative endovascular intervention, apart from patient selection, is the availability of adequate intraoperative imaging. Radiographic imaging for OpTA runs the gamut from the use of a simple C-arm to the construction of a full-service special procedures room in the operating suite to make available all imaging modalities. Some suites even include biplanar imaging and 14 × 14 cut film. The C-arm, conversely, provided marginal imaging capacity for more sophisticated procedures. For this reason, some surgeons have relocated their OpTA cases to preexisting full-service special procedures rooms. Between these two extremes are two highly useful imaging devices, one portable and one dedicated. The portable C-arm made by OEC-Diasonics (Fig. 33–7) provides an adequate 5-inch × 9-inch field of view, a rotating head anode for sustained imaging, digital subtraction imaging, road mapping, and multiple formats for permanent records including videotape, Polaroid, and color dot-matrix images. All of these features come packaged in a highly portable and convenient-to-use configuration. Also attractive is the dedicated International Surgical Systems (ISS) imaging system built into a lead-lined room (Fig. 33–8). This imaging system has all of the features of the portable machine but is more easily deployed on an overhead traveling arm. It also incorporates a radiolucent table with multiple positions and ease of patient positioning. This is a highly desirable unit, but is three times as expensive as the OEC-Diasonics device.

The choice of lesions for OpTA is based upon the preoperative arteriogram. These should again be localized intraoperatively with a repeat arteriogram. Under fluoroscopy, the site of the lesion can be marked with a hemostat. The balloon catheter can then be advanced to the side of the hemostat in anticipation of the angioplasty. If more sophisticated equipment with road mapping is available, these digital subtraction images can be used to position the balloon catheter. Alternatively, bony landmarks, hemostats, or a sterile radiopaque ruler may be used. Balloon diameter is selected from the preoperative angiogram. Common iliac artery lesions require 7-, 8-, 9-, and rarely 10-mm balloon catheters. External iliac arteries are generally 1 to 2 mm smaller. Superficial femoral and popliteal artery dilatation usually requires balloon catheters in the

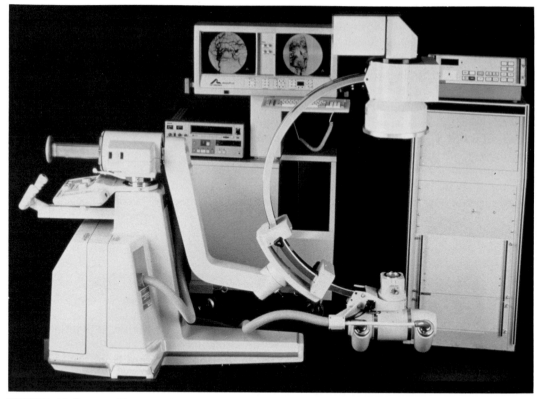

FIGURE 33–7. Portable OEC-Diasonics C-arm for intraoperative balloon angioplasty. Device has rotating anode, road mapping, and multiple formats for image reproduction.

4- to 5-mm range (± 1 mm). We recommend that a permanent x-ray image with the balloon inflated be taken and included in the patient's record. It is helpful to measure the inflated balloon size with the artery size above and below the stenotic lesion. Such measurements help to improve the operator's skill and selection of appropriately sized balloons.

Intraoperative Assessment and Record Keeping

Intraoperative assessment of OpTA and record keeping of the details of the procedure are as important as the operative note for any open revascularization procedure. There are several types of intraoperative assessment of OpTA. These include measurements of pressure gradients across iliofemoral stenoses before and after balloon angioplasty, arteriographic imaging, ankle-brachial indices with a sterile Doppler probe after each of the two components of the procedure, and finally, clinical assessment including palpation of pulses, evaluation of venous and capillary refill and evidence of atheroembolization.

The operative record should be both detailed and explicit. A partial list of the particulars to be mentioned includes the drugs used, the type of entry device, assessment of the punctured artery, types of guide wires and balloons, locations of stenoses, duration of inflation periods as well as the ease with which the "waist" of the arterial lesion was eliminated by the balloon catheter. If possible, a diagram of the entire procedure affixed to the chart enhances later recollection of the procedure.

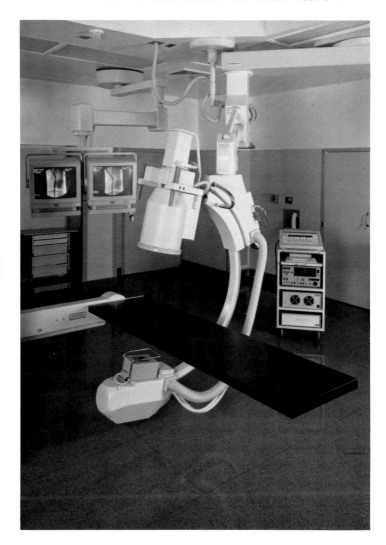

FIGURE 33–8. International Surgical Systems (ISS) dedicated vascular suite.

Management of Complications

Complications of OpTA at the angioplasty site resemble those of PTA in all ways including the infrequency of their occurrence. Although the concept appears rudimentary, virtually every acute complication of balloon angioplasty can be averted by proper patient selection and the use of balloon angioplasty catheters of appropriate size and length. Inadequate dilatation, particularly of an iliac artery, is suggested by a residual pressure gradient across the lesion of greater than 5 mm Hg. If the predilatation gradient is large (i.e., greater than 50 mm Hg), we accept a residual gradient of 15 per cent or less of the proximal systolic pressure. Intraluminal stents have been advocated for cases in which a residual iliac stenosis remains. When a residual gradient is observed, it is tempting to step up to a larger sized balloon to increase the extent of dilatation. Generally speaking, if the inflated balloon (as measured radiographically) is equal to the diameter of the artery above and below the stenosis, there is little to be gained by increasing balloon size to overdilate the artery. Acute arterial occlusion at the site of balloon angioplasty is disquieting. Occasionally, this may be corrected by repeated inflation of the catheter for several minutes if the guide wire has not been removed; more often than not the occlusion is permanent. This may result in a stenosis becoming an occlusion; bypass is the usual outcome. One must try to differentiate an acute occlusion caused by intraluminal thrombus and occlusion caused by dissection of the arteriosclerotic plaque.

Arterial rupture is preventable, although it is occasionally unavoidable, when calcific aortic bifurcation lesions rupture the iliac artery. If an iliac artery is to be dilated before a distal bypass, the entire abdomen must be sterilely prepared and draped as for an aortobifemoral bypass graft. This precaution prevents delays in exploration of the dilated iliac artery should the blood pressure decrease unexpectedly. Finally, the complication of distal atherosclerotic embolism has been observed in PTA series to be less than 1 per cent. We have not, as yet, seen this complication in any of our OpTA patients. One should be wary of these potential complications and have prepared a fall-back position in the event they do occur.

Puncture-site complications such as acute occlusion and arteriovenous fistula are effectively precluded by the use of OpTA. Wound hematoma does occur with both OpTA and PTA. If continued surgical bleeding is anticipated following the OpTA, it is advisable to use a suction drain in the surgical wound.

Patient Management and Follow-up

Only vascular surgeons can provide comprehensive management of the endovascular surgery. All patients are pretreated with aspirin for 3 days prior to surgery; this is continued for 3 months postoperatively. Dextran-40 (Rheomacrodex) is infused following the balloon angioplasty and is continued for 24 to 48 hours postoperatively. Intraoperative heparin is not reversed with protamine. Unless a complication is suspected, patients are not subjected to routine postangioplasty arteriography before discharge from the hospital. We follow balloon angioplasty patients more closely than bypass patients because of the risk of restenosis. Office visits are scheduled every 3 months for the first 2 years, and every 6 months thereafter. Ankle-brachial indices are obtained, if possible, at the time of each visit. A decline of an ankle-brachial index of 0.15 and decrease in peripheral pulses or deterioration in the patient's clinical status are indications for repeat arteriography. Because restenosis may be eccentric, it is often necessary to obtain more than one view of the suspicious arterial segment. Duplex graft surveillance may be employed for both the OpTA and the bypass portions of the revascularization.

DISCUSSION

"It is more important to do the right thing than to do things right." This axiom of Peter Drucker captures the essence of the decision-making process of perioperative balloon angioplasty and concomitant surgical revascularization. We have been thwarted in our attempts to systematize these two procedures into useful algorithims because of the large number of variables in the decision-making process. Nevertheless, OpTA is a useful strategy in the management of chronic arteriosclerotic tandem lesions and must be continuously kept in mind for the treatment of patients with severe peripheral ischemia, resulting from multisegment disease.

Because much of our knowledge of OpTA has been gained empirically, certain theoretical issues remain ambiguous. For example, the concept of the hemodynamic stent to maintain the dilated segment at normal effective flow and diameter is speculative. No studies to date have shown that perioperative arterial defects such as dissections have an adverse effect on long-term patency of the dilated segment. This problem may be understood as our knowledge of the mechanism of balloon angioplasty improves in the future. Practical questions require answers as well. Can one anticipate a restenosis rate in the OpTA-dilated segments equal to that seen with PTA?[13] What criteria should one use to abandon the concomitant downstream procedure after inflow OpTA or bypass has been performed? The effectiveness of revascularizing only one level of multisegment disease has been well demonstrated in the past.[14] Finally, we recommend that OpTA be limited to stenoses rather than occlusions if the balloon procedure is adjunctive. It remains to be seen whether or not this criterion is too restrictive.

REFERENCES

1. Cole SEA, Baird RN, Horrocks M, Jeans WD: The role of balloon angioplasty in the management of lower limb ischemia. Eur J Vasc Surg 1987;*1*(1):61.
2. Hinohara T, Selmon MR, Robertson GC, et al: Direction Atherectomy: New Approaches for treatment of obstructive coronary and peripheral vascular disease. Circulation 1990;*81:*(IV):79–91.
3. Snyder SO, Jr, Wheeler JR, Gregory RT, et al: Kensey catheter—early results with a transluminal endarterectomy tool. J Vasc Surg 1988;*8:*541–543.
4. Ahn SS, Auth D, Marcus DR, et al: Removal of focal atheromatous lesions by angioscopically guided high-speed rotary atherectomy. J Vasc Surg 1988;*7:*292–300.
5. Strandness DE Jr, Barnes RW, Katzen B, Ring E: Indiscriminate use of laser angioplasty. Radiology 1989;*172:*945–946.
6. Murray A, Wood RFM, Mitchell DC, et al: Peripheral laser angioplasty with pulsed dye laser and ball-tipped optical fibres. The Lancet 1989;*2:*1471–1477.
7. Palmaz JC, Richter GM, Noeldge G, et al: Intraluminal stents in atherosclerotic iliac artery stenosis: Preliminary report of a multicenter study. Radiology 1988;*168:*727–731.
8. Puel J, Rousseau P, Joffre F, et al: Intravascular stent to prevent restenosis after transluminal angioplasty. Circulation 1987;*76*(IV):27.
9. Dalman RL, Taylor LM, Porter JM: Current status of extracoronary endovascular procedures. *In* Goldstone J, ed: Perspectives in Vascular Surgery. Quality Medical Publishers, Inc, St. Louis, MO, 1990;1–34.
10. Fogarty TJ, Chin A, Shoor PM, et al: Adjunctive intraoperative arterial dilation, simplified instrumentation technique. Arch Surg 1981;*116:*1391–1398.
11. Kohler TR, Andros G, Porter JM, et al: Can duplex scanning replace arteriography for lower extremity arterial disease? Ann Vasc Surg 1990;*4:*280–287.
12. Andros G, Harris RW, Dulawa LB, et al: Balloon angioplasty of iliac, femoral, and infrainguinal arteries: Percutaneous and intraoperative strategies and techniques. *In* Bergan JJ, Yao JST, eds: Techniques in Arterial Surgery. Philadelphia, WB Saunders Co., 1990;381–398.
13. Harris RW, Dulawa LB, Andros G, et al: Percutaneous transluminal angioplasty of the lower extremities by the vascular surgeon. Ann Vasc Surg 1991;*5:*345–353.
14. Brewster DC, Darling RC: Optimal methods of aortoiliac reconstruction. Surgery 1978;*84*(6):739–748.

34

PHARMACOLOGIC CONTROL OF MYOINTIMAL HYPERPLASIA

MICHAEL D. COLBURN and WESLEY S. MOORE

The number of procedures performed annually for occlusive vascular disease continues to increase. Currently, approximately 500,000 patients undergo reconstructive vascular surgery each year; half are coronary bypass procedures and the remainder are operations on the peripheral vascular tree. These peripheral interventions encompass a wide assortment of procedures including autologous and prosthetic bypass grafts, endarterectomies, as well as a variety of new endovascular procedures. The last 10 years of surgical innovation have resulted in an explosion of new technologies and applications; most of which have proven to be both technically feasible and safe. The value of any surgical procedure, however, should be measured not only by the success by which it can be initially preformed, but also in terms of the durability of the results. Although the in-hospital success rates are excellent, the long-term durability of most of these new endovascular procedures has been disappointing.

The common culprit accounting for most early failures is myointimal hyperplasia. The 3-year primary patency for infrainguinal bypass grafts ranges from 40 to 60 per cent with prosthetic conduits, and 60 to 80 per cent when an autologous graft is utilized.[1] Of those grafts that fail between 6 months and 2 years, most are due to this hypercellular reaction.[2,3] Likewise, this process accounts for a 15 per cent 1-year occlusion rate in coronary artery bypass grafts and up to a 20 per cent restenosis rate following carotid endarterectomies.[4]

Endovascular surgery is a relatively new field that originated with the development of percutaneous transluminal balloon angioplasty (PTA) and has evolved to include angioscopy, laser and mechanical atherectomy, as well as intravascular stents. Together, these techniques have provided impressive initial success rates. However, with the test of time, complications such as dissections, perforations, and especially restenosis, have limited their application. Recent advances such as over–guide-wire catheter systems and "smart" laser technology have reduced the incidence of the early technical complications. Unfortunately, the problem of restenosis remains the Achilles heel of endovascular interventions and threatens to limit their ultimate usefulness.

Results following PTA in the lower extremity have been published by several authors. The combined failure rate after 1 year follow-up ranges from

2 to 40 per cent.[5] Some of these recurrences are no doubt due to either a progression of atherosclerosis or other mechanisms such as intraplaque hemorrhage. However, the majority are the result of intimal hyperplasia. Likewise, long-term results following laser-assisted angioplasty have not been encouraging. In one representative study, White et al. reported on their results of laser-assisted balloon angioplasty for advanced lesions of the lower extremity.[6] In this study, both Argon neodymium:yttrium aluminum garnet (Nd:YAG) and metal hot-tip systems were used. Although the initial recanalization rate was 67 per cent, only 11 per cent remained patent at 1 year. Results from other investigators have been similar. The results of peripheral atherectomy vary depending on the device used and the anatomic location of the lesion. At UCLA, we have had experience treating 41 arteries with the Auth Rotablator.[7] Initial success was achieved in 92 per cent of the cases and the primary patency was 67 per cent at 6 months. However, follow-up at 24 months noted only a 9.5 per cent patency rate. Unfortunately, the long-term outcomes of other devices have not reported any significant improvement on these results. Again, the majority of these failures can be attributed to intimal hyperplasia. Clearly, this process is a significant cause of morbidity in patients undergoing procedures on the vascular system, and investigation into methods to prevent or reverse this process is of great importance.

Currently, the only available option for the treatment of intimal hyperplasia is reoperation. This involves either revision of the affected vascular bypass graft or patch angioplasty of the previously endarterectomized vessel. Often, when the affected graft or vessel has thrombosed, this is not technically possible and thus results in the loss of the vascular conduit. The ability of various pharmacologic agents to suppress the development of intimal hyperplasia has been well documented. Particularly striking is the large variety of medications that have been effective in limiting this response. At least five different classes of drugs have been studied and shown to be at least partially successful in this regard: antiplatelet agents,[8-10] anti-inflammatory agents,[11,12] antihypertensive agents,[13-15] anticoagulants,[16] and lipid metabolites[17-19] (Table 34-1). This

TABLE 34–1. PHARMACOLOGIC AGENTS REPORTED TO BE EFFECTIVE IN SUPPRESSING THE FORMATION OF INTIMAL HYPERPLASIA

Antiplatelet agents
  Aspirin
  Dipyridamole
  Thromboxane synthetase inhibitors
Anti-inflammatory agents
  Dexamethasone
  Azathioprine
  Cyclosporin
Antihypertensive agents
  ACE inhibitors
    Cilazapril
  Calcium channel blockers
    Verapamil
  α_1-Adrenergic inhibitors
    Prazosin
Anticoagulant agents
  Heparins and Heparinoids
Others
  Omega-3 polyunsaturated fatty acids
  Angiopeptin, an octapeptide
  Porphyrin compounds

clearly attests to the complexity of the pathways leading to this lesion and implies that no one agent will likely be totally effective in its elimination. Unfortunately, the nonuniformity of the models of intimal hyperplasia studied, and the doses and duration of the agents investigated, make comparison of the results of these trials unreliable. Therefore, the clinical usefulness of pharmacologic therapy, in this setting, remains undetermined. Nevertheless, if effective pharmacologic therapy could be developed to suppress the growth of intimal hyperplasia and prevent the associated recurrent arterial stenoses, this would have a major impact on the durability of vascular procedures and lower their associated morbidity, mortality, and cost. Also, in addition to suppressing the development of intimal hyperplasia, if these medications prove to be effective in reducing established hyperplastic lesions, this would be an alternative therapy for the patient with a failing vascular procedure and would represent a significant advance in the management of this highly morbid and potentially lethal complication of peripheral vascular surgery.

PATHOPHYSIOLOGY OF INTIMAL HYPERPLASIA

Intimal hyperplasia is the abnormal sustained proliferation of cells and extracellular connective tissue matrix that occurs as the result of injury to the arterial wall. Grossly, these lesions appear firm, pale, and homogeneous. The involved area is smooth and uniformly located beneath the endothelium. Histologically, the important cell in this proliferative response is the myofibroblast.[20] It is probable, but not definite, that these cells originate in the media as differentiated smooth muscle cells (SMC). In response to injury, these smooth muscle cells undergo a series of distinct changes, the earliest of which is replication. This is followed by migration from the media across the internal elastic lamina into the intima. In the intima they proliferate and finally synthesize and secrete extracellular matrix.[21] This cellular proliferation, and deposition of connective tissue elements, forms the basis of the observed intimal changes in the lumen of a traumatized vessel.

Since the cellular component of intimal hyperplasia is derived from smooth muscle cells, an understanding of the normal physiology of these cells, and their role in the healing response of a vascular wound, is crucial to our understanding of intimal hyperplasia. The normal arterial wall consists primarily of three layers: the intima, media, and adventitia. Normally, SMCs are located within the media along with a connective tissue mixture of collagen, elastin, and possibly some fibroblasts. The SMCs are responsible for maintaining the configuration and tone of the vascular wall. The intima is generally considered to consist of a single layer of endothelial cells at the luminal surface and a thin basal lamina. One striking characteristic of the normal healthy vessel wall is the slow growth rate of both the intimal endothelial cells and their underlying medial smooth muscle cells. Damage to the vascular endothelium somehow triggers a complex series of events by which the smooth muscle cells undergo a transformation from this resting state to one of great activity. This leads to the migration of SMCs into the intima and ultimately to the lesion of intimal hyperplasia.

Several mechanisms by which injury to the vascular endothelium may lead to activation of the medial smooth muscle cell have been suggested. Postulated theories include hemodynamic factors, alterations in lipid metabolism, as well as complex interactions between the arterial wall and circulating factors such as platelets, and components of the inflammatory system.

Hemodynamic Factors

The effect of hemodynamic forces on the development of intimal hyperplasia has been studied in a variety of models. The forces which have been implicated include flow velocity, shear stress, and wall compliance.[22–25] It is likely that the common endpoint, shared by all of these forces is the resulting damage to the vascular endothelium.[26,27] Taken together, the findings of these studies support the conclusion that flow velocity is not a major factor in the subsequent development of intimal hyperplasia. However, tangential shear stress appears to be an important hemodynamic force leading to the development of this lesion. Confusingly, either high or low shear forces have been demonstrated to contribute, adversely, to the development of intimal hyperplasia. The mechanism, however, by which each end of the shear-stress spectrum stimulates this response, is likely to be very different. Regions of low shear stress may alter the intimal proliferative response by increasing the time for wall contact.[22,28] This would affect both membrane transport of growth factors and lipids, as well as contact with circulating cellular components. Atherosclerotic lesions occur more commonly in areas of low wall shear stress.[29] Conversely, extremely high shear stress may cause a mechanical endothelial injury, which then leads to the development of intimal lesions.[27]

Compliance mismatch has also been suggested to be an important hemodynamic factor in the progression of anastomotic intimal hyperplasia. Compliance is a measure of vessel wall distensibility and can be defined as the percentage of radial change per unit pressure. While experimental and clinical studies have shown that grafts with compliance values approaching that of a native artery demonstrate increased patency, no effect on intimal hyperplasia has been demonstrated. In one such study, autografts were made from one carotid artery and, after preparation, bilateral femoropopliteal grafts were constructed.[30] The compliant graft was treated externally with saline solution for 30 minutes. The "stiff" graft was soaked in 10 per cent glutaraldehyde for 60 minutes. At harvest, only 43 per cent of the stiff grafts were patent compared with 86 per cent of compliant grafts. Unfortunately, there was no difference in intimal thickening observed between the two groups.

In summary, while these numerous hemodynamic forces probably contribute to the evolution of intimal hyperplasia, it is likely that their role is only facilitative and that several other contributing factors are necessary for the development of a full hyperplastic response.

Lipid Metabolism—The Spectrum of Atherosclerosis

Atherosclerotic plaques are a diverse group of lesions that differ in composition depending on their age, anatomic location, and physiologic status of each individual in which they form. The lesions consist of a matrix of connective tissue proteins in which smooth muscle cells and varying amounts of extracellular lipid are embedded. Early lesions are called fatty streaks and consist primarily of lipid-saturated cells and cholesterol deposits. Fibrous plaques are more advanced lesions which are characterized by a necrotic lipid core surrounded by proliferating smooth muscle cells and a connective tissue matrix.

Ultimately, the variant of atherosclerosis which is expressed by each person is determined by the relative proportions of these components.

Histologic examination of hyperplastic intimal lesions reveals an architecture that is strikingly similar to that seen in specimens of atherosclerosis. Both contain abundant lipid, connective tissue elements, as well as smooth muscle cell proliferation. This observation has led to the hypothesis that intimal hyperplasia may in fact be another variant within the spectrum of atherogenesis. In this theory, atherosclerosis and intimal hyperplasia share a common pathophysiologic pathway, but differ in the kinetics of the lesion formation.

Atherosclerosis forms over decades and appears somehow connected to the slow accumulation of lipids. The association of atherogenesis and high levels of plasma low-density lipoproteins (LDL) has long been recognized. Population studies measuring the plasma concentration of LDL among Eskimos have shown much lower levels in this group compared to age-matched Danes.[31] This difference may be related to the very low incidence of atherosclerotic heart disease in the Eskimo population. Lipids are essential components of all cells and they are involved in a number of cellular structures (particularly membranes) and functions. Furthermore, they play an important carrier function; delivering cholesterol for cellular use. Normally, the vascular smooth muscle cell regulates the accumulation of lipid and cholesterol at the level of a surface membrane high-affinity LDL receptor.[32,33] These receptors bind LDL and internalize the bound compounds by endocytosis. The lipids are incorporated by the cellular membranes and the cholesterol is transported to the liposomes where it is degraded and processed for use by the cell. In atherosclerosis, many years of oversaturation with high concentrations of plasma LDL may lead to increased storage of intracellular cholesterol esters and the development of foam cells. Later, necrosis of these cells, liberation of their lipid contents, and finally, calcification, may lead to the necrotic, lipid-rich extracellular debris seen in mature atherosclerosis. Intimal hyperplasia, on the other hand, is characterized by a higher proportion of smooth muscle cell proliferation and less lipid-laden necrosis. This may be the result of a sudden loss of endothelial integrity immediately exposing the underlying smooth muscle cells to large amounts of plasma-bound LDL. The smooth muscles cells respond by both upregulating production of LDL receptors and initiating cellular replication. Low-density lipoprotein has been shown to be a potent smooth muscle cell mitogen.[34] Thus, in this theory, both intimal hyperplasia and atherogenesis are related to alterations in lipid metabolism. However, the rapid kinetics of intimal hyperplasia formation leads to a predominantly cellular lesion with moderate amounts of extracellular matrix, whereas atherosclerosis develops slowly over many decades leading to necrotic, lipid-laden lesions with a relatively sparse cellular component.

Platelets

The activation of platelets by damaged endothelium has been a major focus of research into the etiology of intimal hyperplasia. Removal of the endothelium from an arterial lumen exposes the subendothelial matrix and leads to platelet adherence. This adhesion requires the interaction of subendothelial collagen with a platelet membrane glycoprotein receptor GPIb, plasma von Willebrand factor, and probably, fibronectin.[35] The attached platelet releases adenosine diphosphate (ADP) and activates the arachidonic acid synthesis pathways to produce thromboxane A_2 (TxA_2).[36] The prostaglandin thromboxane A_2 is a potent chemoattractant and leads to additional platelet recruitment. Once activated, platelets also secrete platelet-derived growth factor (PDGF) along with other granule components.[37] Platelet-derived growth factor is a protein with a molecular weight of approximately 30,000 daltons, and consists of two subunits (A and B).[38] It is a chemoattractant as well as a mitogen for SMCs and fibroblasts.[38–40] It is postulated that PDGF may be the signal which attracts the SMCs from the media into the intima and causes their proliferation. Platelets may not be the only source of this growth factor. Platelet-derived growth factor has been isolated from human endothelial cells.[41,42] In fact, injured endothelial cells exhibit a large increase in PDGF production.[43] Furthermore, SMCs themselves produce PDGF-like activity and it has been shown that SMCs from human atheroma contain copies of mRNA coding for PDGF A-chain.[44] Unfortunately, while the cascades leading to the activation of platelets and the subsequent release of PDGF may play a role in the early response of a vessel to injury, attempts to prevent or reduce intimal hyperplasia by interfering with these pathways have yielded disappointing results.

Inflammatory Pathways

The role of inflammatory pathways in the development of intimal hyperplasia is not universally accepted. It has long been appreciated that the two biological responses, cellular proliferation and inflammation, are closely associated. These processes often occur together as part of the normal physiologic reaction to injury. In the case of vascular injury, this association has been demonstrated in an in vivo model of vasculitis.[45] In this study, endotoxin-soaked thread was employed to create an inflammatory response on one surface of a rat femoral artery. This resulted in a profound leukocyte infiltration which occurred exclusively on the treated half of the vessel. Interestingly, after 14 days, intimal lesions composed primarily of smooth muscle cells were found localized to the treated side of the lumen, suggesting an association between the inflammatory and proliferative processes. Furthermore, following a balloon catheter injury, electron microscopic studies have demonstrated that both monocytes and polymorphonuclear neutrophilic leucocytes (PMNs) adhere to the deendothelialized surfaces.[46,47] The mechanism of this adherence and its possible role in intimal hyperplasia remains undetermined.

Until recently, the contribution of leukocytes in the development of intimal hyperplasia has been largely thought to be limited to their role in endothelial cell damage. Neutrophils are activated by components of the complement system, immune complexes, and endotoxin.[48] Within seconds of activation, degranulation and oxidative metabolic pathways begin. These processes lead to the release of oxygen-free radicals and other toxic products.[49] As a result, neutrophils induce endothelial cell damage mediated primarily by the production of toxic metabolites.[50] The importance of these findings may be the role that neutrophils play in denuding arterial injuries. With neutrophil activation, the marginally adherent endothelial cells bordering a lesion may be detached, increasing the magnitude of the injury to the vessel. This further exposure of the subendothelial layer will allow increased inflammatory cell adherence, aggregation, and activation, recruiting more white blood cell mediators and therefore stimulating a continued cycle of endothelial injury and inflammatory activation.

Recently, a more complex view of the role of inflammatory cells in the development of intimal hyperplasia has emerged. After the deposition of inflammatory cells following an endothelial injury, a number of cytokines are elaborated. These include chemotactic and growth factors, complement components, and enzymes. One of these products, macrophage-derived growth factor (MDGF), has been shown to stimulate the proliferation of SMCs and fibroblasts.[51] This growth factor may be similar, if not identical, to PDGF.[52] Therefore, inflammatory cells also possess the chemical ability to stimulate SMC migration and proliferation.

PHARMACOLOGIC THERAPY

Antiplatelet Agents

Antiplatelet drugs inhibit the synthesis of prostaglandins by blocking the arachidonic acid pathways. Aspirin irreversibly acetylates platelet cell cyclooxygenase. Dipyridamole increases platelet cyclic adenosine monophosphate (AMP) and inhibits the precursors thromboxane A_1 and B_2. Thus, both aspirin and dipyridamole inhibit platelet adherence, as well as aggregation, by interfering with the production of thromboxane metabolites. Excitement about the possibility of limiting intimal hyperplasia by interfering with platelet pathways began with the work of Friedman et al., who reported reduced hyperplasia following aortic balloon catheter injury in thrombocytopenic rabbits.[53] Unfortunately, inhibition of intimal hyperplasia using a number of different antiplatelet drugs has yielded mixed results.

Clinically, and in experimental models, aspirin has been shown to decrease platelet adherence to prosthetic vascular grafts.[54-56] The addition of dipyridamole may or may not enhance this effect. Findings from other studies, however, have demonstrated that although antiplatelet agents may decrease subsequent platelet aggregation and thrombus formation, they have no effect on the initial platelet deposition.[57] The effect of these agents on patency and the development of intimal hyperplasia has also been inconsistent. In one study, bilateral vein bypass grafts were placed in ligated iliac arteries in rhesus monkeys.[58] These monkeys were given aspirin (165 mg bid) and dipyridamole (25 mg bid) beginning 3 weeks before the surgical procedure. Sixteen weeks after the procedure, at sacrifice, the intimal area was compared and found to be significantly reduced in the experimental group. On the other hand, in a follow-up study using a balloon catheter injury model in rabbits, no significant difference between the two groups in tritiated thymidine incorporation, nuclear proliferation, or progression of intimal hyperplasia was established.[10] In our laboratory, we found that aspirin significantly increased the patency of an end-to-side iliac anastomosis, but had no effect on the development of intimal hyperplasia.[8]

Thromboxane synthetase converts cyclic endoperoxide precursors from the arachidonic acid pathways into thromboxane. Thromboxane A_2 is synthesized and stored in the developing platelet. It is a powerful mediator of both platelet aggregation and vascular constriction. Inhibitors of thromboxane synthetase block this conversion of intermediate endoperoxide precursors into TxA_2. Furthermore, in doing so, the intracellular prostaglandin metabolic pathways are then shifted towards the production of prostacycline (PGI_2). Thus, theoretically, thromboxane synthetase inhibitors can block platelet-derived TxA_2 while actually enhancing the production of endothelial cell–

derived PGI_2. It is postulated that these agents may therefore be more specific inhibitors of platelet function. In a recent report, the efficacy of thromboxane synthetase inhibition in the prevention of distal anastomotic intimal hyperplasia was investigated and compared to aspirin.[59] A bilateral aortoiliac bypass graft model was used and two different types of grafts were evaluated: thin-walled polytetrafluoroethylene (PTFE) and PTFE seeded with autologous endothelial cells. Treatment groups consisted of antiplatelet therapy with either aspirin or the thromboxane synthetase inhibitor U-63,577A. Interestingly, in both types of grafts, aspirin was significantly more effective in maintaining patency and inhibiting intimal hyperplasia. Within the thromboxane synthetase inhibitor group, however, the agent was more effective when the bypass grafts were seeded; and both types of graft were improved when compared to no therapy at all. In conclusion, theoretically, these agents in combination with other antiplatelet drugs could prove to be potent inhibitors of platelet function. However, no clinical trials are yet available.

To summarize, at the present time, antiplatelet drugs would seem to increase the patency of vein and prosthetic bypass grafts, but probably do not effect the development of intimal hyperplasia. More work is necessary to determine the role of newer agents in complimenting or enhancing these effects.

Anti-inflammatory Agents

Glucocorticoids exert both immunosuppressive and anti-inflammatory effects. In inflammatory states, neutrophils adhere to endothelial linings and penetrate the vascular wall.[60] Steroids have been demonstrated to decrease this endothelial adhesion.[61,62] They also impair the release of granules from PMNs and decrease the production of superoxide anions.[63] The role of the immune system in the evolution of intimal hyperplasia is not clear. Atherosclerotic plaques have been found to contain activated lymphocytes and SMCs that express class II major histocompatibility antigens.[64] Interaction of these antigens and immune cells may propagate the immune response and result in the release of other inflammatory mediators and cytokines. Steroids also prevent leukocyte aggregation to various chemotactic factors.[65,66] For these reasons, it has been suggested that modification of leukocyte function by steroid administration may be effective in the prevention of intimal hyperplasia.

High-dose methylprednisolone (10 mg) has been found to prevent subendothelial and transmural accumulation of neutrophils and endothelial sloughing in vein grafts implanted into low-flow circuits.[67] This effect on endothelial sloughing may decrease the stimuli for the development of intimal hyperplasia.

Using a canine femoropopliteal Dacron bypass graft model, Hoepp et al. found no significant differences in patency or the hyperplastic response between steroid-treated and control groups.[12] However, in this experiment, the dogs were treated with a relatively low dose of methylprednisolone (1 mg/kg given intramuscularly) and the drug regimen was begun only after completion of the procedure rather than preoperatively. Interestingly, this group found a marked improvement when the dogs were treated with azathioprine (1 mg/kg taken orally), an immunosuppressive agent.

We have reported a marked reduction in intimal hyperplasia using dexamethasone (0.1 mg/kg given intramuscularly).[11] This effect was demonstrated in a rabbit carotid balloon catheter injury model. In this study, the drug regimen was begun the day prior to the carotid artery endothelial injury and continued for a period of 8 weeks. No beneficial effects were noted in this model with either cyclophosphamide or azathioprine.

Most recently, a large, randomized, double-blind clinical study (M-HEART project) assessed whether or not a single large dose of methylprednisolone (1 gram) given intravenously prior to angioplasty could alter the incidence of restenosis.[68] The results found no significant difference between steroid- and placebo-treated groups. In should be recognized, however, that methylprednisolone is a relatively short-acting steroid compared to dexamethasone, and it was given as a single dose. Clowes et al. have demonstrated that the period of maximal intimal proliferation is approximately 2 weeks after an arterial injury.[69] This may explain the disparity between this study and our results in which a longer acting agent was used, and continued for 8 weeks. Furthermore, pilot work in our laboratory has suggested that starting the steroid treatment prior to the arterial injury may be important.

The effect of treatment with cyclosporin was studied in a rat common iliac artery injury model.[70] Prior to undergoing the arterial injury, rats were administered parenteral cyclosporin at a dose of 5 mg/kg/day which was continued for 2 and 6 weeks. The results showed that those arteries treated with cyclosporin demonstrated significantly less medial thickening at each time interval. This data provides further evidence that immunologic mechanisms may be important in the development of intimal hyperplasia.

Antihypertensive Agents

Angiotensin-converting enzyme (ACE) inhibitors, calcium channel blockers, and α_1-adrenergic antagonists, are all agents used clinically in the treatment of systemic hypertension. Each of these categories of antihypertensive drugs has been reported to be effective in suppressing intimal hyperplasia.

Angiotensin-converting enzyme inhibitors prevent the conversion of circulating angiotensin I into the active derivative angiotensin II. Angiotensin II is a potent vasoactive substance and causes a rapid constriction of most arterial beds. The mechanism of this action has been extensively studied and is thought to be mediated through stimulation of medial smooth muscle cells.[71] Furthermore, enhanced collagen-induced platelet activation has been reported to be mediated by specific binding sites for angiotensin II.[72] Recently, the effect of the angiotensin-converting enzyme inhibitor cilazapril on the development of intimal hyperplasia was investigated.[14] In this study, rats were subjected to an endothelial denudation injury by a balloon catheter. Experimental animals received 10 mg/kg of cilazapril beginning 6 days before the endothelial injury. Therapy was continued daily for 14 days. The results showed a significant inhibition of intimal hyperplasia in the treated group, and supports the possibility that this proliferative response is at least partially mediated by angiotensin II receptors.

Calcium channel antagonists are effective agents used in a variety of cardiovascular disorders. In general, the common mechanism of action of all these agents is an interruption of membrane calcium channels, thereby reducing the availability of this cation for a variety of intercellular processes. Calcium has been implicated in a number of events involved in the development of intimal hyperplasia including platelet activation, release of PDGF, medial SMC proliferation, and the formation of extracellular matrix. Treatment with calcium antagonists has been shown to significantly reduce the development of intimal hyperplasia after a mechanical arterial injury.[73] In addition, verapamil was effective in reducing intimal hyperplasia in at least one vein bypass graft model.[15]

Another important mediator of vascular tone is the α_1-adrenergic receptor. These receptors are found on vascular smooth muscle cells and, when stimulated, result in profound contraction. The cytoplasmic secondary messenger system for this receptor response has recently been reported to involve an increase in the turnover of the intracellular phosphatidylinositol cycle.[74] Also, experimental studies have demonstrated that endothelial denudation is accompanied by a selective increase in the sensitivity of the α_1-adrenergic receptor.[75] Furthermore, PDGF function has also been linked to an upregulation of the intracellular phosphatidylinositol cycle. Intermediates of this cycle stimulate protein kinase C to initiate a series of phosphorylating reactions which ultimately lead to cellular mitosis.[76] Therefore, the intracellular mechanisms of SMC proliferation and contraction are connected through a common cytoplasmic pathway: the phosphatidylinositol cycle. Prazosin is a selective α_1-adrenergic receptor blocker and has been studied for its ability to prevent intimal hyperplasia. In a balloon catheter injury model of the rabbit aorta, prazosin was shown to produce a statistically significant reduction in the development of intimal hyperplastic lesions.[13] No clinical trials utilizing this agent have been reported.

Anticoagulants

Heparin is a naturally occurring polymer containing chains of sulfonated mucopolysaccharides. In vivo, it is concentrated in mast cells and found in several different tissues, including the endothelium. The length, and thus molecular weight of heparin polymers, is highly variable. Furthermore, different size polymers have different anticoagulant potency.[77] Because of this variability, heparin has unpredictable biological activity and is therefore quantified in international units rather then by weight.

Heparin works through its inhibition of the plasma-bound proteolytic clotting cascades. Antithrombin III is a potent naturally occurring anticoagulant that inhibits several of the activated coagulant proteins. Certain size heparin polymers combine with antithrombin III. This binding greatly enhances the enzymatic action of antithrombin III. Also, because these bound cofactors are not consumed by the inhibition reaction, only a small amount of heparin is required when the plasma load of activated coagulant proteins is moderate. This forms the basis of low-dose heparin therapy for prophylaxis.

Clinically, heparin has been used most frequently in the prophylaxis and treatment of venous thrombosis and pulmonary emboli. A few studies have concluded that perioperative high-dose heparin can prevent early thrombosis in peripheral bypass grafts.[78] This action is presumably due to the drugs' ability to shift the balance of the coagulation cascade and counteract the thrombotic forces of low flow states and thrombogenic surfaces.

Recently, heparin has been shown to prevent SMC migration and proliferation in vivo and in vitro.[16] The mechanism of this action has not yet been established. In addition, available data also indicate that both anticoagulant and nonanticoagulant fractions of heparin possess this antiproliferative activity.[16] Low molecular weight (LMW) heparin is a combination of short-chain heparin polymers with significantly lower anticoagulant activity than standard heparin preparations. Interest in this heparin derivative stems from its potential in modulating intimal hyperplasia without affecting the coagulation system. At least one recent study has shown that LMW heparin may be effective in this regard.[16]

Lipid Metabolites

As mentioned before, Eskimos have extremely low plasma levels of LDL and this may explain their low incidence of atherosclerotic heart disease.[31] Further, characterization of Eskimo plasma lipid composition has demonstrated low levels of circulating arachidonic acid and unusually high concentrations of eicosapentaenoic acid (EPA).[79] Eicosapentaenoic acid is an omega-3 polyunsaturated fatty acid that is present in large amounts in fish, but which cannot be synthesized de novo by humans. Following ingestion, EPA enters the prostaglandin synthesis pathway and competes directly with arachidonic acid. As mentioned before, one by-product of arachidonic acid metabolism is TxA_2, a potent stimulator of platelet aggregation. Eicosapentaenoic acid, however, is converted to TxA_3, which has no effect on platelet function.

Several studies have tested the hypothesis that high levels of EPA present at the time of an endothelial injury may inhibit the production of intimal hyperplasia. Both Cahill et al. and Landymore et al. have reported the ability of small doses of marine oils to reduce intimal thickening in vein graft models.[17,18] Most recently, O-hara et al. has reported a marked suppression in intimal hyperplasia following treatment with EPA in a rabbit PTFE grafting model.[19]

Further investigation is needed to establish both the precise mechanism by which EPA prevents intimal hyperplasia, and at which dose and duration of exposure is this effect optimal.

NEW HORIZONS

Angiopeptin

A universal theme, recurring in all the postulated mechanisms of intimal hyperplasia, is the promotion of vascular smooth muscle cell growth by peptide mitogens. Examples include PDGF and MDGF. Likewise, intimal hyperplasia can be seen as a hemodynamic response of the vessel wall to the endogenous trophic actions of angiotensin II, another peptide mitogen. Emerging from this idea is the concept of the vascular wall as a complex integrated organ complete with its own endogenous local autocrine system. In this model, intimal hyperplasia can be viewed as the result of an imbalance of these local hormonal systems. This may be due to an excess of trophic peptides or, alternatively, the smooth muscle cell proliferation could be the result of the absence or reduction of the suppressive effects of inhibitory hormones.

Somatostatin is a widely occurring peptide hormone that acts as a modulator of a diverse class of endogenous growth promoters. It has been postulated that if intimal hyperplasia is the result of an imbalance in local vascular autocrine systems following an endothelial injury, somatostatin may be effective in limiting this response. Unfortunately, somatostatin is unsuitable for use in in vivo models because of storage instability and a very short half-life. Angiopeptin is a stable octapeptide somatostatin analog that has been shown to be an effective long-acting somatostatin receptor agonist. This analog has been extensively studied as a potential inhibitor of intimal hyperplasia.

Several authors have reported the success of this peptide in suppressing the development of intimal hyperplasia in animal models.[80–82] In one publication, angiopeptin was also shown to significantly reduce the degree of post-transplant coronary artery intimal hyperplasia in rabbits.[83] This study was complicated, however, by the fact that these rabbits also received cyclosporin immunosuppression which, as discussed above, has also been reported to effect the development of intimal hyperplasia. Whether or not, in this setting, angiopeptin is actually antagonizing the trophic effects of growth mitogens is not clear. In vitro work has also demonstrated the ability of angiopeptin to inhibit the proliferation of smooth muscle cells.[84] This suggests that the action of angiopeptin may be a direct effect on the smooth muscle cell and not related to the inhibition of a somatostatin receptor. This is further supported by the fact that some somatostatin analogs have not been successful in limiting the intimal hyperplastic response.[82] Nonetheless, the concept of the vascular tree functioning in a complex local hormonal system and the possibility of altering and controlling this balance with pharmacologic therapy remains an exciting area of investigation.

Photodynamic Therapy

Another way to view the intimal hyperplastic response is as a process akin to that of a benign neoplastic lesion. In this scheme, the proliferating intimal smooth muscle cell is pictured as an undifferentiated pluripotent medial myofibroblast whose growth continues in the absence of normal cellular controls. The resulting lesion can be considered a form of "vascular keloid." Recently, photodynamic therapy has been shown to be safe and effective in the treatment of several rapidly growing benign neoplasms. Photofrin-II is a hematoporphyrin derivative that has been shown to be absorbed by atherosclerotic plaques.[85] Furthermore, laser phototherapy directed at these photofrin-bound hyperplastic cells has significantly inhibited their growth in vitro.[86] The ability of intimal hyperplastic lesions to selectively absorb porphyrin compounds in vivo has not been demonstrated. However, photodynamic therapy remains an intriguing area of investigation in the treatment of intimal hyperplasia.

Modulation of the Immune System

The contribution of the inflammatory mediators in the pathophysiology of intimal hyperplasia has already been discussed. It is possible that these same pathways could be manipulated to control these very same processes. Immunotherapy for a variety of neoplastic conditions has emerged as an exciting new area of research. The basic idea of programming the body's own immune defenses against specific antigens located on the surface of offending tumor cells is likely to be applicable to other conditions as well.

Activated T-lymphocytes have already been detected in atherosclerotic plaques.[64] These lymphocytes produce gamma interferon and various interleukins that promote expression of class II major histocompatibility antigens and perpetuate the immune response. Future work in directing this response against specific SMC antigens expressed within intimal hyperplastic lesions may provide an exciting new research direction.

REFERENCES

1. Dalman RL, Taylor LM Jr: Basic data related to infrainguinal revascularization procedures. Ann Vasc Surg 1990;*3*(3):309–312.
2. Imparato AM, Bracco A, Kim GE, Zeff RZ: Intimal and neointimal fibrous proliferation causing failure of arterial reconstruction. Surgery 1972;*72*:1107–1117.
3. Szilagyi DE, et al: Biologic fate of autologous vein implants as arterial substitutes: Clinical, angiographic and histologic observations in femoropopliteal operations for atherosclerosis. Ann Surg 1973;*178*:232–246.
4. Healy DA, Clowes AW, Zierler RE, et al: Immediate and long-term results of carotid endarterectomy. Stroke 1989;*20*:1138–1142.
5. Wilson SE, Sheppard B: Results of percutaneous transluminal angioplasty for peripheral vascular occlusive disease. Ann Vasc Surg 1990;*4*(1):94–97.
6. White RA, White GH, Mehringer MC: A clinical trial of laser thermal angioplasty in patients with advanced peripheral vascular disease. Ann Surg 1990;*211*:257–265.
7. Ahn SS, Yeatman LR, Deutsch LS, et al: Intraoperative peripheral atherectomy: Preliminary clinical results. 1991 (in submission).
8. Quiñones-Baldrich W, Ziomek S, Henderson T, Moore W. Patency and intimal hyperplasia: The effect of aspirin on small arterial anastomosis. Ann Vasc Surg 1988;*2*(1):50–56.
9. Landymore RW, Karmazyn M, MacAulay MA, Sheridan B, Cameron CA: Correlation between the effects of aspirin and dipyridamole on platelet function and prevention of intimal hyperplasia in autologous vein grafts. Can J Cardiol 1988;*4*(1):56–59.
10. Radic ZS, O'Malley MK, Mikat EM, et al: The role of aspirin and dipyridamole on vascular DNA synthesis and intimal hyperplasia following deendothelialization. J Surg Res 1986;*41*(1):84–91.
11. Chervu A, Moore WS, Quiñones-Baldrich WJ, Henderson T: Efficacy of corticosteroids in suppression of intimal hyperplasia. J Vasc Surg 1989;*10*:129–134.
12. Hoepp LM, Elbadawi A, Cohn M, et al: Steroids and immunosuppression: Effect on anastomotic intimal hyperplasia in femoral arterial Dacron bypass grafts. Arch Surg 1979;*114*:273–276.
13. O'Malley MK, McDermott EW, Mehigan D, O'Higgins NJ: Role for prazosin in reducing the development of rabbit intimal hyperplasia after endothelial denudation. Br J Surg 1989;*76*(9):936–938.
14. Powell JS, Clozel JP, Muller RK, et al: Inhibitors of angiotensin-converting enzyme prevent myointimal proliferation after vascular injury. Science 1989;*245*:186–188.
15. El-Sanadiki MN, Cross KS, Murray JJ, et al: Reduction of intimal hyperplasia and enhanced reactivity of experimental vein bypass grafts with verapamil. Ann Surg 1990;*212*(1):87–96.
16. Dryjski M, Mikat E, Bjornsson TD: Inhibition of intimal hyperplasia after arterial injury by heparins and heparinoid. J Vasc Surg 1988;*8*(5):623–633.
17. Cahill PD, Sarris GE, Cooper AD, et al: Inhibition of vein graft intimal thickening by eicosapentaenoic acid: Reduced thromboxane production without change in lipoprotein levels or low-density lipoprotein receptor density. J Vasc Surg 1988;*7*:108–117.
18. Landymore RW, Manku MS, Tan M, MacAulay MA, Sheridan B: Effects of low-dose marine oils on intimal hyperplasia in autologous vein grafts. J Thorac Cardiovasc Surg 1989;*98*(5 Pt 1):788–791.
19. O-hara M, Esato K, Harada M, et al: Eicosapentaenoic acid suppresses intimal hyperplasia after expanded polytetrafluoroethylene grafting in rabbits fed a high cholesterol diet. J Vasc Surg 1991;*13*:480–486.
20. Spaet TH, Stemerman MB, Veith FJ, Lejnieks I: Intimal injury and regrowth in the rabbit aorta: Medial smooth muscle cells as a source of neointima. Circ Res 1975;*36*:58–70.
21. Clowes AW, Clowes MM, Fingerle J, Reidy MA: Regulation of smooth muscle cell growth in injured artery. J Cardiovasc Pharmacol 1989;*14*(suppl. 6):S12–S15.
22. Rittgers SE, Karayannacos PE, Guy JF, et al: Velocity distribution and intimal proliferation in autologous vein grafts in dogs. Circ Res 1978;*42*:792–801.
23. Morinaga K, Okadome K, Kuroki M, et al: Effect of wall shear stress on intimal thickening of arterially transplanted autogenous veins in dogs. J Vasc Surg 1985;*2*:430–433.
24. Lyon RT, Runyon-Hass A, Davis HR, et al: Protection from atherosclerotic lesion formation by reduction of artery wall motion. J Vasc Surg 1987;*5*:59–67.
25. Sottiurai VS, Kollros P, Glagov S, et al: Morphological alteration of cultured arterial smooth muscle cells by cyclic stretching. J Surg Res 1983;*35*:490–497.
26. Chervu A, Moore WS: An overview of intimal hyperplasia. Surg Gynecol Obstet 1990;*171*:433–447.
27. Fry DL: Acute vascular endothelial changes associated with increased blood velocity gradients. Circ Res 1968;*22*:165–167.
28. Berguer R, Higgins RF, Reddy DJ: Intimal hyperplasia: An experimental study. Arch Surg 1980;*115*:332–335.
29. Caro CG, Fitz-Gerald JM, Schroter RC: Arterial wall shear: Observation, correlation and proposal of a shear dependent mass transfer mechanism for atherogenesis. Proc R Soc Lond 1971;*177*:109–159.

30. Abbott WM, Megerman J, Hasson JE, et al: Effect of compliance mismatch on vascular graft patency. J Vasc Surg 1987;5:376–382.

31. Bang HO, Dyerberg J, Nielsen A: Plasma lipid and lipoprotein pattern in greenlandic westcoast Eskimos. Lancet 1971;1:1143–1145.

32. Brown MS, Faust JR, Goldstein JL: Role of the low density lipoprotein receptor in regulating the content of free and esterified cholesterol in human fibroblasts. J Clin Invest 1975;55:783.

33. Goldstein JL, Brown MS: The low-density lipoprotein pathway and its relation to atherosclerosis. Ann Rev Biochem 1977;46:879.

34. Wissler RW: Biochemistry of Artherosclerosis, Vol 7. New York, Marcel Dekker, 1979;345.

35. George J, Nurden A, Phillips D: Molecular defects in interactions of platelets with the vessel wall. N Engl J Med 1984;311:1084–1098.

36. Bell R, Kennerly D, Stanford N, Majerus P: Diglyceridelipase: A pathway for arachidonate release from human platelets. Proc Natl Acad Sci USA 1979;76:3238–3241.

37. Scharf R, Harker L: Thrombosis and atherosclerosis: Regulatory role of interactions among blood components and endothelium. Blut 1987;55:131–144.

38. Ross R, Glomset J, Kariya B, Harker L: A platelet-dependent serum factor that stimulates the proliferation of arterial smooth muscle cells in vivo. Proc Natl Acad Sci USA 1974;71:1207–1210.

39. Grotendorst G, Chang T, Seppa H, et al: Platelet derived growth factor is a chemoattractant for vascular smooth muscle cells. J Cell Physiol 1982;113:261–266.

40. Rutherford R, Ross R: Platelet factors stimulate fibroblasts and smooth muscle cells quiescent in plasma serum proliferate. J Cell Biol 1976;69:196–203.

41. Collins T, Ginsburg D, Boss J, et al: Cultured human endothelial cells express platelet-derived growth factor B chain: cDNA cloning and structural analysis. Nature 1985;316:748–750.

42. Limanni A, Fleming T, Molina R, et al: Expression of genes for platelet-derived growth factor in adult human venous endothelium: A possible nonplatelet dependent cause of intimal hyperplasia in vein graft and perianastomotic areas of vascular prostheses. J Vasc Surg 1988;7:10–20.

43. Di Corleto P, Chisolm G: Participation of the endothelium in the development of the atherosclerotic plaque. Prog Lipid Res 1986;25:365–374.

44. Libby P, Warner S, Salomon R, Birinyi L: Production of platelet-derived growth factor-like mitogen by smooth muscle cells from human atheroma. N Engl J Med 1988;318:1493–1498.

45. Prescott MF, McBride CK, Venturini CM, Gerhardt SC: Leukocyte stimulation of intimal lesion formation is inhibited by treatment with diclofenac sodium and dexamethasone. J Cardiovasc Pharmacol 1989;14(suppl 6):S76–S81.

46. Lucas J, Makhoul R, Cole C, et al: Mononuclear cells adhere to sites of vascular balloon catheter injury. Curr Surg 1986;12–115.

47. Cole C, Lucas J, Mikat E, et al: Adherence of polymorphonuclear leukocytes to injured rabbit aorta. Surg Forum 1984;440–442.

48. Weissmann G, Smole J, Korchak H: Release of inflammatory mediators from stimulated neutrophils. N Engl J Med 1980;303:27–34.

49. Babior B: Oxygen-dependent microbial killing by phagocytes. N Engl J Med 1978;298:659–668.

50. Sacks T, Moldow C, Craddock P, Bowers T: Oxygen radicals mediate endothelial cell damage by complement-stimulated granulocytes: An in vitro model of immune vascular damage. J Clin Invest 1978;61:1161–1167.

51. Leibovich S, Ross R: A macrophage-dependent factor that stimulates the proliferation of fibroblasts in vitro. Am J Pathol 1976;84:501–513.

52. Shimokado K, Raines E, Madtes D, et al: A significant part of macrophage-derived growth factor consists of at least two forms of PDGF. Cell 1988;43:277–286.

53. Friedman RJ, Stemerman MB, Wenz B, Moore S, Gauldie J: The effect of thrombocytopenia on experimental arteriosclerotic lesion formation in rabbits: Smooth muscle cell proliferation and re-endothelialization. J Clin Invest 1977;60:1191–1201.

54. McCollum C, Crow M, Rajah S, Kester R: Anti-thrombotic therapy for vascular prosthesis. An experimental model testing platelet inhibitory drugs. Surgery 1980;87:668–676.

55. Oblath R, Buckley F, Green R, et al: Prevention of platelet aggregation to prosthetic vascular grafts by aspirin and dipyridamole. Surgery 1978;84:37–44.

56. Zammit M, Kaplan S, Sauvage L, et al: Aspirin therapy in small-caliber arterial prostheses: Long-term experimental observations. J Vasc Surg 1984;1:839–851.

57. Plate G, Stanson A, Hollier L, Dewanjee M: Drug effects on platelet deposition after endothelial injury of the rabbit aorta. J Surg Res 1985;39:258–266.

58. McCann R, Hagen P-O, Fuchs J: Aspirin and dipyridamole decrease intimal hyperplasia in experimental vein grafts. Ann Surg 1980;191:238–243.

59. Graham LM, Brothers TE, Darvishian D, et al: Effects of thromboxane synthetase inhibition on patency and anastomotic hyperplasia of vascular grafts. J Surg Res 1989;46:611–615.

60. Atherton A, Born G: Quantitative investigations of the adhesiveness of circulating polymorphonuclear leukocytes to blood vessels. J Physiol 1972;222:447–474.

61. Mishler J: The effects of corticosteroids on mobilization and function of neutrophils. Exp Hematol 1977;5:15–32.
62. MacGregor R, Spagnuolo P, Lentnek A: Inhibition of granulocyte adherence by ethanol, prednisone, and aspirin measured with a new assay system. N Engl J Med 1974;29(81):642–646.
63. Goldstein I, Roos D, Weissmann G, Kaplan H: Influence of corticosteroids on human polymorphonuclear leukocyte function in vitro enzyme release and superoxide production. Inflammation 1976;1:305–315.
64. Hansson GK, Holm J, Jonasson L: Detection of activated T lymphocytes in the human atherosclerotic plaque. Am J Pathol 1989;135:169–175.
65. Hammerschmidt D, White J, Craddock P, Jacob H: Cortico-steroids inhibit complement-induced granulocyte aggregation: A possible mechanism for their efficacy in shock states. J Clin Invest 1979;63:798–803.
66. Oseas R, Allen J, Yang H-H, et al: Mechanism of dexamethasone inhibition of chemotactic factor induced granulocyte aggregation. Blood 1982;59:265–269.
67. Pearce WJ, Dujovny M, Ho K, et al: Acute inflammation and endothelial injury in vein grafts. Neurosurgery 1985;17:626–634.
68. Pepine C, et al: A controlled trial of corticosteroids to prevent restenosis after coronary angioplasty. Circulation 1990;81:1753–1761.
69. Clowes AW, Reidy MA, Clowes MM: Kinetics of cellular proliferation after arterial injury. I. Smooth muscle growth in the absence of endothelium. Lab Invest 1983;49:327–333.
70. Wengrovitz M, Selassie LG, Gifford RRM, Thiele BL: Cyclosporine inhibits the development of medial thickening after experimental arterial injury. J Vasc Surg 1990;12(1):1–7.
71. Griendling K, et al: Angiotensin II stimulation of vascular smooth muscle. J Cardiovasc Pharmacol 1989;14(suppl 6):S27–S33.
72. Moore T, Williams G: Angiotensin II receptors on human platelets. Circ Res 1982;51:314–320.
73. El-Sanadiki M, Cross K, Mikat E, Hagen P-O: Verapamil therapy reduces intimal hyperplasia in balloon injured rabbit aorta. Circulation 1987;76(suppl):314.
74. O'Malley M, Cotecchia S, Hagen P-O: Receptor mediated noradrenaline supersensitivity in rabbit aortic intimal hyperplasia. Eur Surg Res 1986;18:43.
75. O'Malley M, Mikat E, McCann R, Hagen P-O: Increased vascular sensitivity to norepinephrine following injury. Surg Forum 1984;35:445–447.
76. Mark J: The polyphosphoinositides revisited. Science 1985;228:312–313.
77. Cifonelli J: The relationship of molecular weight, and sulfate content and distribution to anticoagulant activity of heparin preparations. Carbohydr Res 1974;37:145.
78. Schweiger H, Klein P, et al: Avoiding early failure of tibial prosthetic bypass grafts. Thorac Cardiovasc Surg 1987;35:148–150.
79. Dyerberg J, Bang HO, Stoffersen E, Moncada S, Vane JR: Eicosapentaenoic acid and prevention of thrombosis and atherosclerosis. Lancet 1978;2:117–119.
80. Calcagno D, Conte JV, Howell MH, Foegh ML: Peptide inhibition of neointimal hyperplasia in vein grafts. J Vasc Surg 1991;13:475–479.
81. Conte JV, Foegh ML, Calcagno D, Wallace RB, Ramwell PW: Peptide inhibition of myointimal proliferation following angioplasty in rabbits. Transplant Proc 1989;21:3686–3688.
82. Lundergan C, Foegh ML, Vargas R, et al: Inhibition of myointimal proliferation of the rat carotid artery by the peptides, angiopeptin and BIM 23034. Atherosclerosis 1989;80:49–55.
83. Foegh ML, Khirabadi BS, Chambers E, Amamoo S, Ramwell PW: Inhibition of coronary artery transplant atherosclerosis in rabbits with angiopeptin, an octapeptide. Atherosclerosis 1989;78(2-3):229–236.
84. Vargas R, Bormes GW, Wroblewska B, et al: Angiopeptin inhibits thymidine incorporation in rat carotid artery in vitro. Transplant Proc 1989;21:3702–3704.
85. Spears JR, Serur J, Shopshire D, et al: Fluorescence of experimental atheromatous plaque with hematoporphyrin derivative. J Clin Invest 1983;71:395–399.
86. Hundley RF, Weinstein R, Spears JR: Photodynamic cytolysis of rat arterial smooth muscle cells with hematoporphyrin derivative in vitro. Lasers Life Sci 1988;2:19–27.

35

PERIPHERAL PERCUTANEOUS TRANSLUMINAL ANGIOPLASTY WITH ULTRASOUND IMAGING

LARRY H. HOLLIER, BRUCE J. BRENER, SCOTT R. CLULEY,
CHRISTOPHER J. WHITE, and STEPHEN R. RAMEE

Endovascular techniques have gained increasing popularity over the last decade. The use of balloon angioplasty,[1-5] laser recanalization,[6-7] percutaneous atherectomy,[8] and intraluminal stents[9] are now widely accepted. In the early days of development of these techniques, vascular surgeons were generally opposed to their use, since they believed that the immediate and long-term success of nonoperative procedures would be inferior to conventional surgical revascularization techniques. However, increasing experience with endovascular techniques and improvements in technology have allowed steady improvement both in immediate success and long-term patency. Nonetheless, vascular surgeons have been slow to adopt nonoperative angioplasty, while radiologists and cardiologists have aggressively adopted these techniques. Today, most endovascular procedures are done by nonvascular surgeons. Nonsurgical intervention will have impact on the practice of vascular surgery.[10]

One of the major reasons for the paucity of endovascular procedures done by vascular surgeons is the fact that they generally do not have ready access to radiographic suites. Thus, they have limited ability to perform angiographic directed endovascular procedures. Recently, the development of intravascular ultrasound has allowed adequate visualization of the lumen of an artery.[11-12] This chapter discusses a new, and perhaps superior, approach to endovascular procedures—ultrasound-guided angioplasty. This technique, and the facilities required to implement it, are readily available to all vascular surgeons and may provide an additional avenue of participation in the ever-expanding field of vascular disease management.

A new catheter has been developed that can accurately and precisely be positioned using duplex ultrasonography alone.[13] This catheter has been successfully tested in animals and, following FDA approval, has been utilized in human clinical trials.

ULTRASOUND-GUIDED CATHETER SYSTEM

Standard 7-F angioplasty catheters of varying balloon diameters were modified for ultrasound guidance. A spherical brass bead 2.49 mm in diameter was mounted on the shaft of each catheter in the mid-balloon region. The bead had been coated with a 70-μm layer of polyvinylidene difluoride and copolymer, a compound with piezoelectric properties. This spherical structure functions as an omnidirectional receiver, with its signal carried by a wire to the proximal end of the catheter. The receiver was then integrated electronically to a duplex ultrasound system via a catheter-system interface (CSI), as diagrammed in Figure 35–1.

As an ultrasound pulse hits the sensor, a signal is transmitted through the wire in the catheter to a CSI. The time delay for transmission of the imaging ultrasound pulse from the scan head to the receiver is measured. The particular ultrasound ray (i.e., ray 54 in Fig. 35–1) which hits the sensor is determined by monitoring the transmissions at the scan head as shown. This information then places the receiver on a particular ray at a particular distance. This positional data is transmitted from the CSI to the scan head, where it is electromagnetically injected into the image at exactly the position of the receiver. The position of the receiver is shown by a flashing bright arrow superimposed on the ultrasound B-mode image of the tissue (Fig. 35–2).

ANIMAL STUDIES

Twenty 5-kg adult female mongrel dogs were anesthetized with intravenous thiamylal (Biotal) and intubated. Anesthesia was maintained by an inhalation mixture of 1 to 2 per cent halothane and 4 L/min oxygen. Respiration was maintained by mechanical ventilation. Electrocardiogram and blood pressure were monitored continuously. All dogs were anticoagulated with intravenous heparin (100 U/kg). Animal care was in compliance with the Principles of Laboratory and Animal Care (formulated by the National Society for Medical

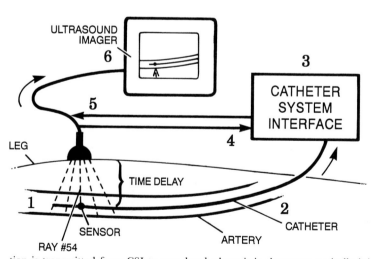

FIGURE 35–1. Echo-Mark ultrasound-guided catheter system. 1, Imaging ultrasound pulse strikes omnidirectional receive attached to the midballoon region of the catheter. 2, Signal is transmitted through wire in catheter to catheter-system interface (CSI). 3, CSI measures time delay for transmission of imaging ultrasound pulse from the scan head to the receiver. 4, CSI determines the particular ultrasound ray (i.e., ray 54) which strikes the receiver by monitoring the transmissions at the scan head. 5, Information tabulated from steps 3 and 4 is used to determine the location of the receiver in horizontal and vertical planes. This positional information is transmitted from CSI to scan head where it is electromagnetically injected into the B-mode image and displayed on the duplex monitor. 6, The location of the receiver is represented by a flashing bright arrow superimposed on the ultrasound B-mode image. (Reprinted with permission from Cluley SR, Brener BJ, Hollier LH, et al: Ultrasound-guided balloon angioplasty is a new technique for vascular surgeons. Am J Surg 1991;162:18.)

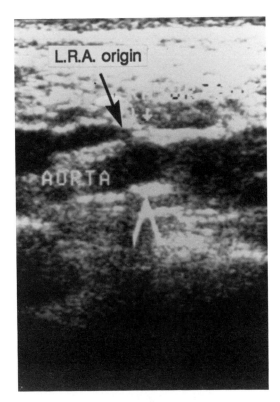

FIGURE 35–2. Longitudinal duplex ultrasound view. The arrow, created by the Echo-Mark system, points to the receiver attached to the midballoon region of the catheter.

Research) and the Guide for the Care and Use of Laboratory Animals (NIH publication #80-23, revised 1985).

The Echo-Mark catheter was introduced via a sheath in the carotid artery and advanced into the abdominal aorta. Using duplex ultrasonography alone, the catheter was positioned using various vessels (e.g., renal artery, inferior mesenteric artery, iliac trifurcation) as points of reference. Arteriograms were then performed with the Echo-Mark catheter in place at each ultrasound-guided position to document the accuracy of placement. These early studies confirmed the feasibility of using ultrasound guidance alone as a technique for accurate placement of balloon catheters.

Fistulas between the femoral artery and femoral vein were then created in nine dogs using 4-mm polytetrafluoroethylene (PTFE) grafts. This reliably produced the formation of stenotic lesions near the anastomotic sites within 6 to 10 weeks. These fistulas were able to be monitored by duplex ultrasonography, and when a stenosis was detected, the animals were appropriately anesthetized and cannulated. The Echo-Mark catheter was then introduced and the catheter was advanced to the appropriate stenotic area and the lesions were dilated. Angiography was then performed, and confirmed the accuracy and the success of the angioplasty. In two additional animals, a balloon-expandable intravascular Medtronic-Wiktor stent was placed at the site of the lesion using the Echo-Mark catheter for stent delivery and angioplasty. Duplex flow velocity data on these animal studies are presented in Table 35–1. Measurable reductions in flow velocity were seen at the stenotic sites postdilatation in 9 of the 11 cases; success indicated by these duplex studies were confirmed by angiography. The two dilatations deemed unsuccessful by duplex scan proved not successful on arteriogram.

TABLE 35–1. DUPLEX FLOW VELOCITY DATA

		Flow Velocity (m/sec[a])	
Treatment	**Site of Stenosis**	*Predilatation*	*Postdilatation*
Angioplasty	Venous	5.00	1.59
Angioplasty	Venous	5.30	.84
Angioplasty	Venous	4.49	4.45
Angioplasty	Arterial	1.59	1.59
Angioplasty	Arterial	5.13	1.89
Angioplasty	Arterial	4.21	1.95
Angioplasty	Arterial	5.94	4.00
Angioplasty	Arterial	2.99	1.33
Angioplasty	Arterial	1.74	.64
Angioplasty + stent	Arterial	1.04	.36
Angioplasty + stent	Arterial	1.54	.84

[a] m/sec, meters per second.

Following these initial animal studies, carefully controlled human studies were initiated. Thus far, we have utilized this technique for the treatment of short-segment lesions in five patients, achieving both anatomic and hemodynamic success in each case. One such case is illustrated by Figure 35–3. Clinical trials continue.

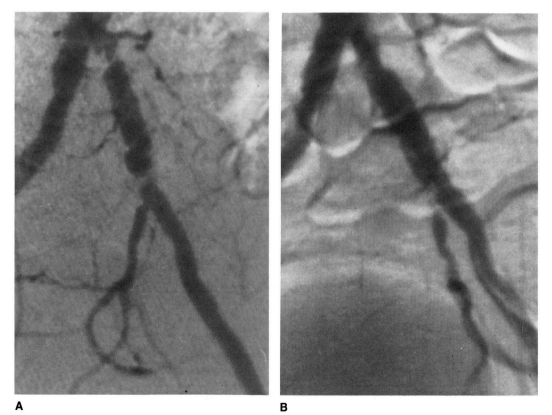

A   **B**

FIGURE 35–3. *A,* Preoperative angiographic confirmation of ultrasound detected and localized arterial stenosis. *B,* Angiographic confirmation of arterial stenosis after ultrasound-guided balloon angioplasty of arterial stenotic lesion.

DISCUSSION

The Echo-Mark catheter can be positioned accurately without angiography and used to perform angioplasty and deploy stents. In our initial studies, duplex ultrasonography and arteriography appear equally effective for catheter positioning and performance of balloon angioplasty. Duplex imaging is an accurate predictor of outcome compared to arteriography,[14–16] and duplex imaging allows visualization in both transverse and longitudinal planes. Balloon expansion and vessel wall separation can be visualized at the time of dilatation, and dynamic data pertaining to anatomy and flow physiology provide immediate information predictive of outcome.

One of the main reasons that vascular surgeons have not become more involved in percutaneous angioplasty, even though it is evident that endovascular techniques will undoubtedly become increasingly utilized, is the lack of ready availability to the vascular surgeon of catheterization laboratories and good biplanar angiographic equipment. Although angiographic facilities are available in some operating rooms, at least with the use of portable equipment, these facilities are not conducive to the development of an endovascular practice. The operating room is a more expensive milieu in which to work and the lack of biplanar fluoroscopy, freeze-frame capabilities, and review-loop video place the surgeon at a disadvantage when attempting to perform angioplasty. Additionally, the political climate in most hospitals, as well as financial considerations, have generally prevented the vascular surgeon from having access to the cardiology or radiologic catheterization suites and have left hospital administrators unwilling to develop additional catheterization laboratories for the vascular surgeon. Although the vascular surgeon, because of his familiarity with direct exposure of blood vessels and his in-depth knowledge of vascular disease, would be able to readily master endovascular techniques, he simply has not generally had the facilities in which to develop these skills.

The domain of the vascular surgeon has generally been the vascular laboratory and the operating room. As previously mentioned, endovascular procedures can be done in the operating room, but are done with more difficulty and with more expense. Most vascular laboratories have ultrasound equipment, but no angiographic facilities. However, if endovascular procedures could be safely and reliably performed with high-resolution ultrasonography and without the need for fluoroscopy, surgeons might be more able to be actively involved in the performance of endovascular procedures. The limitation to this development appears to have been the development of high-resolution ultrasonography and the development of an angioplasty catheter that is readily visualized on ultrasound.

Today, color flow duplex ultrasonography is readily able to identify vessels and accurately localize stenoses within peripheral arteries.[15] Additionally, duplex ultrasonography is a dynamic modality that provides both anatomic and physiologic real-time data. This, therefore, potentially allows not only the identification of the lesion, but an immediate analysis of whether or not interventional techniques (e.g., balloon angioplasty) can effect hemodynamic improvement.[16]

Several workers have reported the therapeutic potential of intravascular ultrasound-guided technique.[17–20] The implementation of ultrasound-guided angioplasty by the peripheral vascular surgeon in his clinical practice appears readily achievable. After initial history and physical examination, a patient might be suspected of having superficial femoral artery occlusive disease. This patient might then be referred for routine angiography for visualization of the lesion or may simply be directed to the vascular laboratory for duplex ultrasonography and identification of the lesion. If a short-segment stenosis were identified in the superficial femoral artery, the patient could then have percutaneous angioplasty performed in an expanded vascular laboratory with direct, continuous ultrasound duplex guidance and monitoring. This technique would not only eliminate the risk associated with radiographic imaging, but would also enable the collection of physiologic data on the success of the angioplasty procedure.

SUMMARY

A new balloon angioplasty catheter has been demonstrated that can be positioned and manipulated accurately and precisely using duplex ultrasonography alone. This system was tested successfully in dogs and in humans. It eliminates the risks associated with radiographic imaging, and allows for monitoring of procedures in real time. Dynamic data pertaining to anatomy and physiology is obtained using a format familiar to the vascular surgeon. Clinical trials are currently in progress. Future applications depend on further advances in the fields of duplex ultrasonography and interventional catheter technology. Catheters and guide wires of all types and sizes can be modified to permit ultrasound guidance. This might allow for therapeutic applications in other areas such as introduction of caval filters, central venous pressure monitors, thrombectomy, and placement of abdominal drainage catheters. The full scope of this technology is clearly increasing.

REFERENCES

1. Johnston KW, Rae M, Hogg-Johnston SA, et al: Five-year results of a prospective study of percutaneous transluminal angioplasty. Ann Surg 1987;206:403.
2. Rutherford RB, Patt A, Kumpe DA: The current role of percutaneous transluminal angioplasty. In Greenlagh KM, ed: Vascular Surgery: Issues in Current Practice. New York, Grune and Stratton, 1986;229–244.
3. Schneider E, Gruntzig A, Bollinger A: Long-term patency rates after percutaneous transluminal angioplasty for iliac and femoropopliteal obstructions. In Dotter CT, Gruntzig AR, Schoop W, et al., eds: Percutaneous Transluminal Angioplasty. Technique, Early and Late Results. Berlin, Springer-Verlag, 1983;175–180.
4. Krepel VM, van Andel GJ, van Erp WFM, et al: Percutaneous transluminal angioplasty of the femoropopliteal artery: Initial and long-term results. Radiology 1985;156:325.
5. Murray RR, Hewes RC, White RI, et al: Long-segment femoropopliteal stenoses: Is angioplasty a boon or a bust? Radiology 1987;162:473.
6. McCarthy WJ, Vogelzang RL, Nemcek AA Jr, et al: Excimer laser-assisted femoral angioplasty: Early results. J Vasc Surg 1991;13:607–614.
7. Perler BA, Osterman FA, White R, et al: Percutaneous laser probe femoropopliteal angioplasty: A preliminary experience. J Vasc Surg 1989;10:351–357.
8. Simpson JB, Selman MR, Robertson CC, et al: Transluminal atherectomy for occlusive peripheral vascular disease. Am J Cardiol 1988;61:96–101.
9. Brener BJ, Parsonnet V, Eisenbud DE, et al: The Medtronic-Wiktor stent: A new balloon-expandable, flexible, tantalum stent. In Greenhalgh R, Hollier LH, eds: The Maintenance of Arterial Reconstruction. London, WB Saunders Co., 1991.
10. Hollier LH: Presidential address: Influence of nonsurgical intervention on vascular surgical practice. J Vasc Surg 1989;9(5):627.
11. Crowley RJ, von Behren PL, Couvillon LA Jr, et al: Optimized ultrasound imaging catheters for use in the vascular system. Int J Card Imaging 1989;4:145–151.
12. Garg AK, Houston AB, Laing JM, et al: Positioning of umbilical arterial catheters with ultrasound. Arch Dis Child 1983;58:1018.

13. Cluley SR, Brener BJ, Hollier LH, et al: Ultrasound-guided balloon angioplasty is a new technique for vascular surgeons. Am J Surg 1991;*162*:117–121.

14. Kohler TR, Nance DR, Cramer MM, Vanderburghe N, Strandness DE Jr: Duplex scanning for diagnosis or aortoiliac and femoropopliteal disease: A prospective study. Circulation 1987;*76*:1074–1080.

15. Cossman DV, Ellison JE, Wagner WH, et al: Comparison of contrast arteriography to arterial mapping with color-flow duplex imaging in the lower extremities. J Vasc Surg 1989;*10*:522–529.

16. Edwards JM, Coldwell DM, Goldman ML, Strandness DE Jr: The role of duplex scanning in the selection of patients for transluminal angioplasty. J Vasc Surg 1991;*13*:69–74.

17. Van Wormer ME: Ultrasonographically guided angioplasty in a flow phantom. J Vasc Tech 1991;*15*(1):33–36.

18. Langberg JJ, Franklin JO, Landzberg JS, et al: The echotransponder electrode catheter: A new method for mapping the left ventricle. J Am Coll Cardiol 1988;*12*:218–223.

19. Cikes I, Breyer B, Ernst A, Costovic F: Interventional echocardiography. *In* Holm HH, Kristensen JK, eds: Interventional Ultrasound. Copenhagen, Munksgaard, 1985;164–168.

20. Cikes I, Breyer B, Ernst A: Cardiac Catheterization guided by ultrasound (abstr). J Am Coll Cardiol 1984;*3*:564.

VI
THROMBOLYTIC THERAPY

36

ADVANCES IN PERIPHERAL VASCULAR THROMBOLYSIS: Recombinant Technology and Methodologies to Enhance Lysis

ARTHUR A. SASAHARA, JACK HENKIN, WALTER M. BARKER,
JAMES P. LEWKOWSKI, SANDRA E. BURKE, JOHN C. SOBOLSKI,
CECILIA C. St.MARTIN, and GREGORY A. SCHULZ

The existence of substances capable of fibrinolytic activity has been known for many years. Indeed, the autolysis of clotted blood must have been observed for centuries. In a review of the mechanisms of fibrinolysis, MacFarlane and Biggs[1] stated that over 100 years earlier, Denis and Zimmerman had observed the dissolution of fibrin in human blood after standing for 12 to 24 hours. In 1933, Tillett and Garner[2] demonstrated that some strains of beta-hemolytic streptococci produced a substance that rapidly dissolved the fibrin in human plasma clots. This material was later found to be incapable of dissolving purified fibrin without the presence of a "lytic factor" associated with the euglobulin component of human serum[3] and was subsequently shown to be an activator for a proenzyme (plasminogen) normally found in blood.[4,5] The material produced by the beta-hemolytic streptococci [streptokinase (SK)] was later shown to be a single-chain polypeptide with a molecular mass of 47,000 daltons.

Tillett and Sherry[6] ushered in the therapeutic use of fibrinolytic agents in 1946 when they injected concentrated, partially purified broth cultures of hemolytic streptococci into the pleural cavities of patients suffering from pleural exudations. Subsequent clinical trials which explored the use of streptokinase in pulmonary embolism, peripheral vascular thrombosis, thrombotically occluded arteriovenous cannulae, and acute myocardial infarction led to the approval of the agent for treating these indications.

Streptokinase, however, possesses several negative clinical properties. Being a foreign protein, it is antigenic, and severe allergic reactions have been reported in about 0.1 per cent of the patients treated. Moreover, patients who have had recent streptococcal infections have high antibody titers to streptokinase, which can inactivate substantial amounts of the drug, thus decreasing its efficacy. The efficacy of streptokinase is further jeopardized by its plasminogen depleting property; streptokinase combines stoichiometrically with plasminogen to form an active complex. The decrease in circulating plasminogen can become evident as a decreased efficacy in some patients, particularly during long infusions. Despite these shortcomings, streptokinase is relatively inexpensive and remains the most commonly used thrombolytic agent.

MacFarlane and Pilling[7] described the fibrinolytic activity of normal urine, and in 1952, Astrup and Sterndorff[8] demonstrated that this activity was due to a plasminogen activator present in the urine. Sobel et al.[9] designated the new plasminogen activator "urokinase" (UK). This material was a naturally occurring enzyme of human origin, and as a result had a major therapeutic advantage over the streptococcal-derived material, SK. It did not induce the production of antibodies, and therefore could be administered repeatedly without loss of activity owing to antigen-antibody reactions or concern about allergic reactions.

Although a number of investigators conducted small clinical studies to evaluate the use of the two thrombolytic agents (UK and SK) in various disease states, the first large, controlled trial was the Urokinase-Pulmonary Embolism Trial (UPET)[10] organized and supervised by the National Heart and Lung Institute (NHLI). This trial, which compared the use of UK and heparin in the treatment of pulmonary embolism, was followed by another NHLI trial, the Urokinase-Streptokinase Pulmonary Embolism Trial (USPET),[11] which compared UK and SK. As a result of these trials, both UK and SK were approved by the FDA for use in pulmonary embolism in 1978.

Urokinase was subsequently approved for intracoronary administration in acute myocardial infarction and for clearing thrombosed venous catheters. In addition to these approved claims, a number of investigators have used UK for the treatment of peripheral arterial occlusive disease, deep vein thrombosis, and as intravenous therapy for acute myocardial infarction.

SECOND GENERATION AGENTS

Anisoylated Plasminogen Streptokinase Activator Complex

All of the naturally occurring thrombolytic agents are rapidly cleared by the liver; the half-life of streptokinase is about 23 minutes, urokinase about 13 minutes or less, and tissue-type plasminogen activator (tPA), about 5 minutes. Because of these short half-lives, the agents must be infused over extended periods of time. During the 1980s cardiologists perceived a need for a thrombolytic agent which could be administered as a single bolus to acute myocardial infarction patients.

Anisoylated plasminogen streptokinase activator complex (APSAC) was developed in an attempt to acquire such a single-dose agent. By acylating the active site on the plasminogen portion of the streptokinase-plasminogen complex, the molecule was rendered inactive. Gradual removal of the anisoyl blocker by in vivo hydrolysis provided a gradual release of the active complex. The half-life of APSAC was found to be about 90 minutes, and fibrinolytic activity was apparent for 4 to 6 hours after administration.[12] In clinical trials, APSAC achieved reperfusion rates similar to streptokinase. As could be predicted by its mode of action, APSAC offered some protection against reocclusion;

the reocclusion rate for APSAC-treated patients was about 10 per cent compared to about 15 per cent for streptokinase-treated patients.[13] Unfortunately, except for the occurrence of hypotension during rapid administration, the adverse event profile for APSAC is essentially identical to that of streptokinase. Anisoylated plasminogen streptokinase activator complex was approved for use in acute myocardial infarction in 1989.

Tissue-Type Plasminogen Activator

Streptokinase-plasminogen complex and urokinase act directly on plasminogen and produce significant systemic lytic states by activating circulating plasminogen as well as clot-bound plasminogen. In contrast, tissue-type plasminogen activator (tPA) per se is very inefficient in activating plasminogen. However, tPA readily binds to fibrin and undergoes a conformational change which increases its catalytic efficacy about 1500-fold. Thus tPA is a clot-selective plasminogen activator which produces minimal systemic effects at low concentrations. At high concentrations, tPA produces a systemic lytic state approaching that induced by streptokinase and urokinase. Tissue-type plasminogen activator, like urokinase, is a natural occurring protease with a molecular mass of about 65,000 daltons. Following initial studies, which indicated a potential use for tPA as a thrombolytic agent, an intensive effort to express the protein by recombinant DNA techniques ensued.[14] The current product marketed in the United States is expressed from Chinese hamster ovary cells using complementary DNA from a human melanoma cell line. Tissue-type plasminogen activator was approved for use in acute myocardial infarction in 1987 and for pulmonary embolism in 1990.

Prourokinase

Another activator of the fibrinolytic system which is normally found in human plasma is a precursor of UK, prourokinase (proUK). The first suggestion that urokinase might be secreted in an inactive form was made by Bernik et al.[15] The latent material described by these workers was found in cultures of kidney, lung, spleen, and thyroid, and appeared to be activated by plasmin. Subsequent work completed by Nolan et al.[16] reported that UK derived from human neonatal kidney cell cultures also occurred as a proenzyme form in the culture media. Later, in 1976, Bernik[17] partially purified such a precursor from neonatal and adult lung cultures, referring to it as "preurokinase."

In 1983, Husain, Gurewich, et al.[18] purified and described a 56-kd precursor of UK from urine, naming it prourokinase. Several groups have also isolated a homogeneous single-chain form of UK from urine,[19] plasma,[20] or conditioned cell culture media.[21] Prourokinase, also called single-chain urokinase-type plasminogen activator (scu-PA), is a glycoprotein containing 411 amino acids. Hydrolysis of the lysine-158–isoleucine-159 peptide bond by plasmin or kallikrein converts the molecule to UK, a two-chain molecule with one interconnecting disulfide bridge.

Like tPA, this activator catalyzes the conversion of the proenzyme plasminogen to plasmin, which hydrolyzes fibrin into soluble breakdown products. Both proUK and tPA have fibrin-dependent modes of action, showing higher activity against fibrin-bound plasminogen and less systemic generation of plasmin than UK or SK. However, the mechanisms responsible for fibrin-specific fibrinolysis by proUK and tPA are distinctive.

MECHANISMS OF FIBRINOLYSIS

The fibrinolytic agents commonly used or under development all function by catalyzing the hydrolysis of a single peptide bond in the 93-kd inert proenzyme, plasminogen (Pg). Specific cleavage creates the two-chain plasmin (Pm), which is an active trypsin-like protease that attacks a variety of proteins at various arginine and lysine sites. Its primary targets in the circulation are fibrinogen and fibrin. The plasminogen activators (PAs) have unique properties as discussed below, but all have some clot specificity and will degrade polymeric fibrin more rapidly than fibrinogen.

There are two reasons for this specificity, the first having to do with the structural deformability[22] of Pg (Fig. 36–1). More than 99 per cent of circulating Pg begins with glutamic (Glu) as the first amino acid (Glu-Pg) and has a very compact structure in which the five "kringle" subdomains of the N-terminal region protect the activation site from the action of PAs. When Glu-Pg binds to fibrin, the latter acts as a rack and spreads out the Pg into an open structure where access of PAs to their target site is unimpeded. Thus, clot-bound Pg is a much better substrate than free Pg for all PAs. This mechanism focuses activity on the clot rather than in the circulation.

The second reason for clot specificity derives from the quenching of Pm by a fast-acting inhibitor in plasma, α_2-antiplasmin. This protein inactivates circulating Pm within a fraction of a second, but inactivates fibrin-bound Pm slowly, requiring several seconds or sometimes minutes as fibrin occupies a critical Pm interaction site. Thus, under normal physiological conditions, plasmin in plasma is neutralized, again focusing activity on the clot. Typically there are about half as many antiplasmin molecules as Pg molecules in blood. If lysis continues to a point where antiplasmin is significantly depleted, clot specificity can rapidly disappear. This occurs not only because of the loss of differential buffering, but also because of the increased flux of unquenched Pm. Accumulating Pm can cleave Glu-Pg to yield Lys-Pg. The latter has an intrinsically open structure and binds more readily to fibrin than does Glu-Pg. A small amount of Lys-Pg can therefore actually enhance clot specificity and PA efficacy.[23] However, increased amounts of circulating, unbound Lys-Pg can further degrade clot specificity.[24] With these common features of all PAs as background, the distinctive properties and mechanisms of the individual PAs, can be understood.

Streptokinase

Streptokinase is the only PA which is not an enzyme or proenzyme. It is a bacterial protein of about 46 kd that binds tightly to Pg. The SK-Pg complex which is formed will efficiently activate additional Pg molecules (Fig. 36–2). Thus SK is an indirect Pg activator. As SK is probably the least fibrin-specific PA, continuous treatment depletes circulating Pg so that the major lytic activity eventually becomes that of free Pm (mainly Lys-Pm). This free Pm functions less efficiently than Pm generated in situ on the clot surface, and administration of additional SK then yields little increase in clot lysis. Being a foreign bacterial

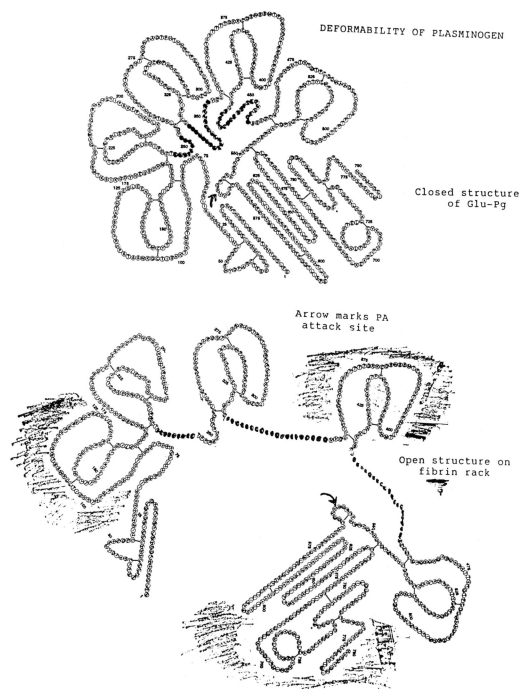

FIGURE 36–1. The top structure shows the compact, closed structure of Glu-plasminogen, which "protects" the activation site (see arrow) from the action of plasminogen activators, making Glu-plasminogen a poor substrate. The bottom panel depicts the "open" conformational change of Glu-plasminogen into the open Lys-plasminogen configuration. The interaction between lysine residues of fibrin (shaded areas) and kringles 1 and 4 of Glu-plasminogen maintain the open conformation, exposing the activation site to plasminogen activators. Thus, plasminogen activation is focused on fibrin-bound Glu-plasminogen. Removal of the first 76 amino acids, forming Lys-plasminogen, also allows similar opening of the structure, exposing the activation site. Thus, Lys-plasminogen is a much better substrate for plasminogen activators.

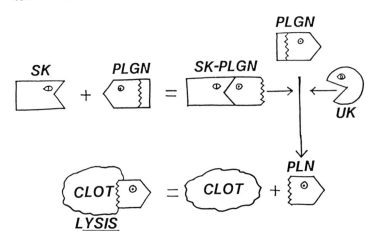

FIGURE 36-2. Graphic depiction of the formation of the streptokinase-plasminogen (SK-PLGN) complex that is necessary before other plasminogen molecules can be converted to plasmin. Streptokinase, therefore, is an indirect plasminogen activator. Urokinase (UK), in contrast, is a direct activator, activating plasminogen to plasmin (PLN) on a stoichiometric basis.

protein, SK can elicit an antibody response. Circulating anti-SK antibody can neutralize SK activity in presensitized individuals.

Anisoylated Plasminogen Streptokinase Activator Complex

Because of the rapid surge in plasmin activity following SK administration, it is not usually feasible to give SK as a bolus injection or rapid infusion. A high flux of Pm can activate kallikreins, releasing bradykinin and causing hypotension.[25] Maximum clot lysis can be achieved by gradual intravenous (IV) infusion, maintaining the SK activity at a level not greatly exceeding the rate at which circulating Pg binds to newly exposed sites on the dissolving clot.

In order to remove the need for continuous infusion, a time-release prodrug form of the SK-Pg complex has been developed, in which the pseudoactive site is blocked, forming APSAC. Upon contact with plasma, the blocking group in the inert prodrug begins to be removed by hydrolysis, with a half-life of about 90 minutes, and the lytic potency clears with a half-life of about 105 minutes. The activation of the prodrug mimics and replaces the need for infusion so that rapid injection is possible. On the other hand, once injected, it is not possible to subsequently cut off evolution of the active form as would be the case with an IV line. Anisoylated plasminogen streptokinase activator complex may be useful for systemic lytic therapy but probably has no usefulness in locally administered thrombolysis because very little of it is likely to become activated while still concentrated in the clot vicinity.

Urokinase

Urokinase is an enzyme of approximately 54 kd which can also break down enzymatically to a lower molecular weight form of about 32 kd. Both forms can be obtained from human urine or from kidney cell culture; commercial UK in Europe and Asia is urine-derived and is generally a mixture, mainly containing the higher molecular weight (HMW) form. That available in the United States, Abbokinase, is low molecular weight (LMW) and is obtained from cell culture. Urokinase is a two-chain trypsin-family enzyme with high specificity for cleaving only the activation site on plasminogen, yielding plasmin. Of the two chains, all of the catalytic activity of UK resides in the B-chain. In LMW UK, the A-chain is very small (1 to 2 kd), whereas in HMW UK, the A-chain is about 20 kd and has two structural domains, a growth factor domain (GFD) and a kringle domain (Fig. 36–3). The GFD is known to bind with high affinity to specific endothelial cell receptors[26] for UK, and similar receptors have also been found on other circulating cells along with receptors for plasminogen.[27] These receptors may serve as a "reservoir" for UK to concentrate and focus plasmin formation on the cell surface. Their role in clot dissolution is still poorly understood. The kringle of HMW UK can tightly bind heparin, but its physiological role has not been elucidated.

While there appear to be subtle differences between HMW and LMW UKs, these differences have not thus far led to noticeable differences in clot lysis efficacy or fibrin specificity in animal models of thrombolysis or in human clinical trials. Both types of UK are normally given by IV infusion or a combination of bolus plus infusion for reasons similar to those described for SK. Small amounts of UK, of the order of 25 U/ml of plasma are rapidly quenched by circulating inhibitors including plasminogen activator inhibitor-1 (PAI-1) and PAI-3, so that the UK-stimulated lysis shows a small threshold effect equal to about 1 to 2 mg of the enzyme in a patient dosed systemically.

Prourokinase

Prourokinase is the single-chain precursor of urokinase. It is also called single-chain urokinase-type plasminogen activator (Scu-PA). However, the latter name implies enzyme activity and it is now generally agreed that free proUK has little if any activity until cleaved by plasmin into an active two-chain

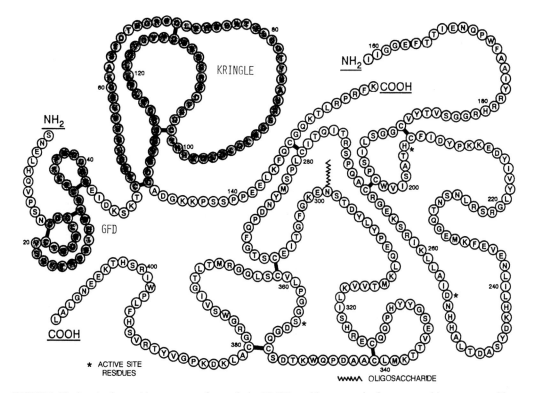

FIGURE 36–3. Amino acid sequence of two-chain HMW urokinase, made from recombinant prourokinase. Note the single kringle and the growth-factor domain.

UK form. The possibility, however, remains that an appropriate ligand or surface contact might evoke UK activity in single-chain proUK, much as SK does to Pg. Both natural and recombinant HMW proUKs have been produced and have undergone some clinical testing.

A mixture of pure Pg and ProUK in buffer solution will produce both UK and Pm at a continuously increasing rate, because of an expanding cycle of mutual activation initiated by the trace amounts of UK in proUK and of Pm in Pg. However, this reaction is short-circuited by quenching inhibitors present in plasma, so that proUK added to plasma is essentially inert. Yet, if a clot is added to plasma containing proUK, after a lag period active fibrin lysis will ensue accompanied by a modest amount of fibrinogenolysis that increases as more UK is formed.

Compared with UK, proUK is quite clot specific; the mechanism by which the clot triggers proUK activation while maintaining specificity remains controversial.[28] An important observation is that very small amounts of tPA, UK, or Pm appear to greatly enhance proUK activity.[29] Also, pretreatment of a clot with any of these agents charges or "primes" the clot so that the lag period is shortened or eliminated. A simple possible explanation may be that some active Pm can persist within the thrombus, protected from fast-acting inhibitors for some time. Collision of proUK with this "protected" Pm leads to formation of UK (Fig. 36–4). This local activation may transiently focus UK activity on the clot. It has also been proposed[30] that minimal lysis generates a new family of Pg binding sites on the clot, and that this special bound Pg is actually a substrate for ProUK. Then the locally formed plasmin activates the same proUK.

Whatever the actual mechanism, proUK is a prodrug form of UK, and only a small portion of the administered dose is converted into UK during its brief circulation lifetime ($t_{1/2}$ 5 to 6 minutes) until such time as significant depletion of antiplasmin occurs. Prourokinase has been shown to be effective, as well as sparing of fibrinogen, even when given by bolus injection in animal models.[31] As a prodrug it is also protected from quenching by circulating PA inhibitors such as PAI-1 or PAI-3. It will also occupy the same uPA receptors as does HMW UK.

Tissue-Type Plasminogen Activator

This enzyme is named for the fact that it is made by the vascular endothelium of many tissues. Two-chain tPA is a Pg-specific protease much like UK, although its maximum catalytic turnover rate is several-fold lower than that of UK. Unlike the great majority of enzymes in this class, however, tPA is nearly as active as a single-chain precursor as in its Pm-cleaved two-chain

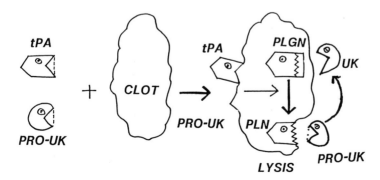

FIGURE 36–4. Graphic depiction of a collision between proUK and a "protected" plasmin within the clot (PLN), converting single-chain proUK to two-chain UK. Tissue-type plasminogen activator, in contrast, binds tightly to fibrin, adjacent to a fibrin-bound plasminogen (PLGN), converting it to plasmin.

form. Tissue-type plasminogen activator is even more clot-specific than proUK, at least during the early stages of clot lysis. The ultimate source of this specificity is the tight binding to fibrin, immediately adjacent to its substrate, fibrin-bound plasminogen (Fig. 36–4). Fibrin binding stimulates the catalytic rate of tPA, further enhancing its specificity.

Because of tenacious clot binding which protects tPA from inactivation by the circulating inhibitor PAI-1, even a small amount of tPA is able to initiate clot lysis immediately with little or no threshold or lag effects. However, because of the limited number of functional tPA sites on the clot surface, and tPA's low catalytic rate, the full theoretical specificity of tPA is not realized in actual clinical practice. Thus a large amount must be infused gradually over several hours to complete lysis, and activity spills over into the circulation, giving some fibrinogenolysis. As fibrin degradation products are released from the dissolving thrombus, they increasingly stimulate tPA activity in the systemic circulation, leading to lowered specificity over time. Nonetheless, in the relatively large doses, infused tPA is an effective thrombolytic agent.

METHODOLOGIES TO ENHANCE THROMBOLYSIS

The Procoagulant State Favoring Reocclusion

Therapeutic lysis of thrombi is opposed by simultaneous prothrombotic processes, and conditions that favored the initial formation of an occlusive clot. These conditions tend to remain after thrombolysis, in the absence of further intervention. A thrombolytic strategy designed to maximize the rate and extent of clot dissolution, and to maintain blood flow until stabilization can be accomplished, would attempt to shift the balance away from coagulation both during and after lytic therapy.

Coagulation is initiated whenever the unmodulated enzyme, thrombin (factor IIa), is generated from its inert precursor, prothrombin, by the action of the protease, factor Xa, in complex with factor Va, Ca^{+2}, and membrane surfaces. Thrombin-catalyzed cleavages remove a peptide (FpA, FpB) from each of the N-termini of the Aα and Bβ chains of fibrinogen, forming fibrin with exposed sites for extended noncovalent polymerization. Thrombin also activates platelets via binding to a specific receptor. The accumulation of Xa and thus of thrombin is the culmination of a number of steps (coagulation cascade) from two convergent possible pathways, both involving the sequential activation of Arg/Lys-specific proteases from their inert proenzyme forms.

Thus, thrombin is the principal procoagulant that needs to be neutralized in order to shift the balance away from the prothrombotic state.

Natural Anticoagulation

The main natural inhibitor of thrombin is antithrombin III (AT III), the activity of which is greatly enhanced by heparin. It is likely that proteoglycans bound to the endothelial surface have heparin-like behavior and thus stimulate normal anticoagulation. Another protein, heparin cofactor II (HC II) behaves similarly to AT III. Dermatan sulfate in extracellular matrix is its likely physiologic activator.[32] Another system for the control of thrombin in the vasculature is the system of thrombomodulin—protein C and protein S. Thrombomodulin (TM) is a thrombin binding protein on the surface of intact endothelium. When bound to TM, thrombin is much less active against fibrinogen or factor V but much more active at cleaving and activating protein C.[33] The latter, a vitamin K-dependent protein, is anchored to endothelial membranes through interaction with S, a membrane-bound protein. Activated protein C (Ca) cleaves and inactivates factors Va and VIIIa. Thus, in complex with TM, thrombin can actually display anticoagulant behavior, breaking the cycle of its own formation.

Lysis-Associated Procoagulant Activity

The need to inhibit thrombin during and after thrombolysis is underscored by observations that fibrinolytic treatment itself causes an apparent increase in thrombin activity, which is then associated with slower clot lysis and frequent reocclusion. Administration of streptokinase or tPA to patients[34,35] has been associated with a surge in the level of fibrinopeptide A (FpA), a clear marker of thrombin activity. Complexes of thrombin with AT III (T-AT III) increase significantly shortly after the onset of therapy with either tPA or combinations of UK/proUK, and persistent high levels of this complex correlated strongly with greater risk of reocclusion after 24 hours.[36] The mechanism of this fibrinolytic induction of thrombin activity is not clear. However, it has been[37] noted that Pm can initially activate factor V, thus displaying procoagulant activity, which is followed by a slower Pm-dependent inactivation of factor Va. Alternatively, lysis may expose active thrombin within a clot that is refractory to AT III and thus especially active. The importance of this observation is illustrated by the enhancement of clinical thrombolysis with SK when patients were pretreated with heparin.[38] If the extent of clot lysis during the period of therapy can be greatly increased by concomitant anticoagulation, less residual clot will be present after therapy.[13] Studies indicate that residual clot is a much greater stimulus for clot formation than is damaged arterial wall.[39] Thus, complete or nearly complete clot dissolution in excess of that just required to establish restoration of blood flow is probably a desirable goal, from the view of preventing reocclusion.[40]

Other factors predisposing toward reocclusion may also be mitigated by achieving a more systemic lytic state. This is supported by studies in the canine model in which rethrombosis 24 hours after clot lysis by tPA was reduced by subsequent UK treatment,[41] and also by the lower reocclusion rates observed in clinical trials where combinations of clot-specific and less-specific agents (e.g., tPA plus UK) have been used.[42] Interestingly, there may be a prolonged prothrombotic effect even when a relatively nonspecific thrombolytic agent is used. It has been reported that patients who have received SK therapy required 5 days of heparin at 37,750 U/day to achieve a specified level of anticoagulation [activated partial thromboplastin time (APTT)] compared with non–thrombolytic treated patients who required only 3 days at 30,294 U/day (mean values).[43] It is not known if this response is unique to SK.

Adjunctive Therapy with Heparin and Heparinoids

Heparin is a complex and heterogeneous mixture of highly sulfated polysaccharide glycosaminoglycans of diverse molecular weights ranging from about 3000 to about 30,000 g/mol. Low molecular weight heparins have been isolated by gel filtration of heparin, or alternatively, generated by chemical or enzymatic degradation of heparin.[44] These LMW heparins or heparinoids tend to have relatively more anti-Xa activity relative to anti-II activity when compared with unfractionated heparin. Thomas and Merton[45] have pointed out that LMW heparins, with their higher anti-Xa activity, still prolonged the APTT or thrombin time. They found unfractionated heparin superior to LMW heparin for therapeutic anticoagulation. These LMW forms are probably most advantageous for subcutaneous administration in the prevention of deep vein thrombosis in patients undergoing major surgery.

Heparin is now a major adjunctive therapy to thrombolytic agents in patients with acute myocardial infarction (MI). However, the exact role as well as dosing, timing of dosage, and the use of LMW forms remain subjects of both pharmacologic and clinical experimentation. In experiments in which canine femoral artery clots were lysed with tPA, Cercek et al.[46] found a greater than threefold increase in the loss of clot weight when animals were pretreated with 200 U/kg of heparin. Fears[47] reported that in a rabbit jugular vein model of thrombolysis using tPA, heparin was ineffective in increasing the extent of lysis at high or low doses of tPA, although it could successfully inhibit regrowth of thrombus subsequent to reperfusion. The controversy as to whether heparin should be given before or after lytic therapy, particularly in peripheral vascular disease, underscores the unsatisfactory nature of animal or other models in simulating clinical conditions, and will only be settled by controlled human trials.

In a rabbit jugular vein thrombosis model[48] LMW heparin fractions were compared with ordinary unfractionated heparin in their ability to augment lysis by tPA or proUK. A particular fraction (CY222) was reported to potentiate lysis by either agent to a greater extent than did ordinary heparin, although the results were not dramatic. Clinical combinations of LMW heparins with thrombolytic agents have not yet been reported, and it will be interesting to see if the advantage suggested above is maintained.

While it remains uncertain to what extent heparin can augment clot lysis in combination with a given lytic agent, heparin clearly has a role in preventing reocclusion as shown in recent canine model studies,[41] and its administration is currently recommended during and after lytic therapy.[49] In clinical trials, there was no difference in the coronary artery patency rate of patients receiving heparin immediately upon initiation of tPA therapy compared to ones in whom heparin was delayed by 90 minutes.[50] Heparin was distinctly superior to aspirin (82 per cent versus 52 per cent) in maintaining patency in the first 24 hours after tPA treatment.[51] Prourokinase may represent a special positive case where heparin actually augments thrombolysis. Gulba et al.[52] found only one of nine unheparinized MI patients to have a patent coronary artery 90 minutes after proUK treatment, while seven of nine others who received concomitant heparin were patent. It was speculated that this may relate to the fact that thrombin can inactivate proUK; however, the mechanism of this apparent heparin stimulation is unknown.

Direct Thrombin Inhibition

The usefulness of heparin to enhance lysis is undoubtedly limited because of the refractory nature of thrombin within a clot to AT III-dependent inhibitors. This was convincingly demonstrated by Weitz et al.[53] who utilized FpA levels as an index of thrombin activity in comparing heparin to direct thrombin inhibitors. Direct agents including, hirudin, hirugen, and PPACK were equally effective against both fluid-phase and clot-bound thrombin, while heparin was about 20-fold less potent at inhibiting the clot-bound form. Thrombin associated with fibrin must therefore be relatively inaccessible to heparin or AT III or both. This being the case, it seems reasonable to postulate that the rebuilding of clots undergoing therapeutic lysis could be better prevented by direct agents and that these may be superior to heparin in augmenting thrombolysis. Such compounds may also be useful posttreatment to prevent rethrombosis, since they can inhibit both free and clot-bound thrombin. Compounds in this family include hirudin and its analogs and reversible inhibitors such as Argatroban.

Hirudin and Analogs

Hirudin is an acidic protein the molecular weight of which is approximately 8000 daltons (66 amino acids) secreted by medicinal leeches. It contains three disulfide bonds and is able to form a very tight essentially 1:1 inactive complex with thrombin.[54] Hirudin (and some analogs) is the most potent and specific inhibitor of thrombin discovered thus far and has no known natural antagonist. Hirudin produced by recombinant technology[55] is virtually identical with the natural material. Both native and r-hirudin were well tolerated by human volunteers given intravenous or subcutaneous single injections of 0.1 mg/kg, and bleeding times were not prolonged while TT and APTT were extended according to drug plasma levels. Hirudin appears to be relatively nonimmunogenic by animal testing.[56] Through in vitro clot lysis experiments, Mirshahi et al.[57] found hirudin superior to heparin in preventing clot buildup during tPA-catalyzed lysis. In a rabbit model in which clot was generated in the presence of damaged endothelium and lysed using streptokinase, low doses of r-hirudin prevented both thrombus formation and reocclusion. Only very high doses of heparin could achieve similar results.

Synthesis of portions of the hirudin molecule gave initial insights into its mode of action. This led to the development of exosite inhibitors of thrombin, which leave the active site accessible to inhibition by AT III.[58] Later, Maraganore used detailed x-ray structure information on the thrombin-hirudin complex to design more potent inhibitors known as hirulogs,[59] which are peptides of about 2000 kd that bind both the active site and the exosite of thrombin. These smaller synthetic analogs of hirudin mimic its action and have comparable high affinity but short half-lives.

Hirugen was examined in a dog femoral artery model of rethrombosis following[60] thrombolysis and was shown to effectively inhibit thrombosis, with fewer side effects than heparin. It will be most interesting to determine whether these agents can augment the lytic activity of plasminogen activators in vivo. A preliminary report by Yao et al.[61] utilizing a copper coil–induced coronary clot in dogs suggested that time to lysis was shortened and delay of reocclusion was prolonged by treating with both heparin and hirugen-1 compared with heparin alone. While hirudin and its analogs are promising from the points of view of potency and a unique site of action, it should be remembered that there is no antidote for these compounds other than allowing their clearance whereas a patient receiving heparin who displays bleeding complications may be treated with heparin-binding compounds.[62] Thus, there may be a virtue in potent but short-lived hirudin analogs that can clear or break down rapidly after discontinuation of infusion. On the other hand, thrombin may rebound when these are removed.

Reversible Inhibition

Few specific and potent reversible inhibitors of the thrombin active site have been discovered. One such compound, Argatroban of 509 kd, is an N- and C-blocked derivative of arginine that has been used clinically as an antithrombotic agent[63] given by intravenous infusion of 30 to 60 mg/day. In a rabbit model of rethrombosis 15 minutes after the end of tPA-mediated lysis of a carotid artery thrombus,[64] intravenous Argatroban from 0.6 to 2.5 mg/kg/ hr maintained 43 to 62 per cent of free flow, while heparin at 160 U/kg gave only 17 per cent of free flow. Such compounds have particular promise as they are expected to have little or no immunogenicity or toxicity, and their use together with plasminogen activators should be anticipated.

Protein C

As described earlier, activated protein C (Ca or APC), itself formed by thrombin bound to thrombomodulin, can powerfully inhibit coagulation via inactivation of factors Va and VIIIa.[65] In addition, it was found that time to lysis by tPA of platelet-free human plasma clots was shortened when APC was added.[66] This enhancement was dependent on calcium ion and on as yet unisolated plasma components. Activated protein C can also rapidly consume a heparin-dependent inhibitor (PCI or PAI-3) which is abundant in plasma, and this inhibitor also inactivates UK.[67] Thus significant amounts of protein C or APC could be both anticoagulant and slightly profibrinolytic. Recombinant protein C has recently become available and is undergoing extensive investigation. The combination of this agent with plasminogen activators in model systems should prove interesting.

Newer Antiplatelet Technologies

Platelets play a critical role in the restoration of vascular integrity after vessel wall damage. Upon exposure to subendothelium, platelet adhesion, the initial event in platelet-mediated hemostasis, proceeds with the subendothelial components, particularly von Willebrand factor (vWF), fibronectin, and collagen, binding to platelet surface receptors. Two phases of adhesion occur; the first a contact phase in which initial binding of platelet membrane occurs, followed by a secondary spreading phase. Von Willebrand factor is required for optimal adhesion of platelets via their surface glycoprotein receptors, binding both platelet glycoprotein (GP) Ib and GPIIb/IIIa.[68,69]

These events are followed by a platelet shape change, in which the cells take on a spheroid configuration, preceding the formation and extrusion of pseudopodia. Under physiological conditions, shape change is followed by aggregation of platelets and secretion of their granular contents. This irreversible phase results in recruitment of greater numbers of platelets, which aggregate and help to stabilize the hemostatic plug.

A large number of physiological mediators act as platelet stimuli. Among these are arachidonic acid, released from membrane phospholipids, which can be metabolized to thromboxane A_2, a potent aggregating agent. Thrombin, the procoagulant protein responsible for the conversion of fibrinogen to fibrin, as well as ADP and serotonin from platelet-dense granules, are also important in producing platelet aggregation. Collagen located in subendothelial layers is important in both platelet adhesion and aggregation.

It has been shown that platelets are activated in patients with unstable angina and in those with acute myocardial infarction.[70,71] In addition, it has been established that at least 20 per cent of patients who undergo successful thrombolytic therapy suffer rethrombosis of the previously reperfused vessels. It has also been suggested that the high rates of reocclusion observed in patients previously treated with thrombolytic agents are due in part to the presence of activated platelets and their subsequent aggregation, contributing to further thrombosis. Some investigators have presented evidence that treatment with plasminogen activators such as streptokinase or tPA is in itself associated with platelet aggregation.[72,73]

In contrast, others have demonstrated that these thrombolytic agents actually inhibit the aggregation process. For example, dose-dependent inhibition of ADP- and collagen-induced aggregation has been observed with urokinase and tPA, and to a lesser extent, with streptokinase.[74] In some cases, tPA has been shown to disperse previously aggregated platelets, as in studies by Loscalzo and Vaughan[75] who showed that disaggregation by tPA was prevented by α_2-antiplasmin. Results from a recent study have shown that tPA and streptokinase produced an initial increase, followed by a reduction in the aggregation response produced by ADP in rabbits.[76] Therefore, previous contradictory data may be explained by different experimental protocols in which the time of sampling and measurement of aggregation would play an important role. It is clear that the interaction of platelets and plasminogen activators is complex and may involve both proaggregatory and antiaggregatory components.

Because platelets play such an integral part in hemostasis, and, especially in the presence of atherosclerotic plaques, can promote thrombus formation, interventions to modulate platelet function have been investigated as preventatives for various thrombotic conditions.[77] Those that will be covered here, particularly as adjuncts to thrombolytic therapy, include specific inhibitors of thromboxane A_2 synthesis, antagonists of endoperoxide/thromboxane A_2 receptors, antibodies to platelet glycoprotein receptors, and peptide inhibitors of binding to these receptors.

Inhibitors of Arachidonic Acid Metabolism

An important pathway in the induction of platelet aggregation involves the conversion of released arachidonic acid to its endoperoxide and thromboxane metabolites, both of which are potent agonists.[78] Inhibition of this conversion might be expected to prevent platelet-mediated thrombus formation, and reduce the incidence of reocclusion observed after thrombolytic therapy. Fitzgerald et al.[79] have shown that thromboxane A_2 synthesis accompanies lysis induced by tPA in a canine model of coronary thrombosis. This finding was also observed in patients who had received intravenous tPA.[80] Aspirin, which irreversibly acetylates the cyclooxygenase of platelets, preventing the further metabolism of arachidonic acid, is often used in conjunction with thrombolytic agents in order to prevent reocclusion. However, the incidence of rethrombosis remains unacceptably high, suggesting other pathways of importance.

Since aspirin treatment also prevents the formation of the desired antiaggregatory metabolite prostacyclin, more selective agents might be used to prevent reocclusion. This was the rationale for studies that utilized inhibitors of thromboxane synthesis or antagonists of the endoperoxide/thromboxane A_2 receptor as adjuncts to thrombolytic therapy. Mickelson et al.[81] used intracoronary streptokinase to lyse thrombi in dogs treated with the thromboxane synthetase inhibitor CGS 13080. In comparison with dogs that did not receive the inhibitor, oscillations in coronary blood flow, indicative of platelet activation, were significantly reduced in CGS 13080-treated animals. This effect was accompanied by a marked reduction in reocclusion of these vessels. The same inhibitor was used to shorten the time to tPA-induced clot lysis, as well as to increase the incidence of reperfusion in a rabbit femoral artery model of thrombosis.[82] The efficacy of combined thromboxane receptor antagonism and synthetase inhibition in enhancing tPA-induced lysis and subsequent reocclusion has been demonstrated in a canine coronary artery thrombosis model.[83] Others have observed similar beneficial results with tPA and streptokinase in the presence of thromboxane A_2 receptor antagonists.[84]

Blockade of GPIIb/IIIa Receptors

Fibrinogen binding to platelet membranes is an important prerequisite for aggregation. Binding is mediated by glycoprotein receptors IIb and IIIa, which must form a complex, in the presence of calcium, in order to bind fibrinogen, fibronectin, and vWF. Thus, the IIb/IIIa receptor plays a central role in the aggregation process, so that inhibition of binding can be expected to prevent aggregation and subsequent thrombus formation. A recent and promising approach to this problem involves the use of monoclonal antibodies to IIb/IIIa. These agents have been used in a number of experimental models and have been shown to prevent platelet aggregation.[85] Gold et al.[86] demonstrated the potential of these agents as adjuncts to thrombolytic therapy in studies using a canine coronary artery thrombosis model. Reperfusion was accomplished using intravenous tPA; however, all dogs that received tPA alone showed evidence of cyclical reflow patterns followed by reocclusion. When the plasminogen activator was combined with the F(ab')$_2$ fragments of the monoclonal antibody 7E3, reocclusion was prevented and bleeding time was prolonged in a dose-related manner. Others had also observed similar results using this antibody. Thus, experimental evidence suggests that this approach may be useful in reducing the incidence of rethrombosis after thrombolytic therapy in humans.

It has been suggested, however, that these antibodies may find limited use in the clinical setting because, as foreign proteins, they may induce an immunogenic response.[87] In contrast, peptide antagonists of the IIb/IIIa receptors may show similar efficacy to the murine antibodies in preventing arterial reocclusion, without being immunogenic. Gartner and Bennett[88] used such as peptide to inhibit both fibrinogen binding to ADP-stimulated human platelets, as well as aggregation in response to this agonist. Furthermore, the combination of heparin and the snake venom peptide bitistatin was efficacious in reducing both the time and incidence of reperfusion after tPA infusion in dogs.[89] Promising as they seem, clinical trials will be necessary to determine their eventual clinical value.

Prostacyclin

Prostacyclin, a metabolite of arachidonic acid that is synthesized in the vessel wall, is a potent vasodilator and inhibitor of platelet aggregation. These characteristics make this mediator or its stable synthetic analogs particularly interesting candidates for adjuncts to thrombolytic therapy, since platelets are integrally involved in clot formation and in reocclusion of vessels which often occurs after successful thrombolysis. Moreover, the vasodilator effects suggest that improvements in blood flow, leading to salvage of ischemic tissue would accompany treatment with prostacyclins.

Patients with arteriosclerosis obliterans who were treated with the sodium salt of prostacyclin demonstrated significant shortening of the euglobulin clot lysis time (ECLT), prompting the authors to suggest that, in addition to the antiaggregatory and vasodilator effects of prostacyclin, the agent also provides direct activation of fibrinolysis.[90] Furthermore, in patients with peripheral arterial disease, both prostacyclin and its analog iloprost, shortened the ECLT, accompanied by an increase in tPA activity, providing further evidence for a possible direct effect of the agent.[91]

Defibrotide, a DNA fragment of mammalian origin, has been shown to increase prostacyclin production. Both antithrombotic and thrombolytic effects of defibrotide were demonstrated in a rabbit femoral vein model; the authors suggest that this agent increases both plasminogen activator and prostacyclin synthesis.[92] However, more recent results, obtained in patients with atherosclerotic disease who showed an increase in tPA activity after defibrotide, were attributed to a significant decrease in the activity of a plasminogen activator inhibitor.[93]

There is limited experimental evidence with the prostacyclin analog taprostene that this agent may be a beneficial adjunct to thrombolytic therapy. In a canine coronary thrombosis model, this agent increased myocardial salvage of tissue after lysis with recombinant prourokinase. In addition, when studied in a stenosis model in rabbits, taprostene prevented the cyclical flow reductions known to be associated with platelet deposition, and produced increases in carotid blood flow.[94]

The prostacyclin analog iloprost, which has a slightly longer half-life than prostacyclin, has received considerable attention as a possible adjunct to thrombolytic therapy. However, recent evidence suggests that this agent may actually exert a detrimental effect. Iloprost increased the time to reperfusion obtained with tPA alone, as well as shortening the duration of tPA-induced reperfusion in dogs with a coronary artery thrombus.[95] In addition, plasma levels of tPA were actually reduced by iloprost when compared to plasma levels in the group of animals that received only tPA. The authors suggest that iloprost may promote hepatic degradation of the lytic agent. Similar results were obtained in a more recent study in which iloprost also increased the time to reperfusion in a dog model, as well as preventing tPA-induced reperfusion in some of the animals.[96] An explanation presented by the authors is that iloprost increases hepatic blood flow, which increases the rate of clearance of the lytic agent, decreasing its efficacy. In patients with acute myocardial infarction, iloprost, in combination with tPA, did not show improvement in coronary artery patency in comparison to those who received tPA alone. In addition, ventricular function was not improved in these patients.[97] Patients with peripheral vascular disease exhibited increases in platelet reactivity after iloprost and showed evidence of enhanced coagulation.[98] Therefore, this prostacyclin analog does not appear to be an appropriate candidate for adjunctive therapy. However, further studies with other candidates may show beneficial effects for prostacyclin analogs in keeping with their known anti-platelet and vasodilator characteristics.

NEW CATHETER DELIVERY TECHNOLOGY

The ultimate goal of thrombolytic therapy for peripheral arterial occlusive diseases is to achieve complete clot lysis expeditiously, while minimizing serious bleeding complications. The latter is critically important in a non–life-threat-ening situation and where many patients are referred for vascular surgery following thrombolytic therapy.

Intravenous thrombolysis for peripheral arterial occlusion was attempted in the late 1950s and in the 1960s.[99,100] Data from those early trials indicated that successful thrombolysis could be achieved in up to 80 per cent of occlusions treated within 12 hours, while no lysis was observed in occlusions presumed to have been present for over 3 months. However, infusions of up to 100,000 U/hr of SK for several days were not uncommon and resulted in an unacceptably high incidence of serious bleeding complications. These observations prompted investigators to turn to local, intra-arterial infusions in order to achieve higher concentrations of the thrombolytic drug on the clot, while minimizing the risk of serious bleeding. In 1974, Dotter modified the intra-arterial technique to position the catheter tip in contact with the proximal portion of the thrombus.[101] Although the study yielded somewhat disappointing results (35 per cent complete clot lysis and 24 per cent incidence of bleeding), it generated substantial interest for intrathrombus administration of thrombolytic agents.

Factors known to influence the outcome of thrombolysis include age of the clot, location (supra- or infrainguinal level), length of the occlusion, as well as its nature (thrombotic or embolic). The consensus among clinicians is that duration of the occlusion is one of the best predictors of success, the highest success rates being observed in acute or subacute occlusions.

As a result, many investigators have adopted clot traversability with a soft-tipped guide wire as a major selection criterion for thrombolytic ther-apy.[102–105] Recent animal and in vitro studies have confirmed the clinician's perception that speed of lysis is increased by direct drug delivery into a penetrable clot rather than in its immediate vicinity, increasing the total contact area between thrombolytic drug and the clot. The latter is achieved by combining chemical thrombolysis with mechanical disruption of the clot.[104,106,107]

Clinical studies comparing high- versus low-dose intrathrombus infusions[103] seem to confirm that contact area between drug and thrombus is more important than total dose administered. These observations led to the development of new delivery techniques. McNamara and Fischer[105] advocate inserting a guide wire as far as possible into the clot, advancing an end-hole catheter over the guide wire, and positioning it several centimeters into the clot. The guide wire is then removed and the drug is infused into the "channel" created by the guide wire. The catheter is then advanced into the clot at 2-hour intervals as lysis progresses. Modifications of this technique include a bolus injection of the fibrinolytic drug into the thrombus during catheter withdrawal to the proximal portion of the thrombus,[103] or use of a coaxial infusion system to "lace" the clot throughout its length prior to initiating the infusion.[108]

Recently, the coaxial infusion system has been adopted by several investigators. The proximal catheter is positioned several centimeters into the clot, while the distal infusion catheter rests within the distal portion of the thrombus, resulting in a reduced need for repositioning of the infusion system as thrombolysis progresses.[109] In an attempt to further disrupt the clot and accelerate thrombolysis, Valji et al.[104] recently reported their experience in 48 patients with peripheral arterial occlusions, using pulsed-spray pharmacomechanical thrombolysis. In this setting, highly concentrated urokinase (250,000 IU/ml) in small volumes (0.2 ml) is injected forcefully (by hand or mechanically) through side-holes in the infusion catheter. Initially, one to two pulses per minutes are injected and a total of 150,000 IU of urokinase are given over 15 to 20 minutes. Additional pulses are given at a rate of about one per minute, until reestablishment of adequate antegrade flow. Initial complete or near complete clot lysis was achieved in all but one patient. Mean time to lysis was dramatically reduced to 65 minutes (native arteries) and to 93 minutes (bypass grafts) in the first 33 patients. Distal embolization (4 of 48) is a relatively frequent complication of this technique. Avoiding infusing into the distal 1 cm of the clot may help reduce the incidence of embolization. Minor modifications of the above technique have recently been proposed. In order to avoid dissecting the vessel wall, Mewissen et al.[110] introduced "over-the-wire" thrombolysis. Urokinase is injected under pressure through side-holes in the catheter, while a guide wire occludes the end hole. This method eliminates the risk of dissection if the lesion can be crossed.

The rapid expansion of interventional vascular radiology has generated a flurry of activity with the use of new catheters, designed to increase the speed of lysis through an increase in contact area between clot and drug. Experimental pump devices are being investigated to disrupt the clot and further increase contact area. Over the last 10 years, these new devices have contributed to substantial reductions in mean time to (complete) clot lysis. Turning to the problem of preventing reocclusion, some investigators have recently reported on the use of double-balloon catheters, which allow infusion of thrombolytic drugs in an isolated space between two inflated balloons. Jorgensen et al.[111] showed that rethrombosis at 30 days was prevented in 6 of 6 patients who had been given 5 mg of rt-PA for 30 minutes in an enclosed space of the superficial femoral artery.

It still remains to be demonstrated whether (adjunctive) thrombolysis has a beneficial effect on long-term patency in chronically occluded peripheral arteries.

RECOMBINANT TECHNOLOGY FOR THROMBOLYTIC AGENTS

The human thrombolytic enzymes, like many important proteins, are normally present in very small amounts. Thus, UK and tPA both usually circulate at concentrations in the vicinity of 10 ng/ml of plasma,[112] and a typical dose of 100 mg of tPA would require the complete circulatory contents of tPA from about 3000 people; clearly not practical! Urokinase is made primarily by kidney cells, and some UK concentrates in the urine to the extent of a few µg/ml. Urokinase has been produced by the processing of hundreds or thousands of gallons of urine, or by the extraction of kidney cell culture medium. Both of these methods are very slow, time consuming, and low in yield. The difficulties in handling also tend to make such products heterogeneous, owing to the action of proteases over time in the urine or media.

The advent of modern recombinant technology (genetic engineering) has recently made possible the enrichment by thousands of times of the cell yield of plasminogen activators (PAs). An ordinary cell will typically have just one copy of the gene for a PA commanding synthesis of the corresponding messenger RNA (mRNA) and thence the protein. Indeed, in most normal cells, the controlling region of the gene will be turned off so that there is little or no production. Many tumor cells (e.g., melanoma) produce considerably more tPA or UK than ordinary tissues because their PA genes are turned on, making a good deal of message. However, even these cells represent only a modest improvement, as they have only one gene copy. Still, they are an enriched source of PA mRNA and were therefore the starting point for cloning and expression of the PAs through isolation of the relevant mRNAs as outlined below.

Because mRNAs in eukaryotic cells contain stretches of poly-A at their 3' ends, a mixture of all mRNA can be readily obtained from a cell extract by adsorption onto a column of oligo-dT cellulose. Complimentary DNAs (cDNA) can then be formed by treating the isolated mRNA mixture with reverse transcriptase, which copies the RNA messages into single strands of DNA. The new mixture of DNAs is then made into double-stranded form by treatment with DNA polymerase. In order to obtain the cDNAs for UK and for tPA, tumor cell extracts were treated in the above way. However this yielded a complex mixture of all active genes, so the next step was to move these into individual prokaryotic cells (*Escherichia coli*) where thousands of cells can be screened for the desired gene. This is accomplished by ligating the mixture of genes, via appropriate splicing enzymes, into plasmids. The latter are independent circular DNAs that can propagate inside a host bacterium alongside the host genome.[113]

An early procedure for locating colonies carrying the appropriate gene was simply to look for an anti-PA antibody reaction in extracts from the colonies. Now, more efficient methods are used. After exposure to plasmids, thousands of individual colonies arising on Petri plates from individual *E. coli* cells can be transferred to nitrocellulose filters for screening. Treatment with detergent and ethanol essentially leaves only a DNA precipitate on the filter from the original colony. Detection of the relevant clones simply requires hybridizing this DNA with an appropriate radioactive probe that can later be detected by autoradiography. The necessary probe can be made once some amino acid sequence information is available on the protein desired. Once urinary UK was sequenced,[114] it was possible to deduce from the genetic code what the corresponding DNA sequence must be. Synthetic radioactive oligonucleotides with the ability to hybridize to the relevant cDNAs were then synthesized as probes to find the PA gene-containing bacteria.[115]

With some proteins, actual productive expression of the mammalian protein can be accomplished in the *E. coli* carrying the above plasmid. In mammalian cells, tPA and UK (proUK) are normally glycosylated at specified asparagine residues through the action of multiple enzyme systems that attach and remove sugars to generate oligosaccharide chains. They are then both secreted through the action of a leader N-terminal sequence, which is removed as the protein leaves the cell. Bacteria can neither glycosylate nor secrete these proteins. Even more formidable difficulties are encountered with bacterial expression, when the desired protein contains multiple disulfide bonds, as do both UK (12 S-S bonds) and tPA (16 S-S bonds). The intracellular environment of mammalian cells is sufficiently oxidizing that disulfide bond formation can follow rapidly in tandem with primary chain elongation, allowing the uniquely evolved sets of cysteine SH groups to pair for proper three-dimensional folding of the protein. In bacteria, the cytoplasm is too reducing, and cysteines remain reduced until the protein escapes into the periplasmic space or is exposed to air after intentional cell disruption. Thus S-S–containing proteins fail to fold and often clump into denatured precipitates or sudden oxidation causes formation of multiple mispaired disulfides. In either case, the protein is not functional.

It has been possible to renature such proteins by exposure to mixtures of low molecular weight thiols and disulfides. This usually requires exquisitely tuned conditions using partial denaturing solvents with gradual progress to a fully oxidized and nondenaturing environment. Small yields of refolded active proUK have been obtained and several manufacturers eventually succeeded in achieving useful production yields of r-proUK from *E. coli* through proprietary refolding processes.[116] The products are nonglycosylated but appear to have enzymatic properties similar to natural proUK. It has not yet been thoroughly proven that all 12 of the disulfide bonds are properly paired in all of the refolded molecules. *Eschericha coli* production has the advantages of high initial yield with low cost medium. Full-size active tPA has not yet been successfully produced in bacteria.

In order to produce PAs in a more "natural way," not requiring refolding, the genes must be moved into mammalian cells. The active plasmids described above are clipped enzymatically and the genes are spliced into mammalian expression vectors which often contain viral elements for genomic insertion and regulation. This method was used to introduce the tPA gene via transfection into Chinese hamster ovary (CHO) tumor cells in which commercial tPA is now manufactured.[117] In order to amplify the production, the gene was placed in tandem with a dihydrofolate reductase (DHFR) gene. This allows selection of clones of cells with intrinsically high spontaneous gene copy number, because these cells will survive exposure to the toxic antifolate, methotrexate (MTX), by producing large amounts of its target enzyme, DHFR. Gradual passage of cells exposed to increasing levels of MTX leads to overproducers of both DHFR and tPA.

The situation is maintained by continued exposure to MTX. Glycosylated PA is thus secreted into the medium, already folded and fully functional. A basically similar approach has also been applied to the manufacture of r-proUK in mouse myeloma cells, a product which is currently under clinical investigation.

r-Urokinase

Only a continuous, single-chain protein such as proUK can be obtained directly from genetic engineering as described. As UK is a two-chain derivative of proUK, additional manipulation is required for its production. Recombinant urokinase is formed by the plasmin activation of HMW r-proUK. Two approaches have been taken with this starting material. If HMW r-UK is desired, controlled gentle exposure to human plasmin can yield a mainly (greater than 90 per cent) HMW product. This is cleaved essentially only at Lys-158 and can be stabilized by removal of plasmin and storage at pH at or below 5.0. If it is desired to form LMW r-UK, then the above product is allowed to autodigest itself at higher pH where the bond at Lys-135 is cleaved releasing the bulk of the N-terminal domain. The product is not precisely identical with natural LMW UK (Abbokinase), but only contains eight additional N-terminal amino acids (out of nearly 300 residues) and is a structure that also occurs naturally. The r-UK will be nonglycosylated or glycosylated according to whether one starts with bacterial- or mammalian-expressed r-proUK.

Thus far, by in vitro and animal clot lysis testing, r-UK appears to be equivalent to natural UK. Nonglycosylated LMW r-UK was compared with natural urine-derived HMW UK, and no significant differences were found by either human plasma clot lysis or in a rabbit model of PE.[118] Likewise, HMW r-UK made by plasmin activation of glycosylated r-proUK expressed in mouse cells was compared with LMW natural cell culture UK. No significant differences were found in human plasma clot lysis or in a canine clot lysis model.

The advantages gained from recombinant production of tPA, proUK, and UK are products that are purer, stable, consistent, homogeneous, and of higher specific activity than the corresponding naturally obtained proteins. There is also elimination of concern over diseases which may be transmitted by human tissue or body fluids. The manufacturing processes also tend to be much more highly controlled. In the long run, recombinant manufacture is also much more economical, although initially there are very significant costs arising from research and development required to establish the product and to insure that no significant nonhuman proteins, nucleic acids, or viruses are carried over from the expression cell,[119] and that correct nonantigenic folding of the product has taken place.

REFERENCES

1. MacFarlane RG, Biggs R: Fibrinolysis. Its mechanism and significance. Blood 1948;*3*:1167–1187.
2. Tillet WS, Garner RL: The fibrinolytic activity of hemolytic streptococci. J Exp Med 1933;*58*:485–502.
3. Milstone H: A factor in normal human blood which participates in streptococcal fibrinolysis, J Immunol 1941;*42*:109–116.
4. Christensen LR: Streptococcal fibrinolysis: A proteolytic reaction due to a serum enzyme activated by streptococcal fibrinolysis. J Gen Physiol 1945;*28*:363–383.
5. Kapslan MH: Nature and role of the lytic factor in hemolytic streptococcal fibrinolysis. Proc Soc Exp Biol Med 1944;*57*:40–43.
6. Tillet WS, Sherry S: The effect in patients of streptococcal fibrinolysin (streptokinase) and streptococcal desoxyribonuclease or fibrinous, purulent and sanguinous pleural exudations. J Clin Invest 1949;*28*:173–190.
7. MacFarlane RG, Pilling J: Fibrinolytic activity of normal urine. Nature 1947;*159*:779.
8. Astrup T, Sterndorff I: An activator of plasminogen in normal urine. Proc Soc Exp Bio Med 1952;*81*:675–678.
9. Sobel GW, Mohler SR, Jones NW, Dowdy ABC, Guest MM: Urokinase: An activator of plasma profibrinolysin extracted from urine. Am J Physiol 1952;*171*:768–769.
10. Urokinase-Pulmonary Embolism Trial Study Group. Urokinase pulmonary embolism trial. Phase I results. JAMA 1970;*214*:2163–2172.

11. Urokinase-Pulmonary Embolism Trial Study Group. Urokinase-streptokinase pulmonary embolism trial. Phase II results. JAMA 1974;*229*:1606–1613.

12. Glatter T: Trends in cardiology: Proper use of the thrombolytic agents. Mod Med 1990;*58*:62–73.

13. Marder VJ, Sherry S: Thrombolytic therapy: Current status. N Engl J Med 1988;*318*:1512–1520.

14. Collen D: Human tissue—type plasminogen activator: From the laboratory to the bedside. Circulation 1985;*72*:18–20.

15. Bernik MB: Increased plasminogen activator (urokinase) in tissue culture after fibrin deposition. J Clin Invest 1973;*52*:823–834.

16. Nolan C, Hall LS, Barlow GH, Tribby IIE: Plasminogen activator from human embryonic kidney cell cultures—evidence for a proactivator. Biochim Biophys Acta 1977;*496*:384–400.

17. Bernik MA, Oller EP: Plasminogen activator and proactivator (urokinase precursor) in lung cultures. J Am Med Woman's Assoc 1976;*31*:465–472.

18. Husain SS, Gurewich V, Lipinski B: Purification and partial characterization of a single-chain, high molecular weight form of urokinase from human urine. Arch Biochem Biophys 1983;*220*:31–38.

19. Stump DC, Thienpont M, Collen D: Urokinase-related proteins in human urine. J Biol Chem 1986;*261*:1267–1273.

20. Wun TC, Schleuning WD, Reich E: Isolation and characterization of urokinase from human plasma. J Biol Chem 1982;*257*:3276–3283.

21. Wijngaards G, Rijken DC, Van Wezel AL, Groeneveld E, van der Velden CAM: Characterization and fibrin-binding properties of different molecular forms of pro-urokinase from a monkey kidney cell culture. Thromb Res 1986;*42*:749–760.

22. Mangel W, Lin B, Ramakrishnan V: Characterization of an extremely large, ligand-induced conformational change in plasminogen. Science 1990;*248*:69–73.

23. Badylak SF, Voytik SL, Henkin J, Burke SE, Sasahara AA, Simmons A: Enhancement of the thrombolytic efficacy of prourokinase by lys-plasminogen in a dog model of arterial thrombosis. Thromb Res 1991;*62*:115–126.

24. Watahiki Y, Scully MF, Ellis V, Kakkar VV: Potentiation by lys-plasminogen of clot lysis by single or two-chain urokinase-type plasminogen activator or tissue-type plasminogen activator. Thromb Haemost 1989;*61*(3):502–506.

25. Green J, Dupe RJ, Smith RAG, Harris GS, English PD: Comparison of the hypotensive effects of streptokinase-plasminogen activator complex and BRL26921 (p-anisoylated streptokinase-plasminogen activator complex) in the dog after high dose, bolus administration. Thromb Res 1991;*36*:29–36.

26. Appella E, Robinson EA, Ullrich SJ, et al: The receptor-binding sequence of urokinase. J Biol Chem 1987;*262*(10):4437–4440.

27. Gonzalez-Gronow M, Stack S, Pizzo SV: Plasmin binding to the plasminogen receptor enhances catalytic efficiency and activates the receptor for subsequent ligand binding. Arch Biochem Biophys 1991;*286*(2):625–628.

28. deMunk GAW, Rijken DC: Fibrinolytic properties of single chain urokinase-type plasminogen activator (pro-urokinase). Fibrinolysis 1990;*4*:1–9.

29. Pannell R, Black J, Gurewich V: Complementary modes of action of tissue-type plasminogen activator and pro-urokinase by which their synergistic effect on clot lysis may be explained. J Clin Invest 1988;*81*:853–859.

30. Gurewich V: The sequential, complementary and synergistic activation of fibrin-bound plasminogen by tissue plasminogen activator and pro-urokinase. Fibrinolysis 1990;*3*:59–66.

31. Badylak SF, Voytik S, Klabunde RE, Henkin J, Leski M: Bolus dose response characteristics of single chain urokinase plasminogen activator and tissue plasminogen activator in a dog model of arterial thrombosis. Thromb Res 1988;*52*(4):295–312.

32. Tollefson DM, Pestka CA, Monafo WJ: Activation of heparin cofactor II by dermatan sulfate. J Biol Chem 1983;*258*:6713–6716.

33. Esmon CT, Esmon NL, Harris KW: Complex formation between thrombin and thrombomodulin inhibits both thrombin-catalyzed fibrin formation and factor V activation. J Biol Chem 1982;*257*:7944–7947.

34. Eisenberg PR, Sherman LA, Jaffe AS: Paradoxic elevation of fibrinopeptide A after streptokinase: Evidence for continued thrombosis despite intense fibrinolysis. J Am Coll Cardiol 1987;*10*:527–529.

35. Owen J, Friedman KD, Grossman BA, Wilkins C, Berke AD, Powers ER: Thrombolytic therapy with tissue plasminogen activator or streptokinase induces transient thrombin activity. Blood 1988;*72*(2):616–620.

36. Gulba DC, Barthels M, Reil GH, Lichtlen PR: Thrombin/antithrombin-III complex level as early predictor of reocclusion after successful thrombolysis. The Lancet 1988;*ii*:97.

37. Lee CD, Mann KG: Activation/inactivation of human factor V by plasmin. Blood 1989;*73*:185–190.

38. Melandri G. Branzi A, Semprini F, Cervi V, Galie N, Magnani B: Enhanced thrombolytic

efficacy and reduction of infarct size by simultaneous infusion of streptokinase and heparin. Br Heart J 1990;*64*(2):118–120.

39. Chesebro JH, Knatterud G, Roberts R, et al: Thrombolysis in myocardial infarction (TIMI) trial, phase I: A comparison between intravenous tissue plasminogen activator and intravenous streptokinase. Circulation 1987;*76*:142–154.

40. Badimon L, Lassila R, Badimon J, Vallabhajosula S, Chesebro JH, Fuster V: Residual thrombosis is more thrombogenic than severely damaged vessel wall. Circulation 1988;*78*:II–118.

41. Voytik S, Badylak SF, Burke S, Klabunde RE, Henkin J, Simmons A: The protective effect of heparin in a dog model of rethrombosis following pharmacologic thrombolysis. Thromb Haemost 1990;*64*(3):438–444.

42. Topol EJ, Califf RM, George BS, et al: Coronary arterial thrombolysis with combined infusion of recombinant tissue-type plasminogen activator and urokinase in patients with acute myocardial infarction. Circulation 1988;*77*:1100–1107.

43. Zahger D, Maaravi Y, Matzner Y, Gilon D, Gotsman MS, Weiss AT: Partial resistance to anticoagulation after streptokinase treatment for acute myocardial infarction. Am J Cardiol 1990;*66*(1):28–30.

44. Fareed J, Walenga JM, Hoppensteadt DA, Messmore HL: Studies on the profibrinolytic actions of heparin and its fractions. Semin Thromb Hemost 1986;*11*:199–207.

45. Thomas DP, Merton RE: A low molecular weight heparin compared with unfractionated heparin. Thromb Res 1982;*28*:343–350.

46. Cercek B, Lew AS, Hod H, Yang J, Reddy NKN, Ganz W: Enhancement of thrombolysis with tissue-type plasminogen activator by pretreatment with heparin. Circulation 1986;*74*(3):583–587.

47. Fears R: Kinetic studies on the effect of heparin and fibrin on plasminogen activators. Biochem J 1988;*249*:77–81.

48. Stassen JM, Juhan-Vague I, Alessi MC, DeCock F, Collen D: Potentiation by heparin fragments of thrombolysis induced with human tissue-type plasminogen activator or human single-chain urokinase-type plasminogen activator. Thromb Haemost 1987;*58*(3):947–950.

49. Webster MWI, Chesebro JH, Mruk JS: Anti-thrombotic therapy during and after thrombolysis for acute myocardial infarction. Coronary Art Dis 1990;*1*:190–198.

50. Topol EJ, George BS, Kereiakes DJ: A multicenter, randomized controlled trial of intravenous tissue plasminogen activator and early intravenous heparin in acute myocardial infarction. Circulation 1989;*79*:281–286.

51. Hsia J, Hamilton WP, Kleiman N, Roberts R, Chaitman BR, Ross AM: A comparison between heparin and low-dose aspirin as adjunctive therapy with tissue plasminogen activator for acute myocardial infarction. New Engl J Med 1990;*323*(21):1433–1437.

52. Gulba DC, Fischer K, Barthels M, et al: Potentiative effect of heparin in thrombolytic therapy of evolving myocardial infarction with natural pro-urokinase. Fibrinolysis 1989;*3*(3):165–173.

53. Weitz JI, Hudoba M, Massel D, Maraganore J, Hirsh J: Clot-bound thrombin is protected from inhibition by heparin-antithrombin III but is susceptible to inactivation by antithrombin III-independent inhibitors. J Clin Invest 1990;*86*:385–391.

54. Markwardt F: Pharmacology of hirudin: One hundred years after the first report of the anticoagulant agent in medicinal leeches. Biomed Biochim Acta 1985;*44*(7/8):1007–1013.

55. Harvey RP, Degryse E, Stefani L, et al: Cloning and expression of a cDNA coding for the anticoagulant hirudin from the blood sucking leech, *Hirudo medicinalis*. Proc Natl Acad Sci USA 1986;*83*:1084–1088.

56. Klocking HP, Guttner J, Fink E: Toxicological studies with recombinant hirudin. Folia Haematol 1988;*115*:75–82.

57. Mirshahi M, Soria J, Soria C, et al: Evaluation of the inhibition of heparin and hirudin of coagulation activation during r-tPA–induced thrombolysis. Blood 1989;*74*(3):1025–1030.

58. Naski MC, Fenton II JW, Maraganore JM, Olson ST, Shafer JA: The COOH-terminal domain of hirudin. J Biol Chem 1990;*265*(23):13484–13489.

59. Maraganore JM, Bourdon P, Jablonski J, Ramachandran KL, Fenton II JW: Design and characterization of hirulogs: A novel class of bivalent peptide inhibitors of thrombin. Biochemistry 1990b;*29*:7095–7101.

60. Badylak SF, Voytik S, Henkin J, Burke S: Hirugen as a safe and effective treatment for prevention of rethrombosis after thrombolysis in a dog model. Arteriosclerosis 1990;*10*(5):A937.

61. Yao SK, McNatt J, Eidt J, Cui K, Maraganore JM: Thrombin inhibitors shorten time to thrombolysis and prolong reocclusion time after treatment with recombinant tissue-type plasminogen activator (abstr) Clin Res 1990;*38*(2)469a.

62. Weiss ME, Nyhan D, Peng ZK, et al: Association of protamine IgE and IgG antibodies with life-threatening reactions to intravenous protamine. New Engl J Med 1989;*320*(14):886–892.

63. Kobayashi S, Kitani M, Yamaguchi S, Suzuki T, Okada K, Tsunematsu T: Effects of an

antithrombotic agent (MD-805) on progressing cerebral thrombosis. Thromb Res 1989;53:305–317.

64. Eisert WG, Koch V, Rigter B, Muller TH: Prevention of rethrombosis after thrombolysis by synthetic thrombin inhibitor argipidine (MD-805) (abstr). Thromb Haemost 1989;62(1):1019.

65. Clouse LH, Comp PC: The regulation of hemostasis: The protein C system. New Engl J Med 1986;314(20):1298–1304.

66. Bajzar L, Fredenburgh JC, Nesheim M: The activated protein C-mediated enhancement of tissue-type plasminogen activator-induced fibrinolysis in a cell-free system. J Biol Chem 1990;265(28):16948–16954.

67. Geiger M, Huber K, Wojta J, et al: Complex formation between urokinase and plasma protein C inhibitor in vitro and in vivo. Blood 1989;74(2):722–728.

68. Fujimura Y, Titani K, Holland LZ, et al: von Willebrand factor. A reduced and alylated 52/48-kDa fragment beginning at amino acid residue 449 contains the domain interacting with platelet glycoprotein Ib. J Biol Chem 1986;261:381–385.

69. Girma J-P, Kalafatis M, Pietu GM, et al: Mapping of distinct von Willebrand factor domains interacting with platelet GPIb and GPIIb/IIIa and with collagen using monoclonal antibodies. Blood 1986;67:1356–1366.

70. Gallino A, Haeberli A, Gaur HR, Straub PW: Fibrin formation and platelet aggregation in patients with severe coronary artery disease: Relationship with the degree of myocardial ischemia. Circulation 1985;72:27–30.

71. Gallino A, Haeberli A, Hess T, Mombelli G, Straub PW: Fibrin formation and platelet aggregation in patients with acute myocardial infarction: Effects of intravenous and subcutaneous low-dose heparin. Am Heart J 1986;112:285–290.

72. Ohlstein EH, Storer B, Fujita T, Shebuski RJ: Tissue-type plasminogen activator and streptokinase induce platelet hyperaggregability in the rabbit. Thromb Res 1987;46:575–585.

73. Vaughan DE, Kirshenbaum JM, Loscalzo J: Streptokinase-induced, antibody-mediated platelet aggregation: A potential cause of clot propagation in vivo. J Am Coll Cardiol 1988;11:1343–1348.

74. Terres W, Umnus S, Mathey DG, Bleifeld W: Effects of streptokinase, urokinase, and recombinant tissue plasminogen activator on platelet aggregability and stability of platelet aggregates. Cardiovasc Res 1990;24:471–477.

75. Loscalzo I, Vaughan DE: Tissue plasminogen activator promotes platelet disaggregation in plasma. J Clin Invest 1987;79:1749–1755.

76. Rudd MA, George D, Amarante P, Vaughan DE, Loscalzo J: Temporal effects of thrombolytic agents on platelet function in vivo and their modulation by prostaglandins. Circ Res 1990;67:1175–1181.

77. Marder VJ: Comparison of thrombolytic agents: Selected hematologic, vascular and clinical events. Am J Cardiol 1989;64:2A–7A.

78. Coller BS: Platelets and thrombolytic therapy. New Engl J Med 1990;322:33–42.

79. Fitzgerald DJ, Wright F, FitzGerald GA: Increased thromboxane biosynthesis during coronary thrombolysis. Evidence that platelet activation and thromboxane A_2 modulate the response to tissue-type plasminogen activator in vivo. Circ Res 1989b;65:83–94.

80. Kerins DM, Roy L, FitzGerald GA, Fitzgerald DJ: Platelet and vascular function during coronary thrombolysis with tissue-type plasminogen activator. Circulation 1989;80:1718–1725.

81. Mickelson JK, Simpson PJ, Gallas MT, Lucchesi BR: Thromboxane synthetase inhibition with CGS 13080 improves coronary blood flow after streptokinase-induced thrombolysis. Am Heart J 1987;113:1345–1352.

82. Shebuski RJ, Storer BL, Fujita T: Effect of thromboxane synthase inhibition on the thrombolytic action of tissue-type plasminogen activator in a rabbit model of peripheral arterial thrombosis. Thromb Res 1988b;52:381–392.

83. Golino P, Rosolowsky M, Yao S, et al: Endogenous prostaglandin endoperoxides and prostacyclin modulate the thrombolytic activity of tissue plasminogen activator. J Clin Invest 1990;86:1095–1102.

84. Kopia GA, Kopaciewicz LJ, Ohlstein EH, Horohonich S, Storer BL, Shebuski RJ: Combination of the thromboxane receptor antagonist, sulotroban (BM 13.177; SK&F 95587), with streptokinase: Demonstration of thrombolytic synergy. J Pharmacol Exp Ther 1989;250:887–895.

85. Coller BS, Folts JD, Smith SR, Scudder LE, Jordan R: Abolition of in vivo platelet thrombus formation in primates with monoclonal antibodies to the platelet GPIIb/IIIa receptor. Circulation 1989;80:1766–1774.

86. Gold HK, Coller BS, Yasuda T, et al: Rapid and sustained coronary artery recanalization with combined bolus injection of recombinant tissue-type plasminogen activator and monoclonal antiplatelet GPIIb/IIIa antibody in a canine preparation. Circulation 1988;77:670–677.

87. Fitzgerald DJ: Platelet inhibition with an antibody to glycoprotein IIb/IIIa. Circulation 1989a;80:1918–1919.

88. Gartner TK, Bennett JS: The tetrapeptide analogue of the cell attachment site of fibronectin inhibits platelet aggregation and fibrinogen binding to activated platelets. J Biol Chem 1985;260:11891–11894.

89. Shebuski RJ, Stabilito IJ, Sitko GR, Polokoff MH: Acceleration of recombinant tissue-type plasminogen activator-induced thrombolysis and prevention of reocclusion by the combination of heparin and the Arg-Gly-Asp containing peptide bitistatin in a canine model of coronary thrombosis. Circulation 1990;82:169–177.

90. Dembinska-Kiec A, Kosta-Trabka E, Gryglewski RJ: Effect of prostacyclin on fibrinolytic activity in patients with arteriosclerosis obliterans. Thromb Haemost 1982;47:190.

91. Musial J, Wilczynska M, Sladek K, Cierniewski CS, Nitzankowski R, Szczeklik A: Fibrinolytic activity of prostacyclin and iloprost in patients with peripheral arterial disease. Prostaglandins 1986;31:61–70.

92. Niada R, Pescador R, Porta R, Mantovani M, Prino G: Defibrotide is antithrombotic and thrombolytic against rabbit venous thrombosis. Haemostasis 1986;16:3–8.

93. Violi F, Ferro D, Alessandri C, Quintarelli C, Saliola M, Balsano F: Inhibition of tissue plasminogen activator by defibrotide in atherosclerotic patients. Semin Thromb Hemost 1989;15:226–229.

94. Groves R, Schneider J, Flohe L: Cooperative action of the prostacyclin analogue taprostene and the fibrinolytic prourokinase (r-scu-PA) in experimental artery thrombosis. Prog Clin Biol Res 1989;301:603–607.

95. Nicolini FA, Mehta JL, Nichols WW, Saldeen TGP, Grant M: Prostacyclin analogue 1-iloprost decreases thrombolytic potential of tissue-type plasminogen activator in canine coronary thrombosis. Circulation 1990;81:1115–1122.

96. Kerins DM, Shuh M, Kunitada S, FitzGerald GA, Fitzgerald DJ: A prostacyclin analog impairs the response to tissue-type plasminogen activator during coronary thrombolysis: Evidence for a pharmacokinetic interaction. J Pharmacol Exp Ther 1991;257:487–492.

97. Topol EJ, Ellis SG, Califf RM, et al: Combined tissue-type plasminogen activator and prostacyclin therapy for acute myocardial infarction. JACC 1989;14:877–884.

98. Kovacs IB, Mayou SC, Kirby JD: Infusion of a stable prostacyclin analogue, iliprost, to patients with peripheral vascular disease: Lack of antiplatelet effect but risk of thromboembolism. Am J Med 1991;90:41–46.

99. Fletcher AP, Alkjaersig N, Shery S: Maintenance of a sustained fibrinolytic state in man. Induction and effects. J Clin Invest 1959;38:1096–1110.

100. Poliwoda H, Alexander K, Buhl V, et al: Treatment of chronic arterial occlusions with streptokinase. N Engl J Med 1969;280:689–692.

101. Dotter CT, Rosch J, Seaman AJ: Selective clot lysis with low dose streptokinase. Radiology 1974;111:31–37.

102. Eisenbud DE, Brener BJ, Shoenfeld R, et al: Treatment of acute vascular occlusions with intra-arterial urokinase. Am J Surg 1990;160:160–165.

103. Cragg AH, Smith TP, Corson JD, et al: Two urokinase regimens in native arterial and graft occlusions: Initial results of a prospective, randomized clinical trial. Radiology 1991;178:681–686.

104. Valji K, Bookstein JJ: Fibrinolysis with intrathrombic injection of urokinase and tissue-type plasminogen activator: Results in a new model of subacute venous thrombosis. Invest Radiol 1987;22:23–27.

105. McNamara TO, Fisher JR: Thrombolysis of peripheral arterial and graft occlusions: Improved results using high dose urokinase. AJR 1985;144:769–775.

106. Bookstein JJ, Saldinger E: Accelerated thrombolysis: In vitro evaluation of agents and methods of administration. Invest Radiol 1985;20:731–735.

107. Kandarpa K, Drinker PA, Singer SJ, et al: Forceful pulsatile local infusion of enzyme accelerates thrombolysis: In vivo evaluation of a new delivery system. Radiology 1988;168:739–744.

108. Sullivan KL, Gardiner GA, Shapiro MJ, et al: Acceleration of thrombolysis with a high-dose transthrombus bolus technique. Radiology 1989;173:805–808.

109. McNamara TO: The use of lytic therapy with endovascular "repair" for the failed infrainguinal graft. Semin Vasc Surg 1990;3:59–65.

110. Mewissen MW, Minor PL, Beyer GA, Lipchik EO: Symptomatic native arterial occlusions: Early experience with "over-the-wire" thrombolysis. JVIR 1990;1:43–47.

111. Jorgensen B, Bullow J, Jorgensen M, et al: Femoral artery recanalisation with percutaneous angioplasty and segmentally enclosed plasminogen activator. Lancet 1989;1:1106–1108.

112. Hersch SL, Kunelis T, Francis RB Jr: The pathogenesis of accelerated fibrinogenolysis in liver cirrhosis: A critical role for tissue plasminogen activator inhibitor. Blood 1987;69(5):1315–1319.

113. Old RW, Primrose SB: Principles of Gene Manipulation. Oxford, Blackwell Scientific Publications, 1989.

114. Gunzler WA, Steffens GJ, Otting F, Buse G, Flohe L: Structural relationship between human high and low molecular mass urokinase. Hoppe-Seyler's Z Physiol Chem 1982;363:133–141.

115. Holmes WE, Pennica D, Blaber M, et al: Cloning and expression of the gene for pro-urokinase in escherischia coli. Bio/Technology 1985;*3*:923–929.

116. Flohe L: Single-chain urokinase-type plasminogen activators: New hopes for clot-specific lysis. Eur Heart J 1985;*6*:905–908.

117. Vehar GA, Spellman MW, Keyt BA, et al: Characterization studies of human tissue-type plasminogen activator produced by recombinant DNA technology. Cold Spring Harbor Symp Quant Biol 1986;*LI*:551–562.

118. Gunzler WA, Cramer J, Frankus E, Friderichs E, et al: Chemical, enzymological and pharmacological equivalence of urokinase isolated from genetically transformed bacteria and human urine. Arzneim-Forsch/Drug Res 1985;*35*:652–662.

119. Petricciani JC: Regulatory considerations for products derived from the new biotechnology. Pharmacol Manuf 1985;*2*(3):31.

37

INTRAOPERATIVE THROMBOLYTIC THERAPY

GREG R. GOODMAN and PETER F. LAWRENCE

Since the Fogarty catheter was introduced in 1963,[1] it has remained the most commonly employed device for extracting emboli and thrombi in the treatment of acute peripheral artery occlusion. Although the catheter has greatly improved the management of thromboembolic disease, this approach is not uniformly successful and is not without complications. Failure to restore adequate perfusion to the ischemic extremity may be related to residual thrombus remaining in the artery after thrombectomy, occurring as often as 36 to 85 per cent of the time[2,3] or to distal thrombus that is inaccessible to this catheter.[4] It is also difficult to remove thrombus when there is coexisting chronic arterial disease which obstructs passage of the catheter. Furthermore, the catheter preferentially travels into the peroneal artery during thrombectomy because of the vascular anatomy,[5] making it difficult to gain access to either the anterior or posterior tibial vessels and reducing effective thrombectomy of these vessels. Finally, the catheter has been shown to induce endothelial damage,[6] with late arterial stenosis and has been associated with perforation of the vessel during repeated passes of the catheter.[7]

Thrombolytic agents have also been used for more than 20 years to treat acute arterial occlusion. Presently, streptokinase (SK) and urokinase (UK) are the agents most frequently used. Streptokinase, first described in 1933, is derived from streptococci and is much less expensive than other agents. The mechanism of action of SK is through indirect activation of plasminogen via formation of an SK-plasminogen cofactor. Once formed, this cofactor converts plasminogen to plasmin. Because SK is a foreign protein, it may be associated with fever, allergic reactions, and anaphylaxis,[8] and most patients will have antibodies to SK, owing to previous exposure to streptococci. Therefore, when using SK, a loading dose must be given to bind these antibodies.[9]

Urokinase, isolated from human urine or fetal kidney cells, is not a foreign protein and therefore has fewer allergic reactions than SK and does not require a loading dose. Studies have shown that use of UK for thrombolytic therapy is associated with fewer hemorrhagic complications[10] (presumably because of a lesser degree of systemic lysis) and has been reported to be equally or more effective at clot lysis.[10,11] Finally, UK may have an added benefit when used intraoperatively. Since arterial inflow is temporarily stopped during this form of therapy, plasminogen in the extremity is limited to that existing in the limb or supplied by the collateral circulation and this may be a limiting factor in fibrinolysis. Since UK acts directly on plasminogen, all of it can be used for the lytic reaction. Streptokinase, however, requires some of the plasminogen for formation of the cofactor, thus limiting the amount available for lysis. In this situation, higher doses of SK may not improve thrombolysis, but might predispose the patient to hemorrhagic complications because of washout into the systemic circulation. Because of these advantages, urokinase is the agent preferred by many,[8,12] despite its greater cost.

Tissue-type plasminogen activator (tPA), one of a group of newer thrombolytic agents, binds preferentially to fibrin-bound plasminogen in the thrombus, with much less affinity for circulating plasminogen. Theoretically, tPA and agents like it would have less of a tendency to cause systemic fibrinolysis. However, tPA has not been shown be more effective clinically or to further reduce hemorrhagic complications despite this theoretical advantage.[13,14] Newer agents, including acylated streptokinase and single-chain urokinase-type plasminogen activator, have only been used to a limited extent intravenously or intra-arterially, and none have been used intraoperatively as an adjunct to balloon catheter thromboembolectomy. Although the experience with these agents is limited, the risk of associated hemorrhage is not reduced.[14] At present, these agents seem to offer no advantage over UK.

Early use of thrombolytic agents (primarily SK) in the treatment of peripheral artery occlusion involved administration of the agent by intravenous (IV) infusion. To achieve effective thrombolysis using this technique, it is necessary to activate circulating plasminogen and develop a systemic lytic state. This approach, however, often requires prolonged infusions, which predispose the patient to bleeding complications. The risk of hemorrhage often precludes the use of thrombolytic agents in patients with a bleeding diathesis, intracranial disease, uncontrolled hypertension, pregnancy, or those who have undergone recent surgery.[15] Intravenous thrombolysis has been only moderately effective and often must be discontinued owing to bleeding complications that develop during treatment. In a summary of six representative trials of IV infusion of lytic agents, the success rates of IV thrombolysis range from 26 to 81 per cent (mean, 56 per cent) with a 6 to 24 per cent (mean, 14 per cent) occurrence of associated major complications.[15]

Based on work demonstrating that activation of fibrin-bound plasminogen rather than circulating plasminogen is most important in successful thrombolysis,[16] a method of intra-arterial infusion of thrombolytic agents was developed.[17] A catheter is placed percutaneously under radiologic guidance directly into the thrombus for infusion of the thrombolytic agents. Theoretically, this technique not only increases the concentration of agent at the site of thrombosis, increasing the ability to effectively lyse thrombus, but also reduces the amount of agent necessary for lysis (by directly activating the fibrin-bound plasminogen in the clot with less inactivation by circulating inhibitors) and therefore reduces the chance of associated bleeding. When used preoperatively, thrombolytic therapy may reveal lesions responsible for the thrombosis. These lesions can then be repaired percutaneously by balloon dilatation or surgically. Furthermore, thrombus which has been propagated into the distal small vessels may also be lysed. This approach is beneficial in two ways; first, distal runoff is recanalized and bypass graft patency may potentially be improved. Second, recanalized distal vessels may enable bypass or reconstruction to be performed with a high patency and where previously it was not thought possible because of poor runoff.[18,19] The intra-arterial infusion technique does improve the efficacy of these agents, and successful thrombolysis occurs in 66 to 89 per cent,[20] but infusions may require as long as 24 to 36 hours. Bleeding as a result of the development of systemic fibrinolysis still complicates this method of delivery in as many as 22 per cent of treatments. Although this technique initially used low doses (5000 U/hr of UK) for long intervals, recent use of higher doses (100,000 U/hr of UK) for shorter infusion periods appear to be more effective, with fewer hemorrhagic complications. The risk of associated hemorrhage, however, continues to limit the use of this technique to patients who have enough collateral circulation to allow limb survival for 24 to 48 hours (the time usually required for a successful infusion of thrombolytic agents) or who are not surgical candidates because of other underlying diseases.

As early as 1962, the successful use of thrombolytic agents in association with surgical treatment of acute arterial occlusion was described by Cotton et al.[21] After an apparently successful embolectomy, a patient required reoperation the following day for recurrent symptoms of ischemia. The patient's surgical wound was opened, and after an intra-arterial loading dose of 50,000 U of SK had been administered, a catheter was placed in the artery for subsequent infusion of SK. The patient's extremity improved 5 hours after infusing 106,000 additional units of SK. The patient sustained no bleeding complications. In this paper, the use of thrombolytic agents is suggested as an adjunct to surgery if there is ongoing ischemia (or no clinical improvement) and a postembolectomy angiogram reveals residual thrombus in the vessel. In 1964[22] and again in 1974,[23] thrombolytic agents were used at the time of incomplete thrombectomy to aid in establishing reperfusion of an occluded vessel. Although only one of these four patients actually achieved successful lysis of the thrombus, none of these patients sustained hemorrhagic complications related to using thrombolytic agents in association with surgery. Reports have continued to support the use of thrombolytic agents in the perioperative period[24] and as an adjunct to surgical intervention.

The same benefits may also be obtained by the use of thrombolytics intraoperatively as an adjunct to balloon catheter thromboembolectomy. The technique involves first using the Fogarty catheter to remove as much of the more proximal thrombus as possible. Then, with the inflow vessel still occluded by a vascular clamp, a catheter is introduced into the artery and thrombolytic agents administered either by infusion (usually over 30 minutes in a small volume) or slow bolus. Commonly, dosages of 20,000 to 50,000 U of SK or UK are used, followed by an angiogram, and the infusion repeated if there is no improvement. Total doses of 200,000 to 375,000 U of thrombolytic agent have been used. Intraoperative thrombolytic therapy has been associated with improved efficacy and fewer bleeding complications than the preoperative percutaneous technique. This may be in part due to several factors. Performing catheter thromboembolectomy prior to infusion of lytic agents reduces the total amount of thrombus that must be lysed, decreasing the amount of thrombolytic agent used and reducing overall infusion time. Additionally, occlusion of the inflow helps to concentrate the agent at the site of the thrombus and reduce washout.[25,26] This helps to minimize the activation of systemic fibrinolysis, theoretically reducing the incidence of hemorrhagic complications. Angiography, duplex scanning, and angioscopy have identified intravascular thrombus in large and medium sized arteries which can be lysed by intraoperative thrombolysis. Furthermore, reports have shown that use of the Fogarty catheter after thrombolytic therapy removes additional thrombus, which was either missed on earlier passes or had been freed by thrombolysis.[27]

Since 1985, eight studies have been published which describe the use of thrombolytic agents in the operating room as an adjunct to thrombectomy. In one study, which examined the technique in dogs[3] (Table 37–1), 40 hind limbs of 20 mongrel dogs were embolized with thrombus. The dogs were then treated with infusions of either 60,000 U of SK in saline, SK and heparin (5000 U), saline alone, or saline and heparin over either a 30 or 60 minute period. Postinfusion angiograms after the 30 minute infusion showed improvement over baseline in 100 per cent of the SK plus heparin group, 80 per cent in the SK only group, and 20 per cent in the control group. In the 60-minute infusion group, only 20 per cent of the SK group showed improvement, indicating that high concentrations administered over shorter periods of time are more efficacious. There were no associated bleeding complications in any of the groups, supporting the safety and efficacy of the technique. Heparinization of the animals apparently increased the efficacy of the thrombolytic agent without increasing the incidence of hemorrhage.

In seven clinical studies (Table 37–2), the same basic technique was used for limb salvage in patients with acutely ischemic extremities. The proximal vessel is dissected free from the surrounding tissue and isolated. An arteriotomy is then created after obtaining proximal control of the vessel, and balloon catheter thromboembolectomy is performed. Once no more thrombus is retrieved after two consecutive passes of the catheter,[3] the vessel is cannulated with a needle or angiocatheter, and the thrombolytic agent infused into the vessel. During the infusion, the superficial femoral artery (SFA) alone[25] or the SFA and profunda femoris[8] are occluded, decreasing inflow. Variations in technique include differences in the agents used (SK or UK), dosage (which is often based on clinical judgement), method of administration (infusion or bolus), and postoperative anticoagulation (Table 37–3). In these studies, a total of 142 patients underwent thrombolytic therapy for limb salvage after balloon catheter thromboembolectomy had failed. Streptokinase was used in 65 patients and UK used in 77 patients. Total dosages ranged from 20,000 to 250,000 U of SK and 35,000 to 375,000 U UK, most often in multiple doses of 20,000 to 50,000 U. The methods of administration included bolus therapy in five studies and infusions over a 30-minute period in two studies. All but one of the studies used postoperative anticoagulation with heparin in at least some of the patients. All studies included patients with thromboembolic disease of native vessels or autogenous grafts (saphenous vein) and three of the studies included patients with synthetic grafts.

Success rates (Table 37–3), defined by clinical or angiographic improvement postoperatively, were reported in 64 to 100 per cent (mean, 87 per cent) of

TABLE 37–1. EXPERIMENTAL STUDY

Test Group	Number of Limbs	Success	Complications
Control			
Saline alone infusion (30 min)	10	3 total $(20\%)^a$	0
Saline + heparin infusion (30 min)	5		
Experiment			
60,000 U SK infusion (30 min)	15	12 (80%)	0
60,000 U SK + heparin infusion (30 min)	5	5 (100%)	0
60,000 U SK infusion (60 min)	5	1 (20%)	0

[a] Represents total success of both control groups combined (3 of a total of 15 limbs).

TABLE 37–2. SUMMARY OF STUDIES

Author	Number of Patients	Thrombolytic Agent	Dosage	Method	Outcome (% Success)	Complications
Quiñones-Baldrich et al.[25] (1985)	5	SK	20,000–100,000	Infusion	100	None
Cohen et al.[28] (1986)	13	SK	25,000–50,000 (250,000 max)	Bolus	85	2 Major 3 Minor
Norem et al.[27] (1988)	19	SK	50,000 (200,000 max)	Bolus	100	1 Death 2 Minor
Comerota et al.[37] (1989)	38	SK-14 UK-24	50,000 max 150,000 max	Bolus	73	None
Parent et al.[8] (1989)	28	SK-7 UK-21	50,000–150,000 35,000–150,000	Bolus	88	2 Major 1 Minor
Quiñones-Baldrich et al.[12] (1989)	23	SK-7 UK-16	20,000–100,000 150,000–375,000	Infusion	74	1 Minor
Garcia et al.[26] (1990)	16	UK	50,000–100,000	Bolus	87	None

patients. Bleeding complications occurred from 0 to 38 per cent and included minor bleeding such as wound hematomas in seven patients (5 per cent) and major hemorrhage requiring surgery in four (2.8 per cent), resulting in the death of one patient (0.7 per cent). Average success rate when SK was used was 87.5 per cent, and 82 per cent when UK was used. Bleeding was more common when SK was used and included all four major hemorrhagic complications (6.2 per cent), three of which required surgical intervention. There were no major bleeding episodes associated with the use of UK. Six wound hematomas occurred in the SK group (9.2 per cent), while only one wound hematoma (1.3 per cent) was associated with administration of UK. When used as an infusion, therapy was successful in 85 per cent, compared with an 83 per

TABLE 37–3. RESULTS

Author	Agent SK	Agent UK	Success SK (%)	Success UK (%)	Infusion/Bolus	Anticoagulation	Complications SK	Complications UK
Quiñones-Baldrich et al.[25] (1985)	5		100		Yes	Heparin postop	0	
Cohen et al.[28] (1986)	13		85			Yes	Heparin after FIB>150	2 Major 3 Minor 38%	
Norem et al.[27] (1988)	19		100			Yes	Heparin in 12 postop patients	2 Minor 10.5%	
Comerota et al.[37] (1989)	14	24	64	73	Yes	Heparin in selected patients	0	0
Parent et al.[8] (1989)	7	21	83	90	Yes	None	2 Major 28.6% 1 Minor 14.3%	1 Minor 4.8%
Quiñones-Baldrich et al.[12] (1989)	7	16	100	75	Yes	Hep/coumadin in selected patients	1 Minor 14.3%	0
Garcia et al.[26] (1990)		16		87	Yes	Heparin postop		0
Total	65	77	87.5	82			15.4%	1.3%

cent success rate for bolus therapy. The incidence of complications seemed to increase with bolus therapy (9 per cent overall, 4 per cent minor, and 5 per cent major), but most were associated with boluses of SK. Infusion therapy was associated with a 3.6 per cent incidence of bleeding.

Many factors, including the agent used, the method of administration, the optimum dosage needed for rapid, complete lysis, and postoperative anticoagulation make comparisons between studies difficult. In the group of patients represented in these studies, SK appears to be slightly more effective (87.5 per cent) than UK (82 per cent), although differences in patient selection may account for this. All of the major bleeding complications were associated with the use of SK, and although bolus therapy was as effective (83 per cent) as 30-minute infusions (85 per cent), it was associated with a higher incidence of bleeding complications, especially when combined with the use of SK. Bolus therapy with UK appears to be safer, however, with only one minor episode of bleeding occurring in this group.

The dosage of the thrombolytic agent and method of administration remain highly variable and are often determined clinically by close monitoring of the fibrinogen level and coagulation parameters[9,27,28] and by personal experience. Previous studies using thrombolytic agents intra-arterially have documented success with both low-dose[29] and high-dose[30,31] infusions, but higher doses have been shown to lyse thrombus more quickly.[32] Low-dose therapy is more often complicated by hemorrhage owing to the prolonged nature of the infusions and the systemic activation of fibrinogen. Although no specific lab tests have been shown to correlate completely, low fibrinogen levels systemically are associated with bleeding complications. In these studies, all four patients who developed major posttherapy hemorrhage were found to have low fibrinogen levels systemically.[8,28] Theoretically, intraoperative use of moderate-dose, low-volume injections with occlusion of inflow into the extremity would allow higher local concentrations of the agent to be achieved and decrease the amount of washout contributing to systemic fibrinolysis. In these studies, systemic fibrinolysis still occurred, owing either to the specific agent, the concentration used, or the method of administration.

Anticoagulation is used after catheter thromboembolectomy because the vessels are thought to be relatively hypercoagulable from thrombus remaining in the vessels or intimal damage from the catheter. Anticoagulation after thrombolytic therapy is thought to reduce the incidence of rethrombosis,[3,12] improving the success of catheter thrombectomy and thrombolytic agents, but is also thought by many to contribute significantly to hemorrhagic complications.[12] In one study, two episodes of minor postoperative hemorrhage were directly attributable to anticoagulation with heparin.[12] Of the four major bleeding complications, however, all occurred in association with low fibrinogen levels and without heparinization (Table 37–3). From these studies there does not appear to be an increased incidence of hemorrhage when thrombolytic therapy is combined with heparin, but it is not possible to draw specific conclusions because there are many procedural differences between these studies.

Presently, the agent and optimum dosage and the method of administration and use of postoperative anticoagulation during intraoperative thrombolytic therapy are determined by personal experience based on follow-up angiogram and clinical outcome. Future prospective studies are indicated to further evaluate each of these variables to optimize this form of therapy.

ISOLATED EXTREMITY THROMBOLYTIC THERAPY

Although intraoperative thrombolytic agents have been shown to be effective in treating acute peripheral artery occlusion, there is often development of a systemic lytic state and associated hemorrhage still occurs, especially when thrombolysis is combined with major surgery. In addition, some patients require such high doses of lytic agents that bleeding complications are virtually assured. In an effort to decrease the incidence of hemorrhage and further improve efficacy, we have developed a technique for isolating the extremity prior to the infusion of the thrombolytic agents, preventing the agents from activating systemic fibrinolysis. This is based on a technique first described in 1950 for the treatment of melanoma that is confined to the extremity.[33] The femoral vessels are cannulated after a tourniquet has been placed on the proximal portion of the extremity, below the femoral incision. The tourniquet is then inflated, preventing blood flow into or out of the extremity. High doses of the chemotherapeutic agents can then be infused into the extremity via the arterial cannula and retrieved via the venous cannula without ever entering the systemic circulation, thereby avoiding the systemic side effects of these agents, even when infused in very high concentrations.

This technique can be adapted for thromboembolic disease of an extremity to protect the systemic circulation from fibrinolysis and its associated potential for hemorrhage during infusion of high doses of lytic agents. Isolated limb perfusion with thrombolytic agents takes intraoperative therapy one step further by allowing delivery of very high doses of the agent and maximum concentration with little or no washout into the systemic circulation. Using this technique, any of the presently available agents could theoretically be used with a lower risk of bleeding complications. Furthermore, because the extremity is completely isolated and the lytic agent never enters the systemic circulation, even those patients with absolute contraindications to thrombolytic therapy might become candidates. This would be particularly applicable to patients who have recently undergone major surgery, which places them at risk for major hemorrhagic complications with thrombolytic therapy. The dosage or length of infusion can be increased further, improving efficacy without increasing the risk of bleeding. Since high doses of these agents have been demonstrated to lyse thrombus more rapidly than lower doses,[32] infusion of ultra high doses might not only reduce the time necessary for infusion (reducing operative time as well), but also further improve success rates. In fact, similar to the original description for chemotherapy, a perfusion technique could be used with high doses of thrombolytic agents infused into and subsequently removed from the extremity by an infusion pump. Intermittent release of the tourniquet could allow reperfusion of the extremity as thrombus is lysed, preventing further ischemia. Flushing the limb with saline prior to reperfusion would also allow removal of some of the toxic products of ischemia as well and reduce their associated systemic side effects (which may be life threatening in this often debilitated group of patients) when reperfusing the ischemic limb.

Animal Studies

In an attempt to demonstrate that these agents could be isolated to the extremity without causing systemic effects, we performed a study in which 11 dogs underwent isolated limb infusion with extremely high doses of UK (20,000 to 50,000 U/kg). Using the technique described previously, one hind limb of each dog was isolated by means of a tourniquet on the proximal portion of the leg after dissection and isolation of the femoral vessels. After inflation of the tourniquet, the urokinase was injected as a bolus, and at 10, 30, and 60 minutes, blood was obtained from both the isolated limb and the systemic circulation and compared for activation of the lytic system. Parameters measured included the fibrinogen levels, fibrin degradation products, plasminogen, thrombin time, prothrombin time, and partial thromboplastin times.[9] There were two major arms to the experiment, one in which the limb was flushed with saline prior to reperfusion, and the second in which reperfusion was performed without first flushing the limb. Another group served as controls and underwent systemic infusion of similar doses of UK without isolation of the extremity to demonstrate systemic lysis.

In all of the dogs undergoing the isolated limb infusion, the prothrombin, partial thromboplastin, and thrombin times were elevated ($p < 0.001$) in the isolated limb compared to the systemic values (Fig. 37–1). The fibrinogen level was undetectable in the isolated limb ($p < 0.001$) (Fig. 37–2). When compared to baseline, none of the systemic values were significantly different, indicating the absence of a systemic effect. In the group of animals in which the isolated limb was not flushed prior to reperfusion, systemic values were not significantly changed after the tourniquet was removed (although they were slightly increased, they remained in the normal range). The most interesting finding in the experiment was that the plasminogen level in the isolated limb (Fig. 37–3) actually increased significantly at 10 and 30 minutes ($p < 0.001$) and remained elevated 60 minutes ($p < 0.005$) after application of the tourniquet and infusion of the UK. There was no corresponding change in the systemic plasminogen levels from their baseline. At present there is no definite explanation for this

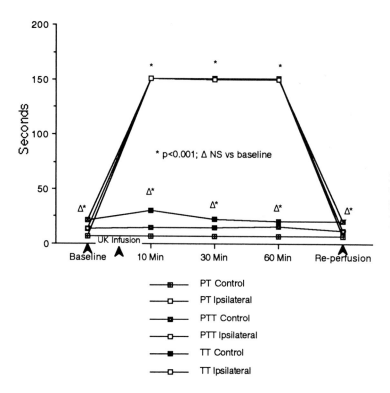

FIGURE 37–1. Prothrombin time, partial thromboplastin time, and thrombin time in the isolated limb (ipsilateral) and systemic (control) circulation.

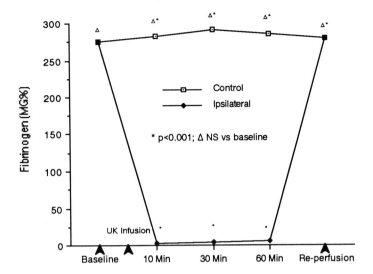

FIGURE 37–2. Fibrinogen concentration in the isolated limb (ipsilateral) and systemic (control) circulation.

finding, which was consistent in all the dogs undergoing the isolated limb therapy.

In the experimental model, urokinase produced a marked lytic state in the isolated limb that was manifested by significant prolongation in the coagulation times and complete depletion of fibrinogen. Corresponding coagulation parameters in the systemic circulation showed no significant changes from baseline, demonstrating that this technique was able to limit the lytic state to the isolated limb. The experiment also demonstrated that the limb could be reperfused without activating systemic fibrinolysis if the isolated limb was first flushed with saline to remove the agent. There is no direct correlation between thrombolysis and the development of a lytic state, but studies have associated clinical success with low fibrinogen levels during thrombolytic therapy.[34] In the same respect, low *systemic* fibrinogen levels have been associated with bleeding complications. The optimum situation then, would be induction of local thrombolysis without creating a systemic reaction; this was attained in this isolated-limb model.

Of the four control animals that underwent high-dose infusions of urokinase systemically (25,000 to 41,000 U), only two showed evidence of systemic

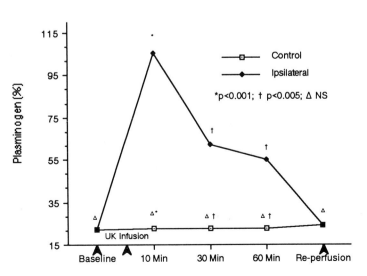

FIGURE 37–3. Plasminogen concentration in the isolated limb (ipsilateral) and systemic (control) circulation.

fibrinolysis. It has been shown in other studies, however, that dogs may be more resistant than humans to the effects of thrombolytic agents on coagulation parameters.[3,35] It is possible that activation of systemic fibrinolysis in the dog model (because of its relative resistance) would require doses of urokinase that are equal to those found in the isolated limb. We did not attempt this during the experiment because these concentrations are much higher than necessary to achieve lysis of clot in the isolated limb.

Clinical Studies

Seven patients (Table 37–4) have undergone high-dose, isolated-limb thrombolytic therapy at our institution. The patients ranged from 39 to 72 years old, and the duration of their preoperative symptoms ranged from several hours to 3 months. All patients had a traditional balloon catheter thrombectomy performed, which was unsuccessful in restoring adequate blood flow to the affected extremity, prior to infusion of the thrombolytic agent. The thrombolytic agent was administered as a slow bolus. Streptokinase was used in two patients (27,000 to 200,000 U) and urokinase (150,000 to 500,000 U) in five patients. This group included two patients who had previously undergone bypass surgery using polytetrafluoroethylene (PTFE) which was no longer patent.

The technique involves placement of a sterile tourniquet, the "banana cuff" disposable pneumatic tourniquet (Zimmer-Jackson, Warsaw, IN) proximal to the arteriotomy used for thrombectomy of the involved limb. If a tourniquet must be placed below a femoral incision, then long cannulas are placed down the vessels, below the tourniquet. The tourniquet is inflated to a pressure at least 50 mm Hg greater than the patient's systemic arterial pressure. The thrombolytic agent, mixed in a small volume of normal saline, is then administered as a slow bolus. The amount of agent used is based clinically on the location and extent of the thrombus, as well as the blood volume. The thrombolytic agent is left in the isolated limb for at most 20 minutes. Prior to reperfusion, as much of the agent as possible is removed by one of two methods. One involves aspiration of blood from the arterial catheter and a large vein (either superficial or deep) while exsanguinating the isolated portion of the limb. The second method involves flushing the agent from the limb by infusing heparinized saline into the arteriotomy until the effluent retrieved from a venous cannula is clear.

One patient had a history of peptic ulcer disease and two patients had undergone major surgery (one, elective coronary revascularization and the second, a carotid-subclavian bypass) within 6 days of thrombolytic therapy. The efficacy of this technique is demonstrated in the description of two patients:

Patient #1

A 66-year-old hispanic man with end-stage renal disease and non–insulin-dependent diabetes mellitus for 20 years underwent cardiac catheterization which revealed severe three-vessel coronary artery disease. Following the procedure, the patient complained of paresthesias and was found to have a cool, pulseless foot. Noninvasive imaging revealed no flow in previously patent posterior tibial or peroneal arteries. The patient was anticoagulated, with improvement in symptoms but without restoration of pulses. The patient underwent uncomplicated coronary revascularization. On the sixth postoperative day, the patient's foot symptoms progressed to severe rest pain. The patient underwent noninvasive vascular studies that suggested left popliteal occlusion (Fig. 37–4A). Subsequent arteriography revealed diffuse

TABLE 37–4. PATIENT SUMMARY

Patient	Age	Duration of Symptom	Etiology	Extremity	Thrombolytic Agent		Systemic Fibrinogen Level		Immediate Outcome	Follow-up
					SK	UK	Before	After		
1.	72	Acute ischemia	Thrombosis distal to fem-pop PTFE graft	Left foot	—	300,000	255	245	Limb salvage	Retrombosed at 1 month (BKA)
2.	71	3 Months	Embolus to tib-peroneal trunk	Left foot	27,000	—	—	—	Limb salvage	Palpable DP pulse at 24 months
3.	59	3 Days	Thrombosis of fem-pop & pop-tib PTFE graft	Left leg	—	500,000	405	405	Limb salvage	Palpable PT pulse at 6 months
4.	39	3 Weeks	Traumatic thrombosis	Right foot	200,000	—	—	—	Initial limb salvage, rethrombosis at 10 days	Amputation at 10 days
5.	66	Acute ischemia	Ax-fem PTFE graft thrombosis, embolus to arm	Right arm	—	150,000	—	400	Limb salvage	Palpable radial pulse at 2 months
6.	66	8 Days	Iliac dissection & popliteal embolus	Left foot	—	250,000	412	412	Limb salvage	Palpable DP pulse at 6 months
7.	56	2 Hours	Subclavian stenosis & embolus to arm	Left arm	—	250,000	460	460	Limb salvage	Hand viable at 6 months

atherosclerotic disease of the distal aorta and iliac vessels bilaterally, with left iliac artery dissection and left popliteal embolus below the knee. The patient was heparinized and underwent popliteal thrombectomy; the popliteal and distal vessels were heavily calcified with diffuse disease, and only a small amount of thrombus could be retrieved, with no clinical improvement in the foot. In an attempt to lyse the remaining distal, small-vessel thrombus, 250,000 U of urokinase was infused into the limb after the leg had been isolated from the systemic circulation by means of a tourniquet. The urokinase was left in the limb for 20 minutes, the venous effluent of the limb was aspirated, and the tourniquet released.

Coagulation studies at baseline, before and after urokinase infusion were measured. Preoperatively the patient's prothrombin time (PT) was 13.1 seconds, the partial thromboplastin time (PTT) was 40 seconds, and the fibrinogen level was 412. After infusion of the urokinase, the PT and PTT were 22.7 seconds and 128.0 seconds in the isolated limb and 16 seconds

Pre-urokinase

Left Thigh

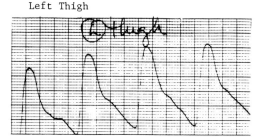

Post-urokinase

Left Thigh

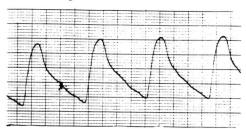

Left Calf

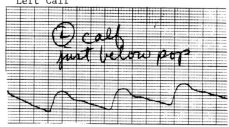

Left Calf

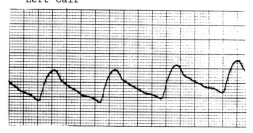

Left Ankle

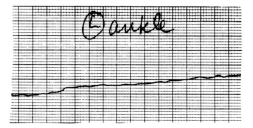

Left Ankle

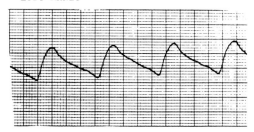

FIGURE 37–4. *A,* Segmental pressures from the left lower extremity before thrombectomy and intraoperative thrombolytic therapy. *B,* Segmental pressures from the left lower extremity 6 months after thrombectomy and intraoperative thrombolytic therapy.

and 56.0 seconds (heparin effect) in the systemic circulation. Two hours postoperatively these values were 14.6 seconds, and 37 seconds, respectively. The fibrinogen level in the isolated limb dropped to 115, while that of the systemic circulation remained at 412. Postoperatively, this patient had no bleeding complications despite the fact that coronary artery bypass grafting had been performed within the previous week. He continues to have a warm foot and has been seen in follow-up at 6 months, doing well and with no symptoms of claudication. He has a palpable dorsalis pedis pulse in this left foot; follow-up noninvasive studies at 6 months postoperatively show marked improvement (Fig. 37–4B).

Patient #7

A 56-year-old woman presented originally to an outside hospital with severe pancreatitis. She responded well initially to rehydration, with decreased abdominal pain and normalization of her amylase level, but subsequently developed pain and cyanosis of the left hand with diminished brachial and radial pulses and necrosis of the tips of the third and fourth digits of that hand. She was transferred to our institution complaining of pain in the left hand extending proximally to the wrist. Physical examination revealed cool, pale fingers with necrosis of the distal third and fourth digits, blistering of the palm, and loss of intrinsic muscle function of the hand. The left brachial pulse was diminished and the radial and ulnar pulses were not palpable.

An angiogram was performed which revealed an ulcerated, high-grade stenosis near the origin of the left subclavian artery and occlusion of the brachial artery with very poor runoff. She subsequently underwent revascularization via a left common carotid to subclavian bypass (using a 6-mm ringed PTFE graft) and thrombectomy of the left brachial, radial, and ulnar arteries. The radial and ulnar pulses were palpable at the end of the procedure and the patient was fully anticoagulated with heparin.

In the early postoperative period, she rethrombosed her left radial artery and required reexploration. After thrombectomy, an intraoperative arteriogram revealed poor distal runoff to the hand (Fig. 37–5). Because the patient had recently undergone major vascular surgery and was at high risk of bleeding due to hemorrhagic pancreatitis, conventional thrombolytic therapy was contraindicated. Therefore, a tourniquet was placed on the proximal left arm and insufflated to 200 mm Hg, effectively isolating the limb from the systemic circulation. Urokinase (250,000 U) was administered by slow bolus into the radial arteriotomy. Fifteen minutes after infusion of the agent, a catheter was placed into a deep vein in the proximal arm, and heparinized saline infused into the arteriotomy until the venous effluent was clear. The tourniquet was then released. Follow-up angiogram demonstrated improved blood flow into the hand (Fig. 37–6).

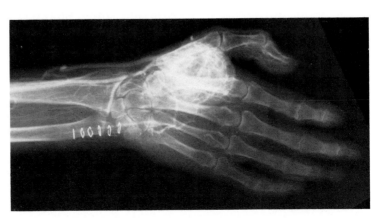

FIGURE 37–5. Intraoperative angiogram demonstrating poor distal runoff to right hand.

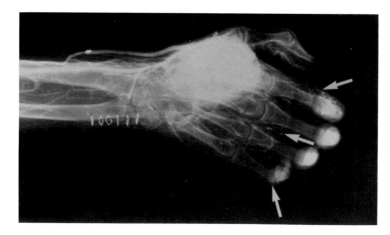

FIGURE 37–6. Intraoperative angiogram following isolated limb infusion of urokinase. Arrows demonstrate improved distal perfusion and vessels not seen on previous angiogram.

Blood samples before surgery revealed a PT of 17.4 (nl = 12.3 to 15.2), a PTT of 55 while heparinized (nl = 32 to 48), a thrombin time (TT) of greater than 150 (control = 15.2), fibrinogen of 460 (nl = 150 to 350), and fibrin degradation products (FDP) of 12 (nl = 0–5). Blood samples obtained from the isolated limb revealed a fibrinogen level of 155, PTT of 38, and FDP of 50 (Table 37–4). After reperfusion of the isolated limb, blood samples from the systemic circulation revealed a PTT of 52, fibrinogen of 460, and FDP of 25. Thrombin time remained unchanged throughout. Postoperatively, the patient's left hand improved except for the stable preexisting dry gangrene of the third and fourth digits. She sustained no systemic or local bleeding complications and after treatment of her pancreatitis, was discharged from the hospital without further problems involving the left upper extremity.

Using the isolated limb perfusion technique, all patients had flow reestablished to the affected limb. Two patients, however, underwent amputation of the affected extremity after they developed recurrent thrombosis which was refractory to further thrombolytic therapy. There were no bleeding complications, even in four patients who were fully anticoagulated, or in the two patients who underwent therapy within 1 week of major surgery. No patients developed a systemic lytic state by fibrinogen levels and coagulation parameters measured postoperatively (Table 37–4).

Plasminogen depletion when high doses of thrombolytic agents are used is a theoretical disadvantage of the isolated-limb technique and might limit complete thrombolysis.[12] Consequently, UK might be a more effective agent in the isolated limb, since it acts directly on plasminogen and does not require additional drug for formation of cofactor. Streptokinase was used successfully in two of the patients in this study, however, without need for additional therapy. In the animal model, there was an unexpected increase in plasminogen levels after the injection of urokinase in all of the isolated limbs of the dogs. Initially suspected to be related to placement of the tourniquet,[36] follow-up studies using the tourniquet without urokinase infusion failed to show an increase in plasminogen in the isolated limb. Currently, there is no explanation for this phenomena, but a rise in plasminogen level during isolated limb thrombolytic therapy would provide increased substrate for thrombolysis. The optimum agent for this technique has yet to be defined and further studies are required for better delineation of the availability and metabolism of plasminogen during isolated-limb thrombolytic therapy.

Since our first description of this technique in 1986, two patients have been reported who underwent isolation of the limb by tourniquet for administration of thrombolytic therapy.[8,37] In one patient, the isolated-limb method was used because the patient had undergone major surgery within the previous 24 hours and she was at increased risk of hemorrhagic complications associated with conventional thrombolytic therapy. One million units of urokinase were infused into her popliteal artery after isolation with a tourniquet and blood flow to the extremity was reestablished without bleeding complications.[37] To overcome the potential for plasminogen depletion, heparinized blood was infused into the leg during treatment, but it is unclear if this was actually necessary or beneficial. In the second patient, despite initial reperfusion, the patient ultimately required amputation.[8] An infusion technique with lower doses of thrombolytic agent (75,000 U over 30 minutes for two infusions) was used in this patient. It is possible that lysis may have been achieved more quickly with higher doses of UK reducing the infusion time and, therefore, total ischemic time.

It is important to realize that the patient population involved in these procedures often has severe underlying chronic atherosclerotic disease. Despite initial reperfusion, many will experience rethrombosis unless the underlying lesion in the diseased vessels can be repaired or bypassed. Anticoagulation postoperatively may help decrease the incidence of rethrombosis, and when the isolated limb technique is used, the risk of associated hemorrhage is reduced because the two drugs have been effectively isolated from each other. Furthermore, use of the newer thrombolytic agents in association with the isolated-limb technique may increase thrombolysis because of their more specific mechanisms of action.

Finally, some surgeons have felt that percutaneous intra-arterial thrombolytic therapy is not cost-effective because the need for intensive care unit (ICU) beds and operative intervention is often required.[38] We believe that the intraoperative methods of thrombolytic therapy, with or without the isolated-limb technique, will be cost-effective despite the use of higher doses of the fibrinolytic agent, primarily because of improved success rates. Reducing operative time, performing concomitant vascular repair or reconstruction at

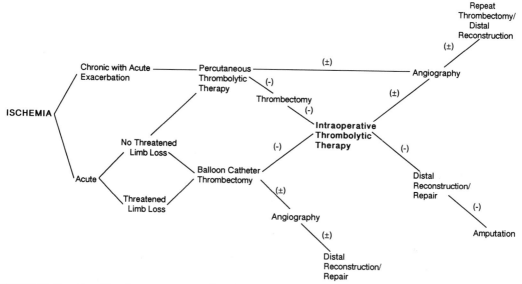

FIGURE 37–7. Algorithm for management of peripheral arterial ischemia. (±) Prior therapeutic step successful, further therapy based on clinical situation. (−) Prior therapeutic step unsuccessful in restoring adequate perfusion.

the time of the infusion will ultimately salvage more limbs, as well as reduce the total number of patient-days in the ICU. Improved success rates with fewer hemorrhagic complications makes intraoperative thrombolytic therapy an effective method of treatment for acute peripheral arterial disease and it should be incorporated as part of the management of these difficult patients (Fig. 37–7).

REFERENCES

1. Fogarty TJ, Cranley JJ, Krause RJ, et al: A method for extraction of arterial emboli and thrombi. Surg Gynecol Obstet 1963;116:241–244.
2. Plecha FR, Pories WJ: Intra-operative angiography in the immediate assessment of arterial reconstruction. Arch Surg 1972;105:902–907.
3. Quiñones-Baldrich JW, Ziomek S, Henderson TC, Moore WS: Intraoperative fibrinolytic therapy: Experimental evaluation. J Vasc Surg 1986;4:229–236.
4. Dunnant JH, Edwards WS: Small vessel occlusion in the extremity after various periods of arterial obstruction: An experimental study. Surgery 1973;73:240–245.
5. Short D, Vaughn GD III, Jachimczyk J, et al: The anatomic basis for the occasional failure of transfemoral balloon catheter thromboembolectomy. Ann Surg 1979;190:555–556.
6. Childi CC, DePalma RG: Atherogenic potential of the embolectomy catheter. Surgery 1978;83:549–557.
7. Foster JH, Carter JH, Graham CP Jr, Edwards WH: Arterial injuries secondary to the Fogarty catheter. Ann Surg 1970;171:971–978.
8. Parent FN, Bernhard VM, Pabst TS III, et al: Fibrinolytic treatment of residual thrombus after catheter embolectomy for severe lower limb ischemia. J Vasc Surg 1989;9:153–160.
9. Shafer KE, Santoro SA, Sobel BE, Jaffe AS: Monitoring activity of fibrinolytic agents. Am J Med 1984;76:879–886.
10. van Breda A, Katzen BT, Deutsch AS: Urokinase versus streptokinase in local thrombolysis. Radiology 1987;165:109–111.
11. Belkin M, Belkin B, Buckman CA, et al: Intra-arterial fibrinolytic therapy. Arch Surg 1986;121:769–773.
12. Quiñones-Baldrich WJ, Baker JD, Busuttil RW, et al: Intraoperative infusion of lytic drugs for thrombotic complications of revascularization. J Vasc Surg 1989;10:408–417.
13. Meyerovitz MF, Goldhaber SZ, Reagan K, et al: Recombinant tissue-type plasminogen activator versus urokinase in peripheral arterial and graft occlusions: A randomized trial. Radiology 1990;175:75–78.
14. Marzelle J, Combe S, Gigou F, Samama M: Results of thrombolysis in the treatment of arterial ischemia of the limbs according to mode of administration. Int Angio 1989;8:179–187.
15. Comerota AJ: Intra-arterial thrombolytic therapy. In Comerota AJ, ed: Thrombolytic Therapy. Orlando, Grune and Stratton, 1988;125–152.
16. Alkjaersig N, Fletcher AP, Sherry S: The mechanism of clot dissolution by plasmin. J Clin Invest 1959;38:1086.
17. McNicol GP, Reid W, Bain WH, Douglas AS: Treatment of peripheral arterial occlusion by streptokinase perfusion. Br Med J 1963;1:1508.
18. Perrson AV, Thompson JE, Patman RD: Streptokinase as an adjunct to arterial surgery. Arch Surg 1973;107:779–784.
19. Hurley JJ, Burrell MJ, Auer AI, et al: Surgical implications of fibrinolytic therapy. Am J Surg 1984;148:830–835.
20. Comerota AJ: Intra-arterial thrombolytic therapy. In Comerota AJ, ed: Thrombolytic Therapy. Orlando, Grune and Stratton, 1988;131.
21. Cotton LT, Flute PT, Tsapogas MJC: Popliteal artery thrombosis treated with streptokinase. Lancet 1962;2:1081–1083.
22. Tsapogas MJ: The role of fibrinolysis in the treatment of arterial thrombosis: Experimental and clinical aspects. Ann R Coll Surg Eng 1964;24:293–313.
23. Fiessinger JN, Vayssairat M, Juillet Y, et al: Local urokinase in arterial thromboembolism. Angiology 1974;31:715–720.
24. Chaise LS, Comerota AJ, Soulen RL, Rubin RN: Selective intra-arterial streptokinase therapy in the immediate postoperative period. JAMA 1982;247:2397–2400.
25. Quiñones-Baldrich WJ, Zierler RE, Hiatt JC: Intraoperative fibrinolytic therapy: An adjunct to catheter thromboembolectomy. J Vasc Surg 1985;2:319–326.
26. Garcia R, Saroyan RM, Senkowsky J, et al: Intraoperative intra-arterial urokinase infusion as an adjunct to Fogarty catheter embolectomy in acute arterial occlusion. Surg Gynecol Obstet 1990;171:201–205.
27. Norem RF, Short DH, Kernstein MD: Role of intraoperative fibrinolytic therapy in acute arterial occlusion. Surg Gynecol Obstet 1988;167:87–91.

28. Cohen LH, Kaplan M, Bernhard VM: Intraoperative streptokinase. Arch Surg 1986;*121*:708–715.

29. Dotter CT, Rosch J, Seaman AJ: Selective clot lysis with low-dose streptokinase. Radiology 1984;*111*:31–37.

30. McNamara TO, Fischer JR: Thrombolysis of peripheral arterial and graft occlusions: Improved results using high-dose urokinase. AJR 1985;*144*:769–775.

31. Gurll NJ, Callahan W, Hufnagel HV: High-dose, short-term local urokinase for clearing femoral thrombi by vasodilation and thrombolysis. J Surg Res 1976;*20*:381–388.

32. Bookstein J, Saldinger E: Accelerated thrombolysis: In vitro evaluation of agents and methods of administration. Invest Radiol 1985;*20*:731–735.

33. Cumberlin R, DeMoss E, Lassus M, Friedman M: Isolation perfusion for malignant melanoma of the extremity: A review. J Clin Oncol 1985;*3*:1022–1031.

34. Conrad J, Meyer SM: Theoretical and practical considerations on laboratory monitoring of thrombolytic therapy. Semin Thromb Hemost 1987;*13*:212–222.

35. Lijnen HR, DeWreede K, Demarsin E, Collen D: Biological and thrombolytic properties of proenzyme and active forms of human urokinase-IV. Variability in fibrinolytic response of plasma of several mammalian species. Thromb Haemost 1984;*52*:31–33.

36. Mullick S: The tourniquet in operations upon the extremities. Surg Gynecol Obstet 1978;*146*:821–825.

37. Comerota AJ, White JV, Grosh JD: Intraoperative intra-arterial thrombolytic therapy for salvage of limbs in patients with distal arterial thrombosis. Surg Gynecol Obstet 1989;*169*:283–289.

38. Dacey LJ, Dow RD, McDaniel MD, et al: Cost-effectiveness of intra-arterial thrombolytic therapy. Arch Surg 1988;*123*:1218–1223.

38

THROMBOLYTIC THERAPY IN ARTERIAL AND GRAFT OCCLUSION

ANTHONY J. COMEROTA

The era of intravascular administration of thrombolytic agents had its true beginning in 1955, when Tillett et al. produced temporary fibrinolytic activity in human blood by using a refined preparation of streptokinase.[1] Subsequently, in a classic study, Sherry and his associates established that the primary and most sensitive mechanism for thrombolysis involves activation of intrinsic clot plasminogen.[2] They described how to induce and maintain a systemic thrombolytic state in humans[3] and applied this method to the treatment of patients with myocardial infarction and venous thromboembolic disorders.[4] Since the most sensitive means of dissolving clot is the activation of plasminogen within the matrix of the clot, which is that portion bound to fibrin, it is reasonable to conclude that delivery of the lytic agent directly to the clot would be the most efficient means of achieving clot dissolution (Fig. 38–1).

If the plasminogen within the thrombus is activated to plasmin, one can expect efficient lysis to occur. This is due to the high concentration of plasmin and the absence of inhibitors of either the activator or plasmin itself (Fig. 38–2). Likewise, systemic activation of plasminogen results in breakdown of fibrinogen, clotting factors, and other plasma proteins. The first attempt at the direct local delivery of a fibrinolytic agent for arterial thrombosis was made by McNicol and colleagues[5] almost 30 years ago. The technique of catheter-directed intra-arterial delivery of thrombolytic agents was promoted by Dotter,[6] and the good results of low-dose streptokinase infusions reported by Katzen and van Breda[7] drew the attention of interventional radiologists and vascular surgeons.

Techniques for the intra-arterial delivery of lytic agents have been refined over the past decade,[6–35] to the point where arterial occlusions can be assessed to predict the likelihood of clot lysis and to insure the most efficient delivery of the lytic agent to the occluding thrombus. Treatment times of 2 to 5 days have been reduced to 8 hours or less.

The issues that remain, regarding catheter-directed lytic therapy, include: (1) whether the occlusion of the vessel or graft can be lysed; (2) whether the risk of thrombolysis has been substantially reduced during recent years; and (3) whether there is long-term benefit from lysis in terms of the patient's ultimate revascularization.

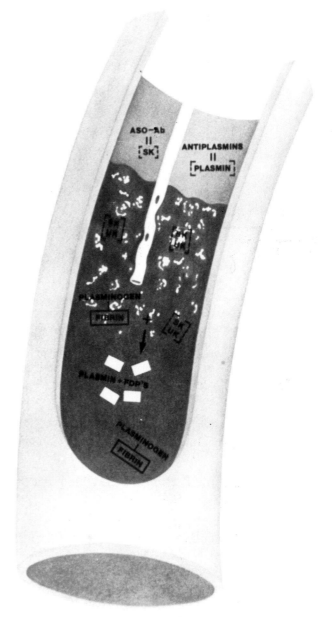

FIGURE 38-1. This schematic illustrates the principle of intra-arterial delivery of thrombolytic agents to the occluding thrombus. The lytic agent interacts with the fibrin-bound plasminogen. If streptokinase is infused, it must bind to plasminogen to form the activator complex, SK-plasminogen, which then acts on the fibrin-bound plasminogen to form plasmin. If urokinase (UK) or recombinant tissue-type plasminogen activator (rt-PA) is used, the fibrin-bound plasminogen will be activated directly. The active agent, plasmin, dissolves fibrin, with the release of fibrin degradation products. If SK is used and escapes into the systemic circulation, it will be bound (at least in part) by antistreptococcal antibodies, thereby inactivating the streptokinase molecule. If small amounts of plasmin escape into the circulation, it will be bound by circulating antiplasmins, thereby inactivating its systemic effect. If, however, appreciable amounts of the lytic agent or appreciable amounts of plasmin escape into the systemic circulation, a systemic fibrinolytic effect will occur.

Can Occluded Arteries and Grafts be Lysed?

The answer to the question, "Can occluded arteries or grafts be lysed?" is undeniably yes. This has been confirmed by numerous investigators (Table 38-1). Factors used to predict lysis in the individual patient are listed in Table 38-2. The importance of the "guide wire test" and proper catheter position cannot be overstated and is further underscored by the data in Table 38-3. In the majority it is possible to predict at the time of angiography whether successful lysis can be achieved. The passage of a guide wire into and through the occlusion indicates that thrombus is at least in part responsible for the occlusion. Seating the infusion catheter into the thrombus insures delivery of the lytic agent to the clot and lysis can be expected. These results have been substantiated by

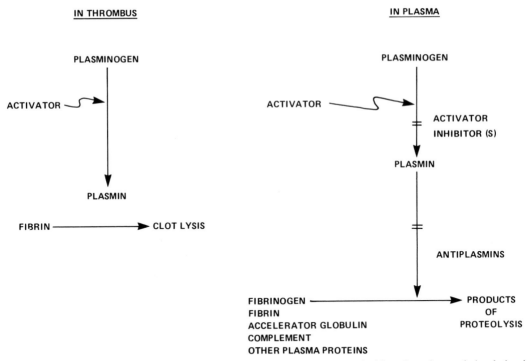

FIGURE 38–2. Schematic of the plasminogen-plasmin system as it occurs inside a thrombus and circulating in plasma. (Reproduced with permission from Comerota AJ, ed: Thrombolytic Therapy. Orlando, Grune & Stratton, 1989.)

numerous investigators and emphasizes that the most effective activation of fibrin-bound plasminogen occurs when the drug is delivered into the thrombus.

Can the Thrombus be Dissolved Safely?

The evolution of the direct infusion techniques over the past decade have increased the efficiency of clot lysis.[29] Increasing the initial dose and the infusion dose has served to decrease infusion time.[21,22,25] Increasing experience with urokinase (UK) has demonstrated improved rates of lysis in addition to fewer complications compared to streptokinase (SK).[20–22] The improved safety may be due to the more direct mechanism of action in addition to shorter infusion times.[30] We have likewise observed improved success rates with fewer complications with the use of UK. Concurrent heparin infusion prevents catheter-associated thrombosis. When heparin was given with SK, however, bleeding complications were excessive. Bleeding complications are the result of lysis of a hemostatic thrombus, the coagulopathy induced by the drugs, or a

TABLE 38–1. SHORT-TERM EFFICACY AND SAFETY OF CATHETER-DIRECTED INTRA-ARTERIAL THROMBOLYSIS[a]

Drug	Number	Authors (refs)	Average Duration of Infusion	Success	Major Complications
SK	542	6–24	41 hours	354 (65%)	112 (21%)
UK	277	18–26	28 hours	222 (80%)	32 (12%)
rt-PA	137	26–28	7 hours	117 (*85%)	11 (8%)

[a] Pooled data from representative studies.

**TABLE 38–2. FACTORS PREDICTIVE OF SUCCESS OF CATHETER-
DIRECTED INTRA-ARTERIAL THROMBOLYSIS**

	Likelihood of Successful Lysis	
Factor	High	Low
Guide wire	Passes into clot	Cannot pass
Duration of occlusion	Short (hours–days)	Long (weeks)
Location of occlusion	Proximal	Distal
Distal vessels (arteriogram)	Visualized	Not visualized
Distal Doppler signals	Audible	None
Relative contraindications	None/few	Some/many

combination of both. We've observed that the most serious bleeding complications have occurred in patients with the most profound induced coagulopathy. Five major bleeding complications, including two fatal intracranial hemorrhages, have occurred in our institution during the past 10 years. In each instance, the patient's fibrinogen was less than 50 mg/dl. No patient who had the fibrinogen maintained above 100 mg/dl had a serious hemorrhagic complication during lytic infusions. I do not think that fibrinogen per se is singularly responsible for hemostasis; rather, it represents the status of the other clotting factors, which are also broken down by the lytic agents. While some of our patients had profound hypofibrinogenemia without suffering a bleeding complication, severe hypofibrinogenemia identified the patient with the most severe coagulopathy induced by the lytic agent and drew attention to those at highest risk of a bleeding complication.

Early experience with tissue-type plasminogen activator (tPA) indicates that lysis can be achieved even more rapidly than that observed with UK.[26–28] Whether this translates into improved patency rates or reduced complications remains to be established. Despite high fibrin affinity, hypofibrinogenemia occurs. Therefore, patients manifest systemic lytic effects with regionally delivered rt-PA, and the same guidelines must be observed when tPA is used as with the other lytic agents.

Is Lysis of an Occluded Artery or Bypass Graft of Significant Benefit to a Patient's Ultimate Revascularization?

This question is most critical when assessing intra-arterial delivery of lytic agents for the treatment of occluded arteries and/or bypass grafts. Regaining

**TABLE 38–3. EARLY RESULTS OF CATHETER-DIRECTED LYTIC
THERAPY AT TEMPLE UNIVERSITY HOSPITAL[a]**

	Success	Failure
Guide-wire test		
Passed	93% (14 of 15)	7% (1 of 15)
Not passed	0% (0 of 5)	100% (5 of 5)
Catheter position		17% (4 of 24)
In thrombus	83% (20 of 24)	86% (6 of 7)
Above thrombus	14% (1 of 7)	

[a] Data indicate results achieved in patients treated prior to use of guide-wire test and catheter position as criteria for therapy.

patency for short periods of time only to have a patient reocclude appears shortsighted, and is of no lasting benefit. On the other hand, if lysis can be achieved and perfusion restored with the subsequent identification and correction of a focal underlying lesion, thereby salvaging the patient's native artery or primary bypass graft, few would argue that dissolving the underlying clot is of benefit. Belkin et al.,[31] Wolfson et al.,[13] and Sicard et al.[32] have reported disappointingly poor long-term patency following lysis of occluded arteries and grafts. Others, however, have reported substantially better long-term results.[21,33]

The key to prolonging patency following catheter-directed thrombolysis is the identification and correction of the underlying lesion (Figs. 38–3 and 38–4). The concept that the underlying etiology of graft failure be corrected must be emphasized. This was initially brought to our attention by McNamara and Bomberger[33] when they showed that after thrombolysis, patients who left the hospital without a persistent stenosis had enviable 6-month patency rates compared to those who had uncorrected underlying disease at the time of discharge. This was true for native arteries and bypass grafts. These results were further confirmed by Gardiner et al.[21] In treating patients with graft failure, it is also important to appreciate the high incidence of an underlying hypercoagulable state. If an underlying coagulopathy is not identified and treated, rethrombosis will occur. Reviewing the literature on intra-arterial delivery of thrombolytic agents, patients are variously treated either with anticoagulation, platelet inhibitors, or without any attention to modifying the hemostatic process. I believe that in the absence of contraindications, all patients suffering graft failure require anticoagulation, unless uncompromised revascularization can be achieved with autogenous tissue.

Graor et al.[36] compared catheter-directed thrombolysis followed by operative graft revision to operative (balloon catheter) thrombectomy, with repair of the lesion presumed to be responsible for the graft thrombosis. Patency rates were significantly higher and amputation rates significantly lower in patients who underwent thrombolysis prior to revision of the bypass graft. These data suggest that preoperative knowledge of the underlying lesion causing thrombosis facilitates definitive correction and might also suggest that pharmacologic thrombectomy is more effective than mechanical thrombectomy. A question that remains, however, is whether any thrombosed bypass graft should undergo thrombectomy (either mechanical or pharmacologic) followed by appropriate operative revision, or; should the patient with a thrombosed bypass be offered an entirely new bypass procedure? We have observed that early failure (1 week to 1 year) of an autogenous infrainguinal bypass can be successfully treated with intra-arterial lytic therapy; however, reocclusions are common (Fig. 38–3). This likely represents extensive underlying arterial disease or a badly compromised graft. This observation has been substantiated by Gardiner et al.[21] In their series, the majority of grafts that failed within 1 month of placement could be recanalized. However, only 33 per cent of those initially lysed were patent at 3 months. It appears that autogenous grafts which fail in the early postoperative period (in the absence of an easily demonstrable and correctable technical problem) are likely doomed to failure. Likewise, it has also been our observation that vein grafts occluding late (2 or more years after placement) are likely to have an underlying lesion which is focal and more easily correctable, with the graft remaining an effective conduit. (Fig. 38–4)

When evaluating the efficacy of "thrombolysis," one must look critically at the technique used to correct the underlying lesion. It is increasingly apparent

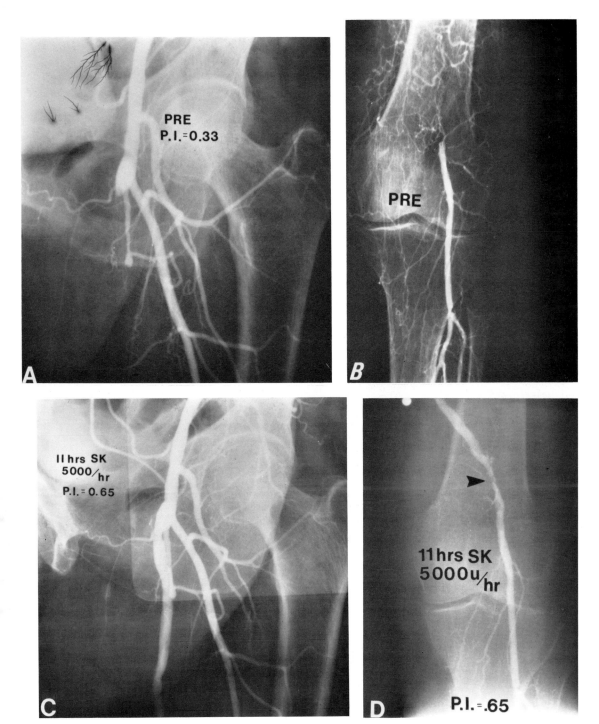

FIGURE 38–3. This is an example of one of the patients treated early in our experience, and is illustrative of data which would subsequently evolve. The arteriogram of this 76-year-old patient is consistent with her clinical presentation of acute occlusion of a femoropopliteal bypass placed 7 months earlier (*A, B*). The patient presented with ischemic rest pain and her ankle-brachial index (ABI) was 0.33. The proximal stump of the occluded graft (*A*) and the patient's popliteal artery (*B*) was visualized. After 11 hours of a low-dose streptokinase infusion, the graft regained patency and the patient achieved an ABI of 0.65 (*C*). A stenosis is noted at the distal anastomosis (*D*) as indicated by the arrow. (*Figure continued*)

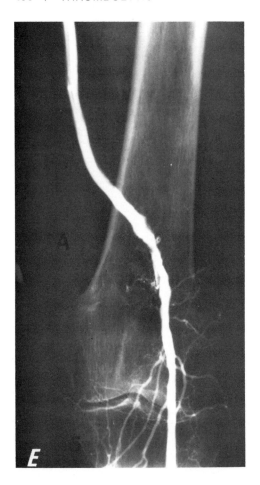

FIGURE 38–3. (*Continued*) A repeat arteriogram following percutaneous balloon dilation indicates a good angiographic result (*E*). The popliteal pulse was easily palpable and the patient's ABI was 0.95. The progressive hemodynamic improvement obtained with dissolution of the thrombus followed by dilation of the associated stenosis is illustrated by the improved ABIs and pulse volume recordings (*F*). Unfortunately, this patient went on to progressive restenosis of her bypass graft over the next 3 months as a result of the distal graft lesion. An operative revision of the patient's bypass was performed and the graft remained patent until the patient's death 5 years later. (Reproduced with permission from Comerota AJ, ed: Thrombolytic Therapy. Orlando, Grune & Stratton, 1989.)

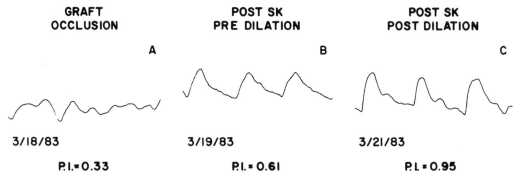

F

that percutaneous techniques are less effective than definitive operative correction of lesions which place grafts in jeopardy of failure.[37-39] It is obvious that the method chosen to correct the underlying lesions is the predominant factor responsible for long-term patency. This is clearly illustrated by the examples shown in Figures 38–3 and 38–4 and the data in Table 38–4. Developing data indicate that percutaneous techniques are inferior to operative revision of the failing autogenous bypass graft.

FIGURE 38–4. This patient illustrates the importance of proper catheter position and reaffirms that regional delivery of a lytic agent dissolves thrombus more effectively than systemic infusion. This patient presented with a 1-week history of ischemic rest pain following occlusion of her femoropopliteal saphenous vein bypass graft (*0*). The catheter was positioned just above the proximal anastomosis at the origin of the profunda femoris artery (arrow). After 20 hours of infusion, only 3 to 4 inches of the proximal thrombus had lysed despite the patient being systemically lytic for at least 16 of the 20 hours. (*20 hr*) The catheter was then advanced into the saphenous vein graft and positioned with the tip at the level of the thrombus. Following an additional 2 hours of infusion, significant lysis had occurred. (*22 hr*) After continuing the infusion overnight, the entire thrombus lysed and the graft regained patency. The distal graft fibrosis responded well to percutaneous balloon dilation. The sclerotic venous valve (arrow) did not respond to balloon dilation, (*postdilation*) however, but was easily excised and a vein patch angioplasty performed. The patient had a good dorsalis pedis pulse at the completion of the operative procedure and had normal pulse waves and ABIs. The patient's graft remained patent until she suffered a fatal myocardial infarction 3.5 years later. (Reproduced with permission from Comerota AJ, ed: Thrombolytic Therapy. Orlando, Grune & Stratton, 1989.)

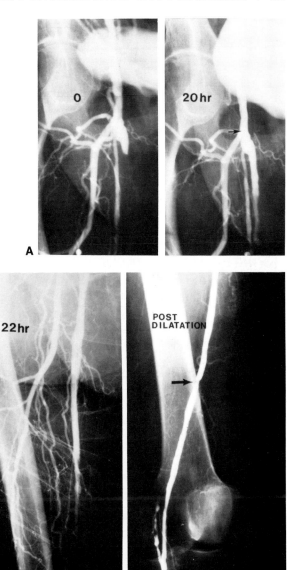

A strong case has been made recently for intra-arterial thrombolysis for the treatment of arterial and graft occlusion.[40,41] It was shown that the initial success of thrombolysis was independent of patient age, graft material, duration of occlusion, or site of distal anastomosis.[37] Although recent results are good, with low complication rates, a control group is not available for comparison to any of the thrombolytic groups. Comparing current thrombolysis results to historical data is not acceptable, and does not answer the question. The low complication rates reported in recent series likewise are not uniformily experienced. Results of a multi-institutional survey was published several years ago that reported treatment failure in 50 per cent of cases, significant hemorrhage in 20 per cent, major amputation in 16 per cent, and a 2.5 per cent mortality.[42] Additionally, Dacey et al.[43] demonstrated that intra-arterial thrombolysis did not result in cost savings when compared with surgical revascularization; and

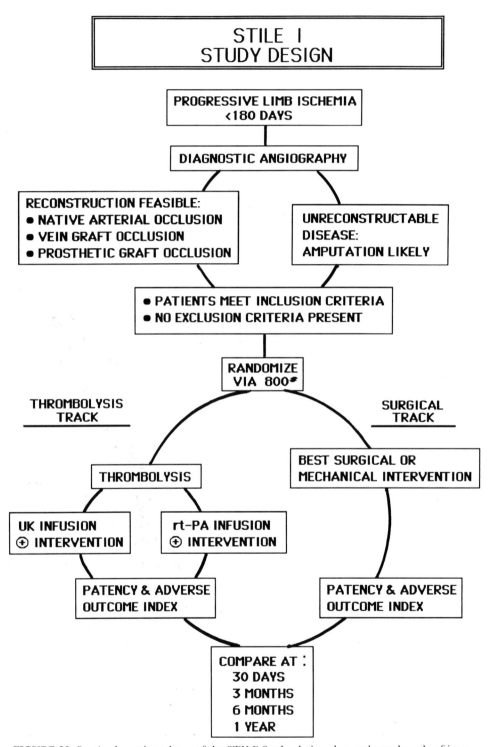

FIGURE 38–5. A schematic pathway of the STILE Study, designed to evaluate the role of intra-arterial thrombolysis for the treatment of patients with arterial and graft occlusion.

TABLE 38–4. THE THREATENED FEMOROPOPLITEAL/TIBIAL AUTOGENOUS BYPASS: COMPARISON OF THE DURABILITY OF TECHNIQUES OF GRAFT REVISION

Author (ref)	5-Year Durability	
	Balloon Dilation	Operative Revision
Bandyk et al.[37] (1991)	50% (9 of 18)	86% (55 of 64)
Perler et al.[38] (1990)	22% (4 of 18)[a]	62% (5 of 9)
Cohen et al.[39] (1986)	43% (3 of 7)	82% (18 of 22)
Total	37% (16 of 43)	82% (78 of 95)

[a] 3-year durability.

when failure rates were considered, thrombolysis was more expensive. None of the above studies are conclusive, but only serve to emphasize the existing questions.

There are clearly instances when intra-arterial thrombolysis offers substantial benefit over available surgical alternatives. Unfortunately, no prospective study is available to assist clinicians in identifying which patients are most appropriately treated by lytic therapy and which should have surgical revascularization. The STILE study (Surgery or Thrombolysis for the Ischemic Lower Extremity), a prospective, randomized, controlled trial, is currently underway and addresses the important question as to whether intra-arterial thrombolytic therapy has a place in the treatment of patients with lower extremity arterial and graft occlusion. If patients do not have contraindications to either thrombolytic therapy or surgical intervention, they will be randomized to either intra-arterial thrombolysis or best surgical/mechanical intervention following complete angiography. Further randomization of the thrombolysis arm will occur, with patients being treated with either rt-PA or urokinase. Endpoints for analysis include patency and an adverse outcome index. This important multi-institutional study is underway, and accrual of 750 patients is expected within the next 18 months. The study design is schematically illustrated in Figure 38–5. The resulting data will likely establish the definitive place of intra-arterial thrombolysis for the treatment of patients with lower extremity arterial and graft occlusion.

REFERENCES

1. Tillett WS, Johnson AJ, McCartey WR: The intravenous infusion of the streptococcal fibrinolytic principle (streptokinase) into patients. J Clin Invest 1955;*34*:169.
2. Alkjaersig N, Fletcher AP, Sherry S: The mechanism of clot dissolution by plasmin. J Clin Invest 1959;*38*:1086.
3. Fletcher AP, Aljaersig N, Sherry S: The maintenance of a sustained thrombolytic state in man: I. Induction and effects. J Clin Invest 1959;*38*:1096.
4. Fletcher AP, Sherry S, Alkjaersig N: The maintenance of a sustained thrombolytic state in man: II. Clinical observations on patients with myocardial infarction and other thromboembolic disorders. J Clin Invest 1959;*38*:1111.
5. McNicol GP, Reid W, Bain WH, Douglas AS: Treatment of peripheral arterial occlusion by streptokinase perfusion. Br Med J 1963;*1*:1508.
6. Dotter CT, Rosch J, Seamen AJ: Selective clot lysis with low dose streptokinase. Radiology 1974;*111*:31.
7. Katzen BT, van Breda A: Low dose streptokinase in the treatment of arterial occlusions. AJR 1981;*36*:1171–1178.
8. Totty WG, Gilula LA, McClennan BL, et al: Low dose intravascular fibrinolytic therapy. Radiology 1982;*143*:59–69.

9. Berni GA, Bandyk DF, Zierler E, et al: Streptokinase treatment of acute arterial occlusion. Ann Surg 1983;*198*:185–191.

10. Mori KW, Bookstein JJ, Heeney DJ, et al: Selective streptokinase infusion: Clinical and laboratory correlates. Radiology 1983;*148*:677–682.

11. Becker GJ, Rabe FE, Richmond BD, et al: Low dose fibrinolytic therapy: Results and new concepts. Radiology 1983;*148*:663–670.

12. Katzen BT, Edwards KC, Albert AS, et al: Low dose fibrinolysis in peripheral vascular disease. J Vasc Surg 1984;*1*:718–722.

13. Wolfson RH, Kumpe DA, Rutherford RB: Role of intra-arterial streptokinase in the treatment of arterial thromboembolism. Arch Surg 1984;*119*:697–702.

14. van Breda A, Robinson JC, Feldman L, et al: Local thrombolysis in the treatment of arterial graft occlusions. J Vasc Surg 1984;*1*:103–112.

15. Kakkasseril JS, Cranley JJ, Arbaugh JJ, et al: Efficacy of low dose streptokinase in acute arterial occlusion and graft thrombosis. Arch Surg 1985;*120*:427–429.

16. Graor ARA, Risius B, Denny KM, et al: Local thrombolysis in the treatment of thrombosed arteries, bypass grafts, and arteriovenous fistulae. J Vasc Surg 1985;*2*:406–414.

17. Fong H, Downs A, Lye C, Morrow I: Low dose intra-arterial streptokinase infusion therapy of peripheral arterial occlusions and occluded vein grafts. Can J Surg 1986;*29*(4):259–262.

18. van Breda A, Katzen BT, Deutsch AF: Urokinase vs streptokinase in local thrombolysis. Radiology 1987;*165*:109–111.

19. Koltun WA, Gardiner GA, Harrington DP, et al: Thrombolysis in the treatment of peripheral arterial vascular occlusions. Arch Surg 1987;*122*:901–905.

20. Belkin M, Belkin B, Bucknam CA, et al: Intra-arterial fibrinolytic therapy. Efficacy of streptokinase vs urokinase. Arch Surg 1986;*121*:7659–773.

21. Gardiner GA, Harrington DP, Koltun W, Wittemore A, Mannick JA, Levin DC: Salvage of occluded bypass grafts by means of thrombolysis. J Vasc Surg 1989;*9*:426–431.

22. Traughber PD, Cook PS, Micklos TJ, Miller FJ: Intra-arterial fibrinolytic therapy for popliteal and tibial artery obstruction: Comparison of streptokinase and urokinase. AJR 1987;*149*:453–456.

23. Price C, Jacocks MA, Tytle T: Thrombolytic therapy in acute arterial thrombosis. Am J Surg 1988;*156*:488–491.

24. O'Donnell TF, Coleman JC, Sentissi J, et al: Comparison of direct intra-arterial streptokinase to urokinase infusion in the management of failed infrainguinal e-PTFE grafts. Medical and Surgical Management of Peripheral Vascular Disease Symposium, Colorado Springs, Colorado, April 20–22, 1990.

25. McNamara TO, Fischer JR: Thrombolysis of peripheral arterial and graft occlusions: Improved results using high dose urokinase. AJR 1985;*144*:769–755.

26. Myerovitz MR, Goldhaber SZ, Reagan K, et al: Recombinant tissue-type plasminogen activator versus urokinase in peripheral arterial and graft occlusions: A randomized trial. Radiology 1990;*175*:75–78.

27. Graor RA, Risius B, Lucas FV, et al: Thrombolysis with recombinant human tissue-type plasminogen activators in patients with peripheral artery and bypass thrombosis. Circulation 1986;74(suppl 1):115–120.

28. Verstraete M, Hess H, Mahler F, et al: Femoro-popliteal artery thrombolysis with intra-arterial infusion of recombinant tissue-type plasminogen activator—report of a pilot trial. Eur J Vasc Surg 1988;*2*:155–159.

29. van Breda A, Katzen BT: Radiologic aspects of intra-arterial thrombolytic therapy. *In* Comerota AJ, ed: Thrombolytic Therapy. Orlando, Grune & Stratton, 1988;99–124.

30. Comerota AJ: Urokinase. *In* Messerli FH, ed: Cardiovascular Drug Therapy. WB Saunders Co., Philadelphia, 1990:1470–1479.

31. Belkin M, Donaldson MC, Wittemore AD, et al: Observations on the use of thrombolytic agents for thrombotic occlusion of infrainguinal vein grafts. J Vasc Surg 1990;*11*:289–296.

32. Sicard G, Schier JJ, Totty WG, et al: Thrombolytic therapy for acute arterial occlusion. J Vasc Surg 1985;*2*:65–78.

33. McNamara TO, Bomberger RA: Factors affecting initial and 6 month patency rates after intra-arterial thrombolysis with high dose urokinase. Am J Surg 1986;*152*:709.

34. Graor RA, Risius B, Young JR, et al: Peripheral artery and bypass graft thrombolysis with recombinant human tissue-type plasminogen activator. J Vasc Surg 1986;*3*:115.

35. Comerota AJ, Rubin R, Tyson R, et al: Intra-arterial thrombolytic therapy in peripheral vascular disease. Surg Gynecol Obstet 1987;*165*:1–8.

36. Graor RA, Risius B, Young JR, et al: Thrombolysis of peripheral arterial bypass grafts: Surgical thrombectomy compared with thrombolysis. J Vasc Surg 1988;*7*:347–355.

37. Bandyk DF, Bergamini TM, Towne JB, Schmitt DD, Seabrook GR: Durability of vein graft revision: The outcome of secondary procedures. J Vasc Surg 1991;*13*:200–210.

38. Perler BA, Osterman FA, Mitchell SE, Burdick JF, Williams GM: Balloon dilation versus surgical revision of infra-inguinal autogenous vein graft stenoses: Long-term follow-up. J Cardiovasc Surg 1990;*31*(5):656–661.

39. Cohen JR, Mannick JA, Couch NP, Wittemore AD: Recognition and management of impending vein-graft failure. Arch Surg 1986;*121*:758–759.

40. Sullivan KL, Gardiner GA, Dandarpa K, et al: Efficacy of thrombolysis in infrainguinal bypass grafts. Circulation 1991;83(suppl I):I-99–I-105.
41. McNamara TO, Bomberger RA, Merchant RF: Intra-arterial urokinase as the initial therapy for acutely ischemic lower limbs. Circulation 1991;*83*(suppl I):I-106–I-119.
42. Ricotta JJ, Green RM, DeWeese JA: Uses and limitations of thrombolytic therapy in the treatment of peripheral arterial ischemia: Results of a multi-institutional questionnaire. J Vasc Surg 1987;*6*:45–50.
43. Dacey LJ, Dow RW, McDaniel MD, Walsh DB, Zwolak RM, Cronenwett JL: Cost effectiveness of intra-arterial thrombolytic therapy. Arch Surg 1988;:1218–1223.

39

THROMBOLYTIC THERAPY IN ACUTE VENOUS THROMBOSIS

ALEXANDER G.G. TURPIE

Deep vein thrombosis usually occurs as a common and serious complication in sick hospitalized patients, but occasionally may affect ambulanting and otherwise healthy individuals. Venous thrombi may propagate, undergo lysis, or embolize to the lungs. The natural history of venous thrombi depends on a balance between factors that promote the formation and extension and those that lead to lysis of the thrombus. Most calf vein thrombi do not extend, but approximately 20 per cent of them, particularly in patients who are immobilized or who have other risk factors, will propagate into the proximal venous system acutely or recur within 3 months if the patients are not treated.[1] Symptomatic pulmonary embolism is, however, uncommon in patients with isolated calf vein thrombosis. In patients with proximal deep vein thrombosis, thromboembolic complications including acute and subacute recurrence are common, particularly in patients who are inadequately treated.[2] Complete spontaneous lysis of large proximal thrombi is uncommon, and even in patients treated with anticoagulants, occurs in less than 20 per cent of cases. Thus, deep vein thrombosis, especially of the proximal veins, may result in chronic venous insufficiency, which is a serious cause of chronic morbidity. Chronic venous insufficiency occurs as the result of valvular incompetence and residual venous outflow obstruction which gives rise to chronic venous hypertension. The postphlebitic syndrome consists of pain, swelling of the legs, pigmentation, varicosities, and less commonly, ulceration. It has been estimated that as many as 50 per cent of patients with proximal vein thrombosis will develop the postphlebitic symptoms.[3] In addition, proximal vein thrombi are the source of most pulmonary emboli, which occur in up to 40 per cent of patients, some of which may be fatal.[4]

TREATMENT OF DEEP VEIN THROMBOSIS

Anticoagulant Therapy

The objectives of treatment of deep vein thrombosis are to relieve symptoms and reduce morbidity of the acute event, to prevent extension or embolization to the lungs, to prevent death from pulmonary embolism, and to prevent chronic venous insufficiency. Since progression and embolization of venous thrombi may occur rapidly and unpredictably, it is important that all patients with deep vein thrombosis should receive antithrombotic therapy as soon as possible. Currently, anticoagulant therapy is the most common treatment of deep vein thrombosis and is effective in almost all patients. Thrombus extension or embolization occurs in less than 5 per cent of patients who are adequately treated with heparin followed by secondary prophylaxis with oral anticoagulants.[2,5] However, anticoagulant therapy is not ideal because it does not produce significant thrombolysis, and although it is effective in reducing the important and immediate complications of deep vein thrombosis, it may be relatively ineffective in preventing the late sequelae, including the postphlebitic syndrome.

Heparin is the initial treatment of choice in most patients with deep vein thrombosis. Heparin may be given by continuous intravenous infusion, intermittent intravenous injection, or by subcutaneous injection. Of the intravenous routes, continuous infusion is preferred over intermittent injection because although both regimens are equally effective in the treatment of deep vein thrombosis, the incidence of hemorrhagic side effects is lower with the continuous infusion.[6] The administration of heparin by subcutaneous injection offers potential advantages over either of the intravenous routes because of its ease of administration, facilitation of early patient mobilization, and the potential for outpatient management. For intravenous administration, heparin should be given initially as a bolus of 3000 to 5000 U followed by a continuous intravenous infusion of 30,000 to 35,000 U/day to maintain the activated partial thromboplastin time (APTT) 1.5 to 2.0 times the control level. For intermittent intravenous administration, since the half-life of heparin is one and one half hours and the effect of a bolus will have cleared within 4 hours, boluses of 10,000 to 12,500 U should be administered every 4 to 6 hours to maintain the preinjection APTT in the therapeutic range. For the subcutaneous administration of heparin, an initial intravenous bolus of 3000 to 5000 U should be administered at the same time that the first subcutaneous dose is given; thereafter, subcutaneous injections of 15,000 to 20,000 U should be given at 12-hourly intervals to maintain the midinterval APTT at 1.5 to 2.0 times the control. Using this regimen, prolongation of APTT and therapeutic plasma heparin concentrations are usually maintained throughout the 24-hour period. The duration of heparin therapy in the treatment of deep vein thrombosis remains controversial. Heparin is usually administered for 7 to 10 days, followed by oral long-term anticoagulant therapy. An alternative approach is to commence heparin and oral anticoagulants at the same time and to discontinue heparin when the prothrombin time reaches the desired therapeutic level on the fourth to fifth day. Two randomized trials comparing this regimen with standard treatment have reported it to be effective and safe.[7,8] Thus, this approach can be recommended for the majority of patients with proximal deep vein thrombosis.

The initial treatment of deep vein thrombosis with heparin should be followed with a period of secondary prophylaxis with oral anticoagulants or adjusted-dose subcutaneous heparin. Oral anticoagulant therapy is the more practical approach and has been shown to prevent recurrence of deep vein thrombosis, extension, or embolization to the lungs.[2,9,10] The duration of secondary prophylaxis with oral anticoagulants for patients with symptomatic calf vein thrombosis is 6 to 8 weeks, and for patients with proximal vein thrombosis and pulmonary embolism, 12 weeks is recommended. The optimal intensity for oral anticoagulant therapy in venous thrombosis has recently been established from the results of a randomized clinical trial comparing two intensities of anticoagulation.[10] The traditionally recommended therapeutic range using commercially prepared rabbit brain thromboplastin was 1.5 to 2.0 times control, equivalent to an international normalized ratio (INR) of 3.0 to 4.5. This level of anticoagulation was highly efficacious in the prevention of recurrences, but was associated with a significant risk of bleeding complications. It has now been established that the risk of bleeding associated with long-term anticoagulant therapy is less than 5 per cent without loss of efficacy using a less intense anticoagulant regimen of 1.3 to 1.5 times the control using rabbit brain thromboplastin, which is equivalent to an INR of 2.0 to 3.0.[10]

Oral anticoagulant therapy with warfarin should be administered in an initial dose of 10 mg/day for the first 3 days along with heparin therapy. The daily dose should then be adjusted according to the results of laboratory monitoring using the prothrombin time. Concurrent heparin therapy and oral anticoagulant therapy should be maintained for 4 to 5 days, at which time the vitamin K coagulation factors will be reduced to therapeutic levels and pro-thrombin time prolonged to the therapeutic range of 1.3 to 1.5 times control or INR 2.0 or 3.0. Depending upon the patient's initial response, the prothrom-bin time should be monitored weekly, and once stable, at intervals of 2 to 3 weeks for the duration of secondary prophylaxis.

Thrombolytic Therapy

Recently, there has been an increased interest in the clinical use of thrombolytic agents in deep vein thrombosis, primarily due to the impressive clinical results in patients with acute myocardial infarction and also to the development of a new generation of plasminogen activators. Thrombolytic therapy has a number of potential advantages over anticoagulant therapy in deep vein thrombosis in preventing the postphlebitic syndrome, which include lysis of the thrombi with restoration of the circulation to normal, and reduction in venous valve damage.

The fibrinolytic agents in clinical use induce thrombolysis by converting the proenzynme plasminogen to the enzyme plasmin, which lyses fibrin and so produces thrombolysis.[11] The first-generation plasminogen activators, strepto-kinase (SK) and urokinase (UK), do not have fibrin specificity, and predictably induce plasma proteolysis when administered systematically in doses that induce thrombolysis. The second-generation plasminogen activators, recombinant tis-sue-type plasminogen activator (rt-PA) and single-chain urokinase-type plas-minogen activator (SCUPA or prourokinase), are much more fibrin specific, while acylated plasminogen-streptokinase activator complex (APSAC), is inter-mediate in fibrin specificity.[12]

Streptokinase is produced by chemical purification of a streptococcal bacterial filtrate. It has a plasma half-life of 30 minutes. Streptokinase is an indirect activator of plasminogen, first combining with plasminogen to form an activator complex, which then cleaves plasminogen to plasmin.[13] Urokinase, which has been purified from human urine and cultured renal cells and can be produced by recombinant DNA technology, is a direct activator of plasmin-ogen.[13] Tissue-type plasminogen activator, initially obtained from cultured melanoma cells and now manufactured by recombinant DNA technology, is a direct activator of plasminogen.[14] Recombinant tissue-type plasminogen activator is fibrin specific because it has a high affinity for fibrin, on which it forms a ternary complex with plasminogen which is protected from the neutralizing effect of antiplasmin through its binding to fibrin. Tissue-type plasminogen activator is produced by recombinant DNA technology. Single-chain urokinase-type plasminogen activator produced by cultured renal cells or by recombinant DNA technology, is clot specific because of its affinity for fibrin-bound plasminogen[15,16] and has a plasma half-life of 5 minutes. Acylated plasminogen-streptokinase activator complex is prepared by chemical modification (acylation) of a complex of SK with human plasminogen which renders the SK-plasminogen complex inactive.[17,18] After injection, APSAC binds to fibrin in the thrombus where in vivo deacylation occurs gradually over a period of hours, at which time it is protected from antiplasmin. However, some deacylation of APSAC occurs in plasma, leading to the production of a plasma proteolytic state.

Although thrombolytic therapy has been approved for over 15 years for the treatment of deep vein thrombosis, thrombolytic therapy is utilized in less than 10 per cent of patients. The reasons for its limited use are multiple and include fear of bleeding, the cost of thrombolytic agents, and uncertainties about the clinical benefits of thrombolytic therapy over anticoagulants in the treatment of venous thromboembolism, in particular in the prevention of the postphlebitic syndrome.

The aims of treating acute deep venous thrombosis are to prevent death from pulmonary embolism, to prevent nonfatal pulmonary embolism, to prevent recurrent venous thrombosis, and to prevent the postphlebitic syndrome. In deep vein thrombosis of the legs, thrombolytic therapy has been shown to be more effective than heparin in producing thrombolysis, particularly in patients with symptoms of less than 5 days. Six randomized controlled trials have compared streptokinase in the treatment of deep vein thrombosis with heparin.[19-24] A pooled analysis of the results[25] has demonstrated that streptokinase is four times more likely to cause clot lysis, but three times more likely to cause major bleeding complications. The comparative effects of streptokinase and heparin on the subsequent development of the postphlebitic syndrome have been evaluated in four studies.[26-29] In three of the studies, the frequency of the postphlebitic symptoms was less in patients treated with streptokinase than in those treated with heparin; in the fourth,[29] there was no difference in the frequency or severity of the postphlebitic syndrome between patients treated with either streptokinase or heparin. However, many patients entered into this latter study had symptoms for a week or more before randomization. Urokinase has been less extensively evaluated in the treatment of deep vein thrombosis.

Streptokinase and urokinase are approved for the treatment of venous thromboembolic disease. Streptokinase should be given in a loading dose of 250,000 U intravenously over 30 minutes followed by 100,000 to 200,000 U/hr. In patients with deep vein thrombosis, the infusion should be maintained for 48 to 72 hours; and in patients with pulmonary embolism, from 12 to 24 hours. The dose of UK is 4400 U/kg by intravenous bolus over 10 minutes, followed by 4400 U/kg/hr by intravenous infusion. The duration of the infusions are identical to streptokinase. Using these regimens, concomitant use of heparin or aspirin should be avoided. Heparin should be commenced 1 to 3 hours after stopping thrombolytic therapy and anticoagulants continued for approximately 3 months.

The major complication of thrombolytic therapy is hemorrhage. Bleeding is caused primarily by dissolution of fibrin in the hemostatic plug.[13] Hemorrhage is also contributed to by plasma proteolysis with its associated depletion of fibrinogen and other coagulation factors and by the production of fibrinogen degradation products, which interfere with fibrin polymerization.

Hemorrhage occurs in 30 to 50 per cent of patients who are treated with

SK or UK infusions for more than 12 hours. The risk of hemorrhage increases with the length of the infusion and occurs most often from sites of vascular invasion, such as needle puncture and cutdown sites or from surgical wounds. Bleeding may also occur from the genitourinary tract, the gastrointestinal tract, and occasionally, into the brain. Oozing from wounds or puncture sites should be treated by local pressure, although this is often unsuccessful. Blood loss should be treated by replacement with whole blood, and if bleeding is associated with hypofibrinogenemia and other coagulation factor deficiencies, fresh plasma or cryoprecipitate should be used. If bleeding is potentially serious and cannot be controlled by these measures, fibrinolytic therapy should be discontinued. If bleeding is life threatening, the fibrinolytic process can be rapidly reversed by the infusion of epsilon amino caproid acid in a dose of 5 g given over 30 minutes, followed by 1 g/hr until hemostasis has been achieved. This may be supplemented with transfusion of fresh plasma or cryoprecipitate.

Other complications include allergic reactions and fever. Allergic reactions rarely occur with UK or rt-PA treatment, but occur in 6 per cent of patients treated with SK. These reactions usually take the form of pruritus or urticaria, but approximately 1 to 2 per cent of patients develop anaphylactic reactions. These allergic reactions can be reversed by epinephrine, parenteral corticosteroids, and antihistamines. Fever occurs in approximately 25 per cent of patients receiving SK and in about 10 per cent of patients receiving UK.

When thrombolytic therapy was used initially, laboratory tests were performed to predict dosage requirements and to document plasma fibrinolytic activity and the consequences of plasma proteolysis. The approach to thrombolytic therapy has now been simplified so that adequate monitoring can be obtained by using tests such as the thrombin clotting time, which reflects hypofibrinogenemia and the levels of fibrinogen/fibrin degradation products (FDP). The thrombin clotting time should be performed approximately 2 hours after initiation of treatment and then every 6 hours as necessary. With UK infusions, the dose of the drug should be decreased by approximately 25 per cent if the thrombin time exceeds 4 to 5 times the control level, and increased by approximately 25 per cent if the thrombin time is less than the control level. Monitoring streptokinase therapy is more complicated. A thrombin time should be performed approximately 2 hours after the onset of the infusion, at which time it would be expected to be prolonged to 2 to 5 times the control value. A lesser degree of prolongation suggests that the patient's SK antibodies have not been adequately neutralized and is an indication for performing a streptokinase resistance test and adjusting the dose accordingly. Once an optimal fibrinolytic state is established, the thrombin time should be maintained at 2 to 5 times the control value. If the thrombin time falls to less than twice the control value, it is an indication that there is excessive plasminogen depletion (because of its conversion to plasmin) and the dose should be decreased by 25 to 50 per cent.

Tests of fibrinolytic activity, such as the euglobulin lysis time, can be performed if available, but are not necessary. It is very important, however, to assess the patients clinically and to monitor routine tests for evidence of bleeding. This is achieved by performing serial hematocrit determinations, at least twice daily, and by observing the urine and stools for evidence of bleeding. After thrombolytic therapy is completed, heparin therapy should be commenced when the thrombin clotting time falls to twice the control or less, to prevent rethrombosis.

Recombinant tissue-type plasminogen activator has recently been evaluated in the treatment of deep vein thrombosis. Investigation in animals and in humans has demonstrated that rt-PA is an effective thrombolytic agent which has potential advantages over the first-generation plasminogen activators (SK and UK) because it has a higher affinity for fibrin and so is able to activate plasminogen on the fibrin surface.[14,30] However, as experience with rt-PA has accumulated, it has become evident that its fibrin selectivity is relative and is influenced by the dose and duration of rt-PA infusion.[31–33]

Two pilot studies designed to determine whether a slow infusion of rt-PA would reduce its hemorrhagic potential while retaining its lytic effect in patients with acute proximal deep vein thrombosis of the legs have been completed at McMaster University.[34] Twenty-four patients were entered into the first study; 12 received rt-PA in a dose of 0.5 mg/kg over 4 hours and 12 received placebo. In addition to rt-PA or placebo, all patients were treated with continuous intravenous heparin for 7 to 10 days. Of the 12 patients who received rt-PA, seven patients (58 per cent) obtained virtually complete lysis of the thrombi, two patients had 0 to 50 per cent lysis, and three patients showed no evidence of thrombolysis. In contrast, only two patients in the placebo group had 0 to 50 per cent lysis, and the remaining patients showed no evidence of lysis. This observed difference in thrombolysis is statistically highly significant ($p < 0.01$). Two patients in the rt-PA group showed evidence of overt hemorrhage compared to one patient in the placebo group who received heparin only. The rt-PA infusion produced a fall in circulating fibrinogen concentration to approximately 50 per cent of the preinfusion value, a fall in plasma plasminogen to 60 per cent of the preinfusion value, a fall in α_2-antiplasmin to almost undetectable levels, and a threefold increase in the concentration of serum FDP. These results indicate that patients with deep vein thrombosis treated with rt-PA infusion in doses of 0.5 mg/kg over 4 hours experience a moderate degree of plasmin-induced proteolysis. Fifty-nine patients were recruited to the second study, of whom 29 received rt-PA and 30 received placebo. Of the 28 patients who received 0.5 mg/kg rt-PA infused over 8 hours, repeated in 24 hours, and who underwent follow-up venography, greater than 50 per cent lysis was achieved in six (21 per cent) compared with two (7 per cent) of the 30 patients who received placebo plus heparin. The between-group difference in the proportion of patients who had greater than 50 per cent lysis favored rt-PA, but was not statistically significant ($p = 0.11$). The results obtained with the two treatment regimens and with placebo are compared in Tables 39–1 and 39–2.

Of the patients who received 0.5 mg/kg rt-PA over 8 hours, repeated once, one patient had significant subcutaneous ecchymosis. In the patients who received placebo plus heparin, one patient had a spontaneous hemarthrosis involving the shoulder, and in one patient, the hemoglobin fell more than 20 g/L without overt bleeding. In the patients who received rt-PA 0.5 mg/kg over 8 hours, there was an 11 per cent reduction in mean plasma fibrinogen concentration, a 36 per cent reduction in mean α_2-antiplasmin levels, and only a moderate increase in serum FDP concentration.

TABLE 39–1. THROMBOLYSIS WITH RT-PA 0.5 MG/KG OVER 4 HOURS OR PLACEBO

% Lysis	rt-PA (n = 12)	Placebo (n = 12)
≥50	7	0
<50	2	2
0	3	10

TABLE 39–2. THROMBOLYSIS WITH RT-PA 0.5 MG/KG OVER 8 HOURS × 2 OR PLACEBO

% Lysis	rt-PA (n = 28)	Placebo (n = 30)
≥50	6	2
<50	7	5
0	15	23

Thus, in these studies, rt-PA administered over 4 hours produced lysis of proximal deep vein thrombosis more often than heparin. The rate of lysis achieved at the higher concentration of rt-PA administered over 4 hours was similar to that reported in previous studies using SK administered over 48 hours to 72 hours.[25] Forty-six patients from both studies were followed-up long term; of the other 37 patients, 22 had died and 15 were not readily available for follow-up. Of these 46 patients, seven received heparin plus rt-PA, 0.5 mg/kg over 4 hours; 20 received heparin plus rt-PA, 0.5 mg/kg over 8 hours (repeated), and 19 received heparin and placebo. Greater than 50 per cent lysis was achieved in 12 patients; in five with 0.5 mg/kg rt-PA infused over 4 hours, in five with 0.5 mg/kg rt-PA infused over 8 hours, repeated once, and in two with placebo. Three (25 per cent) of the twelve patients in whom greater than 50 per cent lysis was achieved had symptoms of the postphlebitic syndrome, compared with 19 (56 per cent) of 34 in whom less than 50 per cent or no lysis was achieved (NS, $p = 0.07$).

In this study, the overall prevalence of the postphlebitic syndrome was 58 per cent at 3-year follow-up. The data suggest, based on a nonsignificant trend ($p = 0.07$), that the incidence of the postphlebitic syndrome is lower in patients in whom greater than 50 per cent lysis is achieved, an observation consistent with reports from other small studies of thrombolysis with SK.[26–29]

Thrombolytic therapy has been shown to produce effective lysis of major deep vein thrombi when evaluated acutely with repeat venography. The results of studies assessing the long-term benefits of thrombolysis in deep vein thrombosis are conflicting, but most suggest benefit in reduction of symptoms of chronic venous insufficiency. Streptokinase and urokinase are approved in the management of deep vein thrombosis, and current studies are evaluating the role of rt-PA in the management of this disorder.

REFERENCES

1. Hull RD, Hirsh J, Carter C, et al: Diagnostic efficacy of impedance plethysmography for clinically suspected deep vein thrombosis: A randomized trial. Ann Intern Med 1985;*102*:21.
2. Hull R, Delmore T, Genton E, et al: Warfarin sodium versus low dose heparin in the long-term treatment of venous thrombosis. N Engl J Med 1979;*301*:855.
3. Negus D: The post-thrombotic syndrome. Ann Roy Coll Surg Engl 1970;*47*:92–105.
4. Kakkar VV, Flanc C, Howe CT: Natural history of postoperative deep vein thrombosis. Lancet 1969;*ii*:230–233.
5. Barrit DW, Jordon SC: Anticoagulant drugs in the treatment of pulmonary embolism. A controlled clinical trial. Lancet 1960;*i*:1309–1312.
6. Salzman EW, Deykin D, Shapiro RM: The management of heparin therapy. Controlled prospective trial. N Engl J Med 1975;*292*:1046–1050.
7. Gallus A, Jackaman J, Tillet, et al: Safety and efficacy of warfarin started early after submassive venous thrombosis or pulmonary embolism. Lancet 1986;*ii*:1293–1296.
8. Hull RD, Raskob G, Rosenbloom D, et al: Heparin for five days as compared with ten days in the initial treatment of proximal venous thrombosis. N Engl J Med 1990;*322*(18):1260–1264.

9. Hull RD, Delmore J, Carter C, et al: Adjusted subcutaneous heparin versus warfarin sodium in the long term treatment of venous thrombosis. N Engl J Med 1982;*306*:189.
10. Hull R, Hirsh J, Jay R, et al: Different intensities of oral anticoagulant therapy in the treatment of proximal deep vein thrombosis. N Engl J Med 1982;*307*:1676.
11. Collen D: On the regulation and control of fibrinolysis. Thromb Haemost 1980;*43*:77.
12. Marder VJ, Bell WR: Fibrinolytic therapy. *In* Colman RW, Hirsh J, Marder VJ, Salzman EW, eds: Haemostasis and Thrombosis: Basic Principles and Clinical Practice. Philadelphia, JB Lippincott Co., 1987;1393–1437.
13. Frantantoni JC, Ness P, Simon TL: Thrombolytic therapy. Current status. N Engl J Med 1975;*293*:1073.
14. Rijken DC, Collen D: Purification and characterization of the plasminogen activator secreted by human melanoma cells in culture. J Biol Chem 1981;*256*:7035.
15. Gurewich V, Pannell R, Louie S: Effective and fibrin-specific clot lysis by a zymogen precursor form of urokinase (pro-urokinase); a study in vitro and in two animal species. J Clin Invest 1984;*73*:1731.
16. Pannel R, Gurewich V: Pro-urokinase: A study of its stability in plasma and of a mechanism for its selective fibrinolytic effect. Blood 1986;*67*:1215.
17. Marder VJ, Rothbard RL, Fitzpatric PG, Francis CW: Rapid lysis of coronary artery thrombi with anisoylated plasminogen: Streptokinase activator complex: Treatment by bolus intravenous injection. Ann Intern Med 1986;*104*:304.
18. Dupe RJ, Green J, Smith RAG: Acylated derivatives of streptokinase-plasminogen activator complex as thrombolytic agents in a dog model of aged venous thrombosis. Thromb Hemost 1985;*53*:56.
19. Robertson BR, Nilsson IM, Nylander G: Value of streptokinase and heparin in treatment of acute deep venous thrombosis: A coded investigation. Acta Chir Scand 1968;*134*:203.
20. Kakkar VV, Flanc C, Howe CT, et al: Treatment of deep vein thrombosis: A trial of heparin, streptokinase and arvin. Br Med J 1969;*1*:806.
21. Robertson BR, Nilsson IM, Nylander G: Thrombolytic effect of streptokinase as evaluated by phlebography of deep venous thrombi of the leg. Acta Chir Scand 1970;*136*:173.
22. Tsapogas MJ, Peabody RA, Wu KT, et al: Controlled study of thrombolytic therapy in deep vein thrombosis. Surgery 1973;*74*:973.
23. Porter JM, Seaman AJ, Common HH, et al: Comparison of heparin and streptokinase in the treatment of venous thrombosis. Am Surg 1975;*41*:511.
24. Elliot MS, Immelman EJ, Jeffery P: A comparative randomized trial of heparin versus streptokinase in the treatment of acute proximal venous thrombosis: An interim report of a prospective trial. Br J Surg 1979;*66*:838.
25. Goldhaber SZ, Burin JE, Lipnick RJ, Hennekens CH: Pooled analyses of randomized trials of streptokinase and heparin in phlebographically documented acute deep venous thrombosis. Am J Med 1984;*76*:393.
26. Common HH, Seaman AJ, Rosch J, Porter JM, et al: Deep vein thrombosis treated with streptokinase or heparin. Follow-up of a randomized study. Angiology 1976;*27*:645.
27. Johansson L, Nylander G, Hedner U, Nilsson IM: Comparison of streptokinase with heparin. Late results in the treatment of deep venous thrombosis. Acta Med Scand 1979;*206*:93.
28. Arnesen H, Hoiseth A, Ly B: Streptokinase or heparin in the treatment of deep vein thrombosis. Acta Med Scand 1982;*211*:65.
29. Kakkar VV, Lawrence D: Hemodynamic and clinical assessment after therapy for acute deep vein thrombosis. A prospective study. Am J Surg 1985;*150*(4A):54.
30. Verstraete M, Bounameaux H, DeCock F, et al: Pharmacokinetics and systemic fibrinogenolytic effects of recombinant human tissue-type plasminogen activator (rtPA) in humans. J Pharmacol Exp Ther 1985;*235*:506.
31. Verstraete M, Bernard R, Bory M: Randomized trial of intravenous recombinant tissue-type plasminogen activator versus intravenous streptokinase in acute myocardial infarction. Lancet 1985;*i*:842.
32. Passamini E, Mueller HS, Braunwald E: The TIMI Study Group: The thrombolysis in myocardial infarction (TIMI) trial. Phase I findings. N Engl J Med 1985;*312*:932.
33. Agnelli G, Buchanan MR, Fernandez F: A comparison of the thrombolytic and haemorrhagic effects of tissue-type plasminogen activator and streptokinase in rabbits. Circulation 1985;*72*:178.
34. Turpie AGG, Levine MN, Hirsh J, et al: Tissue plasminogen activator (rt-PA) vs heparin in deep vein thrombosis. Results of a randomized trial. Chest 1990;*97*:172S–175S.

40

UROKINASE TREATMENT OF OCCLUDED INFRAINGUINAL GRAFTS

ANTHONY D. WHITTEMORE

In spite of many technical advances in infrainguinal arterial reconstruction, approximately 25 per cent of vein and 60 per cent of prosthetic grafts fail during the first 5 years and present the vascular surgeon with a persistent challenge for which a common solution has yet to emerge.[1–10] In our initial review of reversed vein graft failures we were unable to demonstrate a causative lesion in approximately 30 per cent.[11] When the lesion responsible for failure was identified, vein graft stenosis occurring within the first 2 years proved the most common (25 per cent). Early technical errors and delayed progression of distal atherosclerosis were also important factors contributing to graft occlusion. Our more recent review of 90 failures among 455 consecutive in situ saphenous vein grafts demonstrated a causative lesion in all but seven (8 per cent) instances.[12] In the remaining 83 grafts, 102 contributory causes (Table 40–1) were documented and vein graft lesions were again responsible for the majority (40 per cent). It has been repeatedly demonstrated that identification of vein graft lesions and subsequent repair prior to graft thrombosis yields an 80 per cent patency rate after 5 years.[11,13] This favorable result contrasts with the collective experience with occluded grafts which require initial balloon catheter thrombectomy. Even when the causative lesion is properly identified and repaired, the 5-year patency rate is minimal (20 to 30 per cent). The marked discrepancy in these secondary graft patency rates has been attributed to deficiencies associated with balloon catheter thrombectomy including residual laminar thrombus within the graft or within the smaller distal vasculature, and traumatic disruption of the endothelial monolayer, setting the stage for subsequent myointimal hyperplasia. While most vascular centers have therefore instituted some form of surveillance protocol designed to identify failing grafts prior to total occlusion, a significant number of patients continue to present with occluded reconstructions.[6,10,12]

With the availability of thrombolytic agents, an alternative to catheter balloon thrombectomy for occluded grafts was immediately recognized.[14–16] Initial thrombolysis for graft occlusion seemed attractive for several reasons (Table 40–2). Since balloon catheter thrombectomy frequently leaves significant

TABLE 40–1. CAUSES OF VEIN GRAFT FAILURE

Technical failures	20%
Vein graft stenosis	40%
Compromised outflow	21%
Hypercoagulability	9%
Hypotension	6%
Miscellaneous	4%

residual thrombus laminated along the graft, lytic therapy might provide more complete elimination of thrombus.[17,18] The pathologic anatomy is more precisely defined in the angiography suite and surgical repair of the causative lesion therefore more directed. Furthermore, dissolution of thrombus in smaller distal vessels inaccessible to balloon catheters might improve outflow. Trauma to the endothelial surface inherent in balloon thrombectomy is avoided and myointimal hyperplasia potentially minimized.[19–21] Finally, focal venous or anastomotic hyperplastic lesions might be expeditiously repaired with balloon angioplasty thus avoiding surgery altogether.

With respect to intra-arterial thrombolysis, several studies have documented the apparent superiority of urokinase over its clinical predecessor, streptokinase.[14–16,22–24] A higher 75 per cent initial success rate associated with urokinase may be anticipated in a shorter period of time with a lower incidence of bleeding complications when compared with streptokinase. Our earlier experience with 38 vein and prosthetic graft occlusions was encouraging and demonstrated an initial success rate of 81 per cent for grafts treated with urokinase, in contrast to a significantly lower success rate (41 per cent) associated with streptokinase.[16] This success rate was not necessarily dependent on the duration of graft thrombosis; in fact, 89 per cent of grafts felt to be occluded for more than 1 week were successfuly lysed with urokinase. This initial experience was frought with a relatively high rate of complications, 65 per cent associated with streptokinase and 31 per cent with urokinase. Approximately 25 per cent of the complications were defined as major in both groups. The 6-month patency rate achieved with successful thrombolysis of these occluded grafts was 64 per cent, provided a causative lesion was identified and repaired. Without repair, only 15 per cent of these grafts remained patent for 6 months, yielding an unsatisfactory 14 per cent 6-month limb salvage rate.

Based upon this initial preliminary experience, and in view of the dismal results achieved with surgical catheter embolectomy, patients with autogenous vein graft occlusion were initially treated preferentially with urokinase thrombolytic therapy.[25] A total of 35 patients admitted to the Brigham and Women's Hospital underwent thrombolysis for primary infrainguinal vein graft occlusion. Of the 35 vein grafts, 22 were successfully lysed (60 per cent); eight were in situ, and 14 were either reversed or nonreversed, transposed grafts. The distal anastomosis was located in the popliteal artery in 12 grafts and at an infrapo-

TABLE 40–2. THEORETIC ADVANTAGES ASSOCIATED WITH THROMBOLYSIS FOR GRAFT OCCLUSION

Precise definition of causative lesion
Complete lysis of graft thrombus
Minimal trauma to endothelial surface
Maximal lysis of distal outflow thrombus
May avoid necessity for surgery

pliteal level in ten. The average primary patency rate associated with these vein grafts prior to thrombosis was 19 months, and ranged from 1 to 84 months. The somewhat lower 60 per cent successful lysis rate observed in these grafts (Table 40–3) may in part be due to the fact that of the 22 successfully lysed grafts, urokinase was used in 15 and tissue-type plasminogen activator and streptokinase in the remaining seven. The average duration of symptoms prior to thrombolysis was 2 weeks, somewhat longer than in other series.

Following admission to the hospital, patients were taken to the angiography suite and after initial diagnostic studies, the occlusion was traversed with a guide wire which was then exchanged for an appropriately sized catheter. A bolus of urokinase was subsequently delivered throughout the thrombus to acclerate initial lysis. The catheter was then withdrawn and embedded within the most proximal aspect of the thrombus and a constant infusion initiated at 240,000 IU/hr for 2 hours, then 120,000 IU for the following 2 hours, and 60,000 IU/hr thereafter until lysis was achieved. Interval arteriography was carried out every 6 hours early in our experience and more recently at 12-hour intervals. Simultaneous heparin was routinely administered to minimize the incidence of thrombus formation proximal to and upon the delivery catheter.

Following successful lysis, 19 of the 22 grafts underwent subsequent radiologic or surgical intervention to repair the causative lesion. Percutaneous transluminal angioplasty (PTA) was utilized for nine short-segment stenotic lesions within the vein graft or runoff vessels. Surgical vein patch angioplasty of anastomotic lesions was carried out in four grafts, and eight required more extensive reconstruction with distal extension vein grafts. In three patients, no intervention was carried out following thrombolysis, since no causative lesion was identified in two, and the third graft failed owing to inadequate runoff, with no remaining autogenous tissue available for reconstruction. Patients were not routinely placed on long-term anticoagulation, but antiplatelet therapy was always recommended.

The average ankle-brachial index (ABI) in these 22 limbs prior to failure was 0.87, and diminished to 0.32 at the time thrombosis was recognized. Following successful thrombolysis, the average ABI was restored to 0.88. Unfortunately, this gratifying initial result was not sustained in that life-table analysis revealed a 5-year patency limited to 37 per cent. Fifteen of the initial twenty-two grafts failed within 3 years due to recurrent anastomotic lesions in six, inadequate infrapopliteal runoff in five, and recurrent mid–vein-graft stenosis in three. In one instance, the causative lesion could not be ascertained. Analysis of a variety of subgroups failed to identify any significant predictive factors contributing to early failure of thrombolysis.

Despite several theoretic advantages potentially associated with thrombolytic therapy and the encouraging preliminary short-term success rates, the long-term benefits of this approach have not been substantiated and thus far represent no significant improvement over those obtained in the past with

TABLE 40–3. UROKINASE THROMBOLYSIS FOR INFRAINGUINAL GRAFT THROMBOSIS

Material	Author	No. Grafts	Initial Success	Bleeding	Patency (1 yr)
Synthetic	O'Donnell	20	85%	10%	38%
Synthetic/vein	Gardiner	43	84%	10%	49%
Vein	Belkin	35	60%		37%

catheter embolectomy. These results reflect those reported in other series, but contrast with those reported by Gardner utilizing pooled data from three institutions.[22,26] Gardner found a significantly better cumulative patency rate among grafts lysed and subsequently repaired when compared with those without correctable lesions. These grafts included both suprainguinal and infrainguinal reconstructions and a combination of prosthetic as well as autogenous venous conduits.

While the reasons underlying the failure of thrombolytic therapy and balloon catheter thrombectomy may vary, the single common denominator is the presence of thrombus adjacent to the endothelium precluding blood flow through the graft. The alterations in endothelial and vascular wall biology have not been clearly defined, but may include inflammatory and ischemic changes which initiate a cascade of cellular events precluding long-term graft patency despite the complete elimination of luminal thrombus. It is also possible that our particular population, small in number, represented the extreme of peripheral atherosclerosis with advanced tibioperoneal disease. Seven of the twenty-one patients had undergone prior ipsilateral reconstruction that had failed, and 8 of the 15 patients who sustained secondary graft failure required immediate amputation. Thrombolytic therapy with appropriate revision may thus be more effective in patients with less advanced disease. Furthermore, subsequent studies have shown that balloon angioplasty for vein graft lesions has not been particularly effective, such that surgical vein patch angioplasty for all grafts following thrombolytic therapy may significantly improve long-term results.[27] Finally, our results in this group are obscured by the fact that tissue-type plasminogen activator and streptokinase were used in seven patients. Due to the small number of patients in our series, however, we were unable to demonstrate a significant difference between these patients and those treated with urokinase.

It may yet prove that expeditious thrombolysis of occluded grafts using exclusively urokinase followed by specific surgical repair will yield improved secondary patency rates. Fibrinolytic therapy with urokinase can provide rapid dissolution of intraluminal thrombus with increasing efficiency, often within a few hours with the use of a pulsed spray apparatus. Unfortunately, this rapid lysis and identification of the causative lesion with definition of distal anatomy has not as yet translated into improved long-term graft patency rates. The results of this study and others therefore suggest that when a patient has autogenous material available with which to revise a failed vein graft surgically, this course should be undertaken without deliberation. However, in the absence of appropriate autogenous vein, or when goals are limited to short-term patency, thrombolytic therapy utilizing urokinase followed by surgical repair may yet represent a reasonable approach to the patient with an occluded infrainguinal bypass. Thrombolysis may, in fact, result in more adequate resolution of infrapopliteal thrombus which occasionally accompanies proximal graft thrombosis, and may provide a more distal origin for a secondary reconstruction in the setting of limited autogenous tissue. Thus, a short lesser saphenous or arm vein graft might originate from a midsuperficial femoral artery or original vein graft to allow significant secondary limb salvage.

REFERENCES

1. Maini BS, Mannick JA: Effect of arterial reconstruction on limb salvage: a ten-year appraisal. Arch Surg 1978;*1113*:1297.

2. Leather RP, Shah DM, Chang BB, Kaufman JL: Resurrection of the in situ saphenous vein bypass. Ann Surg 1978;*208*:435–442.
3. Kacoyanis GP, Whittemore AD, Couch NP, Mannick JA: Femorotibial and femoroperoneal bypass vein grafts. Arch Surg 1981;*116*:1529–1534.
4. Fogle MA, Whittemore AD, Couch NP, Mannick JA: A comparison on in situ and reversed saphenous vein grafts for infringuinal reconstruction. J Vasc Surg 1987;*5*:46–52.
5. Bandyk DF, Kaehnick FW, Stewart GW, Towne JB: Durability of the in situ saphenous vein arterial bypass: a comparison of primary and secondary patency. J Vasc Surg 1987;*5*:256–268.
6. Taylor LM Jr, Edwards JM, Porter JM: Present status of reversed vein bypass grafting: Five-year results of a modern series. J Vasc Surg 1990;*11*:193–206.
7. Pomposelli FB, Jepsen SJ, Gibbons GW, et al: The efficacy of the dorsalis pedis bypass for limb salvage in diabetic patients. J Vasc Surg 1990;*11*:745–752.
8. Donaldson MC, Mannick JA, Whittemore AD: Femoral-distal bypass with in situ greater saphenous vein: Long-term results using the Mills valvulotome. Ann Surg 1991;*213*:457–465.
9. Whittemore AD, Kent KC, Donaldson MC, Couch NP, Mannick JA: What is the proper role of polytetrafluoroethylene grafts in infrainguinal reconstruction? J Vasc Surg 1989;*110*:299–305.
10. Veith FJ, Gupta SK, Ascer E, et al: A six-year prospective multicenter randomized comparison of autologous saphenous vein and expanded polytetrafluoroethylene grafts in infrainguinal arterial reconstructions. J Vasc Surg 1986;*3*:104–114.
11. Whittemore AD, Clowes AW, Couch NP, Mannick JA: Secondary femoropopliteal reconstruction. Ann Surg 1981;*193*:35–42.
12. Donaldson MC, Mannick JA, Whittemore AD: Causes of primary graft failure after in situ saphenous vein bypass. J Vasc Surg 1991 (In Press).
13. Cohen JR, Mannick JA, Couch NP, Whittemore AD: Recognition and management of impending vein-graft failure. Arch Surg 1986;*121*:758–759.
14. Towne JB, Bandyk DF: Application of thrombolytic therapy in vascular occlusive disease. Am J Surg 1987;*154*:548–559.
15. Belkin M, Belkin BA, Bucknam CA, Straub J, Lowe R: Intra-arterial fibrinolytic therapy. Efficacy of streptokinase vs urokinase. Arc Surg 1986;*121*:769–773.
16. Koltun WA, Gardiner GA, Harrington DP, Couch NP, Mannick JA, Whittemore AD: Thrombolysis in the treatment of peripheral arterial vascular occlusions. Arch Surg 1987;*122*:901–905.
17. Plecha FR, Poires WJ: Intraoperative angiography in the immediate assessment of arterial embolectomy. Arch Surg 1972;*105*:869–874.
18. White GE, White RA, Kopchok GE, Wilson SE: Angioscopic thromboembolectomy: Preliminary observations with a recent technique. J Vasc Surg 1988;*7*:318–325.
19. Chidi CC, DePalma DG: Atherogenic potential of the embolectomy catheter. Surgery 1978;*83*:549–547.
20. Bowles CR, Olcott C, Pakter RL, Lombard C, Mehigan JT, Walter JF: Diffuse arterial narrowing as a result of intimal proliferation: A delayed complication of embolectomy with the Fogarty balloon catheter. J Vasc Surg 1988;*7*:487–494.
21. Foster JH, Carter JW, Graham CP, et al: Arterial injuries secondary to the use of the Fogarty catheter. Ann Surg 1980;*171*:971–978.
22. Gardiner GA, Harrington DP, Koltun WP, Whittemore AD, Mannick JA, Levin DC: Salvage of occluded arterial bypass grafts by means of thrombolysis. J Vasc Surg 1989;*9*:426–431.
23. Van Breda A, Katzen BT, Deutsch AS: Urokinase versus streptokinase in local thrombolysis. Radiology 1987;*165*:109–111.
24. McNamara TO, Fischer JR: Thrombolysis of peripheral arterial and graft occlusions: Improved results using high-dose urokinase. AJR 1985;*144*:769–775.
25. Belkin M, Donaldson MC, Whittemore AD, et al: Observations on the use of thrombolytic agents for thrombotic occlusion of infrainguinal vein grafts. J Vasc Surg 1990;*11*:289–294.
26. Graor RA, Risius B, Young JR, et al: Thrombolysis of peripheral arterial bypass grafts: Surgical thrombectomy compared with thrombolysis. J Vasc Surg 1988;*7*:347–355.
27. Whittemore AD, Donaldson MC, Polak JF, Mannick JA: Limitations of balloon angioplasty for vein graft stenosis. J Vasc Surg 1991;*14*:340–345.

Index

Note: Page numbers in *italics* refer to illustrations; page numbers followed by t refer to tables.